Heart Disease and the Surgical Patient

Heart Disease and the Surgical Patient

EDITED BY

SIMON HOWELL
University of Leeds
Leeds, United Kingdom

CHRIS PEPPER
The General Infirmary at Leeds
Leeds, United Kingdom

DONAT R. SPAHN
University Hospital Zurich
Zurich, Switzerland

informa
healthcare

New York   London

Informa Healthcare USA, Inc.
270 Madison Avenue
New York, NY 10016

© 2007 by Informa Healthcare USA, Inc.
Informa Healthcare is an Informa business

No claim to original U.S. Government works
Printed in the United States of America on acid-free paper
10 9 8 7 6 5 4 3 2 1

International Standard Book Number-10: 0-8493-4091-8 (Hardcover)
International Standard Book Number-13: 978-0-8493-4091-8 (Hardcover)

Visit the Informa Web site at
www.informa.com

and the Informa Healthcare Web site at
www.informahealthcare.com

Preface

The problem of cardiac complications following anesthesia and surgery has taxed clinicians for many decades. Indeed, the death of Hannah Greener under anesthesia in 1848 is attributed to a cardiac cause. The 15-year-old girl was given chloroform for an operation to remove her toenail and probably died from a cardiac arrhythmia induced by chloroform. In 1929, Sprague described a series of 170 patients with cardiac disease who underwent anesthesia and surgery. Forty-two of them (25%) died during or following surgery. With the steady advances that have taken place in anesthesia, surgery, and the management of heart disease, the risk of cardiac complications in the perioperative period has steadily fallen. The risk of death following elective aortic aneurysm surgery is now of the order of 7%. However, this decline in individual risk has been offset by a number of other factors. More people than ever before survive into old age and extreme old age. Cardiac disease is common in old people and, as the population ages, the population burden of cardiac disease is steadily increasing. Improvements in medical technology and care are such that elderly patients who, even a decade ago, would not have been considered candidates for the operating theater can now be offered surgery.

This book is aimed at anesthetists, physicians, surgeons, and intensivists who care for patients at risk of perioperative myocardial injury and infarction. It provides, in one volume, an account of the current state of knowledge about the epidemiology, pathophysiology, and management of this problem.

Perioperative cardiac complications are a major public health issue. The size of the problem is made clear in Chapter 1. The first half of this chapter provides an account of the epidemiology of perioperative myocardial injury and its implications for the individual patient and the population as a whole. In the second half of the chapter, cardiac risk prediction for the individual patient and for the population as a whole are discussed. The strengths and limitations of the various cardiac risk scores, from the Goldman Multifactorial Risk Index to the Revised Cardiac Risk Index of Lee and Colleagues to the Customized Probability Index for vascular surgery, are examined.

The management of ischemic heart disease in the surgical setting rests on our current understanding of the pathophysiology and medical management of this disease. Chapters 2 and 3 provide the non-specialist with an overview of these rapidly advancing fields.

The mechanisms underlying perioperative myocardial infarction are still a subject of debate; is it due to myocardial oxygen supply/demand imbalance or coronary artery plaque rupture? In Chapter 4, Hans Priebe gives an account of our current understanding of the mechanisms of perioperative myocardial infarction and the extent to which pathophysiological mechanisms in the general cardiological population can be extrapolated to the surgical population. Priebe suggests a model that would unify these two mechanisms.

In the following chapter, Foëx and Biccard describe myocardial stunning and hibernation, concepts that are particularly important in light of recent findings concerning the myocardial protective effects of volatile anesthetic agents.

The next five chapters deal with the clinical management of the patient who has ischemic heart disease and who is to undergo non-cardiac surgery. Preoperative risk assessment and investigation are discussed by Chassot and Spahn. The debate about perioperative beta-blockade continues to rage. Wacker, Schaub, and Zaugg give an erudite account of the basic science underlying perioperative beta-blockade and of the place of these treatments in the management of the surgical patient. In the next chapter, Berridge discusses how best to anesthetize patients with ischemic heart disease and asks if the choice of anesthetic can have an impact on outcome. Despite our best efforts, misfortune sometimes befalls us and our patients. In Chapter 9, Lappas and Stafford-Smith discuss the diagnosis of perioperative myocardial ischemia and infarction; and in Chapter 10, Dorsch and McLenachan describe the management of perioperative myocardial ischemia and infarction.

From both an epidemiological and a clinical perspective, perioperative myocardial ischemia and infarction are hugely important problems, but they are not the only cardiac complications that can befall the surgical patient. Chapters 11, by McGavigan and Rankin, and 12, by Skarvan, deal in depth with cardiac arrhythmias in the setting of non-cardiac surgery and heart failure in the surgical patient.

The development and success of surgery for congenital heart disease means that there is now a generation of patients who have survived to adulthood who would previously have died in childhood or early adult life because of their congenital cardiac lesions. This undoubted triumph had brought with it new challenges for the perioperative physician, as these patients present for surgical care of non-cardiac problems. Barnard gives a detailed and insightful account of the care of these patients.

The next chapters examine special cases of the problem of perioperative cardiac risk: the patient with severe coronary artery disease who also requires carotid endarterectomy, and the patient with severe or unstable coronary artery disease who also requires an urgent non-cardiac operation. Both problems are seen with increasing frequency. The benefits of carotid endarterectomy and the hazards of delaying this surgery in patients with symptomatic cerebral embolic disease are now well-recognized. Advances in medical care mean that patients with severe coronary artery disease survive to need surgery for other conditions.

Chapter 16 deals with the issue of non-cardiac surgery in patients with valvular heart disease—yet another problem that is encountered more often with the aging surgical population.

In Chapter 17, we take the long view. In many instances, patients who present for surgery will not have had their cardiac disease assessed for many years, if at all. The opportunity to offer appropriate primary or secondary cardiovascular prevention should not be missed. How and when this should be done is discussed by Zamvar and Hall.

The final chapter draws together the current issues in this field and looks forward to the work that still needs to be done, as well as the studies that are yet to be conducted, and asks what results they will yield.

The care of the non-cardiac surgery patient who has significant cardiac disease is incompletely covered in texts on cardiology, anesthesia, and surgery. In this book, we offer a comprehensive synthesis of the current state of knowledge on this topic. We describe the epidemiology of the problem and the current state of knowledge about the pathophysiology of heart disease in this setting, highlighting both what is known and what is not, and we give advice and instruction on the current best management of these patients. We hope that our readers find the book both enlightening and useful to guide clinical practice.

Simon Howell
Chris Pepper
Donat R. Spahn

Contents

Contributors

Matthew Barnard   The Heart Hospital, London, U.K.

J. Berridge   Department of Anesthesia and Critical Care, The General Infirmary at Leeds, Leeds, U.K.

Bruce Biccard   Department of Anesthetics, Nelson R. Mandela School of Medicine, Congella, South Africa

Kim A. Boost   Department of Anesthesiology, Intensive Care, and Pain Therapy, Johann Wolfgang Goethe-University, Frankfurt, Germany

Pierre-Guy Chassot   Department of Anesthesiology, University Hospital of Lausanne (CHUV), Lausanne, Switzerland

David C. Crossman   Cardiovascular Research Unit, Royal Hallamshire Hospital, University of Sheffield, Sheffield, U.K.

Demosthenes Dellagrammaticas   The Leeds Vascular Institute, The General Infirmary at Leeds, Leeds, U.K.

Micha Dorsch   Yorkshire Heart Centre, The General Infirmary at Leeds, Leeds, U.K.

Pierre Foëx   Nuffield Department of Anesthetics, University of Oxford, Oxford, U.K.

Michael J. Gough   The Leeds Vascular Institute, The General Infirmary at Leeds, Leeds, U.K.

Alistair S. Hall   C-NET Research Group, The General Infirmary at Leeds, Leeds, U.K.

Simon Howell   University of Leeds, Leeds, U.K.

George D. Lappas   Department of Cardiothoracic Anesthesiology, Duke University Medical Center, Durham, North Carolina, U.S.A.

Carlo Marcucci   Department of Anesthesiology, University Hospital of Lausanne (CHUV), Lausanne, Switzerland

Andrew D. McGavigan   Department of Cardiology, Glasgow Royal Infirmary, Glasgow, U.K.

Jim McLenachan   Yorkshire Heart Centre, The General Infirmary at Leeds, Leeds, U.K.

Allison C. Morton   Cardiovascular Research Unit, Royal Hallamshire Hospital, University of Sheffield, Sheffield, U.K.

Chris Pepper   The General Infirmary at Leeds, Leeds, U.K.

Hans-Joachim Priebe   Department of Anesthesia, University Hospital, Freiburg, Germany

Andrew C. Rankin   Department of Cardiology, Glasgow Royal Infirmary, Glasgow, U.K.

Marcus C. Schaub Institute of Pharmacology and Toxicology, University of Zurich, Zurich, Switzerland

Karl Skarvan Department of Anesthesia, University Hospital Basel, Basel, Switzerland

William H. T. Smith Trent Cardiac Centre, Nottingham University Hospital, Nottingham, U.K.

Donat R. Spahn University Hospital Zurich, Zurich, Switzerland

Mark Stafford-Smith Department of Cardiothoracic Anesthesiology, Duke University Medical Center, Durham, North Carolina, U.S.A.

Johannes Wacker Institute of Anesthesiology, University Hospital Zurich, Zurich, Switzerland

Deoraj Zamvar C-NET Research Group, The General Infirmary at Leeds, Leeds, U.K.

Michael Zaugg Institute of Anesthesiology, University Hospital Zurich, Zurich, Switzerland

Bernhard Zwissler Department of Anesthesiology, Intensive Care, and Pain Therapy, Johann Wolfgang Goethe-University, Frankfurt, Germany

1 Epidemiology of Perioperative Cardiac Complications

Simon Howell
University of Leeds, Leeds, U.K.

INTRODUCTION

Cardiac disease is common in developed countries and is becoming common elsewhere in the world (1). In the West, people are living longer and so have greater opportunity to develop coronary artery disease (CAD) or heart failure rather than being carried off by other diseases. Elsewhere in the world, the scourge of tobacco is causing new epidemics of CAD (2). The surgical population has become older and sicker. Surgery, anesthesia, and perioperative care have also advanced. Cancers that were thought to be untreatable are now amenable to combined surgical and chemo- or radiotherapy. Newer anesthetic agents have less effect on the heart and circulation. Sophisticated monitoring, fluid management, and inotropic drugs allow the circulation to be supported during and after surgery. It has become possible to perform operations on patients who 10 or 15 years ago were considered too old or unfit to withstand surgery. It is now felt reasonable to operate on high-risk patients, including those with heart disease, and the benefits to the patient may be substantial (3). However, the risks can also be substantial.

Devereaux et al. (4) identified seven studies that rigorously estimated the risk of cardiac events following noncardiac surgery. To be included in their analysis studies had to include at least 300 patients, have no restriction on the type of surgery studied, and patients had to have at least one cardiac enzyme or biomarker measurement after surgery. Six of these studies evaluated patients who had or were at risk of cardiac disease and one recruited patients with and without cardiac disease. The pooled data from the studies of patients with cardiac disease yielded an incidence of major perioperative cardiac events of 3.9% (95% CI 3.3–4.6%). Lee et al. (5) studied patients aged over 50 years undergoing elective noncardiac surgery that required hospital admission. Patients with and without cardiac disease were included. Their data gave an overall perioperative cardiac complication risk of 1.4% (95% CI 1.0–1.8%). An obvious but nonetheless important truth is that these global estimates of risk are of limited clinical use. The risk of cardiac complications varies widely between patients depending on the severity of their cardiac disease and the nature of the surgery they are to undergo. It would obviously be inappropriate to tell all patients that their overall risk of a myocardial infarction (MI) is about one and a half percent or indeed all patients who have cardiac disease that they have about a 4% risk of perioperative MI.

Leaving aside patients undergoing cardiac surgery, the people at greatest risk of cardiac complications are those presenting for major vascular surgery. Cardiac complications occur in 1% to 5% of unselected patients undergoing major vascular surgery (6). Bayly et al. (7) reported a 7.3% perioperative mortality rate for patients undergoing aortic surgery. This is unsurprising. By the nature of the surgery for which they have presented, these patients have active vascular disease. More often than not, this affects the coronary arteries as well as the aorta or peripheral circulation.

Hertzer et al. (8) reported the results of coronary angiograms performed in 1000 patients who presented for major vascular surgery. Severe correctable CAD was found in 25% of the patients. It is of interest that the incidence was 31% in patients presenting for aortic surgery, but was lower in those with cerebrovascular disease (26%) and lower extremity disease (21%). Although CAD is common in patients having all types of major vascular surgery, it may be that active disease is more common in patients with lower extremity disease. Some authors have reported a higher perioperative cardiac event rate lower limb vascular surgery than after other types of surgery. L' Italien et al. (9) reported a twofold higher risk of cardiac complication rates in infrainguinal procedures as compared with aortic procedures (13% vs. 6%). This finding is not consistent across all studies. Krupski et al. (10) studied 140 patients undergoing aortic or lower limb vascular surgery. They reported a 24% adverse cardiac outcome rate among patients having infrainguinal bypass operations, as compared with a 28% rate among patients undergoing aortic operations. In this study, adverse cardiac outcomes included cardiac death, nonfatal MI, unstable angina, ventricular tachycardia, and congestive heart failure. There seems little doubt, however, that patients with lower limb vascular disease are particularly prone to attrition from cardiac disease in the months and years following surgery. In another paper, Krupski et al. (11) reported on the two-year follow-up results of their study population. Four percent of patients who had undergone aortic surgery suffered a fatal MI in the follow-up period as compared to 16% of the patients who underwent infrainguinal surgery (11). In a study of 115 patients who underwent vascular surgery for abdominal aortic aneurysm or lower extremity pain, the need for nonaortic surgery was a strong independent predictor of mortality at four years (12).

The extent and severity of preexisting CAD is a major consideration in the etiology of perioperative cardiac complications. Patients with vascular disease generally have CAD and often have active CAD. Eagle et al. (13) conducted a nested study based on the Coronary Artery Surgery Study (CASS) registry. The CASS study compared coronary artery surgery and medical treatment for CAD. Patients were entered into this registry if they were considered to be candidates for randomization in the study. Patients underwent coronary angiography and were randomized to medical or surgical treatment. Patients who were found not to have CAD were also followed-up. During the decade or more of follow-up, 3368 of the 24,959 patients in the registry underwent noncardiac surgery. The outcome of these patients is presented in Figure 1. Patients who had unrevascularized CAD and who underwent abdominal, vascular, thoracic, and head and neck surgery had a combined MI and death rate of more than four percent. The perioperative MI and death rate amongst patients who had these types of operations and had undergone coronary revascularization was significantly lower. (It should be remembered that this takes no account of the risk of coronary artery bypass grafting). What is striking is that amongst patients with unrevascularized CAD, those having vascular surgery had a particularly high MI and death rate. Patients undergoing urologic, orthopedic, breast and skin operations had a mortality rate of less than 1% regardless of how their CAD had been treated.

INDIVIDUAL RISK VS. POPULATION BURDEN OF DISEASE

Although the incidence of perioperative cardiac events is higher in patients undergoing vascular surgery than in other types of major noncardiac surgery, vascular surgery patients represent only a small proportion of the surgical population. Howell and Sear (14) examined this implications of this in a recent review. Patients undergoing other

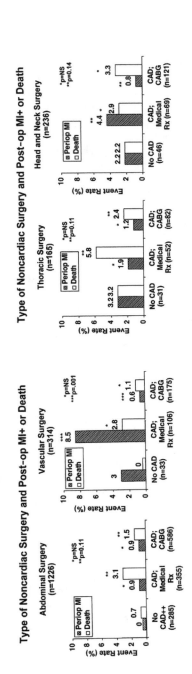

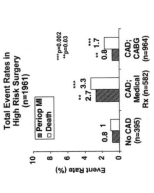

FIGURE 1 Type of noncardiac surgery and incidence of postoperative MI or death among patients undergoing higher-risk procedures (defined as combined MI and death rate ≥4% in medically treated patients). Rates of MI or death among patients undergoing abdominal, vascular, thoracic, and head and neck surgeries are stratified by the presence or absence of CAD and whether it was previously treated medically or with coronary artery bypass surgery. *Abbreviations:* MI, myocardial infarction; CAD, coronary artery disease. *Source:* From Ref. 13.

types of non-cardiac surgery may contribute much to the greater population burden of disease. The Hospital Episode Statistics for England and Wales show that in the year 2002–2003, there were 65,567 operations with codes OPCS4 (Office of Population and Census Surveys) in the range L16 to L31 and L37 to L75. These codes broadly cover major vascular surgical operations on arteries, but exclude operations on the cerebral arteries with codes in the range L33 to L35. In the same period, a total of 5,459,686 operations were reported in patients aged over 59 years (15). The Hospital Episode Statistics report "crude" data and include many minor and diagnostic procedures. Perhaps, only 5% to 10% of the procedures recorded were major operations. However, this is still represents between a quarter and a half a million people aged over 60 years in England and Wales undergoing major surgery each year. It is clear that vascular surgery patients represent only a fraction of the surgical population. Although the cardiac event rate may be higher in patients undergoing major vascular surgery, in any given year, more patients will suffer a perioperative infarction following other types of major noncardiac surgery. This has implications for benefit's to be gained from strategies to reduce perioperative cardiac events. An intervention that reduces risk by half in a vascular surgery patient with a 7% risk of perioperative infarction produces an absolute risk reduction in that patient of 3.5%. The same relative risk reduction in a patient undergoing orthopedic surgery who has a 1% risk of perioperative infarction produces an absolute risk reduction of 0.5%, but may prevent many more events in the population as a whole. There are few more startling results than the reduction in cardiac death and perioperative MI from 34% to 3.4% produced by perioperative beta-adrenergic blockade in the study conducted by Poldermans et al. (16). This represents an absolute risk reduction of 30.6% and a crude odds ratio for the benefit of perioperative beta-blockade of 0.07 (0–0.21). However, this result was obtained in a group of 112 very high-risk patients selected from a total population of 1351 patients. The data on all 1351 patients are reported in a separate paper. A total of 45 patients suffered perioperative cardiac death or MI. Sixteen of these events occurred in the highest risk patients whose risk for a perioperative cardiac event was of the order of 30%. These patients had three or more risk factors for cardiac disease and had inducible wall motion abnormalities on dobutamine stress echocardiography. Twenty-nine of the events occurred in the larger group of intermediate and low risk patients. Among these patients, the perioperative event rate was between 1.2% and 5.8% in patients not taking beta-blockers (17). In this study, the high-risk patients appeared to gain a considerable individual benefit from perioperative beta-blockade, but in absolute terms there were more perioperative MIs in the lower-risk group. A greater reduction in the population burden of disease was achieved by a more modest risk reduction in intermediate and low-risk patients.

PREDICTING PERIOPERATIVE RISK

Clinical risk scoring systems represent an attempt to address the problem of estimating perioperative risk in different patients. Among the best known are those that provide an estimate of the risk of perioperative cardiac complications. Goldman et al. (18) described the eponymous Goldman Risk Score in 1977. Nine cardiac risk factors found to be associated with perioperative cardiac complications were allocated a score (Table 1). By totaling up the risk score for individual patients, the clinician can estimate the risk of perioperative cardiac complications. Despite being carefully and thoughtfully constructed by one of the preeminent researchers in this field, the Goldman Risk Score proved far from perfect and illustrates many of the difficulties that beset clinical risk scoring. The score was constructed by studying a cohort of a

TABLE 1 The Goldman Risk Index

Criteria	Points
History	
Age >70 years	5
MI in previous 6 months	10
Physical examination	
Third heart sound (S3)	11
or jugular venous distension	
Important valvular aortic stenosis	3
Electrocardiogram	
ECG: premature arterial contractions	7
or rhythm other than sinus	
>5 premature ventricular contractions per	7
minute at any time before surgery	
General status	
PaO₂ <60 mmHg (8.0 kPa)	3
or PaCO₂ > 50 mmHg (6.7 kPa)	
K⁺	>3.0 mmol/L or
	HCO₃ <20 mmol/L
Blood urea nitrogen	>50 mg/dL (17.9 mmol/L)
Creatinine	>3.0 mg/dL (265 µmol/L)
Abnormal serum glutamic oxalacetic	
transaminase (aspartate	
aminotransferase or AST)	
Signs of chronic liver disease	
Patient bedridden from noncardiac	
disease	
Operation	
Intrathoracic, intraabdominal,	3
or aortic surgery	
Emergency operation	4

Class	Points total	No or only minor complications number (%) (n =943)	Life-threatening complication number (%) (n =39)	Cardiac deaths number (%) (n =19)
I (n=537)	0–5	532 (99)	4 (0.7)	1 (0.2)
II (n=316)	6–12	295 (93)	16 (5)	5 (2)
III (n=130)	13–25	112 (86)	15 (11)	3 (2)
IV (n=18)	≥26	4 (22)	4 (22)	10 (56)

Abbreviations: MI, myocardial infarction; ECG, electrocardiogram.
Source: From Ref. 18.

1001 patients and noting the presence or absence of over 50 different cardiac risk factors in each patient. Patients were followed-up after surgery, and the occurrence of cardiac complications noted. A complex statistical technique (discriminant function analysis) was then used to identify those risk factors particularly associated with cardiac complications. The stronger the association, the higher the points score awarded to the risk factor. All this sounds simple enough. However, the statistical power of a study of this kind depends not on the number of patients studied but on the number of complications seen. To be statistically robust a study of this type should include at least 10 and ideally 20 patients who suffered a complication for each factor that is in the final risk index (19–21). Fifty-eight patients in Goldman's study suffered cardiac complications and nine risk factors were included in the final index. With just over six risk factors per complication, the model is statistically weak. Furthermore, Goldman et al. made life more difficult for themselves by attempting to study a very large number of risk factors at the outset, many of which were related to each other and therefore not independent. For example, the presence of a third heart sound, the presence of rhales in the lung fields, evidence of cardiomegaly on chest X ray, and many other risk factors are all potential evidence of heart failure. While these may seem severe criticisms of this particular risk index, it should be borne in mind that at the time that it was produced it was the most rigorous study of perioperative cardiac risk available and it represented a significant advance on previous work.

A number of other risk indices have been published, including those of Larsen, Gilbert, and Lee (5,22,23). The most widely used of these is the Lee Score which was published in 1999 and whose authors include Professor Goldman (5). This was derived from a study of over 2893 patients and validated in a study of a further 1422 patients. It includes the risk factors listed in Table 2. Each is allocated one point and as demonstrated in Table 2 the sum of the points gives an estimate of perioperative cardiac risk. It is more robust than the original Goldman Cardiac Risk Index. It was derived in a larger cohort of patients with a larger number of cardiac events. Also, the authors took a more general approach in their definition of cardiac risk factors. For example, the perioperative risk associated with the individual symptoms and signs of congestive heart failure, such as the presence or absence of a third heart sound, was not studied. Instead, congestive heart failure itself was examined as a risk factor. The Lee Index tells us that the two major cardiac pathologies, ischemic heart disease and congestive heart failure, increase perioperative cardiac risk, and that it is further increased by a history of cerebrovascular disease, by the presence of renal impairment or diabetes, and by major surgery, and allows us to estimate the magnitude of the increased risk.

TABLE 2 The Lee Risk Index

Revised cardiac risk index class	Number of risk factors	Cardiac event rate in the validation cohort of the study population ($N = 1422$) events/population	Risk of cardiac complications rate (95% confidence interval)
I	0	2/488	0.4% (0.05–1.5)
II	1	5/567	0.9% (0.3–2.1)
III	2	17/258	6.6% (3.9–10.3)
IV	3 or more	12/109	11% (5.6–18.4)

Note: Risk factors: high-risk type of surgery, history of ischemic heart disease, history of congestive heart failure, history of cerebrovascular disease, preoperative treatment with insulin, preoperative serum creatinine >2.0 mg/dL (177 μmol/L).
Source: From Ref. 5.

Many clinicians feel intuitively that abdominal aortic surgery, with the combined insults of aortic cross-clamping and significant blood loss, subjects the heart to exceptional strain. In their original publication, Lee and colleagues suggested that their system did not offer a reliable prediction of risk in patients undergoing aortic surgery. The Customized Probability Index developed by Kertai et al. is a tool developed to predict cardiac risk in the vascular surgery population. It identified type of vascular surgery, ischemic heart disease, congestive heart failure, previous stroke, hypertension, renal dysfunction, and chronic pulmonary disease as being associated with increased risk, whereas beta-blocker and statin uses were associated with a lower risk of mortality (24).

The Goldman, Larsen, Gilbert, Lee, and customized probability indices all estimate risk in absolute terms. The study population is stratified according to a number of risk factors, and the risk of death or major cardiac complications in each stratum determined. An alternative approach is offered by Bayesian modeling. In this, the effect of various risk factors on baseline risk is estimated. Implicit in this approach is the fact that the baseline risk may vary between institutions. The individual patient's risk score, quantified as a likelihood ratio, is used to adjust the average hospital risk (the pretest probability) to give the risk of complications in that individual (the post-test probability). Two Bayesian cardiac risk indices have been published, those of Detsky and Kumar (25,26). The Detsky index was tested in the study that described the derivation of the Kumar index and shown to perform satisfactorily. However, this is a single validation study and there is a lack of contemporary data on complication rates.

The perfect risk tool would allow the clinician to dichotomize risk. It would give the patient a 95% risk of a major complication or a 95% chance of surviving without mishap. Such tools do not exist! Risk scores such as the Lee Score can take account only of common diseases and common situations. Individual patients are far more complex and frequently have other coexisting diseases that have not been included in the risk calculation. A reliable estimate of risk is a useful epidemiological and audit tool. If a surgeon and anesthetist operate on 100 patients who have a 10% risk of complications and 10 of those patients suffer a complication, the team is performing as expected. However, within those 100 patients will be individuals with a risk of greater than 10% and others with less than 10%.

PREOPERATIVE GUIDELINES

Various guidelines have been published to guide the clinician in the assessment of perioperative cardiac risk. The best known is that promulgated by the American College of Cardiology and the American Heart Association (ACC/AHA Guidelines) (27). In brief, these guidelines suggest that perioperative cardiac risk in the individual patient should be stratified on the basis of the patient's preexisting cardiac disease, their functional capacity, and the severity of the planned surgery. This approach is discussed in detail in chapter 10. Assessing risk can be complex and difficult. The structured analysis of individual perioperative cardiac risk offered by the ACC/AHA Guidelines is immensely valuable to clinicians. Furthermore, the review of the literature offered in the Guidelines is spectacular in both its breadth and depth. Despite this, the limitations of this approach must be appreciated. The ACC/AHA Guidelines have not been fully tested in a randomized controlled trial. Indeed, it is difficult to see how this could be done, as it implies randomizing patients to undergo formal preoperative assessment or not, something that would surely be considered unethical. Specific aspects of the Guidelines have been tested in studies by Samain, Back, and Ali. These yielded equivocal results but were limited by having small sample sizes with relatively few cardiac events (28–30).

DIAGNOSING PERIOPERATIVE MYOCARDIAL INFARCTION

Descriptive epidemiology rests on effective ascertainment. To describe the frequency of a disease or condition in a population, it must be possible to define it precisely and diagnose it reliably. It is well known that perioperative MIs are frequently silent. Devereaux and colleagues attempted to rigorously estimate the frequency of clinically unrecognized MI (31). They evaluated all prospective cohort studies of patients undergoing noncardiac surgery that fulfilled the following criteria:

- Sample size greater than 300 patients
- Surgery restricted to a specific type
- At least one measurement of a cardiac enzyme or biomarker after surgery
- Enumeration of patients suffering a perioperative MI who had no signs or symptoms suggestive of an MI

They identified three eligible studies for this analysis. Their results suggested that only 14% (95% CI 3–25%) of patients experiencing a perioperative MI will have chest pain and only 53% (95% CI 38–68%) will have a clinical sign or symptom that may trigger a physician to consider the diagnosis of perioperative MI.

There are a number of reasons why MI may go unrecognized in the surgical setting. Patients receive potent analgesics that may blunt cardiac pain. The signs and symptoms of MI such as tachycardia, hypotension, and dyspnea may be attributed to other causes. Devereaux et al. (31) proposed that standard diagnostic criteria are required for the diagnosis of perioperative MI in the setting of noncardiac surgery. Their proposed criteria are given in Table 3.

TABLE 3 Proposed Diagnostic Criteria for Perioperative MI in Patients Undergoing Noncardiac Surgery

The diagnosis of preoperative MI requires any one of the following criteria:
A typical rise in the troponin level or a typical fall of an elevated troponin level detected after its peak after surgery in a patient without a documented alternative explanation for an elevated troponin level (e.g., pulmonary embolism); or a rapid rise and fall of CK-MB[a] only if troponin measurement is unavailable. This criterion also requires that one of the following must also exist: ■ Ischemic signs or symptoms, e.g., chest, arm, or jaw discomfort; shortness of breath; pulmonary edema ■ Development of pathological Q-waves on an ECG ■ ECG changes indicative of ischemia ■ Coronary artery intervention ■ New or presumed new cardiac wall motion abnormality on echocardiography, or new or presumed new fixed deficit on radionuclide imaging
Pathological findings of an acute or healing MI
Development of new or pathological Q-waves on an ECG if troponin levels were not obtained or were obtained at times that could have missed the clinical event

[a]CK-MB is less sensitive and specific in the perioperative setting than in other settings and compared with troponin levels. It should be used for diagnostic purposes only when troponin levels are not available.
Abbreviation: MI, myocardial infarction; CK-MB, creatine kinase; ECG, electrocardiogram.
Source: From Ref. 31.

WHAT CONSTITUTES A SIGNIFICANT PERIOPERATIVE
CARDIAC TROPONIN RISE?

It will be seen that the first of Devereaux's criteria is based on perioperative cardiac troponin release. The development of the cardiac troponin assays has driven a change in our understanding of MI. Previous studies used creatine kinase (CK) release for the diagnosis of perioperative infarction (32,33). This enzyme is not specific to the myocardium and is also released from skeletal muscle injured during surgery. It is well known that CK exists in three isoforms CK-MM, CK-MB, and CK-BB of which the CK-MB isoform is predominant in the human heart. However, even with the use of isoforms such as CK-MB, CK is not a specific tool for the diagnosis of perioperative infarction (34). Thus, it is a less than perfect marker for perioperative MI. Unlike CK, cardiac troponin I and T are specific to the myocardium (35). Circulating cardiac troponin has to have come from the heart. Little cardiac troponin I and T are found in normal serum. However, because of assay imprecision at very low levels, the upper limit of normal for serum cardiac troponin is defined as the minimum level of troponin for which the assay can measure with a coefficient of variation of 10% (36).

A patient who has had a large MI will have relatively large amounts of cardiac troponin detectable in the serum. However, in the nonsurgical setting, there is a spectrum of release of cardiac troponin from the heart. Many patients who present with chest pain do not have the full constellation of symptoms and ECG changes that would confirm the diagnosis of an MI but do have a cardiac troponin rise. It has become clear that in medical patients, MI is not a binary event. Instead, there is a spectrum of acute coronary syndromes ranging from unstable angina, through non-ST segment elevation myocardial infarction, to MI with pathological Q-waves (37). It is now understood that patients with cardiac troponin elevation are at increased risk of further cardiac events, but not all of these patients fulfill the criteria for MI (38). This has led to a debate as to whether any cardiac troponin rise above the lower limit of detection should be considered sufficient for the diagnosis of an MI, or if there should be a cut-off based on the prognostic implications of a troponin elevation of a given magnitude (39). Similar considerations may apply in the surgical setting. A number of studies in vascular surgery patients have now confirmed that the release on even small amounts of cardiac troponin in the perioperative period is associated with a worse long-term prognosis. Kim et al. (40) demonstrated that vascular surgery patients who suffer perioperative cardiac troponin I release have an increased risk of death and MI at six months. Landesberg et al. (41) followed-up 447 vascular surgery patients for up to five years after surgery. Patients with perioperative cardiac troponin release had significantly worse survival in the months and years following surgery and there was a clear dose–response effect such that those with the highest levels of perioperative troponin had the worst outlook (Fig. 2). It is less clear, however, that the patient who displays modest amounts of troponin release following with surgery, but who does not have ECG changes diagnostic of MI, should be regarded in the same light as the patient who presents to hospital with chest pain and a transient troponin elevation. The latter would be regarded as having suffered an acute coronary syndrome and would be risk stratified accordingly. Patients who suffer only modest perioperative cardiac troponin release are not classified as having suffered an acute coronary syndrome and the best management of these people had not been defined (42).

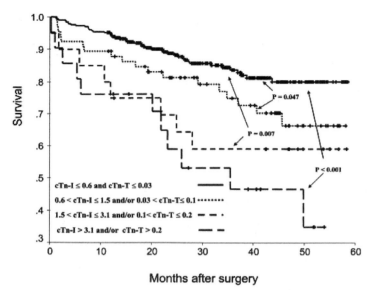

Months after surgery

FIGURE 2 Kaplan–Meier survival curves constructed from survival data on 447 patients who underwent major vascular surgery divided according to their highest postoperative troponin level: Group I—cTn-I≤0.6 ng/ml and cTn-T≤0.03 ng/ml; Group II—0.6 ng/ml<cTn-I≤1.5 ng/ml and/or 0.03 ng/ml<cTn-T≤0.1 ng/ml; Group III—1.5 ng/ml<cTn-I≤3.1 ng/ml and/or 0.1 ng/ml<cTn-T≤ 0.2 ng/ml; Group IV—cTn-I>3.1 ng/ml and/or cTn-T>0.2 ng/ml; Groups II, III, and IV had worse long-term survival than Group I ($p=0.047$, 0.007, and 0.001, respectively, by log-rank test). *Abbreviation*: cTn, cardiac troponin. *Source*: From Ref. 40.

OUTCOME AFTER PERIOPERATIVE MYOCARDIAL INFARCTION

Shah et al. (43) reported an in-hospital mortality rate of 22% in patients who had suffered a perioperative MI. More recent studies suggest little improvement in this figure. In a study of 323 patients, Badner et al. (44) reported a 17% mortality rate among patients who suffered perioperative MI following noncardiac surgery. Kumar et al. (26) reported seven cardiac deaths among 31 patients who suffered a perioperative MI (22%).

The long-term implications of perioperative cardiac troponin release have been alluded to above. However, it has been clear for a decade or more that perioperative MI has long-term implications. In 1992, Mangano et al. (45) reported that patients surviving a postoperative in-hospital MI had a 28-fold increase in the rate of subsequent cardiac complications within six months following surgery, a 15-fold increase within one year, and a 14-fold increase within two years. In a study of 115 patients who underwent vascular surgery for abdominal aortic aneurysm or pain in the lower extremities, perioperative MI was a marginally significant independent predictor of one-year mortality ($p=0.06$) (12).

HEART FAILURE AND ARRHYTHMIA

This review has focused on perioperative myocardial ischemia and infarction. However, these are not the only adverse cardiac events that can occur following surgery.

Both heart failure and arrhythmias may be equally concerning to the clinician and injurious to the patient.

Cardiac failure is well recognized to be a risk factor for perioperative cardiac complications. Robust data on the incidence of heart failure after surgery are more difficult to obtain. Pulmonary edema may be classified as a failure of perioperative fluid management rather than as a cardiac event. In patients who have suffered a perioperative MI, heart failure may be regarded as a consequence of the infarction. The validity of this assumption can be challenged. Increased left ventricular end diastolic pressure may compromise endocardial perfusion and lead to subendocardial infarction, but this does not help us in our quest for robust epidemiological data.

The epidemiology of perioperative arrhythmias is discussed in chapter 10. However, it is reasonable to note here that similar problems arise in determining the incidence of postoperative arrhythmias. It is not always clear if a perioperative arrhythmia is an isolated event or the cause or consequence of other events.

As at other points in this review, it is useful to turn to the large data series accumulated in the derivation and testing of the Lee Modified Cardiac Risk Index. The authors report the incidence of a number of different complications. Complications were not considered to be mutually exclusive, so that a patient could be considered to have suffered more than one complication. Combining the data from the derivation and validation cohorts, 4315 patients were studied. Ninety-two (2%) of these suffered a major cardiac complication. Forty-four (1%) patients developed pulmonary edema, forty-six (1%) patients suffered an acute MI, 16 (0.4%) patients suffered ventricular fibrillation and cardiac arrest, and four (0.1%) patients developed complete heart block (5).

CONCLUSION

The epidemiology of perioperative cardiac complications is not as well defined as might be expected. Perioperative care is evolving rapidly and at the same time the surgical population is changing with many older and higher-risk patients undergoing complex major surgery. Many studies in this field are now a decade or more old. Much has changed in perioperative care since they were conducted; incidence rates for perioperative myocardial infraction and odd ratios for specific risk factors may no longer be valid. These difficulties are compounded by our changing understanding of the pathophysiology of MI and by the redefinition of MI wrought by the development of the cardiac troponin assays. However, amid this uncertainty it remains clear that perioperative cardiac complications are a major cause of death and disability in surgical patients and a considerable challenge to all those involved in perioperative care.

REFERENCES

1. Okrainec K, Banerjee DK, Eisenberg MJ. Coronary artery disease in the developing world. Am Heart J 2004; 148:7–15.
2. Liu BQ, Peto R, Chen ZM, et al. Emerging tobacco hazards in China. 1. Retrospective proportional mortality study of one million deaths. Br Med J 1998; 317:1411–1422.
3. Bouvier AM, Launoy G, Lepage C, Faivre J. Trends in the management and survival of digestive tract cancers among patients aged over 80 years. Aliment Pharmacol Ther 2005; 22:233–241.
4. Devereaux PJ, Goldman L, Cook DJ, Gilbert K, Leslie K, Guyatt GH. Perioperative cardiac events in patients undergoing noncardiac surgery: a review of the magnitude of the

problem, the pathophysiology of the events and methods to estimate and communicate risk. Can Med Assoc J 2005; 173:627–634.

5. Lee TH, Marcantonio ER, Mangione CM, et al. Derivation and prospective validation of a simple index for prediction of cardiac risk of major noncardiac surgery. Circulation 1999; 100:1043–1049.

6. Kertai MD, Klein J, Bax JJ, Poldermans D. Predicting perioperative cardiac risk. Prog Cardiovasc Dis 2005; 47:240–257.

7. Bayly PJ, Matthews JN, Dobson PM, Price ML, Thomas DG. In-hospital mortality from abdominal aortic surgery in Great Britain and Ireland: Vascular Anaesthesia Society audit. Br J Surg 2001; 88:687–692.

8. Hertzer NR, Beven EG, Young JR, et al. Coronary artery disease in peripheral vascular patients: a classification of 1000 coronary angiograms and results of surgical management. Ann Surg 1984; 199:223–233.

9. L' Italien G, Cambria RP, Cutler BS, et al. Comparative early and late cardiac morbidity among patients requiring different vascular surgery procedures. J Vasc Surg 1995; 21:935–944.

10. Krupski WC, Layug EL, Reilly LM, Rapp JH, Mangano DT. Comparison of cardiac morbidity between aortic and infrainguinal operations: Study of Perioperative Ischemia (SPI) Research Group. J Vasc Surg 1992; 15:354–363.

11. Krupski WC, Layug EL, Reilly LM, Rapp JH, Mangano DT. Comparison of cardiac morbidity rates between aortic and infrainguinal operations: two-year follow-up. Study of Perioperative Ischemia Research Group. J Vasc Surg 1993; 18:609–615.

12. McFalls EO, Ward HB, Santilli S, Scheftel M, Chesler E, Doliszny KM. The influence of perioperative myocardial infarction on long-term prognosis following elective vascular surgery. Chest 1998; 113:681–686.

13. Eagle KA, Rihal CS, Mickel MC, Holmes DR, Foster ED, Gersh BJ. Cardiac risk of noncardiac surgery: influence of coronary disease and type of surgery in 3368 operations. CASS Investigators and University of Michigan Heart Care Program. Coronary Artery Surgery Study. Circulation 1997; 96:1882–1887.

14. Howell SJ, Sear JW. Perioperative myocardial injury—individual and population implications. Br J Anaesth 2004; 93:3–8.

15. Department of H. Table 4 Main Operations—Summary 2002–2003. Hospital Episode Statistics 2003.

16. Poldermans D, Boersma E, Bax JJ, et al. The effect of bisoprolol on perioperative mortality and myocardial infarction in high-risk patients undergoing vascular surgery. Dutch Echocardiographic Cardiac Risk Evaluation Applying Stress Echocardiography Study Group. N Engl J Med 1999; 341:1789–1794.

17. Boersma E, Poldermans D, Bax JJ, et al. Predictors of cardiac events after major vascular surgery: role of clinical characteristics, dobutamine echocardiography, and beta-blocker therapy. J Am Med Assoc 2001; 285:1865–1873.

18. Goldman L, Caldera DL, Nussbaum SR, et al. Multifactorial index of cardiac risk in noncardiac surgical procedures. N Engl J Med 1977; 297:845–850.

19. Concato J, Peduzzi P, Holford TR, Feinstein AR. Importance of events per independent variable in proportional hazards analysis. I. Background, goals, and general strategy. J Clin Epidemiol 1995; 48:1495–1501.

20. Peduzzi P, Concato J, Feinstein AR, Holford TR. Importance of events per independent variable in proportional hazards regression analysis. II. Accuracy and precision of regression estimates. J Clin Epidemiol 1995; 48:1503–1510.

21. Peduzzi P, Concato J, Kemper E, Holford TR, Feinstein AR. A simulation study of the number of events per variable in logistic regression analysis. J Clin Epidemiol 1996; 49:1373–1379.

22. Gilbert K, Larocque BJ, Patrick LT. Prospective evaluation of cardiac risk indices for patients undergoing noncardiac surgery. Ann Intern Med 2000; 133:356–359.

23. Larsen SF, Olesen KH, Jacobsen E, et al. Prediction of cardiac risk in non-cardiac surgery. Eur Heart J 1987; 8:179–185.

24. Kertai MD, Boersma E, Klein J, et al. Optimizing the prediction of perioperative mortality in vascular surgery by using a customized probability model. Arch Intern Med 2005; 165:898–904.

25. Detsky AS, Abrams HB, Forbath N, Scott JG, Hilliard JR. Cardiac assessment for patients undergoing noncardiac surgery: a multifactorial clinical risk index. Arch Intern Med 1986; 146:2131–2134.
26. Kumar R, McKinney WP, Raj G, et al. Adverse cardiac events after surgery: assessing risk in a veteran population. J Gen Intern Med 2001; 16:507–518.
27. Eagle KA, Berger PB, Calkins H, et al. ACC/AHA guideline update for perioperative cardiovascular evaluation for noncardiac surgery—executive summary. A report of the American College of Cardiology/American Heart Association Task Force on Practice Guidelines (Committee to Update the 1996 Guidelines on Perioperative Cardiovascular Evaluation for Noncardiac Surgery). Circulation 2002; 105:1257–1267.
28. Samain E, Farah E, Leseche G, Marty J. Guidelines for perioperative cardiac evaluation from the American College of Cardiology/American Heart Association Task Force are effective for stratifying cardiac risk before aortic surgery. J Vasc Surg 2000; 31:971–979.
29. Back MR, Schmacht DC, Bowser AN, et al. Critical appraisal of cardiac risk stratification before elective vascular surgery. Vasc Endovasc Surg 2003; 37:387–397.
30. Ali MJ, Davison P, Pickett W, Ali NS. ACC/AHA guidelines as predictors of postoperative cardiac outcomes. Can J Anaesth 2000; 47:10–19.
31. Devereaux PJ, Goldman L, Yusuf S, Gilbert K, Leslie K, Guyatt GH. Surveillance and prevention of major perioperative ischemic cardiac events in patients undergoing noncardiac surgery: a review. Can Med Assoc J 2005; 173:779–788.
32. Mangano DT, Browner WS, Hollenberg M, London MJ, Tubau JF, Tateo IM. Association of perioperative myocardial ischemia with cardiac morbidity and mortality in men undergoing noncardiac surgery. The Study of Perioperative Ischemia Research Group. N Engl J Med 1990; 323:1781–1788.
33. Raby KE, Goldman L, Creager MA, et al. Correlation between preoperative ischemia and major cardiac events after peripheral vascular surgery. N Engl J Med 1989; 321:1296–1300.
34. Mangano DT. Beyond CK-MB: biochemical markers for perioperative myocardial infarction. Anesthesiology 1994; 81:1317–1320.
35. Apple FS. Tissue specificity of cardiac troponin I, cardiac troponin T and creatine. Clinica Chimica Acta. 1999; 284(2):151–159.
36. Panteghini M, Pagani F, Yeo KT, et al. Evaluation of imprecision for cardiac troponin assays at low-range concentrations. Clin Chem 2004; 50:327–332.
37. Wu AH, Ford L. Release of cardiac troponin in acute coronary syndromes: ischemia or necrosis? Clin Chim Acta 1999; 284:161–174.
38. Myocardial infarction redefined—a consensus document of the Joint European Society of Cardiology/American College of Cardiology Committee for the redefinition of myocardial infarction. J Am Coll Cardiol 2000; 36:959–969.
39. Fox KA, Birkhead J, Wilcox R, Knight C, Barth J. British Cardiac Society Working Group on the definition of myocardial infarction. Heart 2004; 90:603–609.
40. Kim LJ, Martinez EA, Faraday N, et al. Cardiac troponin I predicts short-term mortality in vascular surgery patients. Circulation 2002; 106:2366–2371.
41. Landesberg G, Shatz V, Akopnik I, et al. Association of cardiac troponin, CK-MB, and postoperative myocardial ischemia with long-term survival after major vascular surgery. J Am Coll Cardiol 2003; 42:1547–1554.
42. Howell SJ, Thompson JP, Nimmo AF, et al. Relationship between perioperative troponin elevation and other indicators of myocardial injury in vascular surgery patients. Br J Anaesth 2006; 96:303–309.
43. Shah KB, Kleinman BS, Rao TL, Jacobs HK, Mestan K, Schaafsma M. Angina and other risk factors in patients with cardiac diseases undergoing noncardiac operations. Anesth Analg 1990; 70:240–247.
44. Badner NH, Knill RL, Brown JE, Novick TV, Gelb AW. Myocardial infarction after noncardiac surgery. Anesthesiology 1998; 88:572–578.
45. Mangano DT, Browner WS, Hollenberg M, Li J, Tateo IM. Long-term cardiac prognosis following noncardiac surgery. The Study of Perioperative Ischemia Research Group. J Am Med Assoc 1992; 268:233–239.

2 Pathophysiology of Ischemic Heart Disease

Allison C. Morton and David C. Crossman

Cardiovascular Research Unit, Royal Hallamshire Hospital, University of Sheffield, Sheffield, U.K.

INTRODUCTION

Ischemic heart disease (IHD), the major cause of morbidity and mortality in the Western World, has its basis in the atherosclerosis that affects the epicardial coronary arteries. The term atherosclerosis originates from the Greek, athere (meaning "gruel"), which describes the soft, lipid-rich core of the plaque, and skleros (meaning "hard") that describes the hard fibrous capsule that surrounds the core, a general description that is still useful today. Previously considered as a cholesterol-storage disease, it is now viewed as a chronic inflammatory disorder within the wall of the artery. Inflammation results from a complex interaction between modified lipoproteins, monocyte-derived macrophages, cytokines, and normal components of the arterial wall. In general, disease presentation results either from chronic and gradual reduction of the arterial lumen or instability of the plaque-producing acute luminal obstruction and/or distal vessel embolization. Within the context of IHD, this accounts for presentation as chronic stable angina, acute coronary syndromes (ACS), sudden ischemic coronary death, and heart failure (Table 1). This chapter will describe the fundamental processes involved in atherogenesis and the mechanisms of coronary instability.

ATHEROSCLEROTIC LESION FORMATION—AN OVERVIEW

The lesions of atherosclerosis occur in large- and medium-sized elastic arteries (Table 2). Atheroma formation begins in early childhood with development of a fatty streak, the starting point in the development of an atherosclerotic plaque. Fatty streaks are purely inflammatory lesions consisting of T-lymphocytes and monocyte-derived macrophages, the latter containing fat (1). Streak development occurs following endothelial cell dysfunction which leads to compensatory mechanisms that change the normal homeostatic properties of the endothelium (2). Low-density lipoprotein (LDL) is transcytosed and trapped in the intima, modified by oxidation, recognized by scavenger receptors, and then endocytosed by the monocyte-derived macrophages, giving rise to the hallmark cell of the atherosclerotic lesion, the lipid-filled foam cell.

An essential initial event in atherogenesis is endothelial cell dysfunction and activation. Causes of endothelial cell dysfunction in the context of atherogenesis include elevated blood lipids (especially LDL) (3), genetic predisposition (4), smoking (5), hypertension (6), elevated homocysteine (7), and diabetes (8). In addition, more recent studies have implicated infectious microorganisms such as *Chlamydia pneumoniae* (9), although the relevance of this to human disease progression and presentation is far from clear.

All these processes effectively insult or injure the endothelium. Common pathways of activation exist that may link diverse activating stimuli. One such pathway is increased production of free oxygen radicals [reactive oxygen species (ROS)] from

TABLE 1   Clinical Representation of Coronary Atherosclerosis

Chronic stable angina
ACS
Sudden ischemic coronary death
Heart failure

Abbreviation: ACS, acute coronary syndrome.

endothelial cells. ROS initiate several key processes involved in atherogenesis, including expression of adhesion molecules, vascular smooth muscle cell (VSMC), migration and proliferation, apoptosis in the endothelium, and activation of matrix metalloproteinases (10). Injury to the endothelium also causes an alteration in its permeability and "stickiness" with respect to platelets and leukocytes. The endothelium loses its anticoagulant effect, becoming procoagulant, forming and releasing cytokines (e.g., IL-1) and vasoactive molecules. Complete loss of endothelium leaves a subendothelial matrix that is potently adherent for platelets and white cells.

As in any inflammatory reaction, if the resulting inflammatory response does not remove the stimulus, the process continues indefinitely. Recruited macrophages, platelets, and endothelial cells release chemokines to direct white cell recruitment and growth factors for VSMC which migrate and proliferate within this area. The recruited VSMCs form an abundant collagen-rich, extracellular matrix giving rise to an elevated intimal lesion, the intermediate plaque, or the fibro-fatty plaque. The artery compensates for this accumulating plaque within its wall by gradual dilation (remodeling) which allows the artery lumen diameter to remain essentially unchanged despite a relatively large amount of disease (11).

Continued inflammation results in increased numbers of macrophages and lymphocytes from the blood entering the lesion. Again, activation of these cells leads to further cytokine release, which in turn cause further accumulation and may even result in necrosis. Thus, the cycle of mononuclear cell accumulation, VSMC migration and proliferation, and fibrous tissue formation continues, and the lesion (now termed advanced or complicated) enlarges, eventually becoming covered with a fibrous cap formed from VSMC collagen. The compensatory dilatation of the artery at some point fails to keep up and the plaque then encroaches into the lumen and restricts the flow of blood causing ischemia.

Thinning and rupture of the plaque cap is the most common cause of intracoronary thrombus (12) that results in ACS. This forms the unstable plaque (see below). This can occur on early, nonocclusive fibro-fatty plaques or on more advanced plaques. These steps will be described further below.

ROLE OF LIPOPROTEINS

Lipids and cholesterol are probably obligatory for the formation of arterial atherosclerosis. The lipid hypothesis of atherosclerosis arose from observations of rare

TABLE 2   Hallmark Lesions of Atherosclerosis

Fatty streak—no clinical consequence
Fibro-fatty plaque—chronic stable angina
Unstable plaque—ACS

Abbreviation: ACS, acute coronary syndrome.

hypercholesterolemic conditions that produced very aggressive, early-onset atherosclerosis. The hypothesis, although much debated two to three decades ago, was proven by the overwhelming beneficial effects of the statin-type cholesterol-reducing drugs. It still remains uncertain, however, the exact reason why a raised serum cholesterol is so bad for the arterial wall.

A review of the role of lipids in atherosclerosis is beyond the scope of this chapter. Briefly, serum cholesterol is transported by lipoprotein particles (13). Chylomicrons are the main transporters of dietary lipids; very low-density lipoprotein (VLDL), LDLs, and high-density lipoproteins (HDL) transport endogenous or modified lipids. In humans, the majority of serum cholesterol is transported to peripheral tissues by LDL. LDL is taken up by cells via LDL receptors. Genetic lack or dysfunction of LDL receptors leads to the accumulation of LDL in patients with homozygous familial hypercholesterolemia (14) where atherosclerosis is extensive in untreated individuals by the second decade. In normal individuals, expression of LDL receptors is dependent on feedback control by intracellular cholesterol (15). One of the beneficial effects of statin drugs is to modulate this and cause an upregulation of LDL receptors. In the periphery, LDL becomes oxidized to varying degrees and becomes recognized by scavenger receptors on macrophages. These receptors have evolved to recognize substances that need to be cleared away, in particular, dead cells or bacteria. A key function of this system in macrophages is to ingest modified ingested molecules and present them to cells of the adaptive immune system. This occurs with oxidized LDL, and antibodies may be formed. The role of these in the propagation of atherosclerosis is a subject of continuing research.

HDL cholesterol (often viewed as "good" cholesterol, as low levels of HDL cholesterol are intensely atherogenic) participates in reverse cholesterol transport, taking cholesterol back to the liver from the periphery. The new generation of highly efficacious statins and nicotinic acid have mild HDL-cholesterol-raising properties but there is intense activity in the pharmaceutical industry to identify drugs that more effectively raise HDL cholesterol.

The importance of lipids and the cholesterol pathway in atherosclerosis is also confirmed in genetically modified animals. Genetic manipulation of mice by disruption of the apo-E or LDL receptor gene in combination with a high-cholesterol diet leads to the formation of atherosclerosis in this animal which is normally atherosclerosis resistant. This has proven to be a useful model for research purposes and has afforded mechanistic insights into atherosclerosis.

INITIAL EVENTS IN ATHEROSCLEROTIC PLAQUE FORMATION—FATTY STREAK FORMATION

Atherosclerotic plaques begin as fatty streaks composed of foam cells. The basic atherogenic model for fatty streaks is now well established. At the site of fatty streak formation, endothelial cells become activated and there is upregulation of molecules (adhesion molecules) that tether and recruit circulating monocytes. The monocytes then migrate to the subendothelial layer and differentiate into macrophages. There they ingest lipid and become foam cells.

The modification of LDL by oxidation drives initial fatty streak formation (13,16). The exact site and mechanism of oxidation is still debated. The degree to which LDL is modified and taken up by macrophages varies from minimal, in which the LDL particle can still recognize its receptor (16), to extensive, which results in breakdown of the products of oxidation (13). The particles that result from extensive modification do not bind to the LDL receptor but bind instead to scavenger receptors that are expressed on VSMC and macrophages. After binding to these receptors in vitro, a series of intracellular events results that includes the induction of inflammatory cytokines such as interleukin-1 (IL-1) (17,18). The inflammatory response itself can have effects on lipoproteins within the artery and mediators of inflammation such as IL-1 and tumor necrosis factor alpha (TNF-α) and increases transcription of the LDL receptor gene. Thus, a vicious circle of inflammation and modification of LDL is set up and maintained within the artery.

Many studies have shown that antioxidant treatment reduces the development of atherosclerosis in animal models (19–21). Endothelial NO synthase produces NO that acts as a vasodilator and is protective against atherosclerosis deletion of this gene causes hypertension and atherosclerotic plaque formation (22). It is known that endothelial NO production is sensitive to ROS for complex reasons. ROS not only destroy NO, but also uncouple nitric oxide synthase in such a way that it stops making NO and makes further ROS. In contrast, another isoform of nitric oxide synthase, inducible NO synthase found in macrophages, can cause LDL oxidation directly and increased atherosclerosis (23). It is probable that general reduction in endothelial NO production is pro-atherogenic because of induced endothelial dysfunction, and similarly localized macrophage-derived NO overproduction is also pro-atherogenic through pro-oxidant mechanisms. The complexity of the role of NO in the context of oxidant stress is added to by the observation that downregulation of endothelial cell NO production is linked to upregulation of superoxide generation.

All these pro-oxidant stress mechanisms are potentially important in atherogenesis and thus the role of antioxidants in the treatment of atherosclerosis has been studied. Although epidemiological studies show an inverse relationship between antioxidant vitamin intake and cardiovascular disease, a number of clinical trials have failed to demonstrate the beneficial effects of antioxidants on the risk of cardiovascular events (24). The reason for this is unclear but may in part be a result of the low antioxidant potential of the available compounds at the level of the vessel wall.

MONOCYTE AND MACROPHAGE RECRUITMENT

As outlined above, progressive accumulation of LDL-laden macrophages leads to the development of fatty streaks. The mechanism of monocyte recruitment has therefore been a subject of intense investigation. Early studies using genetically modified mice showed the obligatory role for monocytes in the development of atherosclerosis. Monocyte recruitment appears to be dependent on the adhesion molecules VCAM-1 and ICAM-1, which are expressed on the surface of endothelial cells in response to inflammatory stimuli and are found to be upregulated in atherosclerotic arteries. Deletion of the ICAM-1 gene has been shown to result in significant reductions in monocytes recruitment to atherosclerotic lesions in apo-E-deficient mice (25), although not in all studies. Complete deletion of VCAM-1 is embryonically lethal, but a hypomorphic transgenic animal with reduced amounts of VCAM-1 appears protected from atherosclerosis (26). Oxidized LDL also directly attracts monocytes to the artery wall (27) and induces the expression of chemotactic molecules such as monocyte chemotactic protein (MCP-1) (16). Disruption of the MCP-1 gene reduces atherosclerotic development in apo-E knock-out mice (28). Whether these mechanisms can ever be interrupted in such a way as to block atherosclerosis is uncertain as these are fundamental processes in the regulation of innate immunity, but they prove conclusively the central role of the monocyte/macrophage to atherogenesis.

PLAQUE COMPOSITION AND LESION PROGRESSION

As discussed, foam cells are the "hallmark" cell of the atherosclerotic lesion and are formed following uptake of oxidized LDL by scavenger receptors (29). Oxidized-LDL-derived cholesterol brought into the macrophages by these receptors consists of both cholesterol esters and free cholesterol. Once accumulated, either efflux via membrane transporters, with HDL acting as the main extracellular acceptor, or enzymatic modification into more soluble forms allows macrophages to dispose of excess cholesterol (30) (reverse cholesterol transport). The role of HDL is thought to be critical for this process which may explain why the risk of atherosclerosis is inversely correlated with HDL cholesterol levels (31). Oversaturation of macrophages with cholesterol leads to the formation of foam cells and the immature fatty streak.

The transition from fatty streak to a mature lesion is characterized by migration of VSMC into the intimal space. Cycles of accumulation of macrophages, migration and proliferation of VSMC, and formation of fibrous tissue leads to plaque enlargement and restructuring so that it becomes covered by a fibrous cap which overlies the lipid core. Progression of the plaque is modulated by cytokines and the immune response (12).

NATURE OF THE INFLAMMATORY STIMULUS

Many stimuli are transduced by the arterial wall into an inflammatory response. At these sites, adhesion molecules are expressed on the endothelium which attracts monocytes and T-cells to the artery with consequent formation of an atherosclerotic plaque. The pattern of blood flow at the sites of atheroma formation may be one of the factors that determines whether lesions form or not. Certainly many inflammatory genes have shear response elements in the regulatory parts of their genes that are capable of responding to alteration and disturbance of shear stress.

Chemokines are responsible for chemotaxis and accumulation of macrophages in fatty streaks (32). Activation of monocytes and T-cells leads to upregulation of receptors on their surface that binds chemoattractant molecules. These ligand–receptor interactions cause further monocyte activation, induce cell proliferation, and localize the inflammatory response at the site of lesions (4). Monocytes are found at every stage of plaque development. Macrophages act as both scavenging and antigen-presenting cells secreting, among other things, chemokines and cytokines (e.g., TNF-α and IL-1) and proteolytic enzymes (e.g., metalloproteinases). It is this ability that is critical in the role of these cells in the damage and repair that ensues as lesions progress. The continued survival of macrophages is dependent upon exposure to macrophage colony-stimulating factor but in vivo, in response to other inflammatory cytokines such as interferon gamma, macrophages undergo apoptosis (programmed cell death) and form part of the necrotic core characteristic of an advanced atherosclerotic lesion. Cell-mediated immune responses are involved in atherosclerosis, and the macrophages act as the antigen-presenting cells in this process. T-cells are present in atherosclerotic lesions at all stages and their activation (which occurs when they bind antigen processed and presented by macrophages) results in the secretion of cytokines that amplify the inflammatory response (33). CD40 ligand, an immunoregulatory molecule, and its receptor CD40 are expressed by macrophages, T-cells, and VSMC in atherosclerotic lesions. Both are upregulated in atherosclerotic plaques (34). CD40 ligand induces the release of IL-1β (a potent inflammatory stimulant) enhancing the inflammatory response; inhibition of CD40 with blocking antibodies reduces lesion in apo-E knock-out mice (35).

ROLE OF PLATELETS AND THROMBOSIS

Platelets and thrombosis are involved in plaque instability and plaque progression. Blood-derived products are found within the plaque at all stages of its development. All key cells in human atherosclerotic plaques express the thrombin receptor, including endothelial cells, VSMCs, macrophages, and platelets, indicating that thrombin has the potential to influence the inflammatory and proliferative responses (36). Platelets adhere to injured endothelium, exposed collagen, and macrophages. When activated, they release granules that contain cytokines, chemokines, growth factor vasoconstrictors, and most dangerous of all agonists that stimulate further platelet activation. These, together with thrombin, contribute to the migration and proliferation of VSMC and monocytes (37). Plaque rupture and thrombosis are the commonest complications of the advanced atherosclerotic plaque and result in ACS or myocardial infarction (38). Subclinical episodes of plaque rupture and thrombus formation with healing are probably important as a mechanism of plaque expansion. Antiplatelet agents have shown amazing effectiveness in the prevention and treatment of complications of coronary atherosclerosis and these attest to the critical role of the platelet in IHD.

PLAQUE INSTABILITY

Plaque instability is the basis of the vast majority of ACS. The basic pathophysiological mechanism is that the plaque becomes destabilized to allow formation of an intracoronary thrombus that may grow to occlude the vessel completely, embolize material distally, and block the microcirculation or release potent constrictor mediators that lead to constriction superimposed upon nonocclusive thrombi. All three mechanisms may occur. Plaque instability arises either because of plaque rupture (~70%) or plaque erosion (~30%). Plaque rupture describes the splitting of the cap of the plaque, exposing thrombogenic plaque contents that stimulate the formation of a clot. Plaque erosion is described as a plaque where the surface is intact but there is endothelial erosion and exposure of thrombogenic extracellular matrix that forms the initiating stimulus for clot formation. The cause of the erosion is not clear. Via either mechanism, clot formation results. In arterial thrombosis, the key initial event is platelet adherence with activation. Platelets can participate in coagulation because activation is associated with exposure of the prothrombinase complex. In addition, activated plaques appear to be rich in tissue factor, the essential cofactor for the activation of the extrinsic pathway of coagulation.

Plaque disruption does not always cause a clinical event. Evidence of plaque rupture may be seen in individuals who died for noncoronary reasons. As stated above, subclinical rupture is probably an important mechanism of plaque expansion. There is evidence that in patients presenting with ACS, there may be multiple plaque ruptures, but only one has caused the clinical presentation. These postmortem observations are now confirmed by angiography, intracoronary imaging studies (IVUS and angioscopy), and functional studies that indicate that ACS is more usually associated with activation of plaques throughout the coronary tree.

Why plaques rupture is clearly a very important question. It is clear that this is not a random event; myocardial infarcts are more common at particular times of the day (early hours), particular times of the week (beginning), and particular times of the year (winter months). Infection may be a trigger, and respiratory tract infection appears to increase risk of myocardial infarction by ~5-fold in the three to four weeks following the infection. Biologically, it is clear that unstable plaques have increased levels of matrix metalloproteinases and collagen cleavage products. This suggests that there are specific inflammatory mechanisms that trigger these events which then structurally weaken the cap of the plaque and make it vulnerable to either spontaneous rupture or rupture associated with increased shear forces when there is a surge in blood pressure for environmental reasons.

PATHOLOGICAL–CLINICAL CORRELATES

There are limited opportunities to be able to link the pathological descriptions to clinical syndromes. In general, we see ACS presenting with either ST elevation on the electrocardiogram (ECG; STEMI) or in the absence of ST elevation where there may or may not be evidence of myocyte necrosis. In the presence of myocyte necrosis, this is classified as non-ST elevation myocardial infarction (NSTEMI) and without it is still best described as unstable angina. All of these syndromes have their basis in plaque instability. What determines the nature of the clinical presentation is determined by a number of factors. These will include luminal and extraluminal factors. Luminal factors describe the extent of intravascular thrombus formation. Complete luminal obstruction has the capacity to produce STEMI. Incomplete thrombotic occlusion will lead to non-STEMI although the myocardial necrosis may itself be caused by either distal embolization of platelet-rich thrombus or phasic near-complete occlusion of the epicardial coronary artery. Non-STEMI may also occur following complete luminal obstruction but extraluminal factors determine that STEMI does not occur. These will include: the amount of myocardium subtended, the degree of collateralization, and the territory of the myocardium effected—circumflex occlusions may really be causing STEMI events that are recorded by the ECG as non-STEMI as this is an area is not well scrutinized by the standard ECG.

CONCLUSION

Coronary atheroma is an inflammatory condition and forms the basis of one of the most common and serious of illnesses in the Western world. An understanding of the pathogenesis of this condition has allowed the logical construction of treatment plans for both the prevention and treatment of this condition. An appreciation of the emerging inflammatory mechanism will allow new therapies to be tested in this condition.

REFERENCES

1. Ross R. The pathogenesis of atherosclerosis: a perspective for the 1990s. Nature 1993; 362(6423):801–809.
2. Libby P. Vascular biology of atherosclerosis: overview and state of the art. Am J Cardiol 2003; 91(3A):3A–6A.
3. Diaz MN, et al. Antioxidants and atherosclerotic heart disease. N Engl J Med 1997; 337(6):408–416.
4. Ross R. Atherosclerosis—an inflammatory disease. N Engl J Med 1999; 340(2):115–126.
5. Zhang S, Day I, Ye S. Nicotine induced changes in gene expression by human coronary artery endothelial cells. Atherosclerosis 2001; 154(2):277–283.

6. Sainani GS, Maru VG. Role of endothelial cell dysfunction in essential hypertension. J Assoc Physicians India 2004; 52:966–969.
7. Guthikonda S, Haynes WG. Homocysteine: role and implications in atherosclerosis. Curr Atheroscler Rep 2006; 8(2):100–106.
8. Calles-Escandon J, Cipolla M. Diabetes and endothelial dysfunction: a clinical perspective. Endocr Rev 2001; 22(1):36–52.
9. Libby P, Egan D, Skarlatos S. Roles of infectious agents in atherosclerosis and restenosis: an assessment of the evidence and need for future research. Circulation 1997; 96(11): 4095–4103.
10. Harrison D, et al. Role of oxidative stress in atherosclerosis. Am J Cardiol 2003; 91(3A): 7A–11A.
11. Glagov S, et al. Compensatory enlargement of human atherosclerotic coronary arteries. N Engl J Med 1987; 316(22):1371–1375.
12. Glass CK, Witztum JL. Atherosclerosis: the road ahead. Cell 2001; 104(4):503–516.
13. Steinberg D, a.W., Goldstein JL. In: Chien KR, ed. Lipoproteins, Lipoprotein, Oxidation and Atherogenesis. Philadelphia: WB Saunders, 1999.
14. Goldstein JL, Brown MS. The low-density lipoprotein pathway and its relation to atherosclerosis. Annu Rev Biochem 1977; 46:897–930.
15. Brown MS, Goldstein JL. The SREBP pathway: regulation of cholesterol metabolism by proteolysis of a membrane-bound transcription factor. Cell 1997; 89(3):331–340.
16. Navab M, et al. The Yin and Yang of oxidation in the development of the fatty streak: a review based on the 1994 George Lyman Duff Memorial Lecture. Arterioscler Thromb Vasc Biol 1996; 16(7):831–842.
17. Geng YJ, Libby P. Evidence for apoptosis in advanced human atheroma: colocalization with interleukin-1 beta-converting enzyme. Am J Pathol 1995; 147(2):251–266.
18. Palkama T. Induction of interleukin-1 production by ligands binding to the scavenger receptor in human monocytes and the THP-1 cell line. Immunology 1991; 74(3):432–438.
19. Carew TE, Schwenke DC, Steinberg D. Antiatherogenic effect of probucol unrelated to its hypocholesterolemic effect: evidence that antioxidants in vivo can selectively inhibit low density lipoprotein degradation in macrophage-rich fatty streaks and slow the progression of atherosclerosis in the Watanabe heritable hyperlipidemic rabbit. Proc Natl Acad Sci USA 1987; 84(21):7725–7729.
20. Sasahara M, et al. Inhibition of hypercholesterolemia-induced atherosclerosis in the nonhuman primate by probucol. I. Is the extent of atherosclerosis related to resistance of LDL to oxidation? J Clin Invest 1994; 94(1):155–164.
21. Chang MY, et al. Inhibition of hypercholesterolemia-induced atherosclerosis in the nonhuman primate by probucol. II. Cellular composition and proliferation. Arterioscler Thromb Vasc Biol 1995; 15(10):1631–1640.
22. Knowles JW, et al. Enhanced atherosclerosis and kidney dysfunction in eNOS($-/-$)ApoE ($-/-$) mice are ameliorated by enalapril treatment. J Clin Invest 2000; 105(4):451–458.
23. Behr-Roussel D, et al. Effect of chronic treatment with the inducible nitric oxide synthase inhibitor N-iminoethyl-L-lysine or with L-arginine on progression of coronary and aortic atherosclerosis in hypercholesterolemic rabbits. Circulation 2000; 102(9):1033–1038.
24. Davi G, Falco A. Oxidant stress, inflammation and atherogenesis. Lupus 2005; 14(9):760–764.
25. Collins RG, et al. P-Selectin or intercellular adhesion molecule (ICAM)-1 deficiency substantially protects against atherosclerosis in apolipoprotein E-deficient mice. J Exp Med 2000; 191(1):189–194.
26. Cybulsky MI, et al. A major role for VCAM-1, but not ICAM-1, in early atherosclerosis. J Clin Invest 2001; 107(10):1255–1262.
27. Steinberg D, et al. Beyond cholesterol: modifications of low-density lipoprotein that increase its atherogenicity. N Engl J Med 1989; 320(14):915–924.
28. Boring L, et al. Decreased lesion formation in CCR2$^{-/-}$ mice reveals a role for chemokines in the initiation of atherosclerosis. Nature 1998; 394(6696):894–897.
29. Yamada Y, et al. Scavenger receptor family proteins: roles for atherosclerosis, host defence and disorders of the central nervous system. Cell Mol Life Sci 1998; 54(7):628–640.
30. Bjorkhem I. Mechanism of degradation of the steroid side chain in the formation of bile acids. J Lipid Res 1992; 33(4):455–471.

31. Tall AR, et al. 1999 George Lyman Duff memorial lecture: lipid transfer proteins, HDL metabolism, and atherogenesis. Arterioscler Thromb Vasc Biol 2000; 20(5):1185–1188.
32. Boring L, et al. Impaired monocyte migration and reduced type 1 (Th1) cytokine responses in C–C chemokine receptor 2 knockout mice. J Clin Invest 1997; 100(10):2552–2561.
33. Hansson GK, et al. Immune mechanisms in atherosclerosis. Arteriosclerosis 1989; 9(5): 567–578.
34. Mach F, et al. Activation of monocyte/macrophage functions related to acute atheroma complication by ligation of CD40: induction of collagenase, stromelysin, and tissue factor. Circulation 1997; 96(2):396–399.
35. Mach F, et al. Reduction of atherosclerosis in mice by inhibition of CD40 signalling. Nature 1998; 394(6689):200–203.
36. Nelken NA, et al. Thrombin receptor expression in normal and atherosclerotic human arteries. J Clin Invest 1992; 90(4):1614–1621.
37. Bombeli T, Schwartz BR, Harlan JM. Adhesion of activated platelets to endothelial cells: evidence for a GPIIbIIIa-dependent bridging mechanism and novel roles for endothelial intercellular adhesion molecule 1 (ICAM-1), alphavbeta3 integrin, and GPIbalpha. J Exp Med 1998; 187(3):329–339.
38. Davies MJ. A macro- and microview of coronary vascular insult in ischemic heart disease. Circulation 1990; 82(suppl 3):II38–II46.

3 Management of Ischemic Heart Disease

William H. T. Smith
Trent Cardiac Centre, Nottingham University Hospital, Nottingham, U.K.

Chris Pepper
The General Infirmary at Leeds, Leeds, U.K.

INTRODUCTION

This chapter summarizes the contemporary management of ischemic heart disease (IHD). We address general diagnostic and therapeutic considerations. Issues more specifically relating to the management of IHD around the time of surgery are described in later chapters.

The prevalence of IHD is such that many patients will be diagnosed for the first time by doctors seeing them in the perioperative situation. Existing symptoms may come to light at preoperative assessment, whereas others may develop new symptoms during the postoperative phase. Furthermore, the increasing practice of screening for IHD prior to higher-risk surgery will identify another group of asymptomatic patients with occult IHD. It is, therefore, increasingly important that anesthetists be familiar with modern management of myocardial ischemia.

PRESENTATION OF MYOCARDIAL ISCHEMIA

Myocardial ischemia occurs when there is insufficient coronary blood flow to supply the heart's oxygen demands. This is frequently but not exclusively due to atheromatous coronary artery stenosis. Ischemia may be asymptomatic but will frequently result in either chronic stable angina or an acute coronary syndrome (ACS) depending on the nature of the coronary pathology.

Chronic Stable Angina

In chronic stable angina, the atheromatous process slowly progresses and the coronary lumen gradually narrows over many months and years. The resulting coronary obstruction prevents an adequate increase in oxygen supply when myocardial demand is increased by exercise or other stress. In this situation, the patient frequently presents with chest pain on extra effort which is relieved by rest. With disease progression, symptoms occur with less and less activity as the degree of coronary obstruction increases. The development of angina could thus be viewed as a protective mechanism preventing continuing exertion leading to irreversible myocardial damage. This is not necessarily possible when circulatory demands increase during surgery, and "demand" myocardial infarction is therefore possible without an acute coronary event if the heart's oxygen demands are increased perioperatively in the context of severe coronary artery disease.

Acute Coronary Syndromes

In ACSs, the patient presents acutely with unheralded chest pain at rest or on minimal exertion. This is usually due to fissuring of an atheromatous plaque followed by aggregation of platelets, deposition of fibrin and consequent occlusion or severe obstruction of the coronary artery lumen. Thus, myocardial supply reduces suddenly, whereas the heart's oxygen demands remain fairly constant. If a major epicardial coronary artery occludes completely, there is severe, transmural ischemia, progressing rapidly to infarction, and in general ST segment elevation is evident on the electrocardiogram (ECG). With subtotal coronary occlusion, there can be relative sparing of epicardial blood supply at the expense of endocardial supply. This tends to result in ST segment depression on the ECG. The situation within the coronary artery is dynamic with spontaneous lysis and reformation of thrombus, variable degrees of coronary spasm resulting from the release of vasoactive mediators, and the clinical presentation will depend on the degree and time course of coronary obstruction. Spontaneous resolution of coronary obstruction may result in improvement in the clinical picture by the time of presentation or assessment. This is often the case in patients presenting to emergency departments and may result in a missed diagnosis. If the ischemia was sufficient to cause myocardial necrosis, then myocardial proteins may be released into the circulation in quantities proportional to the extent of myocardial damage and a number of these, including creatinine kinase, troponin I, troponin T, and myoglobin, have been or are used as biochemical markers of infarction and can be used for risk stratification.

DIAGNOSTIC CONSIDERATIONS

Accurate diagnosis of IHD is important for a variety of reasons. These reasons are in principle no different in patients undergoing surgery to those applying to the general population.

- To explain a patient's symptoms
- To guide treatment
- To predict prognosis or level of risk

Clinical Assessment

The classical description with constricting retrosternal discomfort radiating to the upper arms, neck, jaw, or teeth rarely raises too much diagnostic difficulty and further investigation may not be necessary to establish the diagnosis. In many cases, however, particularly in elderly or diabetic individuals, or in the presence of sedative or analgesic drugs, symptoms may be highly variable. Even with modern investigative techniques, it can be very difficult to distinguish between ischemic cardiac, upper gastrointestinal, pleural, or chest wall pain. In practice, any exertional discomfort felt above the diaphragm in an individual potentially susceptible to coronary disease should be viewed with suspicion and prompt further investigation.

The assessment of patients with possible coronary disease should include not only the consideration of possible ischemic symptoms, but also a thorough assessment of concomitant conditions which may impact upon therapy. Features such as obesity, chronic obstructive pulmonary disease (COPD), varicose veins, severe heart failure, and extensive vascular disease make coronary bypass surgery more problematic, whereas bradycardia, hypotension, or asthma may limit the choice of antianginal drugs. Percutaneous coronary intervention (PCI) is more challenging in patients with severe vascular disease and in those with bleeding tendencies that contraindicate the antiplatelet regime necessary after PCI.

Clinical assessment is central to prognostication. Advanced age, heart failure, and diabetes, for example, all point to poorer long-term prognosis. Chronic stable

TABLE 1 Key Features of Investigations for IHD

Test	Key features
Exercise ECG	Readily available and economical with a large body of data supporting its prognostic role Limited by relatively poor sensitivity and specificity and the need for patients to exercise; requires a relatively normal resting ECG
Stress echo	Noninvasive test with greater sensitivity and specificity than Ex ECG; uses widely available equipment without ionizing radiation Limited by interobserver variability, time-consuming interpretation, and dependency on a good echo "window"
Nuclear	Noninvasive test with greater sensitivity and specificity than Ex ECG and a large body of literature supporting its prognostic role Limited by high equipment cost and the need for ionizing radiation
Cardiac MR	Has the potential to be the most accurate noninvasive test, combining both anatomical and physiological information Limited by high equipment cost and availability of trained staff; unsuitable for patients with pacemakers/ICDs or claustrophobia
CT	Fast, high-resolution images of coronary arteries including stents Limited by high radiation exposure and capital equipment cost
Coronary angiography	The reference standard for diagnosing coronary artery disease; potential for therapeutic intervention at the same time as diagnosis Limited by invasive nature and small risk of serious complications; offers only anatomical information; high financial cost

Abbreviations: IHD, ischemic heart disease; ECG, electrocardiogram; MR, magnetic resonance; CT, computed tomography.

angina which is infrequent and occurs only with extra effort points to a more favorable prognosis than recent onset worsening unstable angina occurring with minimal effort or at rest. No further tests may be needed if all the relevant management decisions can be made based on the history and physical examination.

A typical description of exertional chest tightness in association with relevant risk factors may be all that is required to make the diagnosis of chronic stable angina. Frequently, however, the diagnosis is either in doubt or some further diagnostic information is desirable either for stratifying risk or in deciding between the many treatment options. There are a number of diagnostic tests which can help, each with different strengths and weaknesses. A summary of the characteristics of the different tests is given in Table 1.

Exercise Electrocardiogram

This is commonly the first investigation requested in patients complaining of anginal symptoms. It is relatively inexpensive and widely available. It is a functional test and has value both diagnostically and prognostically but is limited by its sensitivity and specificity in comparison to more sophisticated noninvasive imaging modalities.

Typically the development of myocardial ischemia will result in exertional chest tightness associated with ST segment depression. In general, the more profound these changes are and the sooner they occur, the more severe the disease and the worse the prognosis. Significant ventricular arrhythmias or a fall in blood pressure with exercise also increase the likelihood of IHD and are a marker for adverse prognosis. A number of scoring mechanisms, of which the Duke Treadmill Score (Table 2) (1) is the best known, have been developed in an attempt to refine the interpretation of the exercise test.

TABLE 2 The Duke Treadmill Score

Score	Interpretation
≤5	Low risk: 5-yr mortality 3.1%
−10 to 4	Medium risk: 5-yr mortality 9.5%
≤−10	High risk: 5-yr mortality 35%

Score: Example: = Time (min)–(5 × ST depression mm) – (4 × angina index). Angina index: no angina during test = 0; nonlimiting angina = 1; limiting angina = 2.
Source: From Ref. 2.

Unfortunately patients with the highest risk are frequently unable to exercise at all.

Exercise testing is limited in patients with abnormal resting ECGs and those who are unable to exercise sufficient to reach their maximum target heart rate. Some drugs, most importantly digoxin, and conditions such as Wolff–Parkinson–White syndrome also reduce the specificity of the test. In such patients and those with equivocal exercise ECGs, another test should be considered.

Coronary Angiography

Anatomical assessment of coronary arteries by coronary angiography has long been regarded as the gold standard for detecting IHD. In general, a localized stenosis of less than 75% usually does not produce symptoms. This technology allows coronary stenoses to be identified but significant atheroma may be missed if it has not progressed to the point of causing a stenosis (so-called negative remodeling). Furthermore, it has been found that myocardial infarction can occur due to the fissuring of an atheromatous plaque which was either undetected at angiography or produced only mild luminal narrowing (2,3). Angiography is thus an anatomical rather than functional investigation and gives information on the functional significance of an observed stenosis only by inference. Some patients appear to tolerate stenoses which appear quite severe on a two-dimensional angiogram with minimal symptoms, whereas others are symptomatic with seemingly less significant disease. Although an increasingly routine investigation, it is not free of the risk of complication and carries a mortality rate of around 1:1000 and a risk of other serious complication (stroke, myocardial infarction, renal failure, or significant access-site bleeding) of around 1:200. For these reasons, noninvasive tests with greater sophistication than the exercise ECG are very important, especially in the assessment of occult (asymptomatic) ischemia.

Functional Imaging Modalities

Noninvasive (or semi-invasive) imaging modalities, of which the best established are myocardial perfusion scintigraphy and stress echocardiography, provide diagnostic and prognostic information complementary to coronary angiography. This is particularly useful in assisting the interpretation of the functional significance of a coronary stenosis of borderline severity at angiography. They are, in general, more sensitive and specific for the detection of myocardial ischemia than exercise electrocardiography alone. They have the advantages that pharmacologic stress (generally dobutamine or adenosine infusion) may be used in individuals unable to exercise and are unaffected by the presence of an abnormal ECG. U.K. guidelines summarizing the indications for myocardial perfusion scintigraphy have recently been published (www.nice.org.uk/TA073guidance).

Indications
1. Detect ischemia in patients with uninterpretable ECGs.
2. Detect ischemia in patients who cannot exercise maximally.
3. Exclude significant coronary heart disease (CHD) without angiography.
4. Evaluate the significance of anatomically borderline coronary stenoses.
5. Localize ischemia to a particular coronary territory.
6. Detecting the presence of "hibernating" myocardium.

All tests have in the advantage of providing an assessment of left ventricular systolic size and function.

Cardiac MRI perfusion scanning remains a research tool at present but potentially has the added ability to distinguish between infarcted and viable but hypoperfused myocardium. CT coronary angiography is rapidly progressing towards providing an alternative means of anatomical assessment of coronary arteries to angiography but is not yet widely available in the U.K.

The precise technique chosen will depend on local expertise and availability as well as the particular question being asked. The complex nature of these tests and their interpretation make it unlikely that they will replace exercise testing for baseline assessment. The necessity to catheterize the coronary arteries for coronary intervention will ensure that coronary angiography continues but with developments in noninvasive imaging, this may reduce to a test performed only when coronary intervention is likely to be necessary.

THERAPEUTIC CONSIDERATIONS
Medical Treatment of Angina
β-Blockers

Most cardiologists would view β-blockers as the first-line medical treatment for angina based on data suggesting prognostic benefit post-MI (4). β-Blockers help reduce angina by reducing myocardial oxygen demand. By reducing adrenergic tone, they reduce heart rate at rest and on exercise, reduce inotropy, and reduce afterload, the latter predominantly by reducing blood pressure.

In general, β-blockers are well tolerated but are contraindicated in asthma and should be prescribed cautiously and in low doses in the presence of significant left ventricular systolic dysfunction. Common side effects include tiredness, cold extremities, and sleep disturbance, the latter more common with lipid-soluble agents. Tolerability can be improved by commencing at low dose and uptitrating slowly.

A wide range of β-blockers are clinically available. They differ in terms of half-life, solubility in water and lipid, specificity for the β_1 receptor subtype, presence or absence of vasodilator activity, and a variable degree of partial agonism [intrinsic sympathomimetic activity (ISA)]. There is little data available to suggest superiority of one agent over another in terms of their efficacy in reducing angina. In general, β_1 selective agents (so-called cardioselective, although this is misleading as all agents cause some β_2 antagonism) seem to be a little better tolerated. In the chronic situation, it would appear to make sense to use a once-daily agent such as bisoprolol, although short acting agents such as metoprolol have potential advantages in the acute setting or with a potentially unstable patient. "Vasodilating" β-blockers with ISA or nebivolol, which has some nitric oxide-like activity, may have advantages in patients with symptomatic peripheral vascular disease.

Calcium Antagonists

Calcium antagonists are commonly divided into dihydropyridine (e.g., nifedipine, amlodipine) and nondihydropyridine (e.g., diltiazem and verapamil). Dihydropyridines are predominantly arterial vasodilators, whereas the nondihydropyridines have additional negative chronotropic activity by virtue of acting upon the sinus and atrioventricular nodes. If β-blockers are not being given, then, in general, a rate slowing agent should be considered first. In patients taking β-blockers, adding verapamil and to a lesser extent diltiazem can lead to dangerous bradycardia, and dihydropyridines are more safely used in this setting. Their additional antihypertensive effects are helpful in angina patients with high blood pressure but they should be used with caution in patients with heart failure which can be exacerbated by the nondihydropyridines, although amlodipine (and probably nifedipine) is safe in this context (5). Common side effects of calcium antagonists include flushing and ankle edema. The latter is mediated via increased capillary permeability and does not respond to diuretics.

Nitrates

Nitrates cause vasodilatation of coronary arteries, systemic veins, and systemic arteries. In most patients with angina, symptoms occur due to a fixed coronary stenosis which is resistant to vasodilatation. In this setting, it is probably the reduction in preload mediated by venodilatation that is responsible for symptom relief. In ACSs, a degree of coronary spasm is common and this can be helped by nitrate use.

Most nitrates undergo considerable first-pass metabolism in the liver. Isosorbide mononitrate is not metabolized in this way and is the mainstay of oral nitrate therapy. Sublingual, intravenous, or transcutaneous administration can also be used to avoid this problem. Tolerance to nitrates is a well-recognized phenomenon. This can be avoided by ensuring a "nitrate-free period" each day—usually at night when physical activity and likelihood of angina are less. Headache is the most common side effect but usually improves after the first few doses. Hypotension may occur but is usually most noticeable in dehydrated patients in whom venous return is maintained by significant resting venous tone.

Nicorandil

Nicorandil is a potassium channel activator in addition with some nitrate-like activity. There is evidence suggesting some benefit in prognosis in chronic stable angina in addition to symptom relief (6). Headache is the most common side effect.

Ivabradine

This agent inhibits the I_f current that controls diastolic depolarization in the sinus node. Inhibition of the inflow of Na^+ and K^+ leads to a reduction in heart rate without other cardiovascular effects. It is indicated in patients intolerant of β-blockers for the treatment of angina. The most common side effect is visual disturbances with transient flashing lights at the edge of the field of vision being reported (due to inhibition of the structurally similar I_h channel in the eye). Patients may still drive and these effects resolved either during treatment or on withdrawal of therapy.

Combination Drug Therapy for Angina

Antianginal agents can be used concurrently. In practical terms, however, there is a law of diminishing returns with each additional agent added. Drugs all tend to work by reducing the heart's oxygen requirements but do little or nothing to increase supply.

In general, patients who remain limited with angina despite two antianginal agents should be considered for revascularization with either PCI or coronary artery bypass grafting (CABG).

Antithrombotic Therapy

Aspirin

Aspirin reduces platelet activity by inhibiting thromboxane A2-mediated platelet activation. It has a role in the management of both ACSs and chronic stable angina. In acute ST elevation myocardial infarction, its use has been shown to reduce all-cause mortality by 23%, an effect that was largely additive to the 25% reduction from streptokinase, resulting in an overall 42% relative risk reduction in all-cause mortality when the two agents were given together (7). When given acutely, a dose of at least 150 mg should be given which should be chewed to promote absorption through the buccal mucosa. Aspirin is protective in patients with angina or after myocardial infarction, stroke, or CABG (8). Data in primary prevention is less compelling but both the U.S. Preventative Services Task Force and the European Society of Cardiology guidelines indicate the role of low-dose aspirin in those at high risk of developing IHD.

Clopidogrel

Clopidogrel is a thienopyridine which prevents adenosine diphosphate-mediated platelet activation and is a more potent antiplatelet agent than aspirin. It is marginally more effective than aspirin in preventing vascular events in a range of patients with stable atheromatous vascular disease on the basis of the CAPRIE study (9) but its greater cost compared to aspirin results in a marginal cost-efficacy benefit and it has not been widely adopted in this setting. Its lack of gastrotoxicity theoretically makes it an attractive alternative in patients unable to tolerate aspirin, but as these patients were excluded from the CAPRIE study, this indication remains to be validated.

In acute myocardial infarction, the benefit of clopidogrel in addition to aspirin and a thrombolytic has been demonstrated in two recent studies (10,11). Its role in addition to aspirin and heparin in non-ST elevation ACSs was well established by the CURE study (12) where the beneficial effect was greatest in those going on to have PCI. Clopidogrel has a vital role along with aspirin in patients undergoing PCI and should be continued after PCI to prevent within-stent thrombosis. Clopidogrel therapy should be continued for up to one year in this context, and possibly longer in the presence of a drug-eluting stent (DES).

There is no question that clopidogrel increases perioperative bleeding. Its long half-life is such that it should be discontinued at least five days prior to surgery. Patients requiring urgent noncardiac surgery early after PCI raise a clinical dilemma. To operate while clopidogrel is being taken (and for several days after stopping) exposes the patient to a higher risk of bleeding, while stopping it (together with the prothrombotic effects of surgery) increases the risk of stent thrombosis and consequent perioperative myocardial infarction. These decisions are difficult and need to be made in light of the time since PCI and the type and extent of stenting. It is known that noncardiac surgery performed within two weeks of PCI carries a very high risk of death or myocardial infarction. In patients with bare metal stents, the risk has reduced appreciably by six weeks when most stents have endothelialized. DESs endothelialize more slowly, so stopping clopidogrel before three or even six months carries a risk of perioperative MI.

Heparin

Unfractionated heparin along with aspirin is of benefit to patients with unstable angina/NSTEMI (13). The low-molecular-weight heparin Enoxaparin compares favorably to unfractionated heparin (14), whereas other low molecular weight heparins (LMWHs) fail to show superiority.

Glycoprotein 2b3a Inhibitors

These powerful intravenous inhibitors of the final common pathway of platelet aggregation have been shown to be beneficial to patients presenting with ACSs (15,16). The benefit is greatest in those at highest risk, i.e., those with ST segment depression, elevated cardiac markers, diabetics, and those undergoing intervention. They pose a significant bleeding threat when used perioperatively. Abciximab has a very long half-life and redistributes such that its effects are only partially reversed by platelet transfusion. The small molecule agents eptifibatide and tirofiban have rather shorter half-lives, their effects wearing off after four to five hours.

Revascularization

A strategy of undertaking coronary angiography with a view to revascularization via either PCI (angioplasty ± insertion of an intracoronary stent) or coronary artery bypass surgery (CABG) may be considered on either symptomatic (ongoing limiting angina despite antianginal medical therapy) of prognostic grounds. Patients deemed to be at high risk of death or myocardial infarction without revascularization include those with:

1. Severe left ventricular (LV) systolic dysfunction,
2. ACS presentation,
3. Strongly positive, angina limited exercise test at low workload, and
4. Large area of ischemia on other noninvasive testing.

Percutaneous Coronary Intervention

During cardiac catheterization, a fine guide-wire is introduced into the affected coronary artery and steered past the area of narrowing under fluoroscopic guidance. Balloon catheters are advanced over this wire across the stenosis and inflated, expanding the coronary lumen at that point. In most cases, a stent is placed to prevent the stretched artery immediately renarrowing.

PCI has been shown to improve symptoms in chronic stable angina (17) and to reduce major adverse cardiac events after ACSs (18–20). If it can be performed in a timely manner, it can reduce the likelihood of death and reinfarction in patients with ST elevation myocardial infarction compared to thrombolytic therapy (21).

PCI is limited by the necessity to pass a guide-wire down the coronary artery and advance balloons and stents over it. It is therefore more difficult (but not impossible) in arteries that are completely blocked, tortuous, or heavily calcified. The risk of complications including arterial restenosis increases with the extent of intervention. For this reason, patients with extensive and severe lesions in all three coronary territories are more commonly treated by coronary bypass surgery.

The "Achilles heel" of PCI has always been arterial restenosis. Arterial injury results in an exaggerated healing response with smooth muscle hyperplasia and recurrent stenosis. Although reduced to an extent by placement of a stent, it remains a problem in approximately 10% of cases. The risk of restenosis is greater in diabetic patients and following intervention in small caliber coronary arteries and to the proximal left anterior descending or left main stem. The risk of restenosis appears to have been dramatically reduced with the advent of DESs. These devices slowly elute controlled amounts of one of a number of cytotoxic agents reducing smooth muscle overgrowth. This advancement has allowed a greater proportion of patients to benefit from this therapy as it is now possible to treat longer sections of more complex disease with more favorable long-term results. The major adverse effect of DESs is to delay re-endothelialization of the stented segment increasing the risk of late stent thrombosis and mandating prolonged antiplatelet therapy.

Coronary Artery Bypass Grafting

CABG has been shown to have prognostic in addition to symptomatic benefit in patients with disease of the left main coronary artery, proximal left anterior descending coronary artery, or coronary disease associated with reduced LV function when compared to optimal medical therapy (22). Although a major surgical intervention, it is performed with high success rates and very low mortality and morbidity in the absence of major comorbidity and in the presence of favorable anatomy. Graft longevity is better for arterial grafts (typically using the left internal mammary artery). Approximately 50% of saphenous vein grafts will be occluded 10 years following surgery.

Trials of CABG versus PCI in disease amenable to either strategy show similarly favorable outcomes, but repeated procedures are more likely to be necessary following PCI (23). In such patients, the lower morbidity of PCI has to be balanced against the lesser chance of requiring a second procedure with surgery. Currently CABG is generally regarded to be the preferred strategy in the presence of three vessel coronary artery or left main stem disease. Patients with diabetes also appear to fare better with surgery. It is possible that the use of DESs will change this balance. This is currently being assessed by the SYNTAX trial which is randomizing patients with multivessel disease to CABG or PCI with DESs.

Preventative Cardiology

With the identification of risk factors for cardiovascular disease in the 1960s came efforts to change the natural history of the disease by modifying these factors. The five traditional major risk factors are: family history of premature vascular disease, smoking, hypertension, hypercholesterolemia, and diabetes mellitus.

Smoking

Smokers carry a two- to threefold higher risk of coronary artery disease. Conversely, smoking cessation reduces all-cause mortality and nonfatal myocardial infarction by over one-third (24). This is at least as great as any other single intervention in preventative cardiology. Nicotine replacement therapy with transdermal patches and chewing gum has shown increased rates of abstinence and is cost effective (25). Unfortunately, patients who reduce but do not stop smoking only appear to gain a marginal benefit in terms of reduction in coronary artery disease. This is consistent with the finding that even "light" smokers of one to four cigarettes per day have a significantly increased risk, as do those who believe they do not inhale the smoke (26).

Hypertension

Hypertension is frequently underdiagnosed and even when recognized, treatment is often suboptimal. It was clear from the Framingham study that even "high normal" blood pressures of 130 to 139 mmHg systolic or 85 to 89 mmHg diastolic were associated with a doubling of cardiovascular risk compared to those with lower blood pressure. Greater prediction of risk can be achieved by measuring 24-hour ambulatory blood pressure, and the finding of left ventricular hypertrophy in association with hypertension is an even stronger marker for cardiovascular risk (27).

Treatment of hypertension may be frustrating for both patient and physician as often several drugs in combination are required to make any significant impact on blood pressure. This is made more troublesome by the asymptomatic nature of hypertension and the presence of side effects from medication. Nevertheless, there is overwhelming evidence that sustained treatment of hypertension with combination treatment can result in reductions of blood pressure of around 20/10 mmHg with an associated 45% reduction in CHD (28). Even modest reductions of 4 to 5 mmHg have been shown to cause clinically significant reductions in coronary disease in those with other risk factors (29).

The choice of initial antihypertensive agent has been a matter of great debate. Recent evidence (30) suggests that combination with "newer" agents (amlodiopine ± perindopril) is associated with a better outcome than "older" agents (thiazide + β-blocker), although this remains controversial. A detailed discussion of antihypertensive therapy is beyond the scope of this review, but numerous current guidelines exist (31). Usually, several agents in combination are required to bring established hypertension under control.

Dyslipidemia

Hypercholesterolemia [usually driven by high high-density lipoprotein (LDL) cholesterol] has long been established as a causative agent in the pathogenesis of CHD. In its most extreme form, homozygous familial hypercholesterolemia causes coronary disease as early as the first decade of life. More recently, the finding of high triglycerides and low high-density lipoprotein (HDL) cholesterol even in the absence of high LDL cholesterol has been associated with increased risk of coronary disease.

Treatment with hydroxymethylglutaryl coenzyme A reductase inhibitors, or "statins," reliably reduces total and LDL cholesterol levels by at least a quarter, and is associated with a reduction of coronary events by over one-third in both primary (32) and secondary (33) prevention studies. More aggressive strategies of cholesterol reduction appear to produce greater clinical benefit and to date, no level has been identified below which cholesterol cannot be reduced without additional benefit.

The point at which to institute statin therapy has been an area of intensive debate and has led to the concept of global cardiovascular risk as an indicator for the appropriateness of treatment (34). In this regard, patients who have other significant risk factors even with "normal" cholesterol levels have been shown to gain benefit from cholesterol lowering (35).

Other lipid-modulating drugs used in preventative cardiology include fibrates (gemfibrazole, bezafibrate, fenofibrate), nicotinic acid (niacin), cholesterol-absorption inhibitors (ezetimibe), bile-acid-absorption inhibitors (cholestyramine), and fish oils. In addition to these, phytosterols (derivatives of cholesterol from plants) have been added to soft margarines. These naturally found compounds reduce intestinal absorption of cholesterol and may prove useful as adjuvant therapy.

Fibrates have been shown to have a role in secondary prevention in those with high triglycerides and low HDL. This effect was independent of LDL cholesterol which did not change significantly with this therapy (36). Current U.K. guidelines have recently been updated and can be found in Rubins et al. (37).

Diabetes and the Metabolic Syndrome

Patients with diabetes have a threefold greater risk of cardiovascular disease than matched nondiabetic subjects (38). This is compounded by the greater incidence of complications in diabetic patients undergoing revascularization. It has emerged that even before the onset of diabetes these patients are exposed to increased CHD risk almost to the same degree as those with established type 2 diabetes (39). It seems to be the phenomenon of insulin resistance rather than hyperglycemia per se that is responsible for promoting atherosclerosis. This is consistent with data suggesting a disappointingly poor relationship between tight glycemic control and reduction in coronary events (40). Good glycemic control is, however, clearly associated with a reduction in microvascular complications.

The concept of a prediabetic state, termed "metabolic syndrome" has been introduced. This has been defined as the presence of at least three of the following:

1. Waist circumference > 102 cm for men and > 88 cm for women
2. Serum triglycerides > 150 mg/dl (mmol/L) or serum HDL cholesterol < 40 mg/dl in men and < 50 mg/dl in women
3. Blood pressure of at least 130/85 mmHg
4. Serum glucose > 110 mg/dl
5. Age > 45 in men, > 55 in women

Aggressive risk factor management should be considered in this group of patients with both lifestyle modifications such as reduction in dietary fat and increase in physical activity and pharmacological therapy.

REFERENCES

1. Shaw LJ, Peterson ED, Shaw LK, et al. Use of a prognostic treadmill score in identifying diagnostic coronary disease subgroups. Circulation 1998; 98:1622.
2. Naghavi M, Libby P, Falk E, et al. From vulnerable plaque to vulnerable patient: a call for new definitions and risk assessment strategies, Part I. Circulation 2003; 108:1664.
3. Naghavi M, Libby P, Falk E, et al. From vulnerable plaque to vulnerable patient: a call for new definitions and risk assessment strategies, Part II. Circulation 2003; 108:1772.
4. Gottlieb SS, McCarter RJ, Vogel RA. Effect of beta-blockade on mortality among high-risk and low-risk patients after myocardial infarction. N Engl J Med 1998; 339:489–497.
5. Packer M, O'Connor CM, Ghali JK, et al. Effect of amlodipine on morbidity and mortality in severe chronic heart failure. The prospective randomized amlodipine survival evaluation study group. N Engl J Med 1996; 335:1107–1114.
6. The IONA Study Group. Effect of nicorandil on coronary events in patients with stable angina: The Impact of Nicorandil in Angina (IONA) randomised trial. Lancet 2002; 359:1269–1275.
7. ISIS-2 (Second International Study of Infarct Survival) Collaborative Group. Randomised trial of intravenous streptokinase, oral aspirin, both, or neither among 17,187 cases of suspected acute myocardial infarction: ISIS-2. Lancet 1988; 2:349.
8. Antiplatelet Trialists' Collaboration. Collaborative overview of randomised trials of antiplatelet therapy. I. Prevention of death, myocardial infarction, and stroke by prolonged antiplatelet therapy in various categories of patients. Br Med J 1994; 308:81–106.
9. CAPRIE Steering Committee. A randomised, blinded, trial of clopidogrel versus aspirin in patients at risk of ischaemic events (CAPRIE). Lancet 1996; 348:1329–1339.
10. Sabatine MS, Cannon CP, Gibson CM, et al. Effect of clopidogrel pretreatment before percutaneous coronary intervention in patients with ST-elevation myocardial infarction treated with fibrinolytics: the PCI-CLARITY study. J Am Med Assoc 2005; 294(10): 1224–1232.

11. Chen ZM, Jiang LX, Chen YP, et al. Addition of clopidogrel to aspirin in 45,852 patients with acute myocardial infarction: randomised placebo-controlled trial. Lancet 2005; 366(9497):1607–1621.
12. Yusuf S, Mehta SR, Zhao F, et al. Early and late effects of clopidogrel in patients with acute coronary syndromes. Circulation 2003; 7:966.
13. Oler A, Whooley MA, Oler J, et al. Adding heparin to aspirin reduces the incidence of myocardial infarction and death in patients with unstable angina: a meta-analysis. J Am Med Assoc 1996; 276:811.
14. Antman EM, McCabe CH, Gurfinkel EP, et al. Enoxaparin prevents death and cardiac ischemic events in unstable angina/non-Q-wave myocardial infarction: results of the Thrombolysis in Myocardial Infarction (TIMI) 11B trial. Circulation 1999; 100:1593.
15. The Platelet Receptor Inhibition for Ischemic Syndrome Management in Patients Limited by Unstable Signs and Symptoms (PRISM-PLUS) Trial Investigators. Inhibition of the platelet glycoprotein IIb/IIIa receptor with tirofiban in unstable angina and non-Q-wave myocardial infarction. N Engl J Med 1998; 338:1488.
16. The PURSUIT Trial Investigators. Inhibition of platelet glycoprotein IIb/IIIa with eptifibatide in patients with acute coronary syndromes. N Engl J Med 1998; 339:436.
17. The RITA-2 Trial Investigators. Coronary angioplasty versus medical therapy for angina: the second Randomised Intervention Treatment of Angina (RITA-2) trial. RITA-2 trial participants. Lancet 1997; 350(9076):461–468.
18. Fox K, Poole-Wilson P, Henderson R, et al. Interventional versus conservative treatment for patients with unstable angina or non-ST-elevation myocardial infarction: The British Heart Foundation RITA 3 randomised trial. Randomized Intervention Trial of unstable angina. Lancet 2002; 360:743.
19. Cannon C, Weintraub W, Demopoulos L, et al. Comparison of early invasive and conservative strategies in patients with unstable coronary syndromes treated with the glycoprotein IIb/IIIa inhibitor tirofiban. N Engl J Med 2001; 344:1879.
20. The FRISC-II Investigators. Invasive compared with non-invasive treatment in unstable coronary artery disease: FRISC II prospective randomised multcentre study. Lancet 1999; 354:708.
21. Keeley EC, Boura JA, Grines CL. Primary angioplasty versus intravenous thrombolytic therapy for acute myocardial infarction: a quantitative review of 23 randomised trials. Lancet 2003; 361:3.
22. Yusuf S, Zucker D, Peduzzi P, et al. Effect of coronary artery bypass graft surgery on survival: overview of 10-year results from randomised trials by the Coronary Artery Bypass Graft Surgery Trialists Collaboration. Lancet 1994; 344:563–570.
23. Writing Group for the Bypass Angioplasty Revascularization Investigation (BARI) Investigators. Five-year clinical and functional outcome comparing bypass surgery and angioplasty in patients with multivessel coronary disease: a multicenter randomized trial. J Am Med Assoc 1997; 277(9):715–721.
24. Critchley JA, Capewell S. Mortality risk reduction associated with smoking cessation in patients with coronary heart disease: a systematic review. J Am Med Assoc 2003; 290:86.
25. The Tobacco Use and Dependence Clinical Practice Guideline Panel, Staff, and Consortium Representatives. A clinical practice guideline for treating tobacco use and dependence: A U.S. Public Health Service report. J Am Med Assoc 2000; 283:3244.
26. Prescott E, Scharling H, Osler M, et al. Importance of light smoking and inhalation habits on risk of myocardial infarction and all cause mortality: a 22-year follow up of 12,149 men and women in The Copenhagen City Heart Study. J Epidemiol Commun Health 2002; 56:702.
27. Levy D, Salomon M, D'Agostino RB, et al. Prognostic implications of baseline electrocardiographic features and their serial changes in subjects with left ventricular hypertrophy. Circulation 1994; 90(4):1786–1793.
28. Law MR, Wald NJ, Morris JK, et al. Value of low dose combination treatment with blood pressure lowering drugs: analysis of 354 randomised trials. Br Med J 2003; 326:1427.
29. Mehler PS, Coll JR, Estacio R, et al. Intensive blood pressure control reduces the risk of cardiovascular events in patients with peripheral arterial disease and type 2 diabetes. Circulation 2003; 107:753.

30. Dahlof B, Sever PS, Poulter NR, et al., for the ASCOT Investigators. Prevention of cardiovascular events with an antihypertensive regime of amlodipine adding perindopril as required verses atenolol adding bendroflumethiazide as required, in the Anglo-Scandinavian cardiac outcomes trial-blood pressure lowering arm (ASCOT-BPLA): a multicentre randomised controlled trial. Lancet 2005; 366:895–906.
31. Williams B, Poulter N, Brown MJ. Guidelines for management of hypertension: report of the fourth working party of the British Hypertension Society, 2004—BHS IV. J Hum Hypertens 2004; 18:139–185.
32. Shepherd J, Cobbe SM, Ford I, et al. Prevention of coronary heart disease with pravastatin in men with hypercholesterolemia. N Engl J Med 1995; 333:1301.
33. Scandinavian Simvastatin Survival Study Group. Randomised trial of cholesterol lowering in 4444 patients with coronary heart disease: The Scandinavian Simvastatin Survival Study (4S). Lancet 1994; 344:1383.
34. Executive Summary of the Third Report of the National Cholesterol Education Program (NCEP) Expert Panel on Detection, Evaluation, and Treatment of High Blood Cholesterol in Adults (Adult Treatment Panel III). J Am Med Assoc 2001; 285:2486.
35. MRC/BHF Heart Protection Study Investigators. MRC/BHF Heart Protection Study of cholesterol lowering with simvastatin in 20,536 high-risk individuals: a randomised placebo-controlled trial. Lancet 2002; 360:7.
36. JBS 2: Joint British Societies' guidelines on prevention of cardiovascular disease in clinical practice. Heart 2005; 91(suppl 5):1–52.
37. Rubins HB, Robins SJ, Collins D, et al. Gemfibrozil for the secondary prevention of coronary heart disease in men with low levels of high-density lipoprotein cholesterol. Veterans Affairs High-Density Lipoprotein Cholesterol Intervention Trial Study Group. N Engl J Med 1999; 341:410.
38. Stamler J, Vaccaro O, Neaton JD, et al. Diabetes, other risk factors, and 12-year cardiovascular mortality for men screened in the Multiple Risk Factor Intervention Trial. Diabetes Care 1993; 16:434–444.
39. Hu FB, Stampfer MJ, Haffner SM, et al. Elevated risk of cardiovascular disease prior to clinical diagnosis of type 2 diabetes. Diabetes Care 2002; 25:1129.
40. UK Prospective Diabetes Study (UKPDS) Group. Intensive blood-glucose control with sulphonylureas or insulin compared with conventional treatment and risk of complications in patients with type 2 diabetes (UKPDS 33). Lancet 1998; 352:837–853.

4 Mechanisms of Perioperative Myocardial Injury

Hans-Joachim Priebe

Department of Anesthesia, University Hospital, Freiburg, Germany

INTRODUCTION

Perioperative myocardial injury is a major cause of morbidity and mortality after noncardiac surgery (1,2). Unfortunately, the etiology and mechanism(s) of perioperative myocardial injury remain an area of uncertainty and the subject of continued debate and controversy (3–6). However, without knowledge of the causes of perioperative myocardial injury, the design of effective preventive measures to improve perioperative outcome is impossible.

The identification of possible mechanisms and triggers of perioperative myocardial injury requires some basic knowledge: (*i*) of the etiology and pathophysiology of acute coronary syndromes (ACSs) in the nonsurgical setting, (*ii*) of the diagnosis and characteristics of perioperative myocardial injury, and (*iii*) of the factors and interventions that have been shown to affect perioperative myocardial injury. This chapter will address these areas before attempting to define the possible mechanisms of perioperative myocardial injury.

CORONARY ATHEROSCLEROSIS

With the growing effectiveness of coronary revascularization strategies aimed at relieving angiographically demonstrated arterial stenoses, coronary artery disease (CAD) became viewed as a segmental disease, and the risk of an ischemic event was regarded as primarily dependent on the degree of stenosis. During the last decade, however, our understanding of the pathobiology and pathophysiology of CAD has changed dramatically, rendering this traditional viewpoint obsolete. Coronary atherosclerosis is now recognized as the result of multiple complex biochemical and molecular interactions including cells of the vascular wall and blood (7).

During the course of atherogenesis, the atherosclerotic lesion can undergo substantial compensatory outward enlargement (remodeling) (8). As a consequence, even segments of the coronary vasculature that appear angiographically unremarkable may harbor a considerable atherosclerotic burden (9). Such angiographically "hidden" lesions not only escape detection, but also remain asymptomatic until the moment they trigger thrombosis. By the time that atherosclerotic lesions produce stenoses, intimal atherosclerosis is usually diffuse and widespread (10).

Coronary Plaque

The pathophysiology of the ACS embraces a number of factors. These include plaque rupture, the thrombotic/fibrinolytic balance of the plaque's "solid-state" determinants of thrombosis and coagulation, and the blood's "fluid-phase" determinants (e.g., plasminogen activator inhibitor-1, circulating microparticles of tissue factor) (7,11). ACS is associated with structurally as well as functionally complex plaques and coronary artery stenoses, coronary endothelial lesions, and plaque inflammation (12–15). The "vulnerable" or "high-risk" coronary atherosclerotic plaque is a focal lesion that is highly susceptible to fissure, erosion, or disruption. Usually, it is inflamed and is characterized by a lipid-rich, atheromatous core, a thin fibrous cap infiltrated by macrophages and lymphocytes, a decreased smooth muscle content, and outward remodeling (16–18).

Structural morphology, cellular composition, and biological activity of coronary plaques appear to be closely linked (19). Plaque instability correlates more with biological activity and cellular composition than with angiographic findings (20). Myocardial infarctions usually occur at sites that previously caused only angiographically determined mild-to-moderate luminal stenosis (21,22). This confirms that atherosclerotic lesions can progress amazingly quickly, unpredictably, and in a discontinuous fashion (13,23,24). It helps to explain the observation that chronic, stable coronary atherosclerosis can transform into acute, potentially life-threatening coronary events at any time. Sudden rupture of a vulnerable plaque may occur spontaneously without clinical manifestations (silent plaque rupture) and without apparent reason, or it may follow a particular event, such as extreme cardiovascular demand, exposure to cold, or acute infection (25,26).

Such discontinuous progression is often related to episodes of thrombosis (which, in turn, are triggered by plaque rupture, erosion, endothelial activation, or inflammation), and is most often observed in lesions that produce less severe obstruction. The unpredictability of plaque progression is probably related to fluctuations of risk factors and triggers (e.g., physical activity, mental stress, environmental temperature, smoking, infection, hydration, and blood pressure), to heterogeneity of plaque histology, and to differences in the physical forces to which plaques are exposed (12,22,27,28).

In a substantial percentage of culprit lesions, thrombosed plaques without detectable fissures were observed (16). In such cases, plaque vulnerability is probably caused by a thrombogenic tendency or local pro-inflammatory cytokines that trigger thrombosis, sometimes even in the absence of inflammatory cell infiltration and a lipid core. Additional recognition of the importance of fluid-phase factors ("vulnerable blood") enlarged the concept of the "vulnerable plaque" by introducing the concept of the "vulnerable patient" (29,30).

Coronary Thrombosis

The clinical success of antithrombotic and fibrinolytic therapies established the central and causative role of coronary thrombosis in the pathogenesis of ACSs (Fig. 1). Critical coronary artery stenoses are responsible for only a fraction of ACSs (20). On the basis of findings of autopsy studies (which are obviously biased towards fatal outcomes), lethal coronary thrombosis is most often caused by rupture of the plaque's fibrous cap (16,22). Other less frequent causes of lethal coronary thrombosis include superficial plaque erosion, intraplaque hemorrhage, and the erosion of calcium nodules (7,17).

When intraluminal thrombi attach to a ruptured plaque, total occlusion of an epicardial coronary artery may occur resulting in total interruption of nutrient blood flow to the myocardium. The situation may be worsened by distal embolization of the coronary microcirculation by microthrombi that are rich in tissue factor (31). Coronary vasoconstriction can be superimposed by the local release of vasoconstricting substances from platelets (e.g., serotonin, thromboxane A_2) or from the thrombus itself

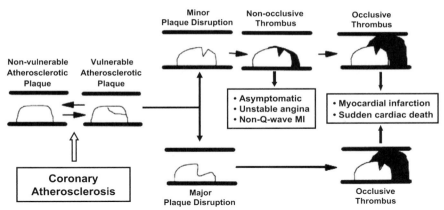

FIGURE 1 Pathophysiology of acute coronary syndrome.

(e.g., thrombin), by reduced production of nitric oxide or increased release of endothelin by the dysfunctional endothelium, or by increased sympathetic tone (32). Especially in the context of the perioperative period, it is important to keep in mind that in the presence of severe but stable CAD, coronary thrombosis may result from a decrease in coronary blood flow and stasis alone (33,34).

The ultimate fate of the thrombus and, thus, the extent of jeopardized myocardium will depend on the duration and degree of coronary occlusion. If the plaque disruption is major with extensive exposure of thrombogenic core material to the blood stream, acute total coronary occlusion with subsequent myocardial infarction or sudden death may develop. If the disruption is minor, the forming thrombus can be nonocclusive and the patient may stay asymptomatic or develop unstable angina or a non-ST-segment elevation infarction (resulting in Q-wave or non-Q-wave infarction). A concomitant increase in coagulability and coronary vasoconstriction (as is common in the perioperative setting) may, however, transform a nonocclusive thrombus into an occlusive thrombus. Ultimately, the balance between thrombosis and thrombolysis, and the flow conditions (affected by coronary vasomotor tone, perfusion pressure, and rheologic properties) are the decisive factors in determining whether the clinical outcome will be myocardial ischemia or infarction.

Inflammation

Inflammation plays a major role at all stages of coronary atherosclerosis (7,35–37). It promotes plaque rupture and thrombus formation by numerous and differing mechanisms (11). Intracoronary ultrasonography (38) and autopsy studies (39) have established that there are often vulnerable plaques at numerous sites in the coronary circulation and the link between inflammation and plaque instability (Fig. 2)

Triggers of Myocardial Injury

The interaction between morphological and functional factors is unpredictable. Exogenous factors (e.g., mechanical stress, vasomotor tone, infection, blood viscosity, coagulability) further modify such interaction, making the final outcome even less predictable. It is, therefore, impossible to predict the time it will take the vulnerable

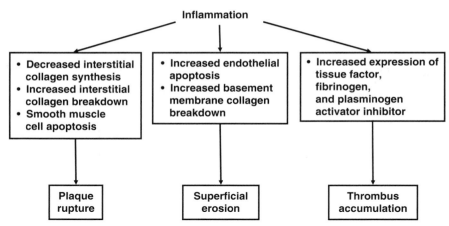

FIGURE 2 Mechanisms by which inflammation promotes plaque disruption and ACS. *Source:* Adapted from Libby P. Act local, act global: inflammation and the multiplicity of "vulnerable" coronary plaque. J Am Coll Cardiol 2005; 45: 1600–1602.

plaque to become unstable, or the trigger that causes the plaque to rupture. Various factors and conditions have the potential to qualitatively alter the stable state of coronary atherosclerosis and to initiate ("trigger") a cascade of events that ultimately results in myocardial injury (18). The triggers may be transient (e.g., hyperadrenergic state, prothrombotic state) or longer lasting (e.g., systemic inflammation). Triggers that facilitate plaque disruption include increased sympathetic tone, increased physical or emotional stress, local or systemic inflammation, and increased local vasomotor tone. Triggers that predispose to thrombosis formation include increased coagulability, inflammation, viscosity, and vasomotor tone. Most of these triggers are present in the perioperative period.

Plaque rupture is more common during various kinds of strenuous physical activity and emotional stress (40). In these situations, the sympathetic nervous system is activated. This leads to increased plasma concentrations of catecholamines, vascular tone (placing additional hemodynamic stress on the plaque), blood viscosity, and of blood pressure and heart rate, accompanied by increases in platelet aggregation and decreases in fibrinolytic activity that both tend to favor thrombosis (41). The increase in heart rate not only increases myocardial oxygen demands and decreases myocardial oxygen supply by decreasing diastolic filling time, but may also predispose to myocardial ischemia by affecting the rheological properties at the site of a plaque and by predisposing the plaque to rupture.

In summary, rupture of the intimal surface of a plaque is the result of a combination of cellular processes that promote plaque instability, and of physical (hemodynamic) processes that influence the magnitude and distribution of stress on the plaque (Fig. 3). The size of the thrombus that forms at the site of plaque rupture and the clinical consequences will depend on several key factors: the degree of plaque disruption (ulceration, fissure, or erosion) and substrate exposure as a major determinant of thrombogenicity at the local coronary artery site, the composition of the plaque, the magnitude of the stenosis, and the extent of platelet activation and intrinsic fibrinolytic activity (42). If coronary blood flow is interrupted for longer

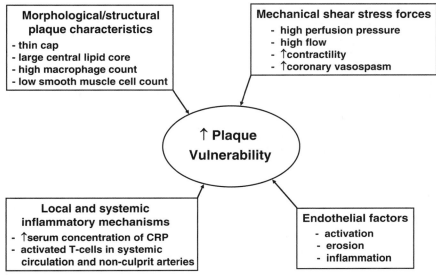

FIGURE 3 Factors increasing plaque vulnerability.

than 30 minutes, a myocardial infarction may result. Persistent coronary artery occlusion will cause a progressive increase in infarct size.

DIAGNOSIS OF PERIOPERATIVE MYOCARDIAL INJURY

A satisfactory explanation of the mechanisms of perioperative myocardial injury depends greatly on reliable data on the associations between various variables and the occurrence of perioperative myocardial injury. Such data can only be obtained if the detection of perioperative myocardial injury is quantitatively and qualitatively reliable.

Myocardial Ischemia

The incidence of perioperative myocardial ischemia and infarction will, obviously, be affected by their definition and method of detection. There is no accepted "gold standard" for the diagnosis of myocardial ischemia. Perioperative myocardial ischemia has predominantly been electrocardiogram (ECG)-detected and defined. The reported incidence of perioperative myocardial ischemia will, thus, greatly depend on choice and number of precordial leads (43), on the definition of "ischemic" ST segment change (extent and duration of ST segment change), and on mode of data acquisition (continuous vs. intermittent) (44). The reported incidence of ECG-defined myocardial ischemia will also depend on the suitability of patients for reliable detection of ischemia-specific ECG changes. In addition, perioperative changes in acid–base balance and electrolytes can affect the ECG in a way that interferes with ischemia detection. Thus, apart from differences in the prevalence of underlying ischemic heart disease and in the type of surgical risk, the high variability in the reported incidence of perioperative myocardial ischemia is likely due to methodological problems.

Myocardial Infarction

Fundamental questions remain regarding definition and diagnostic criteria of myocardial infarction, in general (45), and perioperatively, in particular (2). According to the definition of the World Health Organisation, at least two of three criteria must be fulfilled to diagnose myocardial infarction: (*i*) typical ischemic chest pain; (*ii*) increased serum concentration of creatine kinase (CK)-MB isoenzyme; and (*iii*) typical electrocardiographic findings, including development of pathological Q-waves (46,47). Perioperative myocardial infarction is mostly silent; the ECG is often difficult to interpret, and frequently does not exhibit characteristic ST segment elevation or Q-waves. If the diagnosis of myocardial infarction is based solely on the classical triad, considerable underreporting of the true incidence of perioperative myocardial infarction is to be expected, thereby possibly obscuring the etiology and mechanism(s) of perioperative myocardial injury.

The development of assays for the cardiac troponins T (cTnT) and I (cTnI) that are highly specific and sensitive for myocardial injury formed the basis of a revised definition of myocardial infarction as proposed by the European Society of Cardiology (ESC) and the American College of Cardiology (ACC) (48) (Fig. 4). Any of the two following criteria satisfy the diagnosis of an acute, evolving, or a recent myocardial infarction: (*i*) typical rise and gradual fall in cardiac troponin concentrations or more rapid rise and fall of CK-MB concentration in combination with at least one of the following: (a) typical ischemic symptoms, (b) development of pathological Q-waves in the ECG, (c) ECG changes indicative of myocardial ischemia (ST segment elevation or depression), and (d) coronary artery intervention; and/or (*ii*) pathological findings of an acute myocardial infarction.

Debate continues as to the appropriate cut-off values of troponin concentrations for defining a clinically relevant myocardial infarction. However, it is generally accepted that even small increases in serum concentrations of cardiac troponins are associated with adverse cardiac outcome in patients with or without ST segment elevation ACSs (49,50). Considering the high specificity of cardiac troponins for myocardial cell injury, the recent consensus document of the ESC and the ACC on the redefinition of myocardial infarction states that in the presence of documented myocardial ischemia, even minor increases in troponin serum concentration to greater than the 99th percentile of the normal population should be regarded as myocardial infarction.

In the frequent absence of typical symptoms and ECG signs of acute myocardial infarction, the diagnosis of perioperative myocardial infarction has to rest heavily on changes in biochemical markers. Cardiac troponins appear to be better suited

---

Either one of the following criteria satisfies the diagnosis:

1. **Typical rise and gradual fall (troponin) or more rapid rise and fall (CK-MB) of biochemical markers of myocardial necrosis with at least one of the following:**
   a. **ischemic symptoms**
   b. **development of pathological Q waves on the ECG**
   c. **ECG changes indicative of ischemia (ST-segment elevation or depression)**
   d. **coronary intervention**

2. **Pathological findings of an acute myocardial infarction**

FIGURE 4 Revised definition of acute, evolving myocardial infarction (MI).

to identify perioperative myocardial infarction than CK-MB isoenzyme (51–54). Depending on the biochemical marker and the cut-off values, the overall incidence of perioperative myocardial infarction may vary between 2.8% (CK-MB > 10%), 9% (conventional cut-off values of cTnI > 1.5 ng/mL and/or cTnT > 0.1 ng/mL), and 23% (low level cut-off values of cTnI > 0.6 ng/mL and/or cTnT > 0.03 ng/mL) in the same study (55). Only 5.6% of patients fulfilled the revised definition of myocardial infarction (presence of at least two of three criteria: prolonged chest pain, elevated CK-MB of cTn, ischemic ECG changes). However, without routine measurements of serum concentrations of biochemical markers and continuous ECG monitoring for three postoperative days, myocardial infarction would have been diagnosed in only those 3.6% of patients who experienced prolonged chest pain or symptoms of congestive heart failure. This is just one of several examples which demonstrate the dilemma of defining the "correct" incidence of perioperative myocardial infarction.

The question remains whether a reported incidence of perioperative myocardial injury based on traditional definition underestimates the true incidence of clinically relevant myocardial injury, or whether a reported incidence based on serum concentrations of cardiac troponins overestimates it. When using exclusively biochemical markers, specificity may be sacrificed for sensitivity. Another question is whether biochemical marker-defined myocardial injury carries the same predictive value as traditionally defined infarctions, and whether mechanisms and triggers are identical in both cases. Irrespective of whether one refers to small increases in serum concentrations of troponin as "myocardial infarction" or "subclinical myocardial injury" or "at risk," even minor postoperative increases were associated with adverse long-term outcome following major vascular surgery (56). Thus, existing evidence clearly suggests that even small increases in serum concentrations of cardiac troponins in the perioperative period reflect clinically relevant myocardial injury with short- and long-term consequences on outcome.

CHARACTERISTICS OF PERIOPERATIVE MYOCARDIAL INJURY

The majority of postoperative myocardial ischemia in high-risk patients tends to develop on the day of, or the day after, surgery, with the majority of ischemic episodes starting at the end of surgery and during the emergence from anesthesia (54). The vast majority (more than 90%) of postoperative episodes of myocardial ischemia are silent (57,58). Similarly, most postoperative myocardial infarctions occur early postoperatively and are asymptomatic (59).

Electrocardiogram
Postoperative ST segment changes are almost exclusively episodes of ST segment depression rather than elevation (3,54,57,60,61). The vast majority of perioperative myocardial infarctions are preceded by episodes of ST segment depression (54,58,62–64), and most of them (60–100%) are of the non-Q-wave type (3,43,58,59). Long-duration (single duration >20–30 minutes or cumulative duration >1–2 hours) ST segment change, rather than merely presence of postoperative ST segment depression, seems to be the important factor associated with adverse cardiac outcome (58,62,65). Short-duration ischemic episodes (<10 minutes) do not seem to correlate with postoperative myocardial infarction and cardiac complications (54,58). However, in one study, seven patients with postoperative myocardial ischemia lasting longer than two hours did not sustain an ischemic cardiac event (3).

The findings on the relationship between short-term changes in hemodynamic behavior and the incidence of postoperative ischemic ECG signs are contradictory. However, most studies did not find any association between changes in heart rate and postoperative ST segment changes (57,61,66) or troponin release (67). In one study, however, all episodes of ST segment depression were preceded by increases in heart rate (54). Overall evidence would suggest that heart rate is not a reliable independent predictor of postoperative ST segment depression and troponin release.

The findings of predominantly ST segment depression rather than elevation, and of an association between mostly long-duration ST segment change, rather than merely presence of postoperative ST segment depression with adverse cardiac outcome (58,62,65) have been interpreted as suggestive evidence that prolonged myocardial ischemia rather than coronary plaque disruption and thrombus formation is the primary mechanism of perioperative myocardial injury. However, although ST segment depression usually reflects subendocardial ischemia and is often regarded as reversible injury, it is not inconsistent with an evolving myocardial infarction. During the early evolution of a myocardial infarction, significant ST segment elevation may be lacking (68). Especially elderly patients may present with non-ST segment elevation myocardial infarction (69); in most studies of perioperative cardiac ischemic events, the study populations consisted largely of elderly patients. For these and other reasons, in current clinical practice acute myocardial infarction is divided into ST segment and non-ST segment elevation myocardial infarction (rather than into Q-wave and non-Q-wave myocardial infarction) (68). Thus, prolonged ST segment depression may reflect ongoing myocardial ischemia (ultimately leading to myocardial infarction), or it may reflect the beginning of an evolving myocardial infarction. In one study, ECG evidence of myocardial ischemia (mostly ST segment depression) was strongly associated with postoperative small and conventional increases in serum cardiac troponin concentration (55), suggesting that ST segment depression in the perioperative period frequently reflects irreversible myocardial injury. In contrast, in another study, several patients with prolonged postoperative myocardial ischemia did not sustain an ischemic cardiac event (3), indicating that ST segment depression may also reflect ongoing, reversible myocardial ischemia. Findings of lack of any association between changes in heart rate and postoperative ST segment changes (57,61,66), or troponin release (67), and lack of a consistent association between postoperative cardiac complications and long-duration ST segment depression (3), would argue for either nonischemic causes of ST segment depression in the perioperative period (e.g., hyperventilation, electrolyte changes, drug effects, positional changes), for compensatory mechanisms to myocardial ischemia (e.g., preconditioning as a result of multiple brief episodes of myocardial ischemia and coronary reperfusion), or for functional collateral perfusion (3,70).

The preponderance of non-Q-wave infarctions is clearly different from the nonsurgical setting. This might again suggest that perioperative myocardial infarctions are more often the result of prolonged ischemia than of thrombotic occlusion, similar to the presumed pathophysiology of silent ischemia (71). Abnormal Q-waves were once considered to reflect transmural myocardial infarction, whereas subendocardial (nontransmural) infarctions were thought not to produce Q-waves. However, Q-waves mirror nonphysiological electrical activity but are not identical with irreversible myocardial injury. Accordingly, the absence of Q-waves does not necessarily exclude irreversible myocardial injury. It may merely reflect the insensitivity of the standard 12-lead ECG, especially in the evaluation of the posterior zones of the left ventricle (72). Experimental and clinical ECG–morphological correlative studies have shown that transmural and nontransmural infarctions can occur with or without Q-waves (73). The presence or absence of a Q-wave is not determined primarily by the presence or absence of a myocardial infarction or by the transmural nature of the underlying myocardial infarction but rather by the total size of it (74,75). The probability of a Q-wave infarction increases with the size of the myocardial infarction and the number of transmurally infarcted segments. In a magnetic resonance study, transmural infarctions were of the non-Q-wave type in 29% of 100 consecutive patients with documented previous myocardial infarction (75). In about 25% of patients presenting with acute ST segment elevation, no Q-waves developed (76).

Overall, the ECG lacks sufficient sensitivity and specificity to allow differentiation between transmural and subendocardial (nontransmural) myocardial infarction. Therefore, the categorization of patients into those with and without Q-wave infarction does neither allow us to reliably predict the extent of myocardial injury nor to draw conclusions as to the etiology of the infarct. In addition, Q-waves take time to develop and, accordingly, do not figure strongly in the present acute-management decisions.

Cardiac Troponin

In 106 (10%) of 1136 patients undergoing abdominal infrarenal aortic surgery, postoperative serum cTnI concentrations were between 0.2 and 0.5 ng/mL but always less than 1.5 ng/mL (defined as myocardial injury) (77). A total of 57 (5%) patients showed cTnI concentrations above the threshold value of 1.5 ng/mL (defined as myocardial infarction). In 21 (37%) of these 57 patients with biochemical evidence of myocardial infarction, cTnI serum concentration increased above the threshold value within 24 hours of surgery, lasting for 24 hours or less (defined as early postoperative myocardial infarction). In contrast, in 34 (60%) of the patients, serum concentration of cTnI increased above 1.5 ng/mL later than 24 hours after surgery. All of these 34 patients had at least two abnormal values lower than 1.5 ng/mL within the first 24 hours (defined as delayed postoperative myocardial infarction). In other words, in approximately 60% of patients with perioperative myocardial infarction, infarction was preceded by a prolonged period of myocardial injury (as indicated by increases in cTnI concentrations above the 0.2–0.5 ng/mL threshold values).

The delayed postoperative increases in cTnI concentrations are consistent with the possibility that prolonged ischemia in the presence of severe but stable CAD may have caused the perioperative myocardial infarction. In contrast, the acute early postoperative increases in cTnI concentrations that were not preceded by prolonged low-concentration cTnI increases are consistent with acute coronary occlusion as the cause of the perioperative myocardial infarction. The two patterns of behavior of postoperative cTnI concentrations may thus reflect two distinct pathophysiologies: (*i*) acute coronary occlusion as the cause for early morbidity and (*ii*) prolonged myocardial ischemia as the cause for late events.

Angiography

When compared to a matched control group without perioperative death or myocardial infarction, patients who experienced perioperative myocardial infarctions had more angiographic evidence of extensive CAD (as reflected by a larger number of affected coronary arteries, high-grade stenoses, and collateralized total occlusions) (78). However, high-grade stenoses were an uncommon cause of complications.

Inadequate collateralization of total occlusions seemed to have been the most common cause of infarction. In addition, in a third of the patients with perioperative cardiac events, a "culprit" site could not be identified (i.e., the coronary artery supplying the infarcted territory) (78). In agreement with the latter finding, coronary angiography performed in three patients within seven days of postoperative myocardial infarction revealed chronic, severe CAD but no angiographically visible thrombus or ruptured plaques (54).

The various perioperative angiographic findings are consistent with both perioperative plaque rupture at sites other than critically narrowed coronary artery stenoses, as well as with the possibility that in some patients with severe but stable CAD, perioperative myocardial infarction might have developed primarily on the basis of prolonged myocardial ischemia.

Pathology

In perioperative myocardial infarction, acute plaque disruption and hemorrhage in the infarct-related coronary artery seems to be common (79–81). In an autopsy study from the 1930s, fatal perioperative myocardial infarction was accompanied by thrombosis of the coronary artery supplying the infarcted area (79). Following fatal perioperative myocardial infarction, the vast majority (93%) of 42 autopsy heart specimens showed significant atherosclerotic coronary artery obstruction (80). There was evidence of plaque disruption in 55%, and evidence of plaque hemorrhage in 45% of 42 autopsy heart specimens. Perioperative myocardial infarctions were accompanied by a high incidence of histologically confirmed transmural infarctions (81). However, in more than half the patients, the site of infarction could not have been predicted based on the severity of the underlying stenosis (80).

On the one hand, the pathological findings provide evidence that the etiology of perioperative myocardial infarction resembles that in the nonsurgical setting. Acute plaque disruption in the infarct-related coronary artery seems to be common, but the severity of underlying coronary artery stenoses does not predict the infarct territory (80,81). Such findings are similar to those in autopsies following acute myocardial infarction in the nonoperative setting. The finding of a high incidence of histologically confirmed transmural infarctions is not in contradiction to the electrocardiographic finding of almost exclusively non-Q-wave perioperative myocardial infarctions, when one takes into account that the presence or absence of a Q-wave is not determined primarily by the transmural nature of the underlying myocardial infarction but rather by its total size (74,75).

On the other hand, the presence of circumferential myocardial infarctions (81) is consistent with a myocardial oxygen supply/demand mismatch as being the main trigger of myocardial injury. However, myocardial oxygen supply/demand mismatch and plaque rupture are not mutually exclusive mechanisms, and myocardial infarctions may develop by different mechanisms at different locations in the same patient.

PREVENTIVE MEASURES

Identification of possible mechanisms of perioperative myocardial injury is helped by looking at factors that have been shown to increase, and interventions that have been shown to reduce perioperative cardiac events.

Factors Associated with Postoperative Myocardial Ischemia

Postoperative anemia (82), hypothermia (83,84), and pain (85,86) have been shown to be associated with an increased incidence of postoperative myocardial ischemia. These findings most likely reflect the detrimental effect of accompanying increases in sympathetic tone and catecholamine release on cardiovascular performance and coagulation in the presence of CAD in general. In the absence of simultaneous measurements of biochemical markers (cardiac troponin, in particular), the etiology and nature of the ischemic episodes are difficult to establish. They may or may not have been accompanied by myocardial cell injury. Some episodes of "mere" myocardial ischemia may have been what we refer to today as non-ST segment elevation myocardial infarction.

Interventions Associated with Improved Perioperative Cardiac Outcome

β-Adrenoceptor Antagonists

Several prospective and retrospective studies suggest that perioperative β-blocker therapy improves cardiac outcome in patients with or at risk for CAD undergoing noncardiac surgery (87–90). This protective effect may be related to the ability of β-blockers to reduce the incidence and severity of perioperative myocardial ischemia (91).

Although the exact mechanism(s) by which β-blockers reduce perioperative myocardial injury remain(s) to be determined, numerous cardiovascular and noncardiac effects are likely to account for their cardioprotective effect in the operative (and nonoperative) setting (92,93). β-Blockers can reduce myocardial O_2 consumption (thus improving the myocardial O_2 supply/demand balance) by decreasing sympathetic tone and myocardial contractility, in turn resulting in decreases in heart rate and blood pressure. The reduction in contractility, and in pulse pressure and rate at rest and during cardiovascular stress, may reduce the propensity for plaque disruption by reducing circumferential stress on the fibrous caps of lipid-rich plaques. Furthermore, β-blockers decrease β_2-adrenoceptor-mediated release of intracardiac norepinephrine during ischemia (reducing cardiac toxicity); they attenuate exercise-induced coronary vasoconstriction (improving exercise capacity); and they have antiarrhythmic properties (increasing the threshold for ventricular fibrillation during myocardial ischemia). Additional biochemical and molecular effects of β-adrenoceptor blockade include antiatherogenic (e.g., decreased endothelial injury, decreased affinity of low-density lipoproteins to proteoglycans in the vessel wall) and anti-inflammatory effects (94), increased production of prostacyclins, inhibition of platelet accumulation, altered gene expression and receptor activity, and protection against myocyte apoptosis (92,93).

α_2-Adrenoceptor Agonists

α_2-Adrenoceptor agonists reduce cardiovascular morbidity and mortality following noncardiac and cardiac surgeries (95–100). There are likely to be manifold mechanisms for this protective effect. α_2-Adrenoceptor agonists attenuate perioperative hemodynamic instability (96), inhibit central sympathetic discharge (101), reduce peripheral norepinephrine release (102), and dilate poststenotic coronary vessels (103).

Aspirin

Early postoperative administration of aspirin improves outcome following coronary artery bypass surgery (104). Aspirin has been shown to reduce cardiac events in patients with ACSs and in patients not known to have CAD (105), and to eliminate the diurnal variation in plaque rupture (106). Compared with controls, patients with unstable angina had more than twice the blood concentrations of proinflammatory cytokines (107). Those concentrations decreased after six weeks of aspirin treatment. Aspirin will, of course, reduce platelet aggregability, but its ability to reduce future myocardial infarctions appears greatest in individuals with serologic evidence of increased inflammation (108). Thus, the anti-inflammatory effect of aspirin may be additive to its antithrombotic effect in patients with plaque instability.

Statins

Perioperative use of statins appears to be associated with reduced perioperative mortality in patients undergoing major vascular surgery (109–112). It is noteworthy that the beneficial effect of statins on perioperative outcome was comparable between users and nonusers of β-blockers (109). These findings are consistent with results of a cohort study in almost 20,000 patients with ACSs (113). Patients who were taking statins when experiencing the ACS had fewer myocardial infarctions than those not taking statins. It thus appears that statin therapy may modulate early pathophysiological processes during ischemic cardiac events.

Independent of their lipid-lowering action, statins exert "pleiotropic" effects. Such effects include reversal of endothelial dysfunction (114), modulation of macrophage activation (115), and immunological (115), anti-inflammatory (115), antithrombotic (114), and antiproliferative actions (116). Much of the beneficial effects of statins on cardiac outcome are likely due to these pleiotropic effects and independent of their lipid-lowering action (Fig. 5).

In summary, as perioperative β-blocker, α_2 agonist, aspirin, and statin therapy all appear to be cardioprotective in the perioperative period, and as the different drugs act differently, any of the numerous mechanisms that are blocked by, or interfered with, by these drugs is potentially involved in the etiology of perioperative myocardial injury. Overlapping mechanisms of action include a decrease in sympathetic tone (β-blockers, α_2 agonists), antiatherogenic and anti-inflammatory (β-blockers, statins, aspirin), and antithrombotic effects (aspirin, statins, β-blockers). This is indirect evidence that increased sympathetic, inflammatory, and thrombotic activity mechanisms are involved in the etiology of perioperative myocardial injury. Much of the beneficial effect of all of these drugs on perioperative cardiac outcome in patients with CAD may be due more to their direct (anti-inflammatory, antiatherogenic) or indirect (hemodynamic) stabilizing effect on coronary plaques,

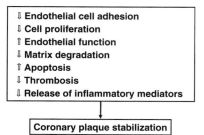

FIGURE 5 "Pleiotropic" (non-LDL-lowering) functions of statins.

than to their effect of lowering myocardial oxygen consumption. Considering the central role of plaque disruption in the etiology of ACSs, this is what would be expected.

MECHANISMS OF PERIOPERATIVE MYOCARDIAL INJURY
Pathophysiology of the Postoperative Period

The immediate postoperative period is accompanied by an activation of the hypothalamus–pituitary–adrenal axis and hypercoagulability that persists for at least one week postoperatively (Fig. 6) (117). Sympathetic nervous-system-induced adrenal medullary activation leads to the release of catecholamines with subsequent stimulation of adrenergic receptors. Adrenergic receptors are located in virtually every organ. In the human heart, they mediate numerous biological responses, including inotropy, chronotropy, myocyte apoptosis, and direct myocyte toxicity. Catecholamines increase each of the four determinants of myocardial oxygen consumption (i.e., heart rate, preload, afterload, and contractility). In addition, the increases in contractility, and in pulse pressure and rate, increase the propensity for plaque disruption by increasing circumferential stress on the fibrous caps of lipid-rich plaques. Furthermore, stimulation of β_2-adrenoceptors releases intracardiac norepinephrine during ischemia (increasing cardiac toxicity) and facilitates exercise-induced coronary vasoconstriction (worsening exercise capacity).

Postoperative hypercoagulability is caused by increased numbers and reactivity of platelets, by increased concentration of fibrinogen and other proteins of the coagulation cascade (factor VIII, von Willebrand factor, α_1-antitrypsin), by impaired deformability of erythrocytes, and by a decrease in the concentration of proteins that are active in the fibrinolytic system (protein C, antithrombin III, α_2-macroglobulin). Consistent with surgery-induced increased sympathetic, pro-coagulant, and antifibrinolytic activity, the majority of ischemic episodes tends to start at the end of surgery and during the emergence from anesthesia (54).

The nonphysiological changes in physical (cardiovascular) factors and the biochemical milieu, and the widespread waxing and waning of systemic (and coronary) inflammation and/or of systemic blood thrombogenicity in the perioperative period

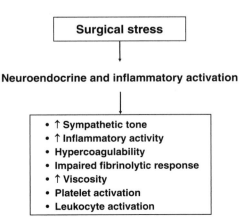

FIGURE 6 Pathophysiology of perioperative period.

induce unpredictable alterations in coronary plaque morphology, function, and progression and predispose the patient with CAD to widespread plaque degeneration and vulnerability, and/or to accelerated subsequent thrombus formation. Frequently, the balance of thrombosis versus thrombolysis is likely to be the decisive factor in determining whether the clinical outcome will be myocardial ischemia or myocardial infarction. The simultaneous pro-coagulant and antifibrinolytic activity may initiate propagation and total occlusion of the coronary artery by a mural thrombus overlying a small plaque erosion that might otherwise have been harmless. Alternatively, it may trigger coronary artery thrombosis during low flow conditions in the presence of underlying stable CAD even in the absence of acute plaque disruption (Fig. 7). Simultaneous perioperative alterations in cardiovascular homeostasis and coronary plaque characteristics may trigger a mismatch of myocardial oxygen supply and demand by numerous mechanisms. If not alleviated in time, it will ultimately result in myocardial infarction, irrespective of its etiology and mechanisms (morphologically, hemodynamically, inflammatory, or coagulation-induced).

Stress-Induced Perioperative Myocardial Injury

Several findings would appear consistent with the possibility that prolonged stress-induced myocardial ischemia rather than coronary plaque disruption followed by thrombus formation is the likely primary cause of perioperative myocardial injury: (*i*) increases in heart rate frequently preceding the ST segment changes, (*ii*) long- rather than short-duration ST segment changes almost universally preceding cardiac events, (*iii*) ST segment depression rather than elevation during literally all ischemic episodes, (*iv*) non-Q-wave rather than Q-wave myocardial infarctions in almost all cases, (*v*) delayed postoperative increases in cTnI concentrations, (*vi*) lack of angiographically visible thrombus or ruptured plaques in some patients who underwent coronary angiography following myocardial infarctions, (*vii*) complete reversal of ECG changes

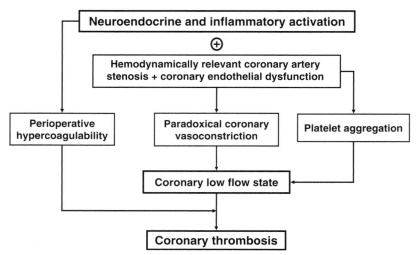

FIGURE 7 Etiology of perioperative coronary thrombosis in the absence of coronary plaque disruption.

to baseline in all but one of the patients with ischemia (including those with infarction) (54), and (*viii*) perioperative cardioprotective effect of anti-ischemic drugs.

Plaque Rupture-Induced Perioperative Myocardial Injury

Several findings would appear consistent with the possibility that plaque rupture and thrombus formation are the primary mechanisms of perioperative myocardial injury: (*i*) no universal association between changes in heart rate and postoperative ST segment changes (57,61,66) or troponin release (67), (*ii*) acute early postoperative increases in cTnI concentrations not preceded by prolonged low-concentration increases (70), (*iii*) pathologic findings of frequent acute plaque disruption and hemorrhage in the infarct-related coronary artery (79–81), and (*iv*) perioperative cardioprotective effect of plaque-stabilizing drugs.

Symbiosis of Mechanisms of Perioperative Myocardial Injury

Several aspects need to be taken into consideration when putting the findings supporting either of the two principal mechanisms into clinical perspective: (*i*) autopsy studies are heavily biased towards fatal outcome; (*ii*) angiographic and autopsy findings of lack of coronary thrombosis in the culprit vessel may be due to early spontaneous lysis and do not exclude primary thrombus formation; (*iii*) on the other hand, coronary thrombus formation may be a preterminal rather than the causative event; (*iv*) ST segment depression is consistent with subendocardial ischemia as well as with an evolving myocardial infarction; (*v*) an absent Q-wave does not exclude a transmural infarction; and (*vi*) even brief but repeatedly occurring ischemic episodes may have a cumulative effect and ultimately cause myocardial necrosis (118).

Taking all uncertainties into consideration, the electrocardiographic and biochemical findings allow several conclusions: (*i*) prolonged perioperative myocardial ischemia leads to myocardial infarction, (*ii*) prolonged myocardial ischemia reflects the onset of permanent myocardial injury, and (*iii*) perioperative myocardial ischemia and infarction are two separate pathophysiologic entities that both develop on the basis of underlying CAD (3). Considering the nature of CAD, and the acutely developing pronounced disturbances in general homeostasis in the perioperative period, it is more than likely that all mechanisms are operative in the etiology of perioperative myocardial injury. The finding that a wide variety of factors (e.g., temperature, hematocrit) and of pharmacological interventions (e.g., β-blocker, α_2 agonists, statins) with vastly different mechanisms (sympatholytic, adrenoceptor-blocking, antithrombotic, anti-inflammatory, plaque-stabilizing) of action influences the incidence of myocardial injury and does this comparably in the nonperioperative and perioperative setting provides strong evidence that the mechanism(s) and trigger(s) (biochemical, physical) of myocardial injury are (*i*) manifold, and (*ii*) comparable in the nonperioperative and perioperative setting (Fig. 8).

Prolonged periods of severe anemia and hypotension (not all that rare in the perioperative period following major surgery) in the presence of limited or absent coronary vasodilator reserve due to underlying CAD will impair myocardial oxygen supply. Any additional increase in oxygen consumption (triggered by increases in blood pressure, heart rate, and cardiac contractility) may acutely provoke subendocardial ischemia. As stenotic atherosclerotic lesions mostly contain segments of dysfunctional endothelium that paradoxically react to vasoactive substances, and as

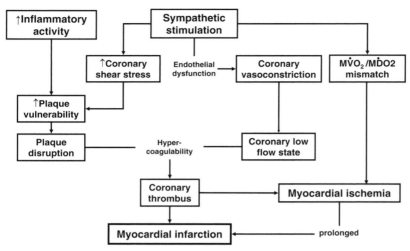

FIGURE 8 Mechanisms leading to perioperative myocardial injury.

sympathetic tone is usually increased in these situations, the critically disturbed myocardial oxygen supply/demand balance may be worsened even further by superimposed coronary vasoconstriction. If not alleviated in time, permanent myocardial injury will result.

It is easy to imagine how some patients with stenotic atherosclerotic lesions may develop acute myocardial infarction even without primary plaque rupture and superimposed thrombus formation. Paradoxical coronary vasoconstriction elicited by perioperatively increased sympathetic tone in the presence of endothelial dysfunction

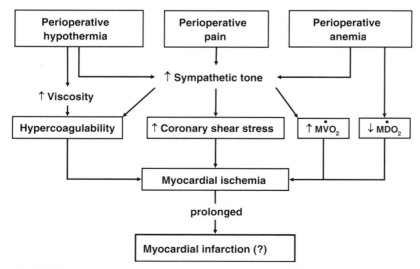

FIGURE 9 Mechanisms leading to perioperative myocardial injury.

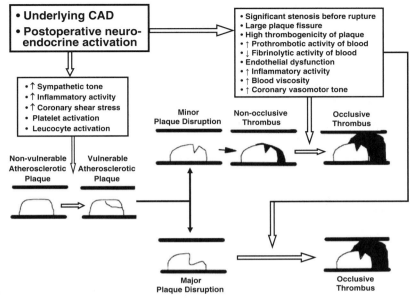

FIGURE 10 Mechanisms of perioperative myocardial injury.

and fixed coronary artery stenosis may lead to a critical reduction in coronary blood flow. The combination of endothelial dysfunction (often accompanied by endothelial erosion), low flow condition, and thrombogenic blood may trigger local thrombus formation. Coronary thrombosis could thus be the consequence rather than the cause of prolonged low coronary flow (Figs. 9 and 10). The ultimate fate of the thrombus and, thus, the extent of jeopardized myocardium will depend on duration and degree of coronary occlusion, which, in turn, will depend on the balance between thrombosis and lysis, and on flow conditions (affected by coronary vasomotor tone, perfusion pressure, and the rheological properties of the blood).

CONCLUSIONS

The overwhelming evidence suggests that the etiology and mechanism(s) of perioperative myocardial injury are as multifactorial as those of myocardial injury in the nonoperative setting. Existing data do not allow a definitive judgment as to whether long-duration subendocardial myocardial ischemia or acute coronary occlusion due to plaque disruption and thrombus formation is the primary mechanism of perioperative myocardial injury in the individual patient. This uncertainty is not surprising considering the enormous structural and functional diversity of coronary atherosclerosis, the unpredictability of plaque progression and vulnerability, and the remaining methodological problems of reliably defining, detecting, and diagnosing perioperative myocardial ischemia and infarction. However, it is almost certain that both mechanisms are involved in the etiology of perioperative myocardial injury. On the basis of increasing knowledge of the etiology and mechanisms of perioperative myocardial injury and the nature of atherosclerotic CAD, and in view of the lack of benefit of preoperative coronary angiography and coronary revascularization in most high-risk patients (119), perioperative plaque stabilization by pharmacological means (statins, aspirin, β-blockers) may be as important (if not more important) in the prevention of perioperative myocardial injury as is an increase in myocardial oxygen supply (by coronary revascularization) or a reduction in myocardial oxygen demand (by β-blockers or α_2-agonists) (5).

REFERENCES

1. Mangano DT. Adverse outcomes after surgery in the year 2001—a continuing odyssey (Editorial). Anesthesiology 1998; 88:561–564.
2. Mangano DT. Perioperative cardiac morbidity. Anesthesiology 1990; 72:153–184.
3. Fleisher LA, Nelson AH, Rosenbaum SH. Postoperative myocardial ischemia: aetiology of cardiac morbidity or manifestation of underlying disease? J Clin Anesth 1995; 7:1–6.
4. Landesberg G. The pathophysiology of perioperative myocardial infarction: facts and perspectives. J Cardiothorac Vasc Anesth 2003; 17:90–100.
5. Priebe H-J. Perioperative myocardial infarction—aetiology and prevention. Br J Anaesth 2005; 95:3–19.
6. Priebe H-J. Triggers of perioperative myocardial ischaemia and infarction. Br J Anaesth 2004; 93:9–20.
7. Libby P, Theroux P. Pathophysiology of coronary artery disease. Circulation 2005; 111: 3481–3488.
8. Clarkson TB, Prichard RW, Morgan TM, Petrick GS, Klein KP. Remodeling of coronary arteries in human and nonhuman primates. J Am Med Assoc 1994; 271:289–294.
9. Arnett EN, Isner JM, Redwood DR, et al. Coronary artery narrowing in coronary heart disease: comparison of cineangiographic and necropsy findings. Ann Intern Med 1979; 91:350–356.
10. Schoenhagen P, Ziada KM, Kapadia SR, et al. Extent and direction of arterial remodelling in stable versus unstable coronary syndromes: an intravascular ultrasound study. Circulation 2000; 101:598–603.
11. Libby P. Act local, act global: inflammation and the multiplicity of "vulnerable" coronary plaques. J Am Coll Cardiol 2005; 45:1600–1602.
12. Maseri A, Fuster V. Is there a vulnerable plaque? Circulation 2003; 107:2068–2071.
13. Casscells W, Naghavi M, Willerson JT. Vulnerable atherosclerotic plaque: a multifocal disease. Circulation 2003; 107:2072–2075.
14. Kereiakes DJ. The emperor's clothes: in search of the vulnerable plaque. Circulation 2003; 107:2076–2077.
15. Corti R, Fuster V, Badimon JJ. Pathogenic concepts of acute coronary syndromes. J Am Coll Cardiol 2003; 41:7S–14S.
16. Davies MJ. Stability and instability: the two faces of coronary atherosclerosis. The Paul Dudley White Lecture, 1995. Circulation 1996; 94:2013–2020.
17. Virmani R, Kolodgie FD, Burke AP, Farb A, Schwartz SM. Lessons from sudden coronary death: a comprehensive morphological classification scheme for atherosclerotic lesions. Arterioscler Thromb Vasc Biol 2000; 20:1262–1275.
18. Stone PH. Triggering myocardial infarction. N Engl J Med 2004; 351:1716–1718.
19. MacNeill BD, Jang I-K, Bouma BE, et al. Focal and multi-focal plaque macrophage distributions in patients with acute and stable presentations of coronary artery disease. J Am Coll Cardiol 2004; 44:972–979.
20. Libby P. Current concepts of the pathogenesis of the acute coronary syndromes. Circulation 2001; 104:365–372.
21. Little WC, Constantinescu M, Applegate RJ, et al. Can coronary angiography predict the site of a subsequent myocardial infarction in patients with mild-to-moderate coronary artery disease? Circulation 1988; 78:1157–1166.
22. Falk E, Shah PK, Fuster V. Coronary plaque disruption. Circulation 1995; 92:657–671.
23. Bruschke AV, Kramer J Jr, Bal ET, et al. The dynamics of progression of coronary atherosclerosis studied in 168 medically treated patients who underwent coronary arteriography three times. Am Heart J 1989; 117:296–305.

24. Yokoya K, Takatsu H, Suzuki T, et al. Process of progression of coronary artery lesions from mild or moderate stenosis to moderate or severe stenosis: a study based on four serial coronary arteriograms per year. Circulation 1999; 100:903–909.
25. Muller JE, Tofler GH, Stone PH. Circadian variation and triggers of onset of acute cardiovascular disease. Circulation 1989; 79:733–743.
26. Willich SN, Maclure M, Mittleman M, et al. Sudden cardiac death: support for a role of triggering in causation. Circulation 1993; 87:1442–1450.
27. Gertz SD, Roberts WC. Hemodynamic shear force in rupture of coronary arterial atherosclerotic plaques. Am J Cardiol 1990; 66:1368–1372.
28. Feldman CL, Stone PH. Intravascular hemodynamic factors responsible for progression of coronary atherosclerosis and development of vulnerable plaque. Curr Opin Cardiol 2000; 15:430–440.
29. Naghavi M, Libby P, Falk E, et al. From vulnerable plaque to vulnerable patient: a call for new definitions and risk assessment strategies, part I. Circulation 2003; 108:1664–1672.
30. Naghavi M, Libby P, Falk E, et al. From vulnerable plaque to vulnerable patient: a call for new definitions and risk assessment strategies, part II. Circulation 2003; 108:1772–1778.
31. Topol EJ, Yadav JS. Recognition of the importance of embolisation in atherosclerotic vascular disease. Circulation 2000; 101:570–580.
32. Lerman A, Zeiher AM. Endothelial function: cardiac events. Circulation 2005; 111: 363–368.
33. Fuster V, Badimon L, Badimon JJ, Chesebro JH. The pathophysiology of coronary artery disease and the acute syndromes (I). N Engl J Med 1992; 326:242–250.
34. Fuster V, Badimon L, Badimon JJ, Chesebro JH. The pathophysiology of coronary artery disease and the acute syndromes (II). N Engl J Med 1992; 326:310–318.
35. Morrow DA, Ridker PM. C-reactive protein, inflammation, and coronary risk. Med Clin North Am 2000; 84:149–161.
36. Buffon A, Biasucci LM, Liuzzo G, et al. Widespread coronary inflammation in unstable angina. N Engl J Med 2002; 347:5–12.
37. Libby P. Inflammation in atherosclerosis. Nature 2002; 420:868–874.
38. Tanaka A, Shimada K, Sano T, et al. Multiple plaque rupture and C-reactive protein in acute myocardial infarction. J Am Coll Cardiol 2005; 45:1594–1599.
39. Mauriello A, Sangiorgi G, Fratoni S, et al. Diffuse and active inflammation occurs in both vulnerable and stable plaques of the entire coronary tree: a histopathologic study of patients dying of acute myocardial infarction. J Am Coll Cardiol 2005; 45:1585–1593.
40. Mittleman MA, Maclure M, Tofler GH, et al. Triggering of acute myocardial infarction by heavy physical exertion: protection against triggering by regular exercise. N Engl J Med 1993; 329:1677–1683.
41. Grignani G, Soffiantino F, Zuchella M, et al. Platelet activation by emotional stress in patients with coronary artery disease. Circulation 1991; 83(suppl II):128–136.
42. Forrester JS. Role of plaque rupture in acute coronary syndromes. Am J Cardiol 2000; 86(suppl):J15–J23.
43. Landesberg G, Mosseri M, Wolf Y, et al. Perioperative myocardial ischemia and infarction: identification by continuous 12-lead electrocardiogram with online ST-segment monitoring. Anesthesiology 2002; 96:262–270.
44. London MJ. Multilead precordial ST-segment monitoring. "The next generation"? (Editorial views). Anesthesiology 2002; 96:259–261.
45. Alpert JS. Defining myocardial infarction: "Will the real myocardial infarction please stand up?" (Editorial). Am Heart J 2003; 146:377–379.
46. Tunstall-Pedoe H, Kuulasmaa K, Amouyel P, et al. Myocardial infarction and coronary deaths in the World Health Organization MONICA Project. Registration procedures, event rates, and case-fatality rates in 38 populations from 21 countries in four continents. Circulation 1994; 90:583–612.
47. WHO MONICA Project Principal Investigators. World Health Organization MONICA Project (monitoring trends and determinants of cardiovascular disease): a major international collaboration. J Clin Epidemiol 1988; 41:105–114.
48. The Joint European Society of Cardiology/American College of Cardiology Committee. Myocardial infarction redefined—a consensus document of the Joint European Society

of Cardiology/American College of Cardiology Committee for the redefinition of myocardial infarction. Eur Heart J 2000; 21:1502–1513.

49. Kaul P, Newby LK, Fu Y, et al. Troponin T and quantitative ST-segment depression offer complimentary prognostic information in the risk stratification of acute coronary syndrome patients. J Am Coll Cardiol 2003; 41:371–380.

50. Lindahl B, Toss H, Siegbahn A, et al. Markers of myocardial damage and inflammation in relation to long-term mortality in unstable coronary artery disease. The Fragmin during Instability in Coronary Artery Disease (FRISC) Study Group. N Engl J Med 2000; 343:1139–1147.

51. Adams JE III, Sicard GA, Allen BT, et al. Diagnosis of perioperative myocardial infarction with measurement of cardiac troponin I. N Engl J Med 1994; 330:670–674.

52. Lee TH, Thomas EJ, Ludwig LE, et al. Troponin T as a marker for myocardial ischemia in patients undergoing major noncardiac surgery. Am J Cardiol 1996; 77:1031–1036.

53. Metzler H, Gries M, Rehak P, et al. Perioperative myocardial cell injury: the role of troponins. Br J Anaesth 1997; 78:386–390.

54. Landesberg G, Mosseri M, Zahger D, et al. Myocardial infarction following vascular surgery: the role of prolonged, stress-induced, ST-depression-type ischemia. J Am Coll Cardiol 2001; 37:1858–1863.

55. Landesberg G, Mosseri M, Shatz V, et al. Cardiac troponin after major vascular surgery: the role of perioperative ischemia, preoperative thallium scanning, and coronary revascularization. J Am Coll Cardiol 2004; 44:569–575.

56. Landesberg G, Shatz V, Akopnik I, et al. Association of cardiac troponin, CK-MB, and postoperative myocardial ischemia with long-term survival after major vascular surgery. J Am Coll Cardiol 2003; 42:1547–1554.

57. Mangano DT, Hollenberg M, Fegert G, et al. Perioperative myocardial ischaemia in patients undergoing noncardiac surgery. I. Incidence and severity during the 4-day perioperative period. J Am Coll Cardiol 1991; 17:843–850.

58. Landesberg G, Luria MH, Cotev S, et al. Importance of long-duration postoperative ST-segment depression in cardiac morbidity after vascular surgery. Lancet 1993; 341:715–719.

59. Badner NH, Knill RL, Brown JE, et al. Myocardial infarction after noncardiac surgery. Anesthesiology 1998; 88:572–578.

60. London MJ, Hollenberg M, Wong MG, et al. Intraoperative myocardial ischemia: localization by continuous 12-lead electrocardiography. Anesthesiology 1988; 69:232–241.

61. Mangano DT, Browner WS, Hollenberg M, et al. Association of perioperative myocardial ischemia with cardiac morbidity and mortality in men undergoing noncardiac surgery. N Engl J Med 1990; 323:1781–1788.

62. McCann RL, Clements FM. Silent myocardial ischemia in patients undergoing peripheral vascular surgery: incidence and association with perioperative cardiac morbidity and mortality. J Vasc Surg 1989; 9:583–587.

63. Ouyang P, Gerstenblith G, Furman WR, et al. Frequency and significance of early postoperative silent myocardial ischemia in patients having peripheral vascular surgery. Am J Cardiol 1989; 64:1113–1116.

64. Pasternak PF, Grossi EA, Baumann G, et al. The value of silent myocardial ischemia monitoring in the prediction of perioperative myocardial infarction in patients undergoing peripheral vascular surgery. J Vasc Surg 1989; 10:617–625.

65. Pasternak PF, Grossi EA, Baumann G, et al. Silent myocardial ischemia monitoring predicts late as well as perioperative cardiac events in patients undergoing vascular surgery. J Vasc Surg 1992; 16:171–180.

66. Raby KE, Barry J, Creager MA, et al. Detection and significance of intraoperative and postoperative myocardial ischemia in peripheral vascular surgery. J Am Med Assoc 1992; 268:222–227.

67. Rapp H-J, Rabethge S, Luiz T, Haux P. Perioperative ST-segment depression and troponin T release. Acta Anaesthesiol Scand 1999; 43:124–129.

68. Keith A, Fox A. Management of acute coronary syndromes: an update. Heart 2004; 90:698–706.

69. Krumholz HM, Friesinger GC, Cook EF, et al. Relationship of age with eligibility for thrombolytic therapy and mortality among patients with suspected acute myocardial infarction. J Am Geriatr Soc 1994; 42:127–131.

70. Sabia PJ, Powers ER, Ragosta M, et al. An association between collateral blood flow and myocardial viability in patients with recent myocardial infarction. N Engl J Med 1992; 327:1825–1831.
71. Singh N, Langer A. Current status of silent myocardial ischemia. Can J Cardiol 1995; 11:286–289.
72. Antman EM, Braunwald E. ST-elevation myocardial infarction: pathology, pathophysiology, and clinical features. In: Zipes DP, Libby P, Bonow RO, Braunwald E, eds. Heart Disease. Philadelphia: Elsevier/Saunders, 2005:1141–1165.
73. Phibbs B, Marcus F, Marriott HJ, et al. Q-wave versus non-Q-wave myocardial infarction: a meaningless distinction. J Am Coll Cardiol 1999; 33:576–582.
74. Arai AE, Hirsch GA. Q-wave and non-Q-wave myocardial infarctions through the eyes of cardiac magnetic resonance imaging (Editorial Comment). J Am Coll Cardiol 2004; 44:561–563.
75. Moon JCC, De Arenaza DP, Elkington AG, Taneja AK, John AS, Wang D, et al. The pathological basis of Q-wave and non-Q-wave myocardial infarction. J Am Coll Cardiol 2004; 44:554–560.
76. Goodman SG, Langer A, Ross AM, et al. Non-Q-wave versus Q-wave myocardial infarction after thrombolytic therapy: angiographic and prognostic insights from the global utilization of streptokinase and tissue plasminogen activator for occluded coronary arteries. I. Angiographic substudy. GUSTO-I Angiographic Investigators. Circulation 1998; 97:444–450.
77. Le Manch Y, Perel A, Coriat P, Godet G, Bertrand M, Riou B. Early and delayed myocardial infarction after abdominal aortic surgery. Anesthesiology 2005; 102:885–891.
78. Ellis SG, Hertzer NR, Young JR, Brener S. Angiographic correlates of cardiac death and myocardial infarction complicating major nonthoracic vascular surgery. Am J Cardiol 1996; 77:1126–1128.
79. Master AM, Dack S, Jaffe H. Perioperative coronary artery occlusion. J Am Med Assoc 1938; 110:1415–1418.
80. Dawood MA, Gutpa DK, Southern J, Walia A, Atkinson JB, Eagle KA. Pathology of fatal perioperative myocardial infarction: implications regarding pathophysiology and prevention. Int J Cardiol 1996; 57:37–44.
81. Cohen MC, Aretz TH. Histological analysis of coronary artery lesions in fatal postoperative myocardial infarction. Cardiovasc Pathol 1999; 8:133–139.
82. Nelson AH, Fleisher LA, Rosenbaum SH. Relationship between postoperative anaemia and cardiac morbidity in high-risk vascular patients in the intensive care unit. Crit Care Med 1993; 21:860–866.
83. Frank S, Beattie C, Christopherson R, et al. Unintentional hypothermia is associated with postoperative myocardial ischemia. The Perioperative Ischemia Randomized Anesthesia Trial Study Group. Anesthesiology 1993; 78:468–476.
84. Frank S, Fleisher L, Breslow M, et al. Perioperative maintenance of normothermia reduces the incidence of morbid cardiac events: a randomized clinical trial. J Am Med Assoc 1997; 277:1127–1134.
85. Mangano DT, Siliciano D, Hollenberg M, et al. Postoperative myocardial ischemia therapeutic trials using intensive analgesia following surgery. Anesthesiology 1992; 76:343–353.
86. Beattie WS, Buckley DN, Forrest JB. Epidural morphine reduces the risk of postoperative myocardial ischaemia in patients with cardiac risk factors. Can J Anaesth 1993; 40:532–541.
87. Mangano DT, Layug EL, Wallace A, Tateo I, for the Multicenter Study of Perioperative Ischemia Research Group. Effect of atenolol on mortality and cardiovascular morbidity after noncardiac surgery: Multicenter Study of Perioperative Ischemia Research Group. N Engl J Med 1996; 335:1713–1720.
88. Poldermans D, Boersma E, Bax JJ, et al., for the Dutch Echocardiographic Cardiac Risk Evaluation Applying Stress Echocardiography Study Group. The effect of bisoprolol on perioperative mortality and myocardial infarction in high-risk patients undergoing vascular surgery. N Engl J Med 1999; 341:1789–1794.
89. Boersma E, Poldermans D, Bax JJ, et al., for the DECREASE Study Group. Predictors of cardiac events after major vascular surgery: role of clinical characteristics, dobutamine echocardiography, and beta-blocker therapy. J Am Med Assoc 2001; 285:1865–1873.

90. Poldermans D, Boersma E, Bax JJ, et al., for the Dutch Cardiac Risk Evaluation Applying Stress Echocardiography Group. Bisoprolol reduces cardiac death and myocardial infarction in high-risk patients as long as 2 years after successful major vascular surgery. Eur Heart J 2001; 22:1353–1358.
91. Wallace A, Layug B, Tateo I, et al., for the McSPI Research Group. Prophylactic atenolol reduces postoperative myocardial ischemia. Anesthesiology 1998; 88:7–17.
92. Kertai MD, Bax JJ, Klein J, Poldermans D. Is there any reason to withhold β blockers from high-risk patients with coronary artery disease during surgery? Anesthesiology 2004; 100:4–7.
93. London MJ, Zaugg M, Schaub MC, Spahn DR. Perioperative β-adrenergic receptor blockade: physiologic foundations and clinical controversies. Anesthesiology 2004; 100: 170–175.
94. Anzai T, Yoshikawa T, Takahashi T, et al. Early use of beta-blockers is associated with attenuation of serum C-reactive protein elevation and favorable short-term prognosis after acute myocardial infarction. Cardiology 2003; 99:47–53.
95. Dorman BH, Zucker JR, Verrier ED, Gartman DM, Slachman FN. Clonidine improves perioperative myocardial ischemia, reduces anesthetic requirement, and alters hemodynamic parameters in patients undergoing coronary artery bypass surgery. J Cardiothorac Vasc Anesth 1993; 7:386–395.
96. McSPI-Europe Research Group. Perioperative sympatholysis: beneficial effects of the α_2-adrenoceptor agonist mivazerol on hemodynamic stability and myocardial ischemia. Anesthesiology 1997; 86:346–363.
97. Oliver MF, Goldman L, Julian DG, Holme I. Effect of mivazerol on perioperative cardiac complications during non-cardiac surgery in patients with coronary heart disease: the European Mivazerol Trial (EMIT). Anesthesiology 1999; 91:951–961.
98. Nishina K, Mikawa K, Uesugi T, et al. Efficacy of clonidine for prevention of perioperative myocardial ischemia: a critical appraisal and meta-analysis of the literature. Anesthesiology 2002; 96:323–329.
99. Wijeysundera DN, Naik JS, Beattie S. Alpha-2 adrenergic agonists to prevent perioperative cardiovascular complications: a meta-analysis. Am J Med 2003; 114:742–752.
100. Wallace AW, Galindez D, Salahieh A, et al. Effect of clonidine on cardiovascular morbidity and mortality after noncardiac surgery. Anesthesiology 2004; 101:284–293.
101. Muzi M, Goff DR, Kampine JP, et al. Clonidine reduces sympathetic activity but maintains baroreflex responses in normotensive humans. Anesthesiology 1992; 77:864–871.
102. Ellis JE, Drijvers G, Pedlow S, et al. Premedication with oral and transdermal clonidine provides safe and efficacious postoperative sympatholysis. Anesth Analg 1994; 79: 1133–1140.
103. Heusch G, Schipke J, Thamer V. Clonidine prevents the sympathetic initiation and aggravation of poststenotic myocardial ischemia. J Cardiovasc Pharmacol 1985; 7:1176–1182.
104. Mangano DT, for the Multicenter Study of Perioperative Ischemia Research Group. Aspirin and mortality from coronary bypass surgery. N Engl J Med 2002; 347:1309–1317.
105. Collaborative Group of the Primary Prevention Project. Low-dose aspirin and vitamin E in people at cardiovascular risk: a randomised trial in general practice. Lancet 2001; 357:89–95.
106. Ridker PM, Manson JE, Buring JE, et al. Circadian variation of acute myocardial infarction and the effect of low-dose aspirin in a randomized trial of physicians. Circulation 1990; 82:897–902.
107. Ikonomidis I, Andreotti F, Economou E, et al. Increased proinflammatory cytokines in patients with chronic stable angina and their reduction by aspirin. Circulation 1999; 100:793–798.
108. Ridker PM, Cushman M, Stampfer MJ, et al. Inflammation, aspirin, and the risk of cardiovascular disease in apparently healthy men. N Engl J Med 1997; 336:973–979.
109. Poldermans D, Bax JJ, Kertai MD, et al. Statins are associated with a reduced incidence of perioperative mortality in patients undergoing major noncardiac vascular surgery. Circulation 2003; 107:1848–1851.
110. Lindenauer PK, Pekow P, Wang K, Gutierrez B, Benjamin EM. Lipid-lowering therapy and in-hospital mortality following major noncardiac surgery. J Am Med Assoc 2004; 291:2092–2099.

111. Kertai MD, Boersma E, Westerhout CM, et al. Association between long-term statin use and mortality after successful abdominal aortic aneurysm surgery. Am J Med 2004; 116:96–103.
112. Kertai MD, Boersma E, Klein J, van Urk H, Poldermans D. Optimizing the prediction of perioperative mortality in vascular surgery by using a customized probability model. Arch Intern Med 2005; 165:898–904.
113. Spencer FA, Allegrone J, Goldberg RJ, et al., for the Grace Investigators. Association of statin therapy with outcomes of acute coronary syndromes: the GRACE study. Ann Intern Med 2004; 140:857–866.
114. Vaughan CJ, Gotto AM Jr. Update on statins: 2003. Circulation 2004; 110:886–892.
115. Almog Y, Shefer A, Novack V, et al. Prior statin therapy is associated with a decreased rate of severe sepsis. Circulation 2004; 110:880–885.
116. Lee T-S, Chang C-C, Zhu Y, Shyy JYJ. Simvastatin induces heme oxygenase-1: a novel mechanism of vessel protection. Circulation 2004; 110:1296–1301.
117. Breslow MJ, Parker SD, Frank SM, et al. Determinants of catecholamine and cortisol responses to lower extremity revascularization: the PIRAT study group. Anesthesiology 1993; 79:1202–1209.
118. Geft IL, Fishbein MC, Ninomyia K, et al. Intermittent brief periods of ischemia have a cumulative effect and may cause myocardial necrosis. Circulation 1982; 66:1150–1153.
119. McFalls EO, Ward HB, Moritz TE, et al. Coronary artery revascularization before elective major vascular surgery. N Engl J Med 2004; 351:2795–2804.

5 Stunning, Hibernation, Preconditioning, Postconditioning, and the Effects of Anesthetic Drugs

Pierre Foëx

Nuffield Department of Anesthetics, University of Oxford, Oxford, U.K.

Bruce Biccard

Department of Anesthetics, Nelson R. Mandela School of Medicine, Congella, South Africa

INTRODUCTION

The effects of myocardial ischemia on the heart have been studied for many years. This is not surprising as myocardial ischemia and its consequences are among the leading causes of morbidity and mortality in an increasingly elderly population. Myocardial ischemia is also a major cause of perioperative morbidity and mortality. Indeed, 60% of the patients who die within 30 days of surgery in England, Wales, and Northern Ireland have evidence of coronary heart disease. The number of cardiac deaths is approximately 9000 per annum (1) to which must be added nonfatal complications. On the basis of the literature, the ratio of severe cardiac complications to cardiac death is approximately one in 10 (2). Therefore, the number of adverse cardiac outcomes is likely to be in the region of 100,000 per annum. In the United States, the number of cardiac complications of anesthesia and surgery was approximately 1 million per annum in 1990 (3). As a result of the high prevalence of coronary heart disease, strategies have been developed to reduce the risk of adverse cardiac events in the general population and in surgical patients.

The most feared complications are cardiac death and nonfatal myocardial infarction. The risk is substantial as fatal and nonfatal myocardial infarction occur in 1% to 5% of unselected patients undergoing noncardiac surgery (4,5). Just over 30 years ago, Braunwald (6) developed the concept of damage control after acute coronary occlusion. He proposed that myocardial tissue within the distribution of an occluded coronary artery may not necessarily die. This led to the development, experimentally first (7), then in patients, of reperfusion of ischemic myocardium. Reperfusion with thrombolytic agents was shown to reduce mortality and to improve postinfarction cardiac function (8). This was followed by the introduction of percutaneous interventions (9). These interventions were, and still are, generally complemented by drug therapy. Many classes of drugs have been proposed; they include antiplatelet agents, β-blockers, glucose–insulin–potassium infusion, adenosine, calcium channel blockers, K_{ATP}^+ channel openers, and, recently, sodium–hydrogen exchange inhibitors (10).

Over the years, it has become obvious that ischemia is a complex phenomenon. Ischemia can cause irreversible damage (myocardial infarction); it can also cause prolonged but slowly reversible dysfunction (stunning), or prolonged dysfunction that can recover after revascularization (hibernation). Paradoxically, ischemia can also be protective: this is the case with ischemic myocardial preconditioning and the more recently described ischemic myocardial postconditioning.

STUNNING

In 1975, Heyndrickx et al. (11) observed prolonged dysfunction after a short period of ischemia followed by reperfusion. The term "myocardial stunning" was coined by Braunwald and Kloner (12). Stunning is characterized by a reduction in cardiac function after a brief period of ischemia followed by reperfusion. Although there is complete restoration of perfusion, dysfunction can last for several hours or days (13). In clinical practice, a number of interventions such as coronary angioplasty and the insertion of stents, coronary bypass surgery, and thrombolysis after acute coronary occlusion are human models of myocardial stunning. As many adult patients experience episodes of silent myocardial ischemia during the perioperative period (14,15), stunning may occur and result in prolonged postoperative acute left ventricular dysfunction.

Paradoxically, in the syndrome of ischemia reperfusion, reperfusion of the myocardium plays a dominant role in the genesis of myocardial dysfunction and damage. Reperfusion injury is particularly relevant to cardiac surgery (16). The mechanisms of stunning include formation of free radicals, accumulation of intracellular Ca^{2+}, and degradation of contractile proteins. During ischemia, and to a greater extent during reperfusion, considerable production of free radicals occurs (17). Free radicals have many intracellular targets including sarcolemmal and the subcellular membranes of organelles (18). Their role in stunning is confirmed by the improved postischemic recovery in the presence of the antioxidant, superoxide dismutase (19). Production of free radicals involves xanthine oxidase, oxidation of catecholamines, mitochondrial respiration, and neutrophil activation.

Calcium overload plays an important role in the reduction of contractile function as the initial calcium overload decreases the sensitivity of contractile proteins to calcium (13). The role of calcium overload is supported by the protective effect of calcium channel antagonists such as nisoldipine (20). Calcium overload results from altered characteristics of the Na^+/Ca^{2+} antiport and from altered Ca^{2+} fluxes at the level of the sarcoplasmic reticulum. The altered Ca^{2+} dynamics may be caused by ischemia-induced intracellular acidosis (21). Calcium overload is accentuated during early reperfusion because the Na^+/H^+ antiport is maximally stimulated causing an increase in myoplasmic Na^+. More Na^+ is therefore available to be exchanged for Ca^{2+}.

Another major consequence of calcium overload is the opening of the mitochondrial permeability transition pore (MPTP). Opening of this pore allows small molecular solutes to move freely across the mitochondrial membrane and renders the membrane permeable to protons. This results in uncoupling of phosphorylative oxidation so that adenosine triphosphate (ATP) synthesis ceases (22).

A few minutes after reperfusion, the effect of calcium overload on contractile function decreases as other factors, such as release of cytokines, activation of neutrophils, and proteolytic enzymes, become more important (23).

There is some evidence that translocation of heat-shock proteins (Hsp-27, αB-cristalline) with covalent binding to myofibrils may be involved in the pathogenesis of stunning, as well as degradation of troponin I as evidenced in a transgenic mouse model with overexpression of troponin I fragments (24).

During reperfusion, an increase in coronary vascular resistance and a reduction in vasodilator response have been reported (13). However, other studies have failed to confirm these changes (25).

It is within the first few minutes of reperfusion that interventions are most likely to decrease the extent of cell death (26).

Anesthetic Agents and Stunning

Most inhalation anesthetics and high-dose opioids confer protection against stunning and increase the rate of myocardial recovery after reperfusion (27,28). In 1988, Warltier et al. (29) demonstrated that prior administration of halothane and isoflurane improved both the speed and extent of recovery of function after a brief (15 minutes) period of ischemia. These observations have generally been confirmed (30,31). However, some studies of isolated heart preparations showed no protection (32,33). However, more recently, sevoflurane and desflurane have been shown to confer protection in such models (34–36).

The most important mechanisms of the effects of inhalation anesthetics on the stunned myocardium include adenosine A_1-receptors, protein kinase C (PKC), and K_{ATP}^+ channels (37,38).

As in many studies, the inhalation anesthetics were given prior to ischemia and reperfusion; protection may have been due essentially to a type of conditioning of the heart. Indeed, as will be described later, pharmacological preconditioning is an important mode of myocardial protection. The possibility of preconditioning rather than an effect of stunning itself is supported by studies during which the inhalation anesthetic was discontinued before ischemia reperfusion and still resulted in reduced infarct size and improved recovery (39,40).

In contrast with inhalation anesthetics, intravenous anesthetics appear to confer little protection (41,42). However, in the isolated heart, as opposed to the intact instrumented heart, propofol has been shown to reduce cellular damage (43–45). Propofol-induced protection was not abolished by blockade of K_{ATP}^+ channels. This suggests that other mechanisms play a role.

Although the effects of opioids on infarct size have been well demonstrated, there are few studies of their effects on myocardial stunning (41,42). In the isolated heart, high concentrations of fentanyl offered significant protection, mediated by delta-opioid receptors, adenosine A_1-receptors, PKC, and K_{ATP}^+ channels (28,46,47). This is not surprising because delta-opioid receptors are known to play an important role in pharmacological preconditioning (48–50). The role of delta-opioid receptors is supported by the abolition of their protective effect by naloxone (49,51,52). As washout of opioids does not prevent their effect, they must act as preconditioning agents rather than protect against stunning (53,54).

Other mechanisms involved in the effects of opioids as protection can be prevented by blockade of Gi proteins and PKC. It is possible that opioids act also by reducing adhesion and migration of neutrophils (55,56).

HIBERNATION

The concept of myocardial hibernation was developed by Rahimtoola (57,58) to describe the reduction of ventricular function attributed to insufficient coronary blood flow. An important feature of myocardial hibernation is that function can improve with an improved oxygen supply–demand balance. Improvement may occur with the administration of β-blockers as they reduce oxygen demand. The benefits of carvedilol in the treatment of heart failure may be due, in part, to recovery of hibernating myocardium (59). More frequently, functional recovery of hibernating myocardium follows coronary revascularization (60,61). In the hibernating myocardium, cardiac metabolism is downregulated and the reduction of contractile performance may result from permanently reduced coronary blood flow. Thus, hibernation can be regarded as a successful adaptation to the prevailing circumstances by active downregulation (62). A porcine experimental model of hibernating myocardium has been developed, based on the chronic reduction of coronary blood flow (63). This suggests that downregulation of cardiac contractility because of low coronary flow is an important cause of myocardial hibernation.

Another hypothesis is that hibernation results from a decrease of the coronary flow reserve. This would expose the myocardium to repeated episodes of myocardial ischemia/reperfusion/stunning leading to chronic stunning or hibernation (64). As coronary artery stenoses of greater than 80% abolish the coronary flow reserve (65), it is easy to imagine that in the presence of such stenoses, an increase in cardiac workload causes ischemia. Clinically, this hypothesis is supported by evidence that exertional angina can lead to persistent postischemic dysfunction (66). Yet, the exact mechanism of hibernation remains partly unclear because some metabolic changes in hibernating myocardium differ from those seen in stunning (67). Another argument in favor of the role of reduced coronary reserve is the observation, obtained by positron emission tomography (PET), that several months after myocardial infarction, patients may show evidence of improved perfusion, whereas metabolism and function are still reduced (68).

Although the stunned myocardium maintains its normal structure, the hibernating myocardium shows loss of myofibrils, disorganization of the cytoskeleton, degeneration of the sarcoplasmic reticulum, and atrophy (69). Active remodeling is present and is an important determinant of potential functional recovery following therapeutic interventions. Remodeling includes the presence of interstitial fibroblasts expressing the embryonal isoform of smooth muscle myosin heavy chain (SMemb) in dysfunctional segments, predominantly located in border areas adjacent to viable myocardial tissue. Continuous remodeling in the cardiac interstitium of the hibernating myocardium appears to be an important predictor of recovery of function after revascularization (70).

As β-adrenergic receptors play a major role in the contractile performance of the heart, the possibility exists that hibernation may be the consequence of altered adrenergic receptor density (ARD). Indeed, in human cardiac biopsies, severely hypokinetic or akinetic segments showed a 2.4-fold increase in alpha-ARD with a concomitant 50% decrease in β-adrenoceptor density (BRD) compared with normal segments. An increase in ARD/BRD ratio was also seen in dysfunctional segments with contractile reserve compared with normal segments (71). The lower β-receptor density may allow the myocardium to conserve energy as its function is downregulated so that recovery remains possible. This, however, is difficult to reconcile with the improvement of function seen after administration of carvedilol, a β-blocker and vasodilator (59), unless it is postulated that improved function results primarily from vasodilatation, whereas β-blockade prevents sympathetically mediated myocardial remodeling.

Tumor necrosing factor (TNF-α) and iNOS appear to play a role in myocardial hibernation (72). Both exert negative inotropic effects. TNF-α causes contractile dysfunction by reducing calcium fluxes in myocytes (73). Excessive NO production acts through a cyclic GMP-dependent mechanism. It attenuates the cyclic AMP-dependent inotropic effect of β-adrenergic stimulation. TNF-α and NO can promote apoptosis, which is a feature of the hibernating myocardium (74).

Heart transplantation is an established therapy for patients with the most severe heart failure. Indeed, for end-stage heart failure cardiac transplantation is the only treatment to provide improvement in quality of life and survival (75). However, its availability is limited by the large mismatch between demand and donor organ availability. As not all ventricular dysfunction secondary to coronary artery disease is irreversible, coronary revascularization is an important treatment option (76). It can be carried out with an acceptable risk, allowing functional improvement to the extent that heart transplantation may become unnecessary (77).

Approximately 40% of patients undergoing coronary artery bypass surgery with preoperative ventricular dysfunction exhibit a significant improvement after successful revascularization (78). This has been confirmed by a meta-analysis based on over 3000 patients with heart failure and coronary artery disease. The study showed a strong association between myocardial viability on noninvasive testing and improved survival after revascularization (79). Thus, patients with left ventricular dysfunction and extensive myocardial hibernation appear to have the potential for improved left ventricular function, symptomatic relief, and survival after revascularization (80). Although patients with a substantial amount of hibernating myocardium seem to have a better outcome with revascularization than medical therapy, those with poor viability fare worse after revascularization in comparison to medical therapy (81).

A retrospective data analysis suggests that patients with impaired left ventricular function who have viable myocardium recover from coronary bypass surgery with a low early mortality and promising short-term survival. Therefore, myocardial viability studies permit selection of patients who are at low risk for serious perioperative complications associated with revascularization, and are likely to derive major functional and survival benefits (82). However, functional improvement is greater for stunned segments than for hibernating segments (83).

The time course of functional recovery after coronary artery bypass graft surgery in patients with chronic left ventricular ischemic dysfunction appears to be progressive; it follows a monoexponential time course with a median time constant of 23 days (range 6–78) (84).

The issue of myocardial hibernation is also important in patients presenting for noncardiac surgery because the risk of adverse cardiac outcome after both cardiac and noncardiac surgery increases with a reduction of the ejection fraction (85). Patients needing major surgery who have a significant amount of hibernating myocardium could benefit from coronary revascularization as their improved cardiac function would reduce the cardiac risk of their operation.

Many techniques are now available to determine the presence of hibernating myocardium. Dobutamine echocardiography (86), intravenous myocardial contrast echocardiography (87), and contrast-enhanced magnetic resonance imaging are effective ways of identifying hibernating myocardium (83).

Although there is a wealth of information on the effects of anesthetic agents and opioids on the stunned myocardium, there are, to our knowledge, no published studies of the effects of anesthetic agents or opioids on the hibernating myocardium. This is not surprising as experimental models of myocardial hibernation are not widely available.

MYOCARDIAL PRECONDITIONING
Ischemic Preconditioning
Ischemic myocardial preconditioning was described by Reimer et al. (88) and Murry et al. (89) in 1986. Reimer et al. (88) demonstrated that short periods of ischemia lasting about five minutes decreased the rate of depletion of ATP during a subsequent prolonged period of ischemia. Murry et al. (89) reported that such short periods of ischemia made the heart more resistant to infarction, reducing the infarct size by 70% to 80%. These authors introduced the term "ischemic preconditioning." Since their seminal work, ischemic preconditioning is now regarded as the most powerful mechanism for myocardial protection. Myocardial preconditioning has been documented in all animal species in which it has been studied, and importantly in human cardiac tissue (90–92).

Mechanisms of Ischemic Preconditioning
Ischemic preconditioning has two windows: an acute memory phase lasting one to three hours and a late memory phase starting 12 to 24 hours after ischemia and lasting from two to four days. Ischemic preconditioning can also result from short periods of remote ischemia involving limbs (93) or viscera (94). Remote preconditioning has been observed in experiments during which hearts were preconditioned by remote ischemia, then explanted, and mounted in a Langendorff apparatus. These hearts were protected against ischemia. This indicates that remote preconditioning was "memorized" in the explanted heart. This remote preconditioning involved mitochondrial K_{ATP}^+ channels (95).

Central to ischemic preconditioning are the mitochondrial K_{ATP}^+ channels (Fig. 1). Activation of these channels can be initiated by stimulation of many sarcolemmal receptors such as those for adenosine and bradykinin. Alpha-adrenoceptors and delta-opioid receptors are also involved in preconditioning; in contrast, kappa-opioid receptors exert an antipreconditioning effect (96).

Adenosine plays an important role in myocardial protection over and above activation of K_{ATP}^+ channels. Adenosine causes vasodilatation, promotes glycolysis, and inhibits neutrophil function, thereby contributing to the attenuation of ischemic

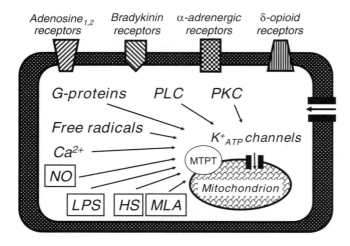

FIGURE 1 Simplified representation of the various mediators involved with ischemic and pharmacological preconditioning. NO (nitric oxide), LPS (lipopolysaccharides), HS (heat stress), and MLA (monophosphoryl lipid A) are more relevant to late than early preconditioning. *Abbreviations*: PLC, phospholipase C; PKC, protein kinase C; MTPT, mitochondrial transition permeability pore.

injury. However, its effects in clinical studies are not as conclusive as those in experimental studies (97).

Bradykinin is an inflammatory stress mediator and a vasodilator. In experimental studies, bradykinin B_2 receptors appear to be important triggers of ischemic preconditioning, whereas their blockade negates the protection offered by ischemic preconditioning (98,99).

Ischemia/reperfusion injury induces renin–angiotensin system activation and increased production of angiotensin in the heart. In experimental studies, both angiotensin II receptors A_1 and A_2 have been shown to play a role as only blockade of both types facilitates recovery from ischemia (100). Subthreshold ischemic interventions can be potentiated by ACE inhibitors probably because they prevent the formation of angiotensin and the degradation of bradykinin (101).

In addition to sarcolemmal receptors, a number of intracellular mediators such as G-proteins, phospholipase C, PKC, free radicals, and calcium are involved in signal transduction for early preconditioning (102–104). The transduction pathway of ischemic preconditioning includes the activation of the kinase cascade represented by PKC, tyrosine kinase, and mitogen-activated protein kinase (MAPK). Reactive oxygen species have also been shown to play an important role (105).

Recently, studies of myocardial preconditioning have included gene expression patterns, made possible by the availability of gene chips. In experimental models, ischemia led to strong upregulation of mRNA transcripts for heat-shock proteins, vascular endothelial growth factor, brain-derived neurotrophic factor, plasminogen activator inhibitor-1, activating transcription factor 3, B-cell translocation gene 2, and growth arrest and DNA-damage-inducible 45α protein (106).

Apoptosis or programmed cell death is genetically controlled. Ischemic preconditioning attenuates apoptosis and decreases neutrophil accumulation in a model of nonlethal ischemia reperfusion: DNA laddering in the area at risk was not observed in any of the ischemic preconditioned animals (107).

The time course of the second window of protection (late preconditioning) is consistent with the concept of activation of genes encoding for cytoprotective proteins such as heat-shock proteins and antioxidant enzymes (108). Indeed, nitric oxide, lipopolysaccharides, heat-shock proteins, and monophosphoryl lipid A are involved in late preconditioning (104).

Myocardial preconditioning exerts beneficial effects in terms of reduced infarct size, ischemia- and reperfusion-induced arrhythmias, myocardial stunning, and vascular dysfunction after ischemia/reperfusion (109). The beneficial effects of ischemic preconditioning on postischemic contractile dysfunction have been demonstrated in animal models (110).

Pharmacological Preconditioning

It is now well established that a number of agents, once they have been administered for a short period of time, typically 15 minutes, protect the myocardium against the effects of a subsequent period of ischemia followed by reperfusion. This phenomenon is termed pharmacological preconditioning. Pharmacological preconditioning is, therefore, one of the mechanisms by which human myocardium can be protected from ischemic insults. Preconditioning-mimetic drugs include adenosine, bradykinin, nitroglycerin, and nicorandil, a K^+_{ATP} channel opener. The development of preconditioning-mimetic drugs is important as such drugs can be expected to increase exercise tolerance, limit infarct size in susceptible patients, and decrease the incidence of sudden cardiac death caused by ventricular tachyarrhythmias. Such drugs would also be expected to reduce the risk of cardiac complications of anesthesia and surgery.

Mechanisms of Anesthetic Preconditioning

Pharmacological preconditioning has been demonstrated for several inhalation anesthetics and has been shown to protect against experimental myocardial infarction (39,40,111–113). As the inhalation anesthetics were administered shortly before a prolonged ischemic episode, their effect is comparable to early ischemic preconditioning (39,40,112,113).

Cardiac protection by inhalation anesthetics is very similar to ischemic preconditioning (36,39,114,115). Improved postischemic recovery (29) and reduction of infarct size (111) have been demonstrated. The cellular mechanisms of myocardial protection are very similar to those of ischemic preconditioning (102–104,116,117). Both sarcolemmal (118,119) and mitochondrial K_{ATP}^+ channels mediate anesthesia-induced preconditioning (38), yet mitochondrial K_{ATP}^+ channels may play a more important role (120). As many anesthetics have profound effects on mitochondrial membranes and can destabilize lipid–protein interactions or induce conformational changes in proteins, a major effect on mitochondrial K_{ATP}^+ channels is not surprising. Protection by barbiturates, isoflurane, and halothane is caused to a large extent by activation of K_{ATP}^+ channels (121).

In addition, anesthetic preconditioning involves stimulation of adenosine receptors (119), mechano-gated channels (37), and formation of reactive oxygen species (105). They are also important in the pharmacological preconditioning induced by flumazenil (122).

Exploration of gene expression has been used to determine whether ischemic and pharmacologically induced preconditioning have similar pathways. In rat hearts, microarray technology showed two distinct phenotypes for ischemic and pharmacologically induced preconditioning (123). Ischemic preconditioning elicits gene expression similar to the unprotected myocardium, whereas pharmacological preconditioning by anesthetic agents elicits gene expression closer to healthy nonischemic myocardium (124). This suggests that pharmacological preconditioning may be more protective than ischemic preconditioning.

Not all anesthetics have the same efficacy as myocardial preconditioners. There is greater reduction of infarct size by halothane, enflurane, and isoflurane by comparison with pentobarbital, ketamine–xylazine, or propofol anesthesia (40) in rabbits. In contrast, in a dog model, halothane was even found to be associated with an increase in infarct size (125). Similarly, dogs anesthetized with barbiturates exhibit larger infarcts than their conscious counterparts (126). This may be explained by the observation that barbiturates competitively antagonize adenosine A_1-receptors, a pivotal signaling pathway in cardiac preconditioning (127). Indeed, adenosine receptor antagonists decrease anesthesia-induced preconditioning (40,119). Reduced preconditioning is also observed in response to PKC antagonists (31).

Depending on the model and modalities of studies, the protective potency of different inhalation anesthetics differs. Anesthesia-induced preconditioning is species-dependent. Halothane preconditions in rabbit (40), but not rat (128) or human (119). Isoflurane preconditions in rabbit (37) and human (119), but not rat (129). Halothane partially blocks sarcolemmal K_{ATP}^+ channels (119), whereas isoflurane does not affect them.

Sevoflurane, isoflurane, halothane, and desflurane have been compared: sevoflurane exerted less protection in rabbits (130). In other studies, sevoflurane was very effective (131).

Anesthetics may also modulate the effects of ischemic preconditioning. For example, ischemic preconditioning is abolished by glibenclamide under ketamine–xylazine anesthesia but not pentobarbital anesthesia (132). In a comparison of the effects of ischemic preconditioning under pentobarbital, isoflurane, and ketamine–xylazine anesthesia, infarct size was not different in the absence of preconditioning, but the magnitude of infarct size limitation by ischemic preconditioning was different depending upon the anesthetic agent (133). In the presence of halothane anesthesia, nicorandil given prior to ischemia did not demonstrate protective effects, whereas ischemic preconditioning did reduce infarct size. Yet a K_{ATP}^+ channel blocker prevented the combined effect of ischemia and nicorandil (134). These observations illustrate the role of anesthetics as preconditioners and modulators of preconditioning. Indeed, pharmacological preconditioning has been shown to reduce myocardial damage in the presence of cardioplegic protection (115,135).

The complexity of mechanisms of pharmacological, anesthesia-induced, preconditioning has been substantiated in a cellular model of simulated ischemia. Modulatory effects of anesthetics were demonstrated by the inhibition of diazoxide-induced mitochondrial K_{ATP}^+ channel opening by R-ketamine, thiopental, and pentobarbital. Conversely, urethane, 2,2,2-trichloroethanol (a main metabolite of α-chloralose), and fentanyl potentiated the channel-opening effect of diazoxide. This potentiation could be blocked by chelerythrine, a specific PKC inhibitor. In contrast, S-ketamine, propofol, xylazine, midazolam, and etomidate do not affect mitochondrial K_{ATP}^+ channel activity (102).

Finally, improved collateral blood flow may play a role. Indeed, sevoflurane increases collateral flow, an effect not reversed by glibenclamide, and reduces infarct size, thus demonstrating pharmacological preconditioning (136).

Thus far there is little data on the possibility of anesthetics conferring late preconditioning. Kehl et al. (137) examined the effect of exposure to isoflurane 24 hours before a 60-minute coronary occlusion followed by a three-hour reperfusion. Although isoflurane exerted early protection, there was no late protection.

Ischemic- and anesthetic-induced preconditioning are not additive, suggesting the same end-effector (128), identified in many studies as K_{ATP}^+ channels (39,118).

Isoflurane

In the absence of ischemia, isoflurane causes opening of K_{ATP}^+ channels, an effect blocked by sulfonylureas (118). Isoflurane reduces infarct size in experimental animals (112) and in human myocardium (119). Sarcolemmal and mitochondrial K_{ATP}^+ channels appear to be involved (31,37,38,118,119,138). Isoflurane increases the open probability of the sarcoplasmic K_{ATP}^+ channel for a given ATP concentration (139).

In a cellular model, the inhalation anesthetics isoflurane and sevoflurane significantly enhanced the diazoxide-mediated activation of mitochondrial K_{ATP}^+ channels. This effect was completely blocked by chelerythrine (PKC inhibitor). Pretreatment with inhalation anesthetics potentiated the diazoxide-mediated protection against ischemia. Cardioprotection was unaffected by the sarcoplasmic K_{ATP}^+ channel blocker HMR-1098, but sensitive to modulations of NO and adenosine-Gi signaling pathways (103).

Does pharmacological preconditioning by isoflurane occur in the human heart? Administration of isoflurane before aortic cross-clamping in patients undergoing coronary artery bypass surgery causes cardiac index to be higher after cardiopulmonary bypass with less changes in ST segments than in the control group. However, there were no differences in terms of arrhythmias (140). Thus, isoflurane may offer some additional protection to cardioplegia. These findings are consistent with the observation of lower levels of CK-MB and troponin reported by Belhomme et al. (135) when isoflurane is used. Moreover, isoflurane (135) causes PKC activation and improves postischemic contractility.

Desflurane
In isolated human atrial trabeculae, desflurane improved the recovery of isometric contraction after a 30-minute period of anoxia. The preconditioning effect of desflurane was abolished by glibenclamide, 5-hydroxydecanoate (5-HD), an adenosine receptor blocker (DPX), phentolamine, and propranolol (141). These observations suggest that preconditioning by desflurane is mediated by mitochondrial K^+_{ATP} channels (141), adenosine A_1-receptors, and α- and β-adrenoceptors. α- and β-Adrenoceptors have been shown to play a role in several studies (142–144) together with delta-opioid receptors (50). In contrast, selective blockade of sarcolemmal K^+_{ATP} channels did not reduce desflurane-induced preconditioning, whereas it abolished anoxia-induced preconditioning.

Desflurane increases sympathetic activity in volunteers (145) and releases catecholamines from myocardial stores in rat (146) and human myocardium (147). α_1-Adrenoceptor stimulation is protective before but detrimental during ischemia (142). Preconditioning also involves a β-adrenoceptor pathway (148) and isoproterenol preconditions the heart via PKC (143). As desflurane induces intramyocardial catecholamine release (147) via stimulation of α- and β-adrenoceptors, desflurane-induced preconditioning may result from this mechanism.

Sevoflurane
Sevoflurane is known to open mitochondrial K^+_{ATP} channels; in dogs, this results in a reduction of infarct size (131). Preservation of myocardial blood flow through collateral circulation, observed with sevoflurane, is independent of K^+_{ATP} channels. In sepsis, ultrastructural changes in the myocardium have been documented and sevoflurane shown to protect cardiac output in septic (cecal ligation and perforation) but not in normal rats (149). In septic shock, K^+_{ATP} channels are known to be activated and to promote vasodilatation (150,151). Thus, sepsis may contribute to protection. More importantly, sevoflurane has been shown to afford protection during coronary bypass surgery (152,153).

Myocardial Preconditioning: Role of Opioids
The involvement of opioid receptors in ischemic preconditioning has been demonstrated in many animal species and in humans. Among opioid receptor subtypes, there is evidence that delta-opioid receptors are responsible for experimental ischemic preconditioning (49,52) and in human myocytes (50). The importance of opioid receptors is confirmed by the observation that naloxone prevents ischemic preconditioning (51).

Protection by opioids had been suggested in observations of increased tolerance to hypoxia (154,155) and has been confirmed in many studies of ischemia (28,47,53,156,157). Interestingly, the protective effect of isoflurane can be potentiated by the administration of morphine in a rat model (158). As two widely used and studied opioids, morphine and fentanyl are capable of binding to delta- and kappa-opioid receptors (although they are preferentially mu-receptor agonists) and they could offer protection. Although the experimental evidence is clear, the clinical relevance is still unclear.

Clinical Relevance of Preconditioning
Spontaneous Ischemic Preconditioning
The relevance of ischemic preconditioning is established. Many studies have shown that patients with angina shortly before myocardial infarction have a better prognosis than those without angina (159–161). Other benefits include a reduction of the risk of ventricular tachycardia or fibrillation (162,163). Whether ischemic preconditioning facilitates functional recovery of stunned myocardium is debatable (164,165). However, new onset angina preceding acute myocardial infarction appears to improve contractile recovery as demonstrated by fewer hypokinetic segments and a more rapid improvement of wall motion scores (160). In addition, prodromal angina has been shown to limit infarct size in the setting of acute anterior myocardial infarction treated with primary percutaneous intervention (166).

Preconditioning in Interventional Cardiology
Ischemic preconditioning is highly relevant to percutaneous coronary intervention. Most studies of preconditioning during percutaneous coronary interventions have examined surrogate markers rather than adverse outcome and shown protection (167). The surrogate markers include ST segment shift, lactate, and creatine kinase release. They have been shown to be diminished with ischemic preconditioning during percutaneous coronary interventions. Indeed, the first coronary occlusion results in larger changes in ST segments than subsequent occlusions. This is observed without any change in the area at risk or collateral flow in the ischemic zone and suggests that ischemic preconditioning occurs rapidly in patients (168).

There is another dimension to ischemic preconditioning during percutaneous coronary interventions: using a surrogate outcome such as ST segment shift during coronary angioplasty, Laskey and Beach (169) observed that 20% of patients failed to manifest preconditioning. This lack of response was more common in female patients and in diabetics. Importantly, lack of evidence of ischemic preconditioning was associated with a significantly poorer long-term event-free survival. The risk of death or nonfatal myocardial infarction was 25.9% versus 11.1% ($p < 0.002$). Conversely, the 80% of patients who developed ischemic preconditioning had a substantially reduced in-hospital morbidity (12.1% vs. 44.1%; $p < 0.0001$) and better long-term outcome (169). This indicates that clinically relevant short- and long-term cardioprotection can be found in association with ischemic preconditioning elicited during percutaneous coronary interventions.

Pharmacological preconditioning may assume an increasing role during percutaneous coronary interventions. In 1999, Leesar et al. (170) showed that an intracoronary infusion of bradykinin prior to coronary angioplasty had no hemodynamic effects but significantly reduced the ST segment shift during three consecutive balloon inflations. The bradykinin-induced protection was similar to that produced by the first balloon inflation in the control group (170). This observation indicates that drug- or mediator-induced preconditioning may afford significant protection in patients undergoing coronary angioplasty. Similarly, previous exposure to a brief episode of ischemia (first balloon inflation) or to adenosine produces concordant decreases in ECG, subjective, mechanical, and metabolic manifestations of ischemia, supporting the view that both ischemic and pharmacological preconditioning exist in humans (171). More recently, nicorandil pretreatment has been shown to induce myocardial preconditioning independent of the severity of ischemia (172). Percutaneous coronary interventions offer a unique opportunity to study the mechanisms and efficacy of drug-induced preconditioning.

Preconditioning in Cardiac Surgery

Ischemic preconditioning is thought to play a role during cardiopulmonary bypass and in off-pump bypass surgery. Yellon et al. (173) were the first to report that ischemic preconditioning offered protection in the context of cardiac surgery. They used the conservation of ATP content as their major endpoint (173). However, some later studies did not show benefits (174,175). For example, a short period of aortocoronary occlusion followed by reperfusion was shown to decrease the release of troponin T but the difference was significant only for the first hour after onset of coronary bypass (176). However, Jenkins et al. (177) and Li et al. (178) reported that patients undergoing coronary artery bypass grafting had significantly less myocardial damage, assessed as reduced troponin release, if they had undergone ischemic preconditioning. More recently, studies have been more conclusive. Very short periods of ischemia/reperfusion applied before coronary artery surgery led to complete recovery of function, absence of postoperative tachycardia, and reduced levels of troponin I (179).

The introduction of off-pump coronary artery bypass surgery has given a new dimension to ischemic preconditioning. Ghosh and Galinanes (180) showed that a cycle of ischemia/reperfusion protected patients undergoing coronary artery bypass on the beating heart but not in those operated under cardiopulmonary bypass. The lack of efficacy of ischemic preconditioning (assessed by the extent of troponin T release), where cardiopulmonary bypass was used suggests that cardiopulmonary bypass induces ischemic preconditioning. Indeed, cardiopulmonary bypass triggers activation of the kinase cascade linked with the opening of K^+_{ATP} channels (181). Thus, drugs that open K^+_{ATP} channels are unlikely to increase kinase activation further and would not be expected to improve markers of cell damage (181).

Ischemic preconditioning is a possible strategy in off-pump coronary bypass surgery because altered cardioplegia is not an option; however, the benefits are limited (182).

Recently, several studies in patients undergoing coronary artery surgery have suggested that pharmacological preconditioning with sevoflurane minimizes cardiac damage (152,153) and may improve the long-term prognosis (152,183).

Interactions Between Drugs and Preconditioning

Some drugs used in clinical practice, such as sulfonylureas, may interfere with the signaling pathway of ischemic and pharmacological preconditioning. For glibenclamide, blockade of protection results from blockade of K^+_{ATP} channels (91). In human cardiac tissue, glibenclamide and gliclazide prevent experimental ischemic preconditioning (184). This is also known to occur with pharmacological preconditioning. Forlani et al. (185) have shown that isoflurane-induced preconditioning was prevented by glibenclamide but was present if glibenclamide therapy was replaced by an insulin regimen.

The effect of sulfonylureas is relevant to diabetic patients. Both diabetes mellitus and sulfonylureas can act in synergism to inhibit activation of K^+_{ATP} channels in patients undergoing coronary angioplasty (186). Not all sulfonylureas are equally potent in inhibiting ischemic preconditioning. The degree of inhibition assessed by metabolic and electrocardiographic parameters is less severe during treatment with glimepiride than with glibenclamide. This may result from lesser inhibition of pre-conditioning in glimepiride-treated patients (187).

With the introduction of new classes of drugs, there may be new interactions. As an example, adenosine receptors are part of the signal transduction of ischemic preconditioning. This signaling pathway may be altered or blocked by adenosine A_1-receptor antagonists. The latter are being developed as diuretics and appear to be promising (188). This raises the possibility that their administration, like that of glibenclamide, may prevent ischemic preconditioning. However, experimental evidence does not support this view, maybe because adenosine receptors other than A_1 type are involved in ischemic preconditioning (189). The role of adenosine receptors other than A_1 type is suggested by the observation that, in an isolated perfused heart model, adenosine A_3-receptor agonist pretreatment before cardioplegic cardiac arrest attenuated cardiac dysfunction and troponin release. However, protection was not superior to that of cold cardioplegia (190).

As nicorandil is a K_{ATP}^+ channel opener, the myocardium of patients chronically treated with nicorandil cannot be preconditioned either by ischemia or pharmacologically, because the mitochondrial K_{ATP}^+ channels become unresponsive. However, protection can be obtained by PKC and p38 MAPK activation, which are downstream of mitochondrial ATP-dependent potassium channels in the signaling transduction pathway of preconditioning (191).

POSTCONDITIONING

Recently, Zhao et al. (117) have shown that reperfusion injury can be minimized by very short sequences of ischemia imposed during reperfusion. This is beneficial because, after a period of ischemia, reperfusion can cause myocardial damage leading to increased cell death or prolonged dysfunction (myocardial stunning).

Experimentally, in a canine model, postconditioning was shown to confer significant protection, similar to that of preconditioning as attested by a marked reduction in infarct size. The reperfusion injury salvage kinase (RISK) pathway is a common target for both ischemic preconditioning and postconditioning (192). A very recent review addresses the issue of postconditioning (193). In addition, reperfusion elicits endothelial dysfunction and an inflammatory response that contributes to reperfusion injury. Pre- and post-ischemic conditioning reduce the consequences of the inflammatory response as attested by decreased markers of oxidant injury (194).

Early restoration of myocardial blood flow after coronary occlusion during percutaneous interventions or coronary artery bypass surgery is critical to myocardial salvage. Avoidance of myocardial damage is critical as infarct size is the decisive determinant of the extent of remodeling and of the prognosis after acute myocardial infarction (195). Timely reperfusion is therefore essential but, as it can cause damage, interventions during reperfusion such as postconditioning may offer benefits.

Postconditioning has been observed to reduce infarct size and apoptosis to the same extent as the gold standard of protection, ischemic preconditioning. Ischemic postconditioning reduced endothelial cell activation and dysfunction, tissue superoxide anion generation, neutrophil activation and accumulation in reperfused myocardium, microvascular injury, tissue edema, and intracellular and mitochondrial calcium accumulation (196). Multiple triggers and pathways contribute to ischemic postconditioning. Adenosine, e-NOS, nitric oxide and guanylyl cyclase, opening of K^+_{ATP} channels, and closing of the MPTP are involved as well as the activation of intracellular survival pathways such as ERK1/2 and PI3 kinase-Akt pathways (196).

In contrast to preconditioning, which requires a prior knowledge of the ischemic event, postconditioning can be applied at the onset of reperfusion at the point of clinical service, i.e., angioplasty, cardiac surgery, and heart transplantation (196). In such situations, ischemic postconditioning may offer protection that is not available by other means, as shown in an experimental model (117). The possible impact of postconditioning has been demonstrated in a canine model. Little was gained by combining pre- and postconditioning: the same protective effects were noted with postconditioning alone (194).

Similar to remote preconditioning, there is now evidence of remote ischemic postconditioning in animal models. Ischemic postconditioning caused by ischemia/reperfusion of the kidney reduced the size of myocardial infarction that had preceded the postconditioning protocol. This inter-organ remote postconditioning phenomenon is likely to be mediated, at least in part, by adenosine with activation of cardiac adenosine receptors (197).

Experimentally, pharmacological postconditioning by isoflurane has been described (183). In addition, a few clinical studies in cardiac surgery indicate that anesthetic agents may protect the human heart (153,198,199).

Although preconditioning and postconditioning have been observed in response to the administration of sevoflurane, the administration of this agent throughout coronary artery surgery offers better protection as assessed by better hemodynamics and reduced postoperative troponin I (153).

Anesthetic pre- and postconditioning have many common signaling pathways including the RISK pathway (200) and provide equivalent protection in experimental models. However, the transcriptional responses are completely different. Importantly, anesthetic postconditioning was unable to prevent the activation of genes involved in myocardial remodeling (201).

CONCLUSIONS

There are many facets to myocardial ischemia. The clinical relevance of myocardial stunning is that some interventions including the administration of inhalation anesthetics and opioids may accelerate recovery. Moreover, it is clinically important to know that recovery of function after ischemia may be slow. Therefore, supportive treatment may be needed for several days or even weeks, after which recovery of function may be much greater than initially expected.

Myocardial hibernation may be responsible for poor cardiac function in myocardium that is still capable of recovery if the oxygen balance improves, generally by coronary revascularization. As myocardial hibernation can be detected by several techniques, including dobutamine echocardiography, a subset of patients with heart failure caused partly by myocardial hibernation can be identified. These patients can benefit from revascularization. This is relevant to their long-term quality of life and may reduce the risk of major surgery.

Ischemic myocardial preconditioning is a complex phenomenon that involves many mediators. It has both an early and late phase. It can be caused by ischemia in the heart itself or in tissue remote from the heart. It is the strongest mechanism for myocardial protection. There is some evidence that ischemic preconditioning reduces ischemic damage during coronary angioplasty and cardiac surgery.

Many pharmacological agents, for example, nicorandil and opioids, mimic ischemic preconditioning, thereby affording cardiac protection. Inhalation anesthetics, especially isoflurane, desflurane, and sevoflurane, minimize infarct size by causing "early" preconditioning of the heart. However, inhalation anesthetic agents do not appear to cause late preconditioning.

Finally, myocardial postconditioning may offer a new approach to the reduction of postischemic damage. This may be of relevance to interventional cardiology, to coronary bypass surgery, and to the perioperative management of ischemic events as inhalation anesthetics appear to be mimicking ischemic postconditioning.

REFERENCES

1. NCEPOD. Then and Now: The 2000 Report of the National Confidential Enquiry into Postoperative Deaths. The National Confidential Enquiry into Postoperative Deaths, 2001.
2. Devereaux PJ, Beattie WS, Choi PT, et al. How strong is the evidence for the use of perioperative beta blockers in non-cardiac surgery? Systematic review and meta-analysis of randomised controlled trials. Br Med J 2005; 331:313–321.
3. Mangano DT. Perioperative cardiac morbidity. Anesthesiology 1990; 72(1):153–184.
4. Mangano DT, Goldman L. Preoperative assessment of patients with known or suspected coronary disease. N Engl J Med 1995; 333:1750–1756.
5. Gilbert K, Larocque BJ, Patrick LT. Prospective evaluation of cardiac risk indices for patients undergoing noncardiac surgery. Ann Intern Med 2000; 133:356–359.
6. Braunwald E. Editorial: Reduction of myocardial-infarct size. N Engl J Med 1974; 291:525–526.
7. Reimer KA, Lowe JE, Rasmussen MM, Jennings RB. The wavefront phenomenon of ischemic cell death. 1. Myocardial infarct size vs. duration of coronary occlusion in dogs. Circulation 1977; 56:786–794.
8. Simoons ML, Serruys PW, van den Brand M, et al. Early thrombolysis in acute myocardial infarction: limitation of infarct size and improved survival. J Am Coll Cardiol 1986; 7:717–728.
9. Zijlstra F, de Boer MJ, Hoorntje JC, Reiffers S, Reiber JH, Suryapranata H. A comparison of immediate coronary angioplasty with intravenous streptokinase in acute myocardial infarction. N Engl J Med 1993; 328:680–684.
10. Kloner RA, Rezkalla SH. Cardiac protection during acute myocardial infarction: where do we stand in 2004? J Am Coll Cardiol 2004; 44:276–286.
11. Heyndrickx GR, Millard RW, McRitchie RJ, Maroko PR, Vatner SF. Regional myocardial functional and electrophysiological alterations after brief coronary artery occlusion in conscious dogs. J Clin Invest 1975; 56:978–985.
12. Braunwald E, Kloner RA. The stunned myocardium: prolonged, postischemic ventricular dysfunction. Circulation 1982; 66(6):1146–1149.
13. Bolli R. Mechanism of myocardial "stunning". Circulation 1990; 82(3):723–738.
14. Raby KE, Barry J, Creager MA, Cook EF, Weisberg MC, Goldman L. Detection and significance of intraoperative and postoperative myocardial ischemia in peripheral vascular surgery. J Am Med Assoc 1992; 268(2):222–227.
15. Landesberg G, Luria MH, Cotev S, et al. Importance of long-duration postoperative ST-segment depression in cardiac morbidity after vascular surgery. Lancet 1993; 341(8847):715–719.
16. Garcia-Dorado D. Myocardial reperfusion injury: a new view. Cardiovasc Res 2004; 61:363–364.
17. O'Neill CA, Fu LW, Halliwell B, Longhurst JC. Hydroxyl radical production during myocardial ischemia and reperfusion in cats. Am J Physiol 1996; 271(2, pt 2):H660–H667.

18. Movahed A, Nair KG, Ashavaid TF, Kumar P. Free radical generation and the role of allopurinol as a cardioprotective agent during coronary artery bypass grafting surgery. Can J Cardiol 1996; 12(2):138–144.

19. Triana JF, Li XY, Jamaluddin U, Thornby JI, Bolli R. Postischemic myocardial "stunning": identification of major differences between the open-chest and the conscious dog and evaluation of the oxygen radical hypothesis in the conscious dog. Circ Res 1991; 69(3):731–747.

20. Ehring T, Bohm M, Heusch G. The calcium antagonist nisoldipine improves the functional recovery of reperfused myocardium only when given before ischemia. J Cardiovasc Pharmacol 1992; 20(1):63–74.

21. Grinwald PM. Calcium uptake during post-ischemic reperfusion in the isolated rat heart: influence of extracellular sodium. J Mol Cell Cardiol 1982; 14(6):359–365.

22. Halestrap AP, Clarke SJ, Javadov SA. Mitochondrial permeability transition pore opening during myocardial reperfusion—a target for cardioprotection. Cardiovasc Res 2004; 61:372–385.

23. Piper HM, Meuter K, Schafer C. Cellular mechanisms of ischemia-reperfusion injury. Ann Thorac Surg 2003; 75:S644–S648.

24. Murphy AM, Kogler H, Georgakopoulos D, et al. Transgenic mouse model of stunned myocardium. Science 2000; 287:488–491.

25. Duncker DJ, McFalls EO, Krams R, Verdouw PD. Pressure–maximal coronary flow relationship in regionally stunned porcine myocardium. Am J Physiol 1992; 262(6, pt 2): H1744–H1751.

26. Piper HM, Abdallah Y, Schafer C. The first minutes of reperfusion: a window of opportunity for cardioprotection. Cardiovasc Res 2004; 61:365–371.

27. Ross S, Foex P. Protective effects of anaesthetics in reversible and irreversible ischaemia-reperfusion injury. Br J Anaesth 1999; 82:622–632.

28. Kato R, Ross S, Foex P. Fentanyl protects the heart against ischaemic injury via opioid receptors, adenosine A1 receptors and KATP channel linked mechanisms in rats. Br J Anaesth 2000; 84:204–214.

29. Warltier DC, al Wathiqui MH, Kampine JP, Schmeling WT. Recovery of contractile function of stunned myocardium in chronically instrumented dogs is enhanced by halothane or isoflurane. Anesthesiology 1988; 69:552–565.

30. Coetzee A, Moolman J. Halothane and the reperfusion injury in the intact animal model. Anesth Analg 1993; 76(4):734–744.

31. Toller WG, Montgomery MW, Pagel PS, Hettrick DA, Warltier DC, Kersten JR. Isoflurane-enhanced recovery of canine stunned myocardium: role for protein kinase C? Anesthesiology 1999; 91:713–722.

32. Oguchi T, Kashimoto S, Yamaguchi T, Nakamura T, Kumazawa T. Comparative effects of halothane, enflurane, isoflurane and sevoflurane on function and metabolism in the ischaemic rat heart. Br J Anaesth 1995; 74(5):569–575.

33. Sahlman L, Waagstein L, Haljamae H, Ricksten SE. Protective effects of halothane but not isoflurane against global ischaemic injury in the isolated working rat heart. Acta Anaesthesiol Scand 1995; 39:312–316.

34. Preckel B, Schlack W, Comfere T, Obal D, Barthel H, Thamer V. Effects of enflurane, isoflurane, sevoflurane and desflurane on reperfusion injury after regional myocardial ischaemia in the rabbit heart in vivo. Br J Anaesth 1998; 81:905–912.

35. Preckel B, Thamer V, Schlack W. Beneficial effects of sevoflurane and desflurane against myocardial reperfusion injury after cardioplegic arrest. Can J Anaesth 1999; 46(11):1076–1081.

36. Schlack W, Preckel B, Stunneck D, Thamer V. Effects of halothane, enflurane, isoflurane, sevoflurane and desflurane on myocardial reperfusion injury in the isolated rat heart. Br J Anaesth 1998; 81:913–919.

37. Piriou V, Chiari P, Knezynski S, et al. Prevention of isoflurane-induced preconditioning by 5-hydroxydecanoate and gadolinium: possible involvement of mitochondrial adenosine triphosphate-sensitive potassium and stretch-activated channels. Anesthesiology 2000; 93:756–764.

38. Toller WG, Gross ER, Kersten JR, Pagel PS, Gross GJ, Warltier DC. Sarcolemmal and mitochondrial adenosine triphosphate- dependent potassium channels: mechanism of desflurane-induced cardioprotection. Anesthesiology 2000; 92:1731–1739.

39. Cason BA, Gamperl AK, Slocum RE, Hickey RF. Anesthetic-induced preconditioning: previous administration of isoflurane decreases myocardial infarct size in rabbits. Anesthesiology 1997; 87(5):1182–1190.
40. Cope DK, Impastato WK, Cohen MV, Downey JM. Volatile anesthetics protect the ischemic rabbit myocardium from infarction. Anesthesiology 1997; 86:699–709.
41. White JL, Myers AK, Analouei A, Kim YD. Functional recovery of stunned myocardium is greater with halothane than fentanyl anaesthesia in dogs. Br J Anaesth 1994; 73(2): 214–219.
42. Ross S, Munoz H, Piriou V, Ryder WA, Foex P. A comparison of the effects of fentanyl and propofol on left ventricular contractility during myocardial stunning. Acta Anaesthesiol Scand 1998; 42(1):23–31.
43. Ko SH, Yu CW, Lee SK, et al. Propofol attenuates ischemia-reperfusion injury in the isolated rat heart. Anesth Analg 1997; 85(4):719–724.
44. Kokita N, Hara A, Abiko Y, Arakawa J, Hashizume H, Namiki A. Propofol improves functional and metabolic recovery in ischemic reperfused isolated rat hearts. Anesth Analg 1998; 86(2):252–258.
45. Mathur S, Farhangkhgoee P, Karmazyn M. Cardioprotective effects of propofol and sevoflurane in ischemic and reperfused rat hearts: role of K(ATP) channels and interaction with the sodium–hydrogen exchange inhibitor HOE 642 (cariporide). Anesthesiology 1999; 91:1349–1360.
46. Kato R, Foex P. Myocardial protection by anesthetic agents against ischemia-reperfusion injury: an update for anesthesiologists [La protection myocardique contre les lesions d'ischemie-reperfusion par des anesthesiques: une mise a jour pour les anesthesiologistes]. Can J Anaesth 2002; 49(8):777–791.
47. Kato R, Foex P. Fentanyl reduces infarction but not stunning via delta-opioid receptors and protein kinase C in rats. Br J Anaesth 2000; 84(5):608–614.
48. Tsuchida A, Miura T, Tanno M, Nozawa Y, Kita H, Shimamoto K. Time window for the contribution of the delta-opioid receptor to cardioprotection by ischemic preconditioning in the rat heart. Cardiovasc Drugs Ther 1998; 12:365–373.
49. Schultz JJ, Hsu AK, Gross GJ. Ischemic preconditioning is mediated by a peripheral opioid receptor mechanism in the intact rat heart. J Mol Cell Cardiol 1997; 29:1355–1362.
50. Bell SP, Sack MN, Patel A, Opie LH, Yellon DM. Delta opioid receptor stimulation mimics ischemic preconditioning in human heart muscle. J Am Coll Cardiol 2000; 36:2296–2302.
51. Chien GL, Mohtadi K, Wolff RA, Van Winkle DM. Naloxone blockade of myocardial ischemic preconditioning does not require central nervous system participation. Basic Res Cardiol 1999; 94:136–143.
52. Takasaki Y, Wolff RA, Chien GL, van Winkle DM. Met5-encephalin protects isolated adult rabbit cardiomyocytes via delta-opioid receptors. Am J Physiol 1999; 277:H2442–H2450.
53. Liang BT, Gross GJ. Direct preconditioning of cardiac myocytes via opioid receptors and KATP channels. Circ Res 1999; 84:1396–1400.
54. Aitchison KA, Baxter GF, Awan MM, Smith RM, Yellon DM, Opie LH. Opposing effects on infarction of delta and kappa opioid receptor activation in the isolated rat heart: implications for ischemic preconditioning. Basic Res Cardiol 2000; 95:1–10.
55. Wang TL, Chang H, Hung CR, Tseng YZ. Attenuation of neutrophil and endothelial activation by intravenous morphine in patients with acute myocardial infarction. Am J Cardiol 1997; 80:1532–1535.
56. Szekely A, Heindl B, Zahler S, Conzen PF, Becker BF. Nonuniform behavior of intravenous anesthetics on postischemic adhesion of neutrophils in the guinea pig heart. Anesth Analg 2000; 90:1293–1300.
57. Rahimtoola SH. A perspective on the three large multicenter randomized clinical trials of coronary bypass surgery for chronic stable angina. Circulation 1985; 72:V123–V135.
58. Rahimtoola SH. The hibernating myocardium. Am Heart J 1989; 117:211–221.
59. Cleland JG, Pennell DJ, Ray SG, Coats AJ, Macfarlane PW, Murray GD, Mule JD, Vered Z, Lahiri A. Myocardial viability as a determinant of the ejection fraction response to carvedilol in patients with heart failure (CHRISTMAS trial): randomised controlled trial. Lancet 2003; 362:14–21.
60. Louie HW, Laks H, Milgalter E, et al. Ischemic cardiomyopathy: criteria for coronary revascularization and cardiac transplantation. Circulation 1991; 84:III290–III295.

61. Bax JJ, Visser FC, Poldermans D, et al. Time course of functional recovery of stunned and hibernating segments after surgical revascularization. Circulation 2001; 104:I314–I318.
62. Hearse DJ, Bolli R. Reperfusion induced injury: manifestations, mechanisms, and clinical relevance. Cardiovasc Res 1992; 26:101–108.
63. St Louis JD, Hughes GC, Kypson AP, et al. An experimental model of chronic myocardial hibernation. Ann Thorac Surg 2000; 69:1351–1357.
64. Camici PG, Rimoldi OE. The contribution of hibernation to heart failure. Ann Med 2004; 36:440–447.
65. Uren NG, Melin JA, De Bruyne B, Wijns W, Baudhuin T, Camici PG. Relation between myocardial blood flow and the severity of coronary-artery stenosis. N Engl J Med 1994; 330:1782–1788.
66. Rinaldi CA, Masani ND, Linka AZ, Hall RJ. Effect of repetitive episodes of exercise induced myocardial ischaemia on left ventricular function in patients with chronic stable angina: evidence for cumulative stunning or ischaemic preconditioning? Heart 1999; 81:404–411.
67. Luss H, Schafers M, Neumann J, et al. Biochemical mechanisms of hibernation and stunning in the human heart. Cardiovasc Res 2002; 56:411–421.
68. Adams JN, Trent RJ, Norton M, Mikecz P, Walton S, Evans N. The persistence of hibernating myocardium after acute myocardial infarction. Eur Heart J 1998; 19:255–262.
69. Schwarz ER, Schaper J, vom Dahl J, et al. Myocyte degeneration and cell death in hibernating human myocardium. J Am Coll Cardiol 1996; 27:1577–1585.
70. Frangogiannis NG, Shimoni S, Chang SM, et al. Active interstitial remodeling: an important process in the hibernating human myocardium. J Am Coll Cardiol 2002; 39:1468–1474.
71. Shan K, Bick RJ, Poindexter BJ, et al. Altered adrenergic receptor density in myocardial hibernation in humans: a possible mechanism of depressed myocardial function. Circulation 2000; 102:2599–2606.
72. Kalra DK, Zhu X, Ramchandani MK, et al. Increased myocardial gene expression of tumor necrosis factor-alpha and nitric oxide synthase-2: a potential mechanism for depressed myocardial function in hibernating myocardium in humans. Circulation 2002; 105:1537–1540.
73. Oral H, Dorn GW II, Mann DL. Sphingosine mediates the immediate negative inotropic effects of tumor necrosis factor-alpha in the adult mammalian cardiac myocyte. J Biol Chem 1997; 272:4836–4842.
74. Kim PK, Zamora R, Petrosko P, Billiar TR. The regulatory role of nitric oxide in apoptosis. Int Immunopharmacol 2001; 1:1421–1441.
75. Westaby S. Coronary revascularization in ischemic cardiomyopathy. Surg Clin N Am 2004; 84:179–199.
76. Lewis ME, Pitt MP, Bonser RS, Pagano D. Coronary artery surgery for ischaemic heart failure: the surgeon's view. Heart Fail Rev 2003; 8:175–179.
77. Tjan TD, Kondruweit M, Scheld HH, et al. The bad ventricle—revascularization versus transplantation. Thorac Cardiovasc Surg 2000; 48:9–14.
78. Rocchi G, Poldermans D, Bax JJ, et al. Usefulness of the ejection fraction response to dobutamine infusion in predicting functional recovery after coronary artery bypass grafting in patients with left ventricular dysfunction. Am J Cardiol 2000; 85:1440–1444.
79. Allman KC, Shaw LJ, Hachamovitch R, Udelson JE. Myocardial viability testing and impact of revascularization on prognosis in patients with coronary artery disease and left ventricular dysfunction: a meta-analysis. J Am Coll Cardiol 2002; 39:1151–1158.
80. Bonow RO. Myocardial hibernation: a noninvasive physician's point of view. Ital Heart J 2002; 3:285–290.
81. Beller GA. Myocardial hibernation: a clinician's perspective. Ital Heart J 2002; 3:291–293.
82. Haas F, Haehnel CJ, Picker W, et al. Preoperative positron emission tomographic viability assessment and perioperative and postoperative risk in patients with advanced ischemic heart disease. J Am Coll Cardiol 1997; 30:1693–1700.
83. Haas F, Jennen L, Heinzmann U, et al. Ischemically compromised myocardium displays different time-courses of functional recovery: correlation with morphological alterations? Eur J Cardiothorac Surg 2001; 20:290–298.
84. Vanoverschelde JL, Depre C, Gerber BL, et al. Time course of functional recovery after coronary artery bypass graft surgery in patients with chronic left ventricular ischemic dysfunction. Am J Cardiol 2000; 85:1432–1439.

85. Halm EA, Browner WS, Tubau JF, Tateo IM, Mangano DT. Echocardiography for assessing cardiac risk in patients having noncardiac surgery. Study of Perioperative Ischemia Research Group. Ann Intern Med 1996; 125(6):433–441.
86. Afridi I, Kleiman NS, Raizner AE, Zoghbi WA. Dobutamine echocardiography in myocardial hibernation: optimal dose and accuracy in predicting recovery of ventricular function after coronary angioplasty. Circulation 1995; 91:663–670.
87. Shimoni S, Frangogiannis NG, Aggeli CJ, et al. Identification of hibernating myocardium with quantitative intravenous myocardial contrast echocardiography: comparison with dobutamine echocardiography and thallium-201 scintigraphy. Circulation 2003; 107: 538–544.
88. Reimer KA, Murry CE, Yamasawa I, Hill ML, Jennings RB. Four brief periods of myocardial ischemia cause no cumulative ATP loss or necrosis. Am J Physiol 1986; 251:H1306–H1315.
89. Murry CE, Jennings RB, Reimer KA. Preconditioning with ischemia: a delay of lethal cell injury in ischemic myocardium. Circulation 1986; 74:1124–1136.
90. Carr CS, Hill RJ, Masamune H, et al. Evidence for a role for both the adenosine A1 and A3 receptors in protection of isolated human atrial muscle against simulated ischaemia. Cardiovasc Res 1997; 36:52–59.
91. Tomai F, Crea F, Chiariello L, Gioffre PA. Ischemic preconditioning in humans: models, mediators, and clinical relevance. Circulation 1999; 100:559–563.
92. Cain BS, Meldrum DR, Meng X, Pulido EJ, Banerjee A, Harken AH. Therapeutic antidysrhythmic and functional protection in human atria. J Surg Res 1998; 76:143–148.
93. Oxman T, Arad M, Klein R, Avazov N, Rabinowitz B. Limb ischemia preconditions the heart against reperfusion tachyarrhythmia. Am J Physiol 1997; 273:H1707–H1712.
94. Clavien PA, Yadav S, Sindram D, Bentley RC. Protective effects of ischemic preconditioning for liver resection performed under inflow occlusion in humans. Ann Surg 2000; 232:155–162.
95. Kristiansen SB, Henning O, Kharbanda RK, et al. Remote preconditioning reduces ischemic injury in the explanted heart by a KATP channel-dependent mechanism. Am J Physiol Heart Circ Physiol 2005; 288:H1252–H1256.
96. Coles JA Jr, Sigg DC, Iaizzo PA. Role of kappa-opioid receptor activation in pharmacological preconditioning of swine. Am J Physiol Heart Circ Physiol 2003; 284: H2091–H2099.
97. Vinten Johansen J, Zhao ZQ, Corvera JS, Morris CD, Budde JM, Thourani VH, Guyton RA. Adenosine in myocardial protection in on-pump and off-pump cardiac surgery. Ann Thorac Surg 2003; 75:S691–S699.
98. Brew EC, Mitchell MB, Rehring TF, et al. Role of bradykinin in cardiac functional protection after global ischemia-reperfusion in rat heart. Am J Physiol 1995; 269: H1370–H1378.
99. Goto M, Liu Y, Yang XM, Ardell JL, Cohen MV, Downey JM. Role of bradykinin in protection of ischemic preconditioning in rabbit hearts. Circ Res 1995; 77:611–621.
100. Ryckwaert F, Colson P, Guillon G, Foex P. Cumulative effects of AT1 and AT2 receptor blockade on ischaemia-reperfusion recovery in rat hearts. Pharmacol Res 2005; 51:497–502.
101. Morris SD, Yellon DM. Angiotensin-converting enzyme inhibitors potentiate preconditioning through bradykinin B2 receptor activation in human heart. J Am Coll Cardiol 1997; 29:1599–1606.
102. Zaugg M, Lucchinetti E, Spahn D-R, Pasch T, Garcia C, Schaub M-C. Differential effects of anesthetics on mitochondrial K(ATP) channel activity and cardiomyocyte protection. Anesthesiology 2002; 97(1):15–23.
103. Zaugg M, Lucchinetti E, Spahn DR, Pasch T, Schaub MC. Volatile anesthetics mimic cardiac preconditioning by priming the activation of mitochondrial K(ATP) channels via multiple signaling pathways. Anesthesiology 2002; 97:4–14.
104. Zaugg M, Schaub MC, Foex P. Myocardial injury and its prevention in the perioperative setting. Br J Anaesth 2004; 93:21–33.
105. Ludwig LM, Tanaka K, Eells JT, Weihrauch D, Pagel PS, Kersten JR, Warltier DC. Preconditioning by isoflurane is mediated by reactive oxygen species generated from mitochondrial electron transport chain complex III. Anesth Analg 2004; 99:1308–1315.

106. Simkhovich BZ, Marjoram P, Poizat C, Kedes L, Kloner RA. Brief episode of ischemia activates protective genetic program in rat heart: a gene chip study. Cardiovasc Res 2003; 59:450–459.
107. Wang NP, Bufkin BL, Nakamura M, et al. Ischemic preconditioning reduces neutrophil accumulation and myocardial apoptosis. Ann Thorac Surg 1999; 67:1689–1695.
108. Yellon DM, Baxter GF. A "second window of protection" or delayed preconditioning phenomenon: future horizons for myocardial protection? J Mol Cell Cardiol 1995; 27:1023–1034.
109. Miura T. Myocardial response to ischemic preconditioning: is it a novel predictor of prognosis? J Am Coll Cardiol 2003; 42:1004–1006.
110. Cohen MV, Liu GS, Downey JM. Preconditioning causes improved wall motion as well as smaller infarcts after transient coronary occlusion in rabbits. Circulation 1991; 84:341–349.
111. Davis RF, Sidi A. Effect of isoflurane on the extent of myocardial necrosis and on systemic hemodynamics, regional myocardial blood flow, and regional myocardial metabolism in dogs after coronary artery occlusion. Anesth Analg 1989; 69:575–586.
112. Kersten JR, Schmeling TJ, Pagel PS, Gross GJ, Warltier DC. Isoflurane mimics ischemic preconditioning via activation of K(ATP) channels: reduction of myocardial infarct size with an acute memory phase. Anesthesiology 1997; 87:361–370.
113. Kersten JR, Orth KG, Pagel PS, Mei DA, Gross GJ, Warltier DC. Role of adenosine in isoflurane-induced cardioprotection. Anesthesiology 1997; 86:1128–1139.
114. Coetzee JF, le Roux PJ, Genade S, Lochner A. Reduction of postischemic contractile dysfunction of the isolated rat heart by sevoflurane: comparison with halothane. Anesth Analg 2000; 90:1089–1097.
115. Preckel B, Schlack W, Thamer V. Enflurane and isoflurane, but not halothane, protect against myocardial reperfusion injury after cardioplegic arrest with HTK solution in the isolated rat heart. Anesth Analg 1998; 87:1221–1227.
116. Warltier DC, Kersten JR, Pagel PS, Gross GJ. Editorial view: anesthetic preconditioning: serendipity and science. Anesthesiology 2002; 97:1–3.
117. Zhao ZQ, Corvera JS, Halkos ME, Kerendi F, Wang NP, Guyton RA, Vinten Johansen J. Inhibition of myocardial injury by ischemic postconditioning during reperfusion: comparison with ischemic preconditioning. Am J Physiol Heart Circ Physiol 2003; 285:H579–H588.
118. Kersten JR, Lowe D, Hettrick DA, Pagel PS, Gross GJ, Warltier DC. Glyburide, a KATP channel antagonist, attenuates the cardioprotective effects of isoflurane in stunned myocardium. Anesth Analg 1996; 83:27–33.
119. Roscoe AK, Christensen JD, Lynch C III. Isoflurane, but not halothane, induces protection of human myocardium via adenosine A1 receptors and adenosine triphosphate-sensitive potassium channels. Anesthesiology 2000; 92:1692–1701.
120. Gross GJ, Fryer RM. Sarcolemmal versus mitochondrial ATP-sensitive K+ channels and myocardial preconditioning. Circ Res 1999; 84:973–979.
121. Cason BA, Gordon HJ, Avery EGT, Hickey RF. The role of ATP sensitive potassium channels in myocardial protection. J Card Surg 1995; 10(suppl 4):441–444.
122. Zhang Y, Irwin MG, Wong TM. Remifentanil preconditioning protects against ischemic injury in the intact rat heart. Anesthesiology 2004; 101:918–923.
123. Sergeev P, da Silva R, Lucchinetti E, et al. Trigger-dependent gene expression profiles in cardiac preconditioning: evidence for distinct genetic programs in ischemic and anesthetic preconditioning. Anesthesiology 2004; 100:474–488.
124. da Silva R, Lucchinetti E, Pasch T, Schaub MC, Zaugg M. Ischemic but not pharmacological preconditioning elicits a gene expression profile similar to unprotected myocardium. Physiol Genomics 2004; 20:117–130.
125. Mergner GW, Mergner WJ, Stoiko M. Anesthetics influence myocardial infarct size. Adv Myocardiol 1985; 6:593–606.
126. Jugdutt BI. Different relations between infarct size and occluded bed size in barbiturate-anesthetized versus conscious dogs. J Am Coll Cardiol 1985; 6:1035–1046.
127. Lohse MJ, Klotz KN, Jakobs KH, Schwabe U. Barbiturates are selective antagonists at A1 adenosine receptors. J Neurochem 1985; 45:1761–1770.
128. Boutros A, Wang J, Capuano C. Isoflurane and halothane increase adenosine triphosphate preservation, but do not provide additive recovery of function after ischemia, in preconditioned rat hearts. Anesthesiology 1997; 86:109–117.

129. Martini N, Preckel B, Thamer V, Schlack W. Can isoflurane mimic ischaemic preconditioning in isolated rat heart? Br J Anaesth 2001; 86:269–271.
130. Piriou V, Chiari P, Lhuillier F, et al. Pharmacological preconditioning: comparison of desflurane, sevoflurane, isoflurane and halothane in rabbit myocardium. Br J Anaesth 2002; 89:486–491.
131. Toller WG, Kersten JR, Pagel PS, Hettrick DA, Warltier DC. Sevoflurane reduces myocardial infarct size and decreases the time threshold for ischemic preconditioning in dogs. Anesthesiology 1999; 91:1437–1446.
132. Walsh RS, Tsuchida A, Daly JJ, Thornton JD, Cohen MV, Downey JM. Ketamine–xylazine anaesthesia permits a KATP channel antagonist to attenuate preconditioning in rabbit myocardium. Cardiovasc Res 1994; 28(9):1337–1341.
133. Haessler R, Kuzume K, Chien GL, Wolff RA, Davis RF, Van Winkle DM. Anaesthetics alter the magnitude of infarct limitation by ischaemic preconditioning. Cardiovasc Res 1994; 28:1574–1580.
134. Nakae I, Takaoka A, Mitsunami K, et al. Cardioprotective effects of nicorandil in rabbits anaesthetized with halothane: potentiation of ischaemic preconditioning via KATP channels. Clin Exp Pharmacol Physiol 2000; 27:810–817.
135. Belhomme D, Peynet J, Louzy M, Launay JM, Kitakaze M, Menasche P. Evidence for preconditioning by isoflurane in coronary artery bypass graft surgery. Circulation 1999; 100:II340–II344.
136. Kersten JR, Schmeling T, Tessmer J, Hettrick DA, Pagel PS, Warltier DC. Sevoflurane selectively increases coronary collateral blood flow independent of KATP channels in vivo. Anesthesiology 1999; 90:246–256.
137. Kehl F, Pagel P-S, Krolikowski J-G, Gu W, Toller W, Warltier D-C, Kersten J-R. Isoflurane does not produce a second window of preconditioning against myocardial infarction in vivo. Anesth Analg 2002; 95(5):1162–1168.
138. Toller WG, Kersten JR, Gross ER, Pagel PS, Warltier DC. Isoflurane preconditions myocardium against infarction via activation of inhibitory guanine nucleotide binding proteins. Anesthesiology 2000; 92:1400–1407.
139. Han J, Kim E, Ho WK, Earm YE. Effects of volatile anesthetic isoflurane on ATP-sensitive K$^+$ channels in rabbit ventricular myocytes. Biochem Biophys Res Commun 1996; 229:852–856.
140. Haroun Bizri S, Khoury SS, Chehab IR, Kassas CM, Baraka A. Does isoflurane optimize myocardial protection during cardiopulmonary bypass? J Cardiothorac Vasc Anesth 2001; 15:418–421.
141. Hanouz JL, Yvon A, Massetti M, et al. Mechanisms of desflurane-induced preconditioning in isolated human right atria in vitro. Anesthesiology 2002; 97:33–41.
142. Loubani M, Galinanes M. alpha1-Adrenoceptors during simulated ischemia and reoxygenation of the human myocardium: effect of the dose and time of administration. J Thorac Cardiovasc Surg 2001; 122:103–112.
143. Miyawaki H, Ashraf M. Isoproterenol mimics calcium preconditioning-induced protection against ischemia. Am J Physiol 1997; 272:H927–H936.
144. Cleveland JC Jr, Meldrum DR, Rowland RT, Banerjee A, Harken AH. Adenosine preconditioning of human myocardium is dependent upon the ATP-sensitive K$^+$ channel. J Mol Cell Cardiol 1997; 29:175–182.
145. Ebert TJ, Muzi M. Sympathetic hyperactivity during desflurane anesthesia in healthy volunteers: a comparison with isoflurane. Anesthesiology 1993; 79:444–453.
146. Gueugniaud PY, Hanouz JL, Vivien B, Lecarpentier Y, Coriat P, Riou B. Effects of desflurane in rat myocardium: comparison with isoflurane and halothane. Anesthesiology 1997; 87:599–609.
147. Hanouz JL, Massetti M, Guesne G, et al. In vitro effects of desflurane, sevoflurane, isoflurane, and halothane in isolated human right atria. Anesthesiology 2000; 92:116–124.
148. Lochner A, Genade S, Tromp E, Podzuweit T, Moolman JA. Ischemic preconditioning and the beta-adrenergic signal transduction pathway. Circulation 1999; 100:958–966.
149. Serita R, Morisaki H, Ai K, et al. Sevoflurane preconditions stunned myocardium in septic but not healthy isolated rat hearts. Br J Anaesth 2002; 89:896–903.
150. Landry DW, Oliver JA. The ATP-sensitive K$^+$ channel mediates hypotension in endotoxemia and hypoxic lactic acidosis in dog. J Clin Invest 1992; 89:2071–2074.

151. Pickkers P, Jansen Van Rosendaal AJ, Van Der Hoeven JG, Smits P. Activation of the ATP-dependent potassium channel attenuates norepinephrine-induced vasoconstriction in the human forearm. Shock 2004; 22:320–325.
152. Julier K, da Silva R, Garcia C, et al. Preconditioning by sevoflurane decreases biochemical markers for myocardial and renal dysfunction in coronary artery bypass graft surgery: a double-blinded, placebo-controlled, multicenter study. Anesthesiology 2003; 98: 1315–1327.
153. De Hert SG, Van der Linden PJ, Cromheecke S, et al. Cardioprotective properties of sevoflurane in patients undergoing coronary surgery with cardiopulmonary bypass are related to the modalities of its administration. Anesthesiology 2004; 101:299–310.
154. Mayfield KP, D'Alecy LG. Role of endogenous opioid peptides in the acute adaptation to hypoxia. Brain Res 1992; 582:226–231.
155. Mayfield KP, D'Alecy LG. Delta-1 opioid agonist acutely increases hypoxic tolerance. J Pharmacol Exp Ther 1994; 268:683–688.
156. Miki T, Cohen MV, Downey JM. Opioid receptor contributes to ischemic preconditioning through protein kinase C activation in rabbits. Mol Cell Biochem 1998; 186:3–12.
157. Schultz JE, Gross GJ. Opioids and cardioprotection. Pharmacol Ther 2001; 89:123–137.
158. Ludwig LM, Patel HH, Gross GJ, Kersten JR, Pagel PS, Warltier DC. Morphine enhances pharmacological preconditioning by isoflurane: role of mitochondrial K(ATP) channels and opioid receptors. Anesthesiology 2003; 98:705–711.
159. Kloner RA, Shook T, Przyklenk K, et al. Previous angina alters in-hospital outcome in TIMI 4: a clinical correlate to preconditioning? Circulation 1995; 91:37–45.
160. Napoli C, Liguori A, Chiariello M, Di Ieso N, Condorelli M, Ambrosio G. New-onset angina preceding acute myocardial infarction is associated with improved contractile recovery after thrombolysis. Eur Heart J 1998; 19:411–419.
161. Ottani F, Galvani M, Ferrini D, Nicolini FA. Clinical relevance of prodromal angina before acute myocardial infarction. Int J Cardiol 1999; 68(suppl 1):S103–S108.
162. Shiki K, Hearse DJ. Preconditioning of ischemic myocardium: reperfusion-induced arrhythmias. Am J Physiol 1987; 253:H1470–H1476.
163. Lawson CS, Hearse DJ. Anti-arrhythmic protection by ischaemic preconditioning in isolated rat hearts is not due to depletion of endogenous catecholamines. Cardiovasc Res 1996; 31:655–662.
164. Ovize M, Przyklenk K, Hale SL, Kloner RA. Preconditioning does not attenuate myocardial stunning. Circulation 1992; 85:2247–2254.
165. Cave AC, Collis CS, Downey JM, Hearse DJ. Improved functional recovery by ischaemic preconditioning is not mediated by adenosine in the globally ischaemic isolated rat heart. Cardiovasc Res 1993; 27:663–668.
166. Ottani F, Galli M, Zerboni S, Galvani M. Prodromal angina limits infarct size in the setting of acute anterior myocardial infarction treated with primary percutaneous intervention. J Am Coll Cardiol 2005; 45:1545–1547.
167. Mikhail P, Verma S, Fedak PW, Weisel RD, Li RK. Does ischemic preconditioning afford clinically relevant cardioprotection? Am J Cardiovasc Drugs 2003; 3:1–11.
168. Argaud L, Rioufol G, Lievre M, et al. Preconditioning during coronary angioplasty: no influence of collateral perfusion or the size of the area at risk. Eur Heart J 2004; 25:2019–2025.
169. Laskey WK, Beach D. Frequency and clinical significance of ischemic preconditioning during percutaneous coronary intervention. J Am Coll Cardiol 2003; 42:998–1003.
170. Leesar MA, Stoddard MF, Manchikalapudi S, Bolli R. Bradykinin-induced preconditioning in patients undergoing coronary angioplasty. J Am Coll Cardiol 1999; 34:639–650.
171. Leesar MA, Stoddard MF, Xuan YT, Tang XL, Bolli R. Nonelectrocardiographic evidence that both ischemic preconditioning and adenosine preconditioning exist in humans. J Am Coll Cardiol 2003; 42:437–445.
172. Matsuo H, Watanabe S, Segawa T, et al. Evidence of pharmacologic preconditioning during PTCA by intravenous pretreatment with ATP-sensitive K+ channel opener nicorandil. Eur Heart J 2003; 24:1296–1303.
173. Yellon DM, Alkhulaifi AM, Pugsley WB. Preconditioning the human myocardium. Lancet 1993; 342:276–277.
174. Perrault LP, Menasche P, Bel A, et al. Ischemic preconditioning in cardiac surgery: a word of caution. J Thorac Cardiovasc Surg 1996; 112:1378–1386.

175. Kaukoranta PK, Lepojarvi MP, Ylitalo KV, Kiviluoma KT, Peuhkurinen KJ. Normothermic retrograde blood cardioplegia with or without preceding ischemic preconditioning. Ann Thorac Surg 1997; 63:1268–1274.
176. Szmagala P, Morawski W, Krejca M, Gburek T, Bochenek A. Evaluation of perioperative myocardial tissue damage in ischemically preconditioned human heart during aorto coronary bypass surgery. J Cardiovasc Surg 1998; 39:791–795.
177. Jenkins DP, Pugsley WB, Alkhulaifi AM, Kemp M, Hooper J, Yellon DM. Ischaemic preconditioning reduces troponin T release in patients undergoing coronary artery bypass surgery. Heart Br Cardiac Soc 1997; 77:314–318.
178. Li G, Chen S, Lu E, Li Y. Ischemic preconditioning improves preservation with cold blood cardioplegia in valve replacement patients. Eur J Cardiothorac Surg 1999; 15:653–657.
179. Laurikka J, Wu ZK, Iisalo P, et al. Regional ischemic preconditioning enhances myocardial performance in off-pump coronary artery bypass grafting. Chest 2002; 121:1183–1189.
180. Ghosh S, Galinanes M. Protection of the human heart with ischemic preconditioning during cardiac surgery: role of cardiopulmonary bypass. J Thorac Cardiovasc Surg 2003; 126:133–142.
181. Pouzet B, Lecharny JB, Dehoux M, et al. Is there a place for preconditioning during cardiac operations in humans? Ann Thorac Surg 2002; 73:843–848.
182. Penttila HJ, Lepojarvi MV, Kaukoranta PK, Kiviluoma KT, Ylitalo KV, Peuhkurinen KJ. Ischemic preconditioning does not improve myocardial preservation during off-pump multivessel coronary operation. Ann Thorac Surg 2003; 75:1246–1252.
183. Garcia C, Julier K, Bestmann L, et al. Preconditioning with sevoflurane decreases PECAM-1 expression and improves one-year cardiovascular outcome in coronary artery bypass graft surgery. Br J Anaesth 2005; 94:159–165.
184. Loubani M, Fowler A, Standen NB, Galinanes M. The effect of gliclazide and glibenclamide on preconditioning of the human myocardium. Eur J Pharmacol 2005; 515:142–149.
185. Forlani S, Tomai F, De Paulis R, et al. Preoperative shift from glibenclamide to insulin is cardioprotective in diabetic patients undergoing coronary artery bypass surgery. J Cardiovasc Surg 2004; 45:117–122.
186. Meier JJ, Gallwitz B, Schmidt WE, Mugge A, Nauck MA. Is impairment of ischaemic preconditioning by sulfonylurea drugs clinically important? Heart 2004; 90:9–12.
187. Lee TM, Chou TF. Impairment of myocardial protection in type 2 diabetic patients. J Clin Endocrinol Metab 2003; 88:531–537.
188. Gottlieb SS. Renal effects of adenosine A1-receptor antagonists in congestive heart failure. Drugs 2001; 61:1387–1393.
189. Auchampach JA, Jin X, Moore J, et al. Comparison of three different A1 adenosine receptor antagonists on infarct size and multiple cycle ischemic preconditioning in anesthetized dogs. J Pharmacol Exp Ther 2004; 308:846–856.
190. Thourani VH, Ronson RS, Jordan JE, Guyton RA, Vinten Johansen J. Adenosine A3 pretreatment before cardioplegic arrest attenuates postischemic cardiac dysfunction. Ann Thorac Surg 1999; 67:1732–1737.
191. Loubani M, Galinanes M. Long-term administration of nicorandil abolishes ischemic and pharmacologic preconditioning of the human myocardium: role of mitochondrial adenosine triphosphate-dependent potassium channels. J Thorac Cardiovasc Surg 2002; 124:750–757.
192. Hausenloy DJ, Tsang A, Yellon DM. The reperfusion injury salvage kinase pathway: a common target for both ischemic preconditioning and postconditioning. Trends Cardiovasc Med 2005; 15:69–75.
193. Tsang A, Hausenloy DJ, Yellon DM. Myocardial postconditioning: reperfusion injury revisited. Am J Physiol Heart Circ Physiol 2005; 289:H2–H7.
194. Halkos ME, Kerendi F, Corvera JS, et al. Myocardial protection with postconditioning is not enhanced by ischemic preconditioning. Ann Thorac Surg 2004; 78:961–969.
195. Heusch G. Postconditioning: old wine in new bottle. J Am Coll Cardiol 2004; 44:1111–1112.
196. Vinten Johansen J, Zhao ZQ, Zatta AJ, Kin H, Halkos ME, Kerendi F. Postconditioning a new link in nature's armor against myocardial ischemia-reperfusion injury. Basic Res Cardiol 2005; 100:295–310.

197. Kerendi F, Kin H, Halkos ME, et al. Remote postconditioning brief renal ischemia and reperfusion applied before coronary artery reperfusion reduces myocardial infarct size via endogenous activation of adenosine receptors. Basic Res Cardiol 2005;100:404–412.
198. De Hert SG, Cromheecke S, ten Broecke PW, et al. Effects of propofol, desflurane, and sevoflurane on recovery of myocardial function after coronary surgery in elderly high-risk patients. Anesthesiology 2003; 99:314–323.
199. De Hert SG, ten Broecke PW, Mertens E, et al. Sevoflurane but not propofol preserves myocardial function in coronary surgery patients. Anesthesiology 2002; 97:42–49.
200. Hausenloy DJ, Yellon DM. New directions for protecting the heart against ischaemia-reperfusion injury: targeting the reperfusion injury salvage kinase (RISK)-pathway. Cardiovasc Res 2004; 61:448–460.
201. Lucchinetti E, da Silva R, Pasch T, Schaub MC, Zaugg M. Anaesthetic preconditioning but not postconditioning prevents early activation of the deleterious cardiac remodelling programme: evidence of opposing genomic responses in cardioprotection by pre- and postconditioning. Br J Anaesth 2005; 95:140–152.

6 Preoperative Assessment

Pierre-Guy Chassot

*Department of Anesthesiology, University Hospital of Lausanne
(CHUV), Lausanne, Switzerland*

Donat R. Spahn

University Hospital Zurich, Zurich, Switzerland

INTRODUCTION

In Western countries, medicine shows an obvious trend towards more aggressive surgery in older people. In recent years, the management of coronary artery disease (CAD) has evolved with the introduction of new technologies (coronary angioplasty with drug-eluting stents, beating-heart coronary bypass surgery), new medical treatments (statins, antiplatelet therapy), and cardioprotection with β-blockade or preconditioning. Assessing the patients with or at risk for CAD before surgery has become a major task for anesthesiologists and the decisions they make can considerably modify the clinical outcome of the patients. The clinician seeks to identify patients who are fit for the planned operation and those who need preoperative testing and medical treatment or coronary revascularization.

There has been an abundance of studies on this subject during the last decade, and some recommendations have been published (1–3). However, they are mostly based on small series of patients, case reports, expert opinions, and precautionary principles. In an era of evidence-based medicine, the literature on which these guidelines is constructed is lacking large, controlled, randomized trials with clear-cut results (level I of evidence). Such studies are difficult to conduct, because the incidence of perioperative cardiac events is low (<10% of the cases) and thus the number of patients required is high (about 10,000). As most of the published studies are underpowered to answer the key questions, it is tempting to pool multiple small series in a meta-analysis, but this tends to overestimate any slightly positive effect and make it more prominent than it really is.

Most of the studies on preoperative evaluation and preparation are conducted in vascular patients, because they represent a high-risk population for perioperative ischemic events: more than half of them suffer from CAD, and their incidence of postoperative myocardial infarction (MI) is 3.4% to 5.6% (4–6). They are usually male, older than 60 years, and frequently undergo major operations. However, they represent less than 10% of the surgical population; this fact introduces a bias when the results are extrapolated to other surgical cohorts. Data from one population are difficult to generalize, because regional and ethnic differences should be taken into account. The incidence and the severity of CAD are variables in different countries. In the case of patients presenting with abdominal aortic aneurysm, for example, the incidence of angina is 20% in France and 49% in Sweden, and the incidence of a history of MI is 16% and 50%, respectively (7,8). In Japan, the proportion of patients with ischemic heart disease is one-tenth of the rates reported in Europe or the United States, but the incidence of perioperative complications among these patients (average 15%) is not significantly different from one continent to another (9). There are also ethnic differences in the response to treatment between white and non-white populations, particularly for β-blockers (10,11). Molecular biology is beginning to identify the genetic polymorphisms that may predict adverse perioperative outcome and response to specific therapy in individual patients (12). Finally, surgical morbidity and mortality are different between different institutions, because they depend on surgical skills, anesthetic care, and nursing quality. These additional biases become important when one compares the results of different publications.

The purpose of preoperative evaluation is to lower perioperative morbidity and mortality while at the same time making the most cost-effective use of preoperative testing, and to focus resource allocation on high-risk patients where treatment modifications may improve long-term results. Preoperative risk stratification identifies the group of high-risk patients who may benefit from cardiological testing, specific perioperative medical treatment and, perhaps, revascularization. Testing a low-risk population not only increases costs unnecessarily, but may also increase morbidity and cause harm by adverse drug reaction and delays in the noncardiac operation. Recently, the catastrophic results seen in patients who have had only a short delay between coronary revascularization and noncardiac surgery (13,14), and the possibility of perioperative myocardial protection with preoperative β-blockade (15,16) have shifted the paradigm from "investigation and possible revascularization" to "perioperative medication and direct operation."

CLINICAL PREDICTORS

History and physical examination of the patient remain the key process of clinical preoperative assessment. Risk stratification of the patient with or at risk of CAD is based on two elements (2,3): First, the cardiac history of the patient (characterized by the number of risk factors for perioperative cardiac complications the patient has) and his or her functional capacity; secondly, the risk of the operation. Predictors of cardiac risk are additive: the higher their number, the greater the risk of an adverse outcome (17,18). It is important to collect information on the severity of any CAD, its degree of stability versus instability, the response to previous treatment, and the functional reserve of the myocardium. In addition to ischemic heart disease, the presence of non-ischemic comorbidities increases the operative risk in each category of patients. The main comorbidities which are independent predictors of cardiac risk are: severe valvular heart disease, history of congestive heart failure with ejection fraction (EF) < 0.35, history of cerebrovascular disease (stroke within six weeks), renal insufficiency (creatinine > 200 μmol), and insulin-dependent diabetes mellitus (17).

Risk Factors

Risk factors for perioperative cardiac complications are subdivided into three categories (Table 1). Minor risk factors are markers of an increased probability of suffering from CAD, but are not independent predictors of perioperative ischemic events. They are: family history of CAD, hypercholesterolemia, polyvascular status (e.g., CAD and cerebrovascular disease), uncontrolled systemic hypertension, smoking habit, metabolic syndrome, and electrocardiogram (ECG) abnormalities [arrhythmias, left ventricular hypertrophy (LVH), bundle branch block]. Patients who have only these risk factors have an average incidence of perioperative cardiac complications of 0.7% (19). Patients with good functional capacity who are asymptomatic without treatment more than three months after coronary artery bypass graft (CABG) or

TABLE 1 Risk Predictors of the Patient

Minor predictors (markers of increased probability of suffering from CAD)
Familial history of CAD
Smoking habit
Hypercholesterolemia
Uncontrolled arterial hypertension
Metabolic syndrome (hypercholesterolemia, type II diabetes, truncular obesity)
Polyvascular status
Coronary events > 3 mo
Nonsinusal rhythm, bundle branch block
Left ventricular hypertrophy
History of stroke > 3 mo
Intermediate predictors (markers of known but stable CAD)
Stable angina (grades I and II)
Asymptomatic patient with optimal medical treatment
Silent ischemia: coronary event > 6 wk and < 3 mo, or > 3 mo if complications
Documented previous ischemic episode
Compensated heart failure (EF < 0.35)
Compensated valvulopathy
Stroke > 6 wk and < 3 mo
Renal insufficiency (creatinine acatininemia ≥ 200 μmol/L)
Diabetes mellitus (blood glucosee ≥ 11 mmol/L)
Major predictors (markers of unstable coronary syndrome)
Unstable angina (grades III and IV)
New angina, or recent symptom modifications
Coronary event < 6 wk
Residual angina after infarction or revascularization
Congestive heart failure
Decompensated valvulopathy
Malignant arrhythmias

Note: Coronary event: infarction, new angina, modification of previous angina, dilatation, stenting, CABG.
Abbreviations: CABG, coronary artery bypass graft; CAD, coronary artery disease; EF, ejection fraction.

MI fall into this category. After percutaneous coronary intervention (PCI), the risk is related to the adequacy of the reendothelialization of the dilated and stented artery; the delay varies from 8 weeks to 12 months, depending of the technique used (see below). The protection offered by a successful revascularization lasts at least six years for CABG (20) and three to four years for PCI (21).

Intermediate risk factors are markers of well established but stable and controlled CAD. They are: angina class I and II with optimal medical treatment, documented previous perioperative ischemia, silent ischemia (by Holter monitoring), patient asymptomatic after infarction under maximal therapy, prior MI or revascularization more than six weeks but less than three months earlier without sequelae or threatened myocardium, and patients revascularized but asymptomatic on medical treatment. The incidence of perioperative ischemic events is 2% to 6% in patients in this category (19,20). Insulin-dependent diabetes mellitus is usually included in this category because it is frequently associated with silent ischemia, and represents an independent risk factor for postoperative complications (2,3,17). The relevance of advanced age (>70 years), hypertension, and LVH to intermediate or minor risk category is still controversial, and might have a different impact according to the population investigated. Advanced age, which should be estimated by physiological and not chronological age, is considered as a minor risk factor by American guidelines (2,19), but the large spectrum of cardiovascular diseases associated with old age inclines us to consider it to be among the intermediate risk factors (22). The impact of hypertension depends probably on the population considered; as it is an easily controllable factor in the perioperative period, it can be safely considered as a minor risk factor (23). LVH has been considered as an independent marker of ischemic heart disease and cardiac complications, but recent recommendations tend to consider it as a minor factor (2,3,17).

Major predictors are markers of unstable coronary syndromes and include: class III and IV angina, recently modified anginal symptoms, angina persisting despite maximal medical treatment, ongoing ischemia after MI, ischemia and congestive heart failure or malignant arrhythmias, patients less than six weeks after infarction or CABG, and patients with nonendothelialized stents after PCI (< 6 weeks to <12 months depending on the type of stent; see below). A six- to eight-week period is necessary for the myocardium to heal after an infarction or for the coronary artery to be reendothelialized after CABG or PCI (24,25); the delay is even longer with drug-eluting stents (26,27). The fate of the patients with major predictors is linked to the evolution of unstable atheromatous plaques. New or changing symptoms and ST elevation on ECG identify plaque rupture and should be considered to indicate impending infarction until proven otherwise. In this category, the rate of cardiac complications is 10% to 20%, and might even be as high as 30% (2,13,19). It is obvious that only vital or emergency procedures should be considered in these patients. All elective operations should be postponed and the patients properly investigated and treated (3).

Functional Capacity

Exercise tolerance is a major determinant of perioperative risk because it is a marker of the myocardial functional reserve (28,29). It is quantified by the increasing energy requirement of a variety of activities, and graded in metabolic equivalent (MET) on a scale defined by the Duke Activity Status Index (Table 2)(30). One MET represents the oxygen consumption of a resting adult ($VO_2 = 3.5$ mL/kg/min). Patients are classified in three categories following their exercise tolerance: poor (≤ 4 MET: home activities, flat level walk), good (5–9 MET: climbing two flights of stairs, uphill walk), and excellent (>9 MET: strenuous physical activity). The cut-off value between 4 and 5 MET, below which the functional capacity is considered as compromised, corresponds to the capacity of climbing two flights of stairs; the inability to reach this level of exercise (4 MET = VO_2 14 mL/kg/min) has a positive predictive value of 89% for postoperative cardiopulmonary complications (29).

The perioperative mortality increases significantly below the threshold of 4 MET (31). The value of 4 MET is higher than the average postoperative VO_2, which is 5 to

TABLE 2   Activities Corresponding to METs

1 MET	3.5 mL O_2/kg/min
1–4 MET	Homework
	Walk on flat ground, 500 m at average speed (4 km/hr)
5–9 MET	Uphill walk
	Two flights of stairs, or more
	Heavy sedentary work
	Moderate sports (golf, trekking, swimming)
>9 MET	Intensive sports (tennis, mountain climbing, bicycle, running)
	Intense physical work (construction worker, lumberjack)

Abbreviation: MET, metabolic equivalent.

6 mL/kg/min (1–2 MET) (31), because the postoperative period should be considered as equivalent to a sustained exercise lasting one to three days. Investigations on athletes have disclosed that, after 24 hours of sustained exercise, a normal individual can only maintain a cardiac output corresponding to about 45% of his maximal oxygen consumption (VO_2) (32). The calculated 45% of 4 MET is 6.4 mL/kg/min, which corresponds to the actual VO_2 in the postoperative situation. Therefore, a preoperative functional capacity of 4 MET certifies that the individual is able to maintain a VO_2 of approximately 6 mL/kg/min for several days and to withstand the physiological stress of the postoperative period (33).

The sensitivity of stress tests for diagnosing a coronary lesion is significantly compromised in patients with chronic β-blockade, because they have a limited capacity to increase their heart rate and cardiac output in response to exercise (34,35). However, these tests retain their full value as a preoperative prognostic tool, as they demonstrate which level of stress the patients can endure before showing myocardial ischemia under the protection of β-adrenergic antagonists. They show adequately the degree of protection achieved with the β-blockers, although the decreased incidence of ischemic modifications is a diagnostic drawback.

Ergometric measurements on a treadmill show that vascular patients who are able to exercise up to 85% of their maximal theoretical heart rate have a low risk of postoperative cardiac events (36), whereas ischemia appearing at low-level exercise (<5 MET or heart rate<100 per minute) identifies a high-risk group (37). In the absence of valvular pathology, the EF of the left ventricle can be considered as an adequate measurement of cardiac functional reserve (normal value: 0.55–0.7) (38). Patients with good functional capacity who present no angina and do not suffer from diabetes can be considered as free from CAD (39). Despite its obvious predictive value in the perioperative setting, the Duke Activity Status Index has never been tested specifically for ischemic patients (3).

Risk Factors Associated with Surgery

The risk associated with the surgical operation varies with its invasiveness, its duration, and with the degree of its associated hemodynamic and volemic disturbances. When evaluating a patient, one should compare the risk of an operation to the risk of not operating on the patient. In some situations, such as rapidly spreading tumors, impending aneurysm rupture, infections requiring surgical drainage, or disabling bone fractures, the alternative to a risky operation might be hemorrhage, sepsis, thromboembolic disease, intractable pain or bowel obstruction, or death. In orthopedic surgery, an early fracture fixation is frequently the only way to decrease thromboembolic risk, and the incidence of pulmonary complications, pain, and chronic anemia. Sometimes, risk can be lowered by a limited, rapid, or palliative operation. Risk reduction strategies must be applied, such as using β-blockers, antiplatelet agents and volatile anesthetics, avoiding extreme anemia, maintaining normothermia, and controlling postoperative pain. In these situations, the performance of the surgical team, the quality of the anesthetic care, and the postoperative nursing management shall make the difference between success and failure.

Surgical procedures are usually stratified into three categories, according to their level of perioperative physiological stress (Table 3). Minor procedures present a risk of cardiac complications less than 1% (2,19). This category includes: ambulatory and superficial procedures such as herniorrhaphy, eye surgery, plastic surgery, or endoscopic procedures. Intermediate operations comprise abdominal and thoracic procedures, orthopedic surgery, neurosurgery, ear–nose-and-throat (ENT), and

TABLE 3   Operative Risk and Types of Surgery

Minor risk surgery (cardiac complication rate < 1%)
Endoscopic surgery
Ambulatory surgery
Parietal surgery (hernia)
Breast surgery
Plastic and reconstructive surgery
Ophthalmology
Intermediate risk surgery (cardiac complication rate 1–4%)
Carotid surgery
Minor peripheral vascular surgery
Abdominal and thoracic surgery
Neurosurgery
ENT
Orthopedic surgery
Urologic surgery
Major risk surgery (cardiac complication rate > 5%)
Intermediate risk surgery in emergency
Abdominal aortic surgery
Major peripheral vascular surgery
Long-duration and blood-loosing operations
Large intraoperative volume shifts
Surgery in old-age patients
Unstable hemodynamic situations

Abbreviation: ENT, ear, nose, throat.

urologic operations, as long as they are not complicated by unusual duration, hemorrhage, volume shifts, or emergency. Simple peripheral vascular surgery and carotid endarterectomy also belong to this category; the cardiac complications rate is 1% to 5% (2,19). Major procedures comprise aortic and major vascular surgery, prolonged surgical procedures with large fluid shifts or hemorrhage, intermediate operations in emergency, and unstable hemodynamic situations. The risk of cardiac events is above 5% (2,19).

Previous Ischemia
The perioperative complication rate of a patient with a previous MI is traditionally estimated from the delay since the ischemic event. However, it is now well established that the risk is related less to the age of the infarction than to its size and location, to its complications such as arrhythmias, to the functional status of the ventricle, and to the amount of myocardium at risk for further ischemia (40). A patient with a small infarction without residual angina in the context of a good functional status and normal EF can withstand vital noncardiac surgery as soon as six weeks after the ischemic episode (41). On the contrary, a patient with a large infarct, with residual symptoms and an EF below 0.35 has a very high probability of further ischemic complications, even six months after the primary event.

For practical purposes, patients can be allotted into three categories of decreasing risk:

1. The period within six weeks of an infarction is considered as a time of very high risk for perioperative cardiac events because it is the mean healing time of the infarct-related lesion (24,42). Any surgery which is nonvital is contraindicated.

2. The period from six weeks to three months is of intermediate risk; it is reasonable to perform operations that cannot be postponed without compromising long term outcome, if the patient is symptom-free without antianginal medication outside aspirin. Antiplatelet therapy should be continued throughout the operation. This period is extended beyond three months in case of complications such as arrhythmias, ventricular dysfunction, or continued antianginal therapy.
3. Beyond three months, the patient is in a low-risk category, as long as he/she is symptom-free without medication. Persisting angina, arrhythmias, or heart failure maintains the patient in the high or intermediate risk categories. In uncomplicated cases, no benefit can be expected from delaying surgery more than three months (41).

Diabetes Mellitus

Diabetic patients deserve a special mention because they have a risk of CAD two to four times higher than the corresponding normal population (43), and a much poorer outcome after surgery, with an increased probability of cardiac death or MI compared with nondiabetics with equivalent CAD (44). Moreover, they frequently have silent myocardial ischemia, which when diagnosed by Holter monitoring has a 35% positive predictive value for postoperative cardiac events (45). Diabetic patients with neither symptoms of angina nor history of infarction, who are theoretically in the category of low risk patients, have an incidence of perioperative ischemic events identical to patients with stable CAD (category of intermediate risk) (46). Factors that are not markers of CAD in the normal population must be added to the list of minor clinical risk predictors of diabetics: truncal obesity, physical inactivity, albuminuria, dyslipidemia, and age more than 50 years (47). Chronically elevated glucose (>11 mmol/L) and glycosylated hemoglobin levels (>7%) are better predictors of cardiac events than the simple presence of diabetes (47,48).

Clinicians should have a low threshold for preoperative cardiac investigations in diabetics. Asymptomatic patients with two or more risk factors for CAD should be investigated by stress testing if they have a low functional capacity, or if they undergo major or vascular surgery (3). Only individuals with good functional capacity scheduled for minor or intermediate surgery can proceed directly to surgery. If the coronary situation is such that β-blockers are indicated to prevent myocardial ischemia and improve postoperative outcome, the risk of disrupting glycemic control is minor compared to the benefit of the treatment (48). However, a recent trial on 921 diabetic patients finds no difference in mortality and major cardiac complications between patients receiving metoprolol or placebo after a median follow-up of 18 months (49,50).

Vascular Surgery

Vascular atheromatosis concerns all the arterial tree. Even if they are asymptomatic because of limitations in physical activity, 37% of surgical vascular patients have significant coronary disease at angiography, and 15% have lesions that warrant revascularization (51). The mortality for noncardiac vascular surgery in patients with CAD is 5% to 9%, whereas it is only 1% to 2% in patients free of coronary lesions, or in patients who have been successfully revascularized (51,52). The postoperative infarction rate in vascular surgery is almost five times higher than in nonvascular surgery (5). It is 8.5% when the patient has proven CAD, but only 1.6% in patients with no risk factors, and 1.9% in patients who have had a successful CABG more than six months and less than six years before (53,54).

However, there is a wide spectrum of vascular operations, and the rate of fatal or nonfatal MI differs significantly according to the type of vascular surgery. For abdominal aortic surgery, it is 5% to 14% in the most recent series (55,56). Surprisingly enough, endarterectomy is experienced by the body as a peripheral and rather minor vascular operation, including carotid thromboendarterectomy, and has a postoperative MI rate of only 1.4% (57). This is one-tenth of the infarction rate recorded after abdominal aortic surgery.

In patients with advanced vascular disease, β-blockers are not contraindicated because their benefit on cardioprotection outweighs their risk on peripheral arterial vasoconstriction (3). However, it might be advantageous to consider β-blockade in addition to β-blockade (e.g., with carvedilol) in order to reduce peripheral vasoconstriction (58).

PREVIOUS CORONARY REVASCULARIZATION

Successful myocardial revascularization places the patient in the low-risk category, as if his or her CAD was cured. This is true as long as two conditions are fulfilled: (i) the patient is asymptomatic without treatment other than aspirin, and (ii) the time elapsed since the operation is more than three months and less than six years for CABG, or more than three months and less than four years for PCI (20,21). In patients who have undergone coronary artery bypass grafting, the MI rate (0.8%) and mortality (1.7%) after major noncardiac surgery are identical to those of patients without CAD; beyond six years after CABG, the infarction rate raises again (2.2%) (20). After PCI, the benefit is present only in patients with normal ventricular function, and during a shorter period (21,59,60). Landesberg et al. (61) found the 5-year survival rate of revascularized patients to be higher (62%) than that of medically treated patients (34%). In other series, however, previous coronary revascularization (CABG less than five years previously, PCI less than two years previously) provided only modest short-term (30 days) (62) or non-significant long-term (2.7–5 years) (56,63) protection against adverse cardiac events and mortality following major arterial reconstruction. There were no significant differences in outcome between revascularization with CABG or PCI within the time ranges studied (62). The widespread use of β-blockers, antiplatelet agents, ACE-inhibitors, and statins in these studies may have improved the outcome in the medically treated patients and decreased the differences between those revascularized and those under conservative treatment.

These data demonstrate the efficiency of PCI or CABG as a treatment for CAD, but they do not prove that revascularization is beneficial as a prophylactic cardioprotection before noncardiac surgery. There are at least four reasons for this statement:

1. Revascularization is aiming at increasing long-term survival or at salvaging threatened myocardium.
2. Revascularization does not improve the outcome after vascular surgery more than preoperative treatment with β-blockers (56).
3. The revascularization procedures are associated with an average mortality rate of 1.7% for CABG and 0.1% for PCI, and an infarction rate of 2.4% for CABG

Mortality (%)

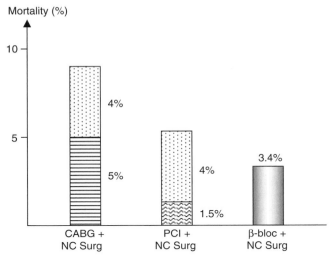

FIGURE 1 Mortality in case of myocardial revascularization before vascular surgery compared to operation without revascularization but under protection of a β-blocker. The mortality of vascular patients in cardiac surgery is 4% to 6% (52,66,67) and 1% to 2% after PCI (64,67). The average mortality after vascular surgery is 4% (5,6,55). The combined mortality rate of revascularization and vascular noncardiac surgery is higher than the mortality of high-risk vascular patients operated without revascularization but under the protection of a β-blocker (16,56). *Abbreviations:* CABG, coronary artery bypass graft; PCI, percutaneous intervention; NC Surg: noncardiac surgery; PCI, percutaneous coronary intervention.

and 0.9% for PCI (64,65). For vascular patients, the mortality in cardiac surgery is 4% to 6% (52,66,67); it is 1% to 2% after PCI (64,67). The average mortality after noncardiac vascular surgery (4%) (6,55,56) must be added to the mortality rates of revascularization (Fig. 1). Therefore, the combined mortality is higher than the mortality of high-risk vascular patients operated on without revascularization but under the protection of perioperative β-blockade (3.4%) (16,56).

4. Every instrumentation of the coronary tree converts a former severe but stable stenosis into a temporarily unstable lesion. A coronary lesion is unstable because a rupture in the endothelial layer allows circulating proteins and blood cells, particularly thrombocytes, to be in contact with interstitial and intracellular structures or materials. This happens when an unstable coronary plaque ruptures, or when the blood is in contact with foreign material like a stent.

Bare metallic stents are covered by a proliferation of endothelium within six to eight weeks (25), but an excessive proliferation might occlude the stent. This disadvantage is prevented by the new drug-eluting stents, which slow down the process in such a way that it takes up to 12 months for the metal to be completely covered by a thin layer of endothelium (26,68). During all this time, the patient needs to be protected by antiplatelet agents, because the situation in the stented coronary artery is equivalent to an unstable lesion, and the patient belongs to the high-risk group of unstable coronary syndrome.

PREVIOUS CORONARY ARTERY BYPASS GRAFTING

Although surgical coronary revascularization reduces cardiac complications associated with subsequent noncardiac surgery, the protection against myocardial ischemia offered by aortocoronary bypasses does not start immediately after the operation. During the first weeks, the recently operated coronary arteries are prone to thrombosis. In a prospective evaluation of patients undergoing sternectomy after CABG, the incidence of ECG changes consistent with ischemia and infarction was fivefold more frequent when the patients were operated on during the first week (24% and 4% of the cases, respectively) than during the second week after revascularization (5% and 0%, respectively) (69). Patients who undergo vascular surgery within one month after CABG suffer significantly greater mortality (20.6%) than case-matched controls operated outside this period (3.9%), although the incidence of nonfatal complications is not significantly different between the groups (70). Beyond three months, the risk of death and nonfatal MI during noncardiac surgery is 1.7% and 0.8%, respectively; these values are similar to the rates observed for major surgery in a population not suffering from CAD (20).

Obviously, the shorter the delay between CABG and noncardiac surgery, the worse is the prognosis. Therefore, one can consider four to six weeks as the minimal safety delay for performing a noncardiac procedure when it is imperative. For a purely elective operation, the safety delay is three months.

PREVIOUS PERCUTANEOUS CORONARY INTERVENTION

In the 1990s, it seemed that percutaneous transluminal coronary angioplasty (PTCA) would provide a good protection against ischemic complications of subsequent noncardiac surgery. In two studies from the Mayo Clinic, major vascular surgery was performed on average 9 to 10 days after simple coronary angioplasty without stenting (71,72); overall mortality of surgery was halved and infarction rate five time less in the groups having previous PTCA compared with nonrevascularized patients. After a median interval of 11 days between PTCA and vascular surgery, the infarction and mortality rate were only 0.5% each (60). However, with the advent of stenting during PCI, more recent studies have shown fundamentally different results. In the first study which served as an alarm signal, there were eight deaths (20% mortality rate) and seven MIs (18%) among 40 patients who underwent coronary stent placement less than two weeks before noncardiac surgery (13). A mortality up to 86% due to stent thrombosis has been recorded when thienopyridine antiplatelet therapy was abruptly discontinued and surgery performed within three weeks of stenting (27). Within 40 days of PCI, patients are nearly three times more likely to have adverse cardiac events than normal controls; their cardiac outcome is improved compared to nonrevascularized patients only beyond 90 days after PCI and stenting (73). In an analysis of the Mayo Clinic Percutaneous Coronary Intervention Registry, eight (4%) among 207 patients who underwent noncardiac surgery during the first months of PCI suffered from MI or died (74); all of them were operated on less than six weeks after stenting. Noncardiac surgery performed within six weeks of PCI present an excessive risk of stent thrombosis if antiplatelet medication is stopped, or of increased bleeding if the treatment is maintained throughout surgery (75).

The guidelines of the American College of Cardiology/American Heart Association specify that the minimal safety delay for noncardiac surgery after PCI and stenting "is ideally 4 to 6 weeks to allow 4 full weeks of dual antiplatelet therapy to allow reendothelialization of the stent to be completed, or nearly so" (2). Two weeks without antiplatelet agents should be added before surgery in order to be free of the anticoagulant effect for the day of the operation. However, this approach does not afford a real guarantee against ischemic accidents. This is illustrated by a case of fatal MI due to stent thrombosis after lung resection in a patient operated on six weeks after PCI, which was followed by four weeks of aspirin and clopidogrel (14).

The situation has further evolved with the introduction of the new drug-eluting stents, because they reduce dramatically the local neo-intimal proliferation that causes restenosis; but their re-endothelialization rate is greatly prolonged. Animal studies have generated concern that they could be prone to late thrombosis, although extrapolation of such findings to human being might be subject to caution (76). Experiments suggest that sirolimus-eluting stent delays but does not impede endothelialization, because almost all the substance has eluted by six weeks, leaving a polymer-coated bare metal stent (77). In contrast, paclitaxel-eluting stent clearly shows very delayed reendothelialization, because only about 10% of the paclitaxel is released by 10 days, the rest remaining in the polymer indefinitely (78). With the bare-metal stents, most of the restenoses requiring repeat PCI occur during the first month at a rate of 0.9%; their infarction rate is 60% and the six-month mortality is 8.9% (64). The peculiar pharmacokinetic profile of drug-eluting stents makes them probably more sensitive to late thrombosis, particularly after discontinuation of antiplatelet therapy (68). Therefore, it seems advisable to adapt the anticoagulation after stent placement to the type of stent that has been placed and to recommend the following minimal treatment durations (26,79):

1. Simple bare-metal stents: clopidogrel (75 mg/day) for four to six weeks (76)
2. Sirolimus (Cypher™) eluting stents: clopidogrel for three months (80)
3. Paclitaxel (Taxus™) eluting stents: clopidogrel for six months (81)
4. Clopidogrel has been proven to be beneficial up to 12 months (82)
5. Acetylsalicylic acid (ASA): life-long treatment (100–325 mg/day) (83)

These data are important for anesthetists, because they have to adapt the timing of the operation and the technique of anesthesia to these requirements. If the coronary lesions of a patient require a percutaneous angioplasty, the type of therapy must be adapted to the indications of the noncardiac surgery (26). In case of purely elective surgery, when the operation can be postponed for at least six months, PCI with paclitaxel-eluting stent can be used. If the operation can wait for three months only, the best choice is a PCI with a sirolimus-eluting stent; but if it cannot wait for more than two months, PCI should be performed with a simple bare-metal stent, in which endothelialization will take six to eight weeks. Finally, the surgical procedure can be imperative and vital; the safety delay of the PCI represents an excessive risk in the evolution of the noncardiac disease, as it is for a rapidly spreading cancer or an impending aneurismal rupture. Two options are then possible: (*i*) simple angioplasty and dilatation without stent placement, but with continuous antiplatelet therapy (delay for noncardiac surgery: two weeks) or (*ii*) no revascularization, and cardioprotection with medical treatment (β-blockers, clopidogrel, statins; delay for noncardiac surgery: 24–72 hours).

Of course, the choice for the type of stent, or the decision to perform a simple angioplasty, relies primarily with the cardiologist in charge of the case. Nevertheless, the involvement of anesthesiologists in the preoperative assessment of the patient and their experience in the postoperative period, where ischemic complication rate differs from the nonsurgical setting, make it mandatory for cardiologists, anesthesiologists, and surgeons to work in close collaboration.

PHARMACOLOGICAL PRETREATMENT

The principle of pharmacological cardioprotection is based on two different concepts. First, half of postoperative infarctions occur in myocardial territories not related to an angiographic severe stenosis (84,85) nor to an area which was suspected at preoperative stress testing (86); the culprit lesions are most probably unstable coronary plaques with only moderate (<60%) angiographic stenoses. Second, the perioperative period is characterized by a massive sympathetic stimulation and activation of the inflammatory immune response due to the stress of surgery and postoperative pain, resulting in postoperative hypercoagulability (87). Any medication which can reduce the hemodynamic, thrombogenic, and metabolic/inflammatory excessive stimulation might improve survival. Two main categories of drugs are in use for that purpose: antiplatelet agents and β-blockers.

Antiplatelet Agents

Three classes of antiplatelet drugs are in use for the prophylaxis of coronary artery thrombosis.

Aspirin or Acetylsalicylic Acid

The acetylation of cyclo-oxygenase-1 inhibits the production of thromboxane A2 and platelet adhesiveness. Although there are 20% of nonresponders, aspirin at 75 to 150 mg/day reduces cardiovascular events by 25% and postoperative MI by 50% (88,89). Higher doses (150–325 mg) increase the hemorrhagic risk but not the cardioprotection (90); doses above 350 mg tend to increase the rate of postoperative MI (89,91). The ability to reduce MI appears greatest in patients with evidence of sustained inflammation, an effect particularly relevant to the postoperative period (92). If the treatment is continued throughout the perioperative period, the hemorrhagic risk is slightly increased (2.5–10%) (93). These dosages do not contraindicate regional anesthesia, and epidural or intrathecal techniques can be performed safely (94). After MI, PCI or CABG ASA contributes efficiently to the prevention of recurrent coronary thrombosis and is a life-long therapy (83,95,96).

Clopidogrel

Clopidogrel is the only thienopyridine in use, because ticlopidine has been abandoned because of frequent gastro-intestinal (GI) upset and neutropenia. After an acute coronary syndrome, it reduces the incidence of infarction, stroke, and death by 27%, but increases the hemorrhagic risk by 25% when given with aspirin (97). It is mandatory during the period of re-endothelialization of coronary stents, which lasts from six weeks to six months, but is still beneficial up to 12 months (82). The treatment is moderately expensive (75 mg/day costs about €75 per month).

Antagonists Against Glycoprotein IIb/IIIa

Antagonists against glycoprotein IIb/IIIa decrease the risk of infarction and death from 22% to 2.5% after coronary stenting for acute coronary thrombosis (98). Three different substances are in use: abciximab (ReoPro®), tirofiban (Agrastat®), and eptifibatide (Integrilin®). The half-life of tirofiban and eptifibatide is only two hours, whereas it is 23 hours for abciximab. Therefore, platelet transfusions are necessary in case of operation within 48 hours of abciximab to prevent massive blood losses (99); in contrast, six hours after administration of tirofiban or eptifibatide, the hemorrhagic risk is not increased (100,101).

As bleeding is increased during operation under ASA (+10%) (92) or clopido-grel (+25%) (97), particularly if the patient is fully anticoagulated during surgery (+50%) (102), the routine is to stop the antiplatelet drugs 7 to 10 days before surgery. However, this practice is surprisingly dangerous. Among 1358 patients presenting with acute coronary syndrome, those who were recently withdrawn from oral antiplatelet agents (average 12 days) had an almost doubled rate of death (19.2% vs. 9.9%) or MI (21.9% vs. 12.4%) at 30 days (103). In this study, interruption of treatment was primarily a physician's decision for scheduled noncardiac surgery, and was a highly significant independent predictor of death and major ischemic events. Defective compliance or withdrawal of aspirin in patients with stable coronary disease has been shown to be associated with a fourfold increase in the rate of death compared with patients appropriately treated (104). It is also associated with a higher incidence of ST segment elevation coronary syndrome as compared to the patients who are still taking aspirin (39% vs. 18%) and with a 20% incidence of thrombosis of an uncoated stent implanted on average 15 months previously (105). Stopping oral antiplatelet drugs during the period of stent endothelialization may have dramatic consequences, with perioperative mortality rates from 20% up to 86% (13,27,73). Premature antiplatelet therapy discontinuation has been identified as the major independent predictor of drug-eluting stent thrombosis (hazard ratio 89.78), with a fatality rate of 45% (106). As the intra- and postoperative "acute phase reaction" is associated with hypercoagulability due to an increased platelet adhesiveness and a decreased fibrinolysis, it is not surprising that the risk of native coronary or stent thrombosis is particularly high when the protection of antiplatelet agents is removed (87). The question of antiplatelet drugs and surgery is more thoroughly discussed in chapter 15 (Urgent surgery in patients with severe coronary artery disease).

β-Blockers

β-Blockers are highly beneficial for ischemic patients because they abate the sympathetic reaction and improve the oxygen delivery/consumption ratio on many different levels. They decrease myocardial oxygen consumption (mVO_2) by decreasing heart rate and contractility; they increase O_2 delivery (mDO_2) by lengthening diastole; not only do they decrease the mechanical stress on unstable atheromatous plaques, but they also slow down the release of proinflammatory cytokines and endothelin E1 (107–109). They reduce the downregulation of $β_1$-receptors during the sustained sympathetic stimulation of chronic ventricular failure, therefore leaving the heart more responsive to epinephrine and norepinephrine (110). They decrease the incidence of arrhythmias. In clinical trials, all β-blockers without intrinsic sympathetic activity have been shown to decrease mortality and cardiac complications after MI (average decrease 24%) (111) and in chronic heart failure (average decrease 30%) (112). They diminish the incidence of ischemic events during and after CABG (113). As the cardioprotection they offer outweighs the reduction in heart rate and blood pressure they induce, particularly in the perioperative setting, it can be argued that the attenuation of postoperative inflammatory events, which cause progression of CAD, is a prominent component of their hemodynamic activities (114). Therefore, it seems logical that β-blockers would be very effective for attenuating the harmful and complex operative stress reaction.

The impact of perioperative β-blockade on cardiac outcome has been addressed in 12 controlled randomized studies totalizing 1070 patients, among whom 575 were β-blocked (3). Two of these studies have demonstrated impressive and much discussed results. The first one, published in 1996, examined the benefit of atenolol versus placebo in a cohort of 200 patients with or at risk of CAD scheduled for noncardiac surgery (15). Atenolol was started 30 minutes before anesthesia induction and continued for seven days after the operation. The risk reduction in the atenolol group was 55% for mortality and 67% for cardiac events; at two-year follow-up, the mortality was significantly lower (10%) in the atenolol than in the placebo group (21%); the combined rate of death and nonfatal MI was 17% and 32%, respectively. This study has been heavily criticized because of numerous biases (79): (i) The proportion of high-risk and intermediate-risk patients is unknown, but patients in the control group tend to have a more severe cardiac history. (ii) The in-hospital mortality has been excluded; the only adverse events taken into account are those occurring after hospital discharge. (iii) Some patients in the control group had their cardiac medication, including β-blocker, withdrawn when enrolled in the study. (iv) The full dose of atenolol was tolerated by less than 60% of the patients. (v) Females were underrepresented.

The second study investigated a particularly high-risk population: 112 patients with known CAD and new wall motion abnormalities (WMAs) on dobutamine stress echocardiography undergoing major vascular surgery (16). Bisoprolol was started more than seven days before operation and continued for 30 days after surgery. The mortality dropped from 17% in the control group to 3.4% in the treatment group, and the infarction rate from 17% to 0%, respectively. The study was terminated when it was apparent that the combined rate of death and MI was 10 times lower in the bisoprolol group (3.4% vs. 34%). The difference was still present at 36 months follow-up (12% vs. 48%) (115). Many criticisms can be raised against this investigation: (i) the selected population is at particularly high risk, and a complication rate of 34% in the control group is abnormally elevated, favoring the results of the treatment group; (ii) the number of patients is restricted because the study was terminated earlier than planned, the difference between groups could be biased by chance due to the small number of cases, and there is no proof that the same results would be repeated with larger numbers of individuals; (iii) the study is not double-blinded; (iv) and the standard care of the control group is unknown.

Despite these criticisms, a meta-analysis of 11 controlled randomized clinical trials has clearly shown the benefit of β-blockade compared to placebo (116):

1. Reduction in the incidence of intraoperative ischemia (7% vs. 20%)
2. Reduction in the incidence of postoperative ischemia (15% vs. 29%)
3. Five times reduction in the rate of MI (0.9% vs. 5%)
4. Four times reduction in the cardiac mortality (0.8% vs. 3.9%)

The amount of risk reduction by β-blockers is directly proportional to the incidence of MI in the studied population. The one study with nonsignificant risk reduction was conducted in an average-risk population undergoing intermediate-risk surgery (elective knee arthroplasty) (117), but the tolerated heart rate was 80 bpm and the treatment was of short duration (esmolol IV intraoperative and metoprolol 48 hours postoperative). The maximal efficacy is obtained when the heart rate is very tightly controlled and maintained below 65 bpm or 20% below the ischemic threshold on stress testing (16,118,119). It can be inferred from the present literature that any cardioselective β_1-blocker is an acceptable choice (atenolol, bisoprolol, metoprolol, esmolol). The β-blockade is more effective when started five to seven days before the operation to allow titration to the targeted heart rate (16,120). For the high-risk cases, it keeps its cardioprotective activity for a month and beyond after the surgery (115), but for low-risk cases, one week of treatment may be sufficient (120). The AHA/ACC has enthusiastically encouraged the use of β-blockers and has recommended (2) starting treatment one week before the day of surgery with a dosage progressively adapted in order to reach a heart rate of 60 bpm. The accepted contraindications to the preoperative treatment are (121): bradycardia, hypotension, AV conduction block, heart failure (EF < 0.35), and severe asthma. Selective β_1-blockers do not interfere with FEV1 in case of chronic obstructive lung disease, and the reactivity to β-stimulants is maintained (122). Peripheral arterial disease, even grade IV, is not a contraindication.

However, there remains a question: who should receive perioperative β-blockade? In other words: which category of patients benefits the most from β-blockers? A partial answer can be found in a retrospective study of 1351 patients scheduled for vascular surgery in which risk score was defined by seven factors: age over 70 years, current angina, prior MI, congestive heart failure, prior cerebrovascular event, diabetes mellitus, and renal failure (18). The combination of three categories of clinical score (no factor, <3 factors, ≥3 factors) and the results of dobutamine stress echocardiography (no WMAs, WMA in one to four segments, WMA in ≥5 segments) were used to divide the patients into five groups (Fig. 2). The first group comprises the patients with no risk factors; cardiac event rates were comparably low in patients receiving and not receiving β-blockers. The three intermediate groups were patients

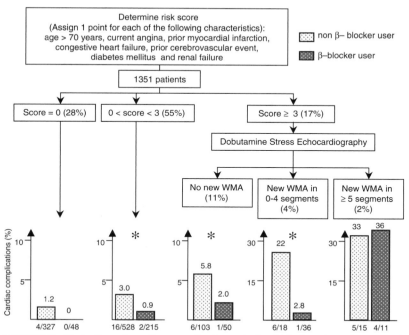

FIGURE 2 Reduction of cardiac complication rate by β-blockers in subgroups of patients with increasing ischemic risk. Numbers in brackets are the percentage of patients in each category of the 1351 patients. Numbers below the bars are the number of patients in each subgroup. Numbers above the bars are the percentage of cardiac complications in each subgroup. The two subgroups at right are on a different scale. Asterisk denotes statistically significant. *Source*: From Ref. 18.

with increasingly higher severity of CAD: fewer than three risk factors, three or more risk factors and no WMA, three or more risk factors and WMA in more than four segments. The protection offered by β-blockers increased in a parallel with the severity of the underlying coronary disease, with a 3- to 10-fold decrease in the incidence of cardiac complications in the β-blocked patients. Finally, the group of highest risk (more than three risk factors and WMA in more than five segments) showed no difference between patients receiving β-blockers or not, probably because these individuals require revascularization and not medical treatment; their cardiac complication rate during noncardiac surgery was between 33% and 36%. Although the numbers in some subgroups are too small to allow a robust statistical analysis, these data suggest that perioperative β-blockers are beneficial in all but subsets of very-low- and very-high-risk patients.

The enthusiasm for β-blockers is slightly tempered by recent evidence, suggesting that they do not benefit every patient, and might even be harmful to some. In a retrospective cohort of 663,635 patients from 329 hospitals, 122,338 of whom were β-blocked, the relationship between β-blockade and mortality, based on matching by propensity analysis, varied directly with the cardiac risk index (123). In low-risk patients (cardiac risk index score of 0 or 1), treatment was associated with an increased mortality. In intermediate- and high-risk patients (cardiac risk index score of 2, 3, and 4 or more), the adjusted odds ratio for in-hospital death were 0.88, 0.71, and 0.57, respectively. In this study, β-blockade was not assigned on random, and was confined to the period of hospitalization. It was presumed that patients who were treated on the first or second hospital day were given the drug for prophylaxis, but some of them might have received the treatment for actual ischemia, and this might incorrectly suggest that β-blockers are harmful in low-risk cases, because they were least likely to receive prophylaxis. Two other trials, smaller but prospective and randomized, did not find significant benefit from perioperative β-blockers in vascular surgery (124) or among diabetics undergoing major noncardiac surgery (odds ratio 0.83) (50).

Pending the availability of data from large prospective randomized trials, the evidence seems clear that perioperative β-blockers are effective in reducing morbidity and mortality of patients at significant risk for myocardial ischemia after noncardiac surgery, and should even be preferred to costly risk stratification and preoperative testing (125). However, one has to remember that these conclusions are based on a small number of patients (2309 patients) with a low total incidence of cardiac events (<10%). The meta-analyses are heavily influenced by the results of the study by Poldermans et al. (16,115), which shows a 10-fold reduction of mortality and MI. Interestingly, the risk reduction offered by the β-blockers in the cardiological studies on MI or chronic heart failure is much lower (20–30%) (111,112). The much higher reduction in the operative setting might be due to statistical biases and artifacts of small series, or to the peculiarities of the perioperative period with an important component of acute phase syndrome and systemic inflammatory response on which β-blockers might be influential independent of their hemodynamic effects (114). This dilemma may be resolved by the ongoing multicentric Canadian Peri-Operative ISchemic Evaluation trial (POISE) which aims to recruit 10,000 patients randomized to receive metoprolol or placebo for 30 perioperative days (126).

Meanwhile, the risk/benefit ratio is in favor of the use of β-blockers. Moreover, the cost effectiveness of the therapy is high because of the low price of the substances. The investment for treating one patient is $45, or 35 to 40 euros, but treating 800 patients should prevent 62 to 89 deaths or MI, costing $21,900 and $15,000, respectively (127). The global financial impact is a net gain of $500 per case (128).

Unfortunately, β-blockers are underused. In a Canadian survey (129), 93% of the anesthetists who responded were well aware that these substances were beneficial for the patient with known CAD. Nevertheless, only 57% used them in the operative period, and 34% for more than one postoperative week. This trend is confirmed by another study on patients requiring cholecystectomy who met the criteria for β-blocker therapy (130); of the 60% of the patients not already β-blocked before hospitalization, only 8% received a prescription by the anesthetist. Use of preoperative β-blockade among suitable candidates appears to be approximately 40% (131). These findings suggest that recommendations should be formulated for the preoperative consultations of the anesthetists, because a wider implementation of this therapy should benefit the patients at risk of, or suffering from, CAD. The place of β-blockade in the perioperative management of CAD patients is summarized in Figure 3.

Chronic β-Blockade

The situation is different when the patient is established on long-term therapy with a β-blocker. In these cases, vascular surgery is associated with an increased rate on

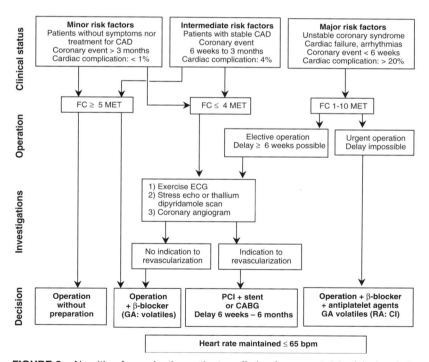

FIGURE 3 Algorithm for evaluating patients suffering from, or at risk of, ischemic heart disease. Coronary event: infarction, new angina, modification of previous angina, angioplasty, stenting, or CABG. Antiplatelet agents: ASA + clopidogrel. *Abbreviations*: FC, functional capacity; MET, metabolic equivalent—the cut-off point between 4 and 5 MET corresponds to the capacity of climbing two flights of stairs; PCI, percutaneous coronary intervention; CABG, aortocoronary bypass graft; GA, general anesthesia; RA, regional anesthesia (neuraxial blockade); CI, contraindicated; ASA, acetylsalicylic acid.

infarction compared to the non-β-blocked individuals (132). The incidence of peri-operative ischemia is not abated by chronic β-blockade (133). There is a lack of asso-ciation between chronic β-blockade and a 30-day cardiac death (134), but the risk of postoperative MI is significantly increased in the chronically β-blocked patients (odds ratio 2.14) (135). This apparent contradiction is probably linked to the fact that β-blockers are efficient as long as the heart rate is tightly controlled. In the above-mentioned studies, the heart rate was similar in the treated and in the control groups. Moreover, the patients already under β-blockade tend to suffer from a more advanced CAD than the nontreated patients. Another explanation can be found in the fact that the individuals receiving β-blockers on a long-term basis display upregulation of their β_1-receptors, which render them exquisitely sensitive to sympathetic stimula-tion. They respond by an excessive tachycardia and hypertension to the operative noxious stimuli (135). A strict control of heart rate is directly associated with a decrease in cardiac complications and death in patients suffering from CAD and in patients after vascular surgery (118,119). Therefore, the ongoing treatment must be continued during the perioperative period, and probably reinforced during the crit-ical periods by the administration of shorter acting drugs in order to keep the heart rate in the 60 to 65 per minute range. As the acute withdrawal of β-blockers is asso-ciated with increased incidence of cardiac events, it is not surprising to find an excess of cardiac complications up to fourfold if the treatment is interrupted in the periop-erative period (136).

Alternative Perioperative Cardioprotection

Other medications might be helpful in addition to the β-blockers or in place of them in case of contraindications, but most of them are less efficient in preventing cardiac complications.

The statins have three different effects: they lower the circulating choles-terol concentration, they stabilize atheromatous plaques, and they have an anti-inflam-matory activity. They are cardioprotective against ischemia in high-risk patients (137). In a retrospective study on 2816 high-risk patients undergoing major vascular sur-gery, atorvastatin reduced perioperative mortality and morbidity in a significant manner. The adjusted odds ratio for perioperative mortality among statin users as compared to nonusers was 0.22 (138). There was only one prospective randomized controlled trial on a small cohort of 100 patients scheduled for vascular surgery tak-ing atorvastatin or placebo on average 30 days before the operation (139); the inci-dence of cardiac events was more than three times higher with placebo (26%) compared with atorvastatin (8%); the six-month survival rate without infarction, angina, or stroke was higher with treatment (91%) than with placebo (73%). These results have been confirmed by a retrospective study on 780,591 patients undergo-ing major noncardiac surgery, among whom 9.9% were on statin therapy (140). Treatment was associated with a 40% reduction of risk for postoperative cardiac death (odds ratio 0.62).

The α2 agonists have been tested in 23 studies (3395 cases), one of which was the large European trial of mivazerol (1897 patients) (141,142). The summarized results of these studies show that mivazerol and clonidine reduce the episodes of intraoperative ischemia by 25% (relative risk 0.76) and cardiac deaths by 50% (rela-tive risk 0.47). They modify the incidence of postoperative infarction only in the sub-set of vascular surgery patients, where the relative risk of MI is 0.66 (116,141–143). A recent randomized study with clonidine on 190 patients for major noncardiac surgery disclosed a significant reduction of perioperative ischemia rate (14% with clonidine and 31% with placebo), and of mortality for up to two years (relative risk 0.43) (144). Clonidine has many advantages: it has sedative and analgesic properties, and reduces severity and incidence of postoperative nausea and vomiting. Its side effects include hypotension and bradycardia, but they occur in the same proportion as with β-blockers. It is the best alternative when the latters are contraindicated (143).

In a meta-analysis of 11 studies (1007 cases) (145), the calcium channel blockers have been found to decrease significantly the incidence of intraoperative tachyarrhythmias (odds ratio 0.52) and major morbid events (odds ratio 0.39), but only marginally the incidence of intraoperative ischemia. These effects were almost entirely due to diltiazem, whereas the other calcium antagonists were less efficacious. The postoperative infarction rate and the mortality were only marginally changed.

There are too few studies in noncardiac surgery to assert that nitrates could offer a protection to the ischemic patient. A prophylactic effect of intra- or perioperative nitroglycerin perfusion has never been proven (146,147). Nicorandil seems to have superior properties to nitrates, because it induces a pharmacologic preconditioning effect on the myocardium which is independent of the severity of ischemia (148). It has been demonstrated in a recent placebo-controlled, randomized trial that nicorandil decreases the rate of major coronary events in patients with stable angina (149), and has a protective effect against ischemic events during major abdominal surgery (150).

Although some substances have a cardioprotective activity, it should be mentioned that others have an adverse effect. Two classes of substances should be avoided because they abolish the cardioprotection of preconditioning: COX-2 inhibitors and sulfonylureas (151,152). They should be withdrawn one week before operation and replaced by other antiinflammatory drugs and by insulin, respectively.

ALGORITHM

Many decisional algorithms have been published during the recent years. The American College of Physicians has based its position on a meta-analysis of studies classified as strong, fair, or poor quality, and proposed an algorithm based on a modified cardiac risk index (1,153); vascular and nonvascular surgery are separated. Unfortunately, it was published before the major studies on β-blockade and the introduction of coated stents; this deprives it from much of its value. The American College of Cardiology/American Heart Association Task Force on practice guidelines have promoted recommendations based on evidence and expert opinions, and summarized them in an algorithm published in 1996 and updated in 2002 (2,19). Other authors have presented their own views on preoperative assessment and have suggested different decisional paradigms which are helpful for the physicians (3,41,154–157). Only the AHA/ACC guidelines have been prospectively tested (62,63,158). In a series of 459 patients undergoing vascular surgery, high cardiac risk ranking (hazard ratio 2.2), adverse perioperative cardiac events (hazard ratio 2.2), and age (hazard ratio 0.33) have been found to be independent prognostic factors for late mortality (63). Type of operation, urgency, noncardiac complications, and presence of diabetes did not affect long-term (five years) survival. Early adverse cardiac events are predicted by preoperative high-risk stratification or presence of severe three-vessel CAD, but not by results of stress imaging (65,158).

The algorithm we propose (Fig. 3) starts with the clinical evaluation of the patients and their stratification in three categories of risk (Table 1): low-risk (indicative of an increased probability of CAD), intermediate-risk (indicative of stable and controlled CAD), and high-risk (indicative of unstable coronary syndromes). Each category is then evaluated through the functional capacity of the patient (cut-off point between 4 and 5 MET, Table 2). For the high-risk category, however, the decision is governed by the possibility of a delay until noncardiac surgery or by the urgent character of the operation.

In elective cases, the algorithm proceeds with specific cardiological investigations such as stress testing or coronary angiogram, and leads to four possible decisions: (*i*) operation without preparation, (*ii*) operation under protection of β-blockade, (*iii*) postponement of surgery because coronary revascularization is indicated, and (*iv*) operation under β-blockade and antiplatelet agents without revascularization because surgery is vital and cannot tolerate the safety delays implied by CABG or PCI.

Patients with minor risk factors and good functional capacity can undergo any kind of operation without further preparation. If they have a poor exercise tolerance (4 MET or less) and are planned for a major operation, we propose that they should receive a β-blocker in the perioperative period. This is not based on strong evidence from the literature, but mainly on a principle of precaution, because the risk/benefit seems in favor of the treatment, as long as the patients do not suffer from severe ventricular dysfunction (EF < 0.35).

Intermediate-risk patients with good functional capacity should be operated under the protection of a β-blocker, as it is evident from the present clinical data (16,18,123); in the recent ACC/AHA Guidelines (159), these patients are considered as a Class IIb indication for β-blocker therapy ("treatment may be considered"); they are in a Class IIa ("treatment is reasonable") if they undergo vascular surgery. Class I indication ("treatment should be administered") is reserved for patients already on β-blocker or patients at high cardiac risk undergoing vascular surgery. Intermediate-risk patients should be investigated by stress tests only if they have a poor functional capacity or if they undergo a major operation. Coronary angiogram is performed as indicated by the results of the stress tests. If a revascularization is indicated, the operation must be postponed by three to six months (see "Previous revascularization"). Some situations, such as impending aneurysm rupture, disabling bone fracture, surgical bowel disease, or rapidly advancing cancer, cannot wait that long because the operation is vital; the patient must then be operated under the protection of β-blockade (18,123). In this case, one can argue that the cardiological investigations were useless because their conclusions cannot modify the therapeutic strategy, which is to perform the noncardiac surgery anyway.

Most of the patients in the major risk category need a revascularization procedure, which is a contraindication for surgery for six weeks to six months, depending on the technique used. Only vital and emergency operations are conceivable in these circumstances. As these patients are threatened by unstable plaques or thrombosis on a loss of continuity of the endothelium (recent PCI or CABG), it is safer to "protect" them with β-blockers and antiplatelet agents continued without interruption throughout the perioperative period, although there is no proof that β-blockers change outcome in the most severe cases (18). If a revascularization is absolutely indicated because of impending infarction, a simple angioplasty (PTCA) without stenting is probably the best choice, because it leaves the possibility to operate safely in a delay of two weeks (see Chapter 15).

These recommendations have not led to a decrease in the incidence of cardiac complications during the perioperative period, but to a decrease in hospital and medical costs, because the number of requests for stress testing and coronary angiogram decrease by 50%, and the indications for revascularization fall to 10% (63,158–160). As they tend to concentrate the cardiac testing on the small subset of high-risk patients who might benefit from coronary revascularization, they might increase the rate of scanning and coronary angiogram in these specific groups, like patients for abdominal aortic surgery (161).

CONCLUSIONS

The preoperative management of patients suffering from CAD is as important as the conduct of intraoperative anesthesia itself. By analyzing the risk factors of patients, their functional capacity, and the risk of the planned surgery, the anesthetist can decide not only if stress testing or coronary angiogram are necessary, but also if it is advisable to start prophylactic medication. It appears now that patients at risk can be protected from ischemia by β_1-blocking agents administered during the perioperative period. Three categories of patients should be β-blocked if they undergo more than minor procedures: all patients in the intermediate category of risk factors (stable CAD), and patients in the low category of risk factors (suspicion of CAD) if their functional capacity is decreased; in case of unstable coronary syndrome, like unstable coronary plaques or recent coronary intervention and stenting, β-blockade should be accompanied by perioperative dual antiplatelet therapy with aspirin and clopidogrel, because they are highly efficacious in preventing recurrent coronary thrombosis. There is clear evidence now that stopping the antiplatelet drugs increases significantly the risk of nonfatal infarction and death; it is even more so during the perioperative period when the platelet adhesiveness is increased and the fibrinolysis is decreased. Therefore, the usual practice of stopping antiplatelet treatment 10 days before operation must be revised. Low-dose aspirin must be continued throughout the operation; it does not preclude performing intrathecal or epidural anesthesia. Clopidogrel, if indicated during the period of re-endothelialization of a stent or for an unstable coronary syndrome, should not be interrupted, and only general anesthesia should be planned.

There is a dramatically increased risk associated with noncardiac surgery during the first six weeks after coronary revascularization; with the new drug-eluting stents, this risk is further increased to six months. The indications to revascularization are the same as in nonoperative setting. If a PCI is indicated, the type of stent must be adapted to the possible delay of noncardiac surgery. After CABG, as after uncomplicated MI, the safe delay before elective surgery should be undertaken is three months. However, each case must be individually considered and discussed between cardiologists, anesthetists, and surgeons, remembering that the risk of hemorrhage is usually easier to circumvent than the risk of coronary thrombosis.

REFERENCES

1. American College of Physicians (ACP). Guidelines for assessing and managing the perioperative risk from coronary artery disease associated with major noncardiac surgery. Ann Intern Med 1997; 127:309–312.
2. Eagle KA, Berger PB, Calkins H, et al. ACC/AHA guidelines update for perioperative cardiovascular evaluation for noncardiac surgery—executive summary. A Report of the American College of Cardiology/American Heart Association Task Force on Practice

Guidelines (Committee to update 1996 guidelines on perioperative cardiovascular evaluation for noncardiac surgery). Circulation 2002; 105:1257–1267.

3. Chassot PG, Delabays A, Spahn DR. Preoperative evaluation of patients with, or at risk of, coronary artery disease undergoing non-cardiac surgery. Br J Anaesth 2002; 89:747–759.

4. Ashton CM, Petersen NJ, Wray NP, et al. The incidence of perioperative myocardial infarction in men undergoing noncardiac surgery. Ann Intern Med 1993; 118:504–510.

5. Khuri SF, Daley J, Henderson W, et al. The National Veterans Administration Surgical Risk Study: risk adjustment for the comparative assessment of the quality of surgical care. J Am Coll Cardiol 1995; 180:519–531.

6. Badner NH, Knill RL, Brown JE, et al. Myocardial infarction after noncardiac surgery. Anesthesiology 1998; 88:572–578.

7. Baron JF, Mundler O, Bertrand M, et al. Dipyridamole-thallium scintigraphy and gated radionuclide angiography to assess cardiac risk before abdominal aortic surgery. N Engl J Med 1994; 330:663–669.

8. Hohner P, Nancarrow C, Backman C, et al. Anesthesia for abdominal vascular surgery in patients with coronary artery disease. Part I. Isoflurane produces dose-dependent coronary vasodilatation. Acta Anaesthesiol Scand 1994; 38:780–792.

9. Seki M, Kashimoto S, Nagata O, et al. Are the incidences of cardiac events during noncardiac surgery in Japan the same as in the United States and Europe? Anesth Analg 2005; 100:1236–1240.

10. Eichhorn E, Domanski M, Krause-Steinrauf H, et al. Beta-blocker Evaluation of Survival Trial (BEST). A trial of the beta-blocker bucindolol in patients with advanced chronic heart failure. N Engl J Med 2001; 344:1659–1667.

11. Yancy CW, Fowler MB, Colucci WS, et al. Race and the response to adrenergic blockade with carvedilol in patients with chronic heart failure. N Engl J Med 2001; 344:1358–1365.

12. Fox AA, Shernan SK, Body SC, Collard CD. Genetic influences on cardiac surgical outcomes. J Cardiothorac Vasc Anesth 2005; 19:379–391.

13. Kaluza GL, Joseph JJ, Lee JR, Raizner ME, Raizner AE. Catastrophic outcomes of noncardiac surgery soon after coronary stenting. J Am Coll Cardiol 2000; 35:1288–1294.

14. Marcucci C, Chassot PG, Gardaz JP, et al. Fatal myocardial infarction after lung resection in a patient with prophylactic preoperative coronary stenting. Br J Anaesth 2004; 92:743–747.

15. Mangano DT, Layug EL, Wallace A, Tateo I. Effect of atenolol on mortality and cardiovascular morbidity after noncardiac surgery. N Engl J Med 1996; 335:1713–1720.

16. Poldermans D, Boersma E, Bax JJ, et al. The effect of bisoprolol on perioperative mortality and myocardial infarction in high-risk patients undergoing vascular surgery. N Engl J Med 1999; 341:1789–1794.

17. Lee TH, Marcantonio TR, Mangione CM, et al. Derivation and prospective validation of a simple index for prediction of cardiac risk of major noncardiac surgery. Circulation 1999; 100:1043–1049.

18. Boersma E, Poldermans D, Bax JJ, et al., for the DECREASE Study Group. Predictors of cardiac events after major vascular surgery: role of clinical characteristics, dobutamine echocardiography, and beta-blocker therapy. J Am Med Assoc 2001; 285:1865–1873.

19. Eagle KA, Brundage BH, Chaitman BR, et al. Guidelines for perioperative cardiovascular evaluation for noncardiac surgery. Report of the American College of Cardiology/American Heart Association Task Force on Practice Guidelines. Circulation 1996; 93:1278–1317.

20. Eagle KA, Rihal CS, Mickel MC, et al. Cardiac risk of noncardiac surgery: influence of coronary disease and type of surgery in 3,368 operations. Circulation 1997; 96:1882–1887.

21. Hassan SA, Hlatcky MA, Boothroyd DB, et al. Outcomes of noncardiac surgery after coronary bypass surgery or coronary angioplasty in the Bypass Angioplasty Revascularisation Investigation (BARI). Am J Med 2001; 110:260–266.

22. Priebe HJ. The aged cardiovascular risk patient. Br J Anaesth 2000; 85:763–778.

23. Howell SJ, Sear YM, Yeates D, et al. Risk factors for cardiovascular death after elective surgery under general anaesthesia. Br J Anaesth 1998; 80:14–19.

24. VanBelle E, Lablanche JM, Bauters C. Coronary angioscopic findings in the infarcted-related vessel within 1 month of acute myocardial infarction: natural history and the effect of thrombolysis. Circulation 1998; 97:26–33.

25. Ueda Y, Nanto S, Komamura K, Kodama K. Neointimal coverage of stents in human coronary arteries observed by angioscopy. J Am Coll Cardiol 1994; 23:341–346.

26. Sattler LF. Recommendations regarding stent selection in relation to the timing of noncardiac surgery postpercutaneous coronary intervention. Catheter Cardiovasc Interv 2004; 63:146–147.

27. Sharma AK, Ajani AE, Hamwi SM, et al. Major noncardiac surgery following coronary stenting: When is it safe to operate? Catheter Cardiovasc Interv 2004; 63:141–121.

28. Morris CK, Ueshima K, Kawaguchi T, Hideg A, Froelicher VF. The prognostic value of exercise capacity: a review of the literature. Am Heart J 1991; 122:1423–1431.

29. Girish M, Trayner E, Dammann O, Pinto-Plata V, Celli B. Symptom-limited stair climbing as a predictor of postoperative cardiopulmonary complications after high-risk surgery. Chest 2001; 120:1147–1151.

30. Hlatky P, Boineau RE, Higginbotham MB, et al. A brief self-administered questionnaire to determine functional capacity (the Duke Activity Status Index). Am J Cardiol 1989; 64:651–654.

31. Older P, Smith R, Courtney P, Hone R. Preoperative evaluation of cardiac failure and ischemia in elderly patients by cardiopulmonary exercise testing. Chest 1993; 104:701–704.

32. Davies CT, Thompson MW. Aerobic performance of female marathon and male supermarathon athletes. Eur J Appl Physiol Occup Physiol 1979; 41:233–245.

33. Biccard BM. Peri-operative β-blockade and haemodynamic optimisation in patients with coronary artery disease and decreasing exercise capacity presenting for major noncardiac surgery. Anaesthesia 2004; 59:60–68.

34. Ferrara N, Longobardi G, Nicolino A, et al. Effect of beta-adrenoreceptor blockade on dipyridamole-induced myocardial asynergies in coronary artery disease. Am J Cardiol 1992; 70:724–727.

35. Weissman NJ, Levangie MW, Guerrero JL, et al. Effect of β-blockade on dobutamine stress echocardiography. Am Heart J 1996; 131:698–703.

36. McPhail N, Calvin JE, Shariatmadar A, Barber GG, Scobie TK. The use of preoperative exercise testing to predict cardiac complications after arterial reconstruction. J Vasc Surg 1988; 7:60–68.

37. Weiner D, Ryan TJ, McCabe CH, Chaitman BR, Sheffield LT, Fisher LD. Prognostic importance of a clinical profile and exercise test in medically treated patients with coronary artery disease. J Am Coll Cardiol 1984; 3:772–779.

38. Robotham JL, Takata M, Berman M. Ejection fraction revisited. Anesthesiology 1991; 74:172–183.

39. Paul SD, Eagle KA, Kuntz KM, Young JR, Hertzer NR. Concordance of preoperative clinical risk with angiographic severity of coronary artery disease in patients undergoing vascular surgery. Circulation 1996; 94:1561–1566.

40. Ryan TJ, Antman EM, Brooks NH. 1999 update: ACC/AHA guidelines for the management of patients with acute myocardial infarction: executive summary and recommendations. Circulation 1999; 100:1016–1030.

41. Tuman KJ. Perioperative cardiovascular risk: assessment and management. Anesth Analg 2001; 92:S106–S112.

42. Mizuno K, Miyamoto A, Satomura K, et al. Angioscopic coronary macromorphology in patients with acute coronary disorders. Lancet 1991; 337:809–812.

43. American Diabetes Association (ADA). Consensus development conference on the diagnosis of coronary heart disease in people with diabetes. Diabetes Care 1998; 21:1551–1559.

44. Cohen MC, Curran PJ, L'Italien GJ, Mittelman MA, Zarich ZW. Long-term prognostic value of preoperative dipyridamole-thallium imaging and clinical indexes in patients with diabetes mellitus undergoing peripheral vascular surgery. Am J Cardiol 1999; 83:1038–1042.

45. Fleisher LA, Rosenbaum SH, Nelson AH, Barash PG. The predictive value of preoperative silent ischemia for postoperative ischemic cardiac events in vascular and nonvascular surgery patients. Am Heart J 1991; 122:980–986.

46. Haffner SM, Lehto S, Rönnemaa T, Pyörälä Laakso M. Mortality from coronary heart disease in subjects with type 2 diabetes and in nondiabetic subjects with and without prior myocardial infarction. N Engl J Med 1998; 339:229–234.

47. Ruiz J, Keller U, Buillard C. Prévention et dépistage de la maladie coronarienne chez le patient diabétique. Bull Méd Suisses 2000; 82:306–310.
48. Grundy SM, Benjamin IJ, Burke GL, et al. Diabetes and cardiovascular disease: a statement for healthcare professionals from the American Heart Association. Circulation 1999; 100:1134–1146.
49. Juul AB, Wetterslev J, Kofoed-Enevoldsen A, et al. The diabetic postoperative mortality and morbidity (DIPOM) trial: rationale and design of a multicenter, randomized, placebo-controlled, clinical trial of metorpolol for patients with diabetes mellitus who are undergoing major noncardiac surgery. Am Heart J 2004; 147:677–683.
50. Juul AB. Randomized, blinded trial on perioperative metoprolol versus placebo for diabetic patients undergoing noncardiac surgery. Presented at Late-breaking Clinical Trials I, American Heart Association Scientific Sessions 2004, New Orleans, Nov 7–10, 2004 (abstract).
51. Hertzer NR. Basic data concerning coronary disease in peripheral vascular patients. Ann Vasc Surg 1987; 1:616–620.
52. Gersh BJ, Rihal CS, Rooke TW, Ballard DJ. Evaluation and management of patients with peripheral vascular and coronary disease. J Am Coll Cardiol 1991; 18:203–214.
53. Eagle KA, Rihal CS, Mickel MC, et al. Cardiac risk of noncardiac surgery: influence of coronary disease and type of surgery in 3,368 operations. Circulation 1997; 96:1882–1887.
54. Vanzetto G, Machecourt J, Blendea D, et al. Additive value of thallium single-photon emission computed tomography myocardial imaging for prediction of perioperative events in clinically selected high cardiac risk patients having abdominal aortic surgery. Am J Cardiol 1996; 77:143–148.
55. LeManach Y, Perel A, Coriat P, Bertrand M, Riou B. Early and delayed myocardial infarction after abdominal aortic surgery. Anesthesiology 2005; 102:885–891.
56. McFalls EO, Ward HB, Moritz TE, et al. Coronary artery revascularization before elective major vascular surgery. N Engl J Med 2004; 351:2795–2804.
57. Assadian A, Senekowitsch C, Assadian O, Ptakovsky H, Hagmuller GW. Perioperative morbidity and mortality of carotid artery surgery under loco-regional anaesthesia. Vasa 2005; 34:41–45.
58. Antman EM. ST-elevation myocardial infarction: management. In: Zipes DP, Libby P, Bonow RO, Braunwald E, eds. Braunwald's Heart Disease. A Textbook of Cardiovascular Medicine. 7th ed. Philadelphia: Elsevier/Saunders, 2005:1167–1226.
59. Rihal CS, Eagle KA, Mickel MC, et al. Surgical therapy for coronary artery disease among patients with combined coronary artery and peripheral vascular disease. Circulation 1995; 91:46–53.
60. Gottlieb A, Banoub M, Sprung J, et al. Perioperative cardiovascular morbidity in patients with coronary artery disease undergoing vascular surgery after percutaneous transluminal coronary angioplasty. J Cardiothorac Vasc Anesth 1998; 12:501–506.
61. Landesberg G, Mosseri M, Wolf Y, et al. Preoperative thallium scanning, selective coronary revascularization, and long-term survival after major vascular surgery. Circulation 2003; 108:177–183.
62. Back MR, Stordahl N, Cuthbertson D, et al. Limitations in the cardiac risk reduction provided by coronary revascularisation prior to elective vascular surgery. J Vasc Surg 2002; 36:526–533.
63. Back MR, Leo F, Cuthbertson D, et al. Long-term survival after vascular surgery: specific influence of cardiac factors and implications for preoperative evaluation. J Vasc Surg 2004; 40:752–760.
64. Cutlip BE, Baim DS, Kalon KL, et al. Stent thrombosis in the modern era: a pooled analysis of multicenter coronary stent clinical trials. Circulation 2001; 103:1967–1971.
65. Nalysnyk L, Fahrbach K, Reynolds NW, et al. Adverse events in coronary artery bypass graft (CABG) trials: a systematic review and analysis. Heart 2003; 89:767–772.
66. Birkmeyer JD, O'Connor FT, Quinton HB, et al. The effect of peripheral vascular disease on in-hospital mortality rates with coronary bypass surgery. J Vasc Surg 1995; 21:445–452.
67. Rihal CS, Sutton-Tyrell K, Schaff HV, et al. Increased incidence of complications among patients with peripheral vascular disease following coronary bypass grafting and angioplasty. Circulation 1997; 96:467–468.
68. McFadden EP, Stabile E, Regar E, et al. Late thrombosis in drug-eluting coronary stents after discontinuation of antiplatelet therapy. Lancet 2004; 364:1519–1521.

69. Glantz L, Ezri T, Cohen Y, et al. Perioperative myocardial ischemia in patients undergoing sternectomy shortly after coronary artery bypass grafting. Anesth Analg 2003; 96:1566–1571.
70. Breen P, Lee JW, Pomposelli F, Park KW. Timing of high-risk vascular surgery following coronary artery bypass surgery: a 10-year experience from an academic medical centre. Anaesthesia 2004; 59:422–427.
71. Huber KC, Evans MA, Bresnahan JF, et al. Outcome of noncardiac operations in patients with severe coronary artery disease successfully treated preoperatively with coronary angioplasty. Mayo Clin Proc 1992; 67:15–21.
72. Elmore JR, Hallett JW, Gibbons RJ, et al. Myocardial revascularization before abdominal aortic aneurysmorrhaphy: effect of coronary angioplasty. Mayo Clin Proc 1993; 68:637–641.
73. Posner KL, Van Norman GA, Chan V. Adverse cardiac outcomes after noncardiac surgery in patients with prior percutaneous transluminal coronary angioplasty. Anesth Analg 1999; 89:553–560.
74. Wilson SH, Fasseas P, Orford JL, et al. Clinical outcome of patients undergoing noncardiac surgery in the two months following coronary stenting. J Am Coll Cardiol 2003; 42:234–240.
75. Vicenzi MN, Ribitsch E, Luha O, et al. Coronary artery stenting before noncardiac surgery: more threat than safety? Anesthesiology 2001; 94:367–368.
76. Schwartz RS, Chronos NA, Virmani R. Preclinical restenosis models and drug-eluting stents: still important, still much to learn. J Am Coll Cardiol 2004; 44:1373–1385.
77. Carter AJ, Aggarwal M, Kopia GA, et al. Long-term effects of polymer-based, slow-release, sirolimus-eluting stents in a porcine coronary model. Cardiovasc Res 2004; 63:617–624.
78. Farb A, Heller PF, Schroff S, et al. Pathological analysis of local delivery of paclitaxel via a polymer-coated stent. Circulation 2001; 104:473–479.
79. Priebe HJ. Perioperative myocardial infarction—aetiology and prevention. Br J Anaesth 2005; 95:3–19.
80. Morice M, Serruys P, Souaa J, et al. A randomized comparison of a sirolimus-eluting stent with a standard stent for coronary revascularization. N Engl J Med 2002; 346:1773–1780.
81. Grube E, Silber S, Hauptman KE, et al. TAXUS I: six- and twelve-month results from a randomized, double-blind trial on a slow-release paclitaxel-eluting stent for de novo coronary lesions. Circulation 2003; 107:38–42.
82. Steinbuhl SR, Berger PB, Mann JT, and CREDO Investigators. Clopidogrel for the reduction of events during observation: early and sustained dual oral antiplatelet therapy following percutaneous coronary intervention: a randomized controlled trial. J Am Med Assoc 2002; 288:2411–2420.
83. Smith SC Jr, Dove JT, Jacobs AK, et al. ACC/AHA guidelines for percutaneous coronary intervention. A Report of the American College of Cardiology/American Heart Association Task Force on Practice Guidelines (Committee to revise the 1993 Guidelines for Percutaneous Transluminal Coronary Angioplasty). J Am Coll Cardiol 2001; 37:2239i–2239txvi.
84. Dawood MM, Gupta DK, Southern J, et al. Pathology of fatal perioperative myocardial infarction: implications regarding physiopathology and prevention. Int J Cardiol 1996; 57:35–44.
85. Ellis SG, Hertzer NR, Young JR, et al. Angiographic correlates of cardiac death and myocardial infarction complicating major non-thoracic vascular surgery. Am J Cardiol 1996; 77:1126–1128.
86. Poldermans D, Boersma E, Bax JJ, et al. Correlation of location of acute myocardial infarct after non-cardiac vascular surgery with preoperative dobutamine echocardiographic findings. Am J Cardiol 2001; 88:1413–1414.
87. Brown MJ, Nicholson ML, Bell PR, et al. The systemic inflammatory response syndrome, organ failure, and mortality after abdominal aortic aneurysm repair. J Vasc Surg 2003; 37:600–606.
88. Merritt JC, Bhatt DL. The efficacy and safety of perioperative antiplatelet therapy. J Thromb Thrombolysis 2004; 17:21–27.
89. Taylor DW, Barnett HJM, Haynes RB, et al. Low-dose and high-dose acetylsalicylic acid for patients undergoing carotid endarterectomy: a randomised controlled trial. Lancet 1999; 353:2179–2184.

90. Peters RJG, Mehta SR, Fox KAA, et al. Effect of aspirin dose when used alone or in combination with clopidogrel in patients with acute coronary syndromes. Circulation 2003; 108:1682–1687.
91. Robless P, Mikhailidis DP, Stansby G. Systematic review of antiplatelet therapy for the prevention of myocardial infarction, stroke or vascular death in patients with peripheral vascular disease. Br J Surg 2001; 88:787–800.
92. Ridker PM, Cushman M, Stampfer MJ, et al. Inflammation, aspirin, and the risk of cardiovascular disease in apparently healthy men. N Engl J Med 1997; 336:973–979.
93. Neilipovitz DT, Gregory L, Nichol B, Nichol G. The effects of perioperative aspirin therapy in peripheral vascular surgery: a decision analysis. Anesth Analg 2001; 93:573–580.
94. Horlocker TT, Wedel DJ, Schroeder DR, et al. Preoperative antiplatelet therapy does not increase the risk of spinal hematoma associated with regional anesthesia. Anesth Analg 1995; 80:303–309.
95. Ridker PM, Manson JE, Gaziano JM, et al. Low-dose aspirin therapy for chronic stable angina: a randomized, placebo-controlled clinical trial. Ann Intern Med 1991; 114:835–839.
96. Mangano DT. Aspirin and mortality from coronary bypass surgery. N Engl J Med 2002; 347:1309–1317.
97. The CURE Trial Investigators. Effects of clopidogrel in addition to aspirin in patients with acute coronary syndromes without ST-segment elevation. N Engl J Med 2001; 345:494–502.
98. Montalescot G, Barragan P, Wittenberg O, et al. Platelet glycoprotein IIb/IIIa inhibition with coronary stenting for acute myocardial infarction. N Engl J Med 2001; 344:1895–1903.
99. Juergens CP, Yeung AC, Oesterle SN. Routine platelet transfusion in patients undergoing emergency coronary bypass surgery after receiving abciximab. Am J Cardiol 1997; 80:74–75.
100. Dyke CM, Bhatia D, Lorentz TJ, et al. Immediate coronary artery bypass surgery after platelet inhibition with eptifibatide. Ann Thorac Surg 2000; 70:866–871.
101. Genoni M, Zeller D, Bertel O, et al. Tirofiban therapy does not increase the risk of hemorrhage after emergency coronary surgery. J Thorac Cardiovasc Surg 2001; 122:630–632.
102. Yende S, Wunderink RG. Effect of clopidogrel on bleeding after coronary artery bypass surgery. Crit Care Med 2001; 29:2271–2275.
103. Collet JP, Montalescot G, Blanchet B, et al. Impact of prior use or recent withdrawal of oral antiplatelet agents on acute coronary syndromes. Circulation 2004; 110:2361–2367.
104. Allen N, Kramer J, Delong E, et al. Patient-reported frequency of taking aspirin in a population with coronary artery disease. Am J Cardiol 2002; 89:1042–1046.
105. Ferrari E, Benhamou M, Carboni P, Marcel B. Coronary syndromes following aspirin withdrawal: a special risk for late stent thrombosis. J Am Coll Cardiol 2005; 45:456–459.
106. Iakovou I, Schmidt T, Bonizzoni E, et al. Incidence, predictors, and outcome of thrombosis after successful implantation of drug-eluting stents. J Am Med Assoc 2005; 293:2126–2130.
107. London MJ, Zaugg M, Schaub MC, Spahn DR. Perioperative β-adrenergic receptor blockade. Anesthesiology 2004; 100:170–175.
108. Duzendorfer S, Wiedermann CJ. Modulation of neutrophil migration and superoxide anion release by metoprolol. J Mol Cell Cardiol 2000; 32:915–924.
109. Garlichs CD, Zhang H, Mügge A, Daniel WG. Beta-blockers reduce the release and synthesis of endothelin-1 in human endothelial cells. Eur J Clin Invest 1999; 29:12–16.
110. Bristow MR. Mechanism of action of beta-blocking agents in heart failure. Am J Cardiol 1997; 80:26L–40L.
111. Freemantle N, Urdahl H, Eastough J, Hobbs FDR. What is the place of β-blockade in patients who have experienced a myocardial infarction with preserved left ventricular function? Evidence and (mis)interpretation. Prog Cardiovasc Dis 2002; 44:243–250.
112. Foody JM, Farrell MH, Krumholz HM. β-Blocker therapy in heart failure: scientific review. J Am Med Assoc 2002; 287:883–889.
113. Ferguson TB, Coombs LP, Peterson ED. Preoperative β-blocker use and mortality and morbidity following CABG surgery in North America. J Am Med Assoc 2002; 287:2221–2227.

114. Yeager MP, Fillinger MP, Hettleman BD, Hartman GS. Perioperative beta-blockade and late cardiac outcomes: a complementary hypothesis. J Cardiothorac Vasc Anesth 2005; 19:237–241.
115. Poldermans D, Boersma E, Bax JJ, et al. Bisoprolol reduces cardiac death and myocardial infarction in high-risk patient as long as 2 years after successful major vascular surgery. Eur Heart J 2001; 22:1353–1358.
116. Stevens RD, Burri H, Tramer MR. Pharmacologic myocardial protection in patients undergoing noncardiac surgery: a quantitative systematic review. Anesth Analg 2003; 97:623–633.
117. Urban MK, Markowitz SM, Gordon MA, et al. Postoperative prophylactic administration of beta-adrenergic blockers in patients at risk for myocardial ischemia. Anesth Analg 2000; 90:1257–1261.
118. Diaz A, Bourassa MG, Guertin MC, Tardif JC. Long term prognostic value of resting heart rate in patients with suspected or proven coronary artery disease. Eur Heart J 2005; 26:967–974.
119. Raby KE, Brull SJ, Timimi F, et al. The effect of heart rate control on myocardial ischemia among high-risk patients after vascular surgery. Anesth Analg 1999; 88:477–482.
120 Auerbach AD, Goldman L. β-Blockers and reduction of cardiac events in noncardiac surgery. J Am Med Assoc 2002; 287:1435–1444.
121. Smith SC, Blair SN, Bonow RO, et al. AHA/ACC Scientific Statement: AHA/ACC guidelines for preventing heart attack and death in patients with atherosclerotic cardiovascular disease: 2001 update. A statement for healthcare professionals from the American Heart Association and the American College of Cardiology. Circulation 2001; 104:1577–1579.
122. Salpeter SR, Ormiston TM, Salpeter EE, et al. Cardioselective beta-blockers for chronic obstructive pulmonary disease: a meta-analysis. Respir Med 2003; 97:1094–1101.
123. Lindenauer PK, Pekow P, Wang K, et al. Perioperative beta-blocker therapy and mortality after major noncardiac surgery. N Engl J Med 2005; 353:349–361.
124. Yang H, Raymer K, Butler R, Roberts R. Metoprolol after vascular surgery (MaVS). Can J Anaesth 2004; 51:A7.
125. Grayburn PA, Hillis LD. Cardiac events in patients undergoing noncardiac surgery: shifting the paradigm from noninvasive risk stratification to therapy. Ann Intern Med 2003; 138:506–511.
126. Leslie K, Devereaux PJ. A large trial is vital to prove perioperative beta-blockade effectiveness and safety before widespread use. Anesthesiology 2004; 101:803–806.
127. Schmidt M, Lindenauer PK, Fitzgerald JL, Benjamin EL. Forecasting the impact of a clinical practice guideline for perioperative β-blockers to reduce cardiovascular morbidity and mortality. Arch Intern Med 2002; 162:63–69.
128. Fleisher LA, Corbett W, Berry C, Poldermans D. Cost-effectiveness of differing perioperative beta-blockade strategies in vascular surgery patients. J Cardiothorac Vasc Anesth 2004; 18:7–13.
129. VanDenKerkhof EG, Milne B, Parlow JL. Knowledge and practice regarding prophylactic perioperative beta blockade in patients undergoing noncardiac surgery: a survey of Canadian anesthesiologists. Anesth Analg 2003; 96:1558–1565.
130. Siddiqui AK, Ahmed S, Delbeau H, et al. Lack of physician concordance with guidelines on the perioperative use of β-blockers. Arch Intern Med 2004; 164:664–667.
131. Rapchuk I, Rabuka S, Tonelli M. Perioperative use of beta-blockers remains low: experience of a single Canadian tertiary institution. Can J Anesth 2004; 51:761–767.
132. Sear JW, Foëx P, Howell SJ. Effect of chronic intercurrent medication with beta-adrenoreceptor blockade or calcium channel entry blockade on postoperative silent myocardial ischaemia. Br J Anaesth 2000; 84:311–315.
133. Sprung J, Abdemalak B, Gottlieb A, et al. Analysis of risk factors for myocardial infarction and cardiac mortality after major vascular surgery. Anesthesiology 2000; 93:129–140.
134. Sear JW, Howell SJ, Sear YM, et al. A nested case–control study of risk factors for perioperative cardiovascular death. Br J Anaesth 2001; 87:669P.
135. Giles JW, Sear JW, Foëx P. Effect of chronic β-blockade on peri-operative outcome in patients undergoing non-cardiac surgery: an analysis of observational and case–control studies. Anaesthesia 2004; 59:574–583.

136. Shammash JB, Trost JC, Gold JM, et al. Perioperative beta-blocker withdrawal and mortality in vascular surgical patients. Am Heart J 2001; 141:148–153.
137. Heart Protection Study Collaborative Group. MRC/BHF Heart Protection Study of cholesterol lowering with simvastatin in 20,536 high-risk individuals: a randomised placebo-controlled trial. Lancet 2002; 360:7–22.
138. Poldermans D, Bax JJ, Kertai MD, et al. Statins are associated with a reduced incidence of perioperative mortality in patients undergoing major noncardiac vascular surgery. Circulation 2003; 107:1848–1451.
139. Durazzo AES, Machado FS, Ikeoka DT, et al. Reduction in cardiovascular events after vascular surgery with atorvastatin: a randomized trial. J Vasc Surg 2004; 39:967–976.
140. Lindenauer PK, Pekow P, Wang K, et al. Lipid-lowering therapy and in-hospital mortality following major noncardiac surgery. J Am Med Assoc 2004; 291:2092–2099.
141. Wijeysundera DN, Naik JS, Beattie WS. Alpha-2 adrenergic agonists to prevent perioperative cardiovascular complications: a meta-analysis. Am J Med 2003; 114:742–752.
142. Oliver MF, Goldman L, Julian DG, et al. Effect of mivazerol on perioperative cardiac complications during non-cardiac surgery in patients with coronary heart disease. Anesthesiology 1999; 91:95–161.
143. Nishina K, Mikawa K, Uesugi T, et al. Efficacy of clonidine for prevention of perioperative myocardial ischaemia: a critical appraisal and meta-analysis of the literature. Anesthesiology 2002; 96:323–329.
144. Wallace AW, Galindez D, Salahieh A, et al. Effect of clonidine on cardiovascular morbidity and mortality after noncardiac surgery. Anesthesiology 2004; 101:284–293.
145. Wijeysundera DN, Beattie WS. Calcium channel blockers for reducing cardiac morbidity after noncardiac surgery: a meta-analysis. Anesth Analg 2003; 97:634–641.
146. Thomson IR, Mutch AC, Culligan JD. Failure of intravenous nitroglycerin to prevent intraoperative myocardial ischemia during fentanyl-pancuronium anesthesia. Anesthesiology 1984; 61:385–393.
147. Dodds TM, Stone JG, Coromillas J, et al. Prophylactic nitroglycerin infusion during noncardiac surgery does not reduce perioperative ischemia. Anesth Analg 1993; 76:705–713.
148. Matsuo H, Watanabe S, Segawa T, et al. Evidence of pharmacologic preconditioning during PTCA by intravenous pretreatment with ATP-sensitive K^+ channel opener nicorandil. Eur Heart J 2003; 24:1296–1303.
149. The IONA study group. Effect of nicorandil on coronary events in patients with stable angina: the impact of nicorandil in angina (IONA) randomized trial. Lancet 2002; 359:1269–1275.
150. Kaneko T, Saito Y, Hikawa Y, et al. Dose-dependent prophylactic effect of nicorandil, an ATP-sensitive potassium channel opener, on intra-operative myocardial ischaemia in patients undergoing major abdominal surgery. Br J Anaesth 2001; 86:332–337.
151. Munch Ellingsen JA, Grover GJ, Gross GJ. Blockade of KATP channel by glibenclamide aggravates ischemic injury and counteracts ischemic preconditioning. Basic Res Cardiol 1996; 91:382–353.
152. Forlani S, Tomai F, De Paulis R, et al. Preoperative shift from glibenclamide to insulin is cardioprotective in diabetic patients undergoing coronary artery bypass surgery. J Cardiovasc Surg 2004; 45:117–122.
153. Palda VA, Detsky AS. Perioperative assessment and management of risk from coronary artery disease. Ann Intern Med 1997; 127:313–328.
154. Fleisher LA, Eagle KA. Lowering cardiac risk in noncardiac surgery. N Engl J Med 2001; 345:1677–1682.
155. Hollenberg SM. Preoperative cardiac risk assessment. Chest 1999; 115:51S–57S.
156. Mangano DT. Assessment of the patient with cardiac disease: an anesthesiologist's paradigm. Anesthesiology 1999; 91:1521–1526.
157. Park KW. Preoperative cardiology consultation. Anesthesiology 2003; 98:754–762.
158. Back MR, Schmacht DC, Bowser AN, et al. Critical appraisal of cardiac risk stratification before elective vascular surgery. Vasc Endovasc Surg 2003; 37:387–397.
159. ACC/AHA 2006 Guideline Update on Perioperative Cardiovascular Evaluation for Noncardiac Surgery: Focused Update on Perioperative Beta-Blocker Therapy. A Report of the American College of Cardiology/American Heart Association Task Force on Practice Guidelines. Circulation 2006; 113:2662–2674.

160. Froehlich JB, Karavite D, Russman PL, et al. ACC/AHA preoperative assessment guidelines reduce resource utilization before aortic surgery. J Vasc Surg 2002; 36:758–763.
161. Licker M, Khatchatourian G, Schweizer A, et al. The impact of a cardioprotective protocol on the incidence of cardiac complications after aortic abdominal surgery. Anesth Analg 2002; 95:1525–1533.

7 Cardioprotection by Modulation of the Adrenergic System

Johannes Wacker
Institute of Anesthesiology, University Hospital Zurich, Zurich, Switzerland

Marcus C. Schaub
Institute of Pharmacology and Toxicology, University of Zurich, Zurich, Switzerland

Michael Zaugg
Institute of Anesthesiology, University Hospital Zurich, Zurich, Switzerland

INTRODUCTION

With increasing life expectancy and improved surgical technology, an increasing number of elderly patients with cardiovascular disease or significant cardiovascular risk factors will undergo major surgery. More than 5% of an unselected surgical population undergoing noncardiac surgery will suffer from severe perioperative cardiovascular complications including myocardial infarction and cardiac death. The incidence of adverse cardiac events may reach 30% in high-risk patients undergoing vascular surgery, causing a substantial financial burden of perioperative health care costs (1). In the United States of America, it is estimated that approximately 1 million patients suffer a major cardiac complication annually, including 500,000 myocardial infarctions. In the United Kingdom, there are approximately 20,000 deaths within 30 days of surgery every year, 9000 of which have a cardiac cause (2,3). Thus, therapeutic measures to lower the incidence of perioperative cardiovascular complications are justified.

Blunting the adrenergic response to the surgical trauma is an important aspect of anesthetic practice (4). Although moderate changes in sympathetic nervous system activity function as a servo-control mechanism and are required to maintain and optimize cardiac performance, undue liberation of substances such as catecholamines and inflammatory cytokines, particularly during emergence from anesthesia and in painful postoperative period, facilitates the occurrence of cardiovascular complications (5,6). The fight-or-flight-response becomes a hazardous and life-threatening maladaptation. The beneficial effects of antiadrenergic treatment in perioperative medicine have been confirmed in observational studies, meta-analyses (7–9), and randomized controlled clinical trials (1,10–14). However, the established concept of "sympatholysis" as an effective treatment modality needs refinement in the light of the new experimental and clinical findings. Sympatholytic protection implies annihilation of any type of adrenergic stimulation and should be replaced with "sympatho-modulatory" protection.

This chapter summarizes findings from large-scale heart failure trials, reviews the principles of adrenergic signaling in the myocardium, and discusses basic and clinical aspects of individual sympatho-modulatory therapies in perioperative medicine, including β-adrenergic antagonism, α_2 agonism, and regional anesthetic techniques. Implications of adrenergic genomics for perioperative medicine will be briefly outlined. The authors have previously reviewed these topics in articles in *Anesthesiology* and the *British Journal of Anaesthesia* (5,15–18).

ADRENERGIC ACTIVITY IN THE HEART: A DOUBLE-EDGED SWORD

Our understanding of the role of the sympathetic nervous system in the delicate equilibrium of health and disease has continuously changed over the last decades and should be briefly summarized. In 1960, increased adrenergic drive in patients with heart failure was regarded as a life-supportive adaptation because of the observed reduced norepinephrine levels in failing myocardium and the detrimental short-term effects of high doses of antiadrenergic agents (19). In the late 1970s, new findings led to a radical change (20,21). First, it was noted that chronic β-adrenergic antagonism increased survival in idiopathic dilated cardiomyopathies. Secondly, β-adrenergic receptor downregulation was recognized as a direct result of the excessive adrenergic drive. Thirdly, coronary sinus blood exhibited increased norepinephrine release despite decreased norepinephrine stores. These findings led to a new "counterintuitive" therapeutic strategy whereby antiadrenergic treatment was considered beneficial in the failing heart. This concept has dominated therapeutic thinking in cardiology for almost 20 years. However, recently results from basic science and clinical studies again questioned this dogma and called for further refinement of the concept (20). Moxonidine, a centrally active imidazoline/α_2 agonist, which lowers norepinephrine spillover and reverses remodeling in the myocardium, increased mortality by over 50% in the Moxonidine Congestive Heart Failure Trial (22). This is in accordance with experimental results from a canine heart failure model where dopamine β-hydroxylase inhibition resulting in decreased noradrenaline levels did not improve left ventricular function (23). Moreover, in the β-Blocker Evaluation of Survival Trial (BEST), bucindolol increased mortality disproportionately in African-American New York Heart Association (NYHA) class IV patients, although the overall benefit of bucindolol still prevailed in the whole bucindolol cohort when compared to placebo (24). It was suggested that excessive reduction in presynaptic norepinephrine release due to β_2-adrenergic antagonism, in conjunction with unopposed α_1-blockade, was responsible for the adverse effects of bucindolol. Irreversible withdrawal of adrenergic activity with the inability to recruit compensatory adrenergic drive when required to maintain adequate cardiac function is obviously detrimental. These changing therapeutic philosophies reflect the complexity of adrenergic activity and challenge the simple dogma of "sympatholytic equals beneficial." Also, these observations highlight the fundamentally different consequences of unselective inhibition of adrenergic drive, which may be achieved by central inhibition of sympathetic tone versus selective peripheral receptor-targeted blockade.

IMPLICATIONS FOR PERIOPERATIVE MEDICINE

Excessive adrenergic drive is a hallmark of the perioperative stress response. Maladaptive changes in the autonomic nervous system, such as downregulation of adrenergic receptors and autonomic imbalance, persist for weeks after surgery (25). Activation of the sympathetic nervous system, particularly β-adrenergic receptors, dramatically increases heart rate and oxygen consumption, and plays a central role in the development of perioperative ischemia (17). Patients with coronary artery disease, risk factors for coronary artery disease, or specific genetic polymorphisms may be particularly sensitive to catecholamine toxicity and prone to perioperative ischemia and cardiovascular complications. Current knowledge suggests significant selective inhibition and/or activation of specific alpha and beta receptor subtypes may offer protection from maladaptive adrenergic activity (5). At present, the pharmacological armamentarium is limited with respect to receptor-subtype selectivity. Identification of patients with genetic polymorphisms (see last paragraph of this chapter) associated with adverse outcome may improve patient management by allowing timely pharmacological intervention (26). As discussed in the following paragraphs, the usefulness of β-receptor antagonists in perioperative medicine rests on a limited number of studies with relatively small sample sizes. However, there is a substantial base of large clinical studies in the cardiology literature supporting the use of β-blockers in acute coronary syndromes, myocardial infraction, congestive heart failure, and arrhythmias. This does not exist for the α_2 agonists. In chronic heart failure, downregulation of β_1-receptor and upregulation of the inhibitory Gαi signaling protein (5,18), together with changes in the intracellular Ca^{2+} handling (27) lead to progressive contractile dysfunction. Contractile impairment is also found as an acute response during the perioperative period due to a variety of ischemia/reperfusion-injury-related mechanisms such as hibernation, stunning, and myocardial β-receptor desensitization (28). In fact, the markedly increased catecholamine levels found during cardiac surgery result in agonist-induced desensitization. Acute administration of a β-receptor antagonist in an open chest dog model of coronary artery bypass graft (CABG) surgery was shown to attenuate β-receptor desensitization (29). On the other hand, neither chronic oral nor intraoperative intravenous administration of β-blockers attenuated β-receptor desensitization in patients undergoing CABG surgery (28).

In summary, pan-adrenergic inhibition of the sympathetic nervous system may not be an optimal cardioprotective treatment modality in perioperative medicine, because irreversible removal of adrenergic support with the inability to maintain adequate cardiac function may be detrimental.

PRINCIPLES OF ADRENERGIC SIGNALING AND FUNCTION IN THE HEART

Acute and long-term regulation of myocardial function including heart rate, systolic and diastolic function, and metabolism is primarily governed by the β_1- and β_2-receptor signaling pathways. A functional role for the α-adrenergic receptors is less well established, although positive and negative inotropic effects have been attributed to specific α-receptor subtypes, particularly in cardiomyopathies and heart failure (18,30–35).

The human adrenergic receptor family consists of nine subtypes originating from different genes: α_{1A}, α_{1B}, α_{1D}, α_{2A}, α_{2B}, α_{2C}, β_1, β_2, and β_3. These receptors comprise seven trans-membrane α-helices and couple to signal transferring guanine nucleotide-binding G-proteins (G-protein-coupled receptors, called GPCRs) (18,30,36–40). The adrenergic receptors belong to a GPCR superfamily with over 1500 members (18,41–43). The three-dimensional structure has not yet been resolved for any of the GPCRs except for the bovine photoreceptor rhodopsin. Figure 1 shows a schematic representation of the predicted structure of the β_2-AR, based on its amino acid sequence homology with that of rhodopsin. All three extracellular loops between TM2–TM3, TM4–TM5, and TM6–TM7 are thought to contribute to ligand binding. Similarly, all intracellular loops as well as the C-terminal region are structurally involved in the interaction with the heterotrimeric G-protein complex. The GPCRs couple at the inner side of the cell membrane to the heterotrimeric G-protein complex (Gα, Gβ, and Gγ), of which Gα binds guanosine triphosphate (GTP). On receptor activation, the Gα subunit releases guanosine diphosphate in exchange for GTP,

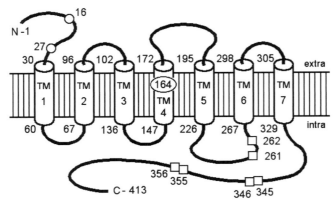

FIGURE 1 Predicted structure of the human β₂-adrenergic receptor based on protein sequence homology with the bovine photoreceptor rhodopsin, displaying the approximate location of the polymorphisms at amino acid positions 16, 27, and 164 (*circles*) as well as the serine phosphorylation sites (*squares*) for receptor desensitization by protein kinase-A (261, 262, 345, 346) and by GRK (355, 356). The seven transmembrane alpha-helices (*cylinders labeled TM1 through TM7*) contain around 30 amino acid residues each (number of first and last residues given for each helix). Agonists are thought to bind to the extracellular domains of TM3–TM4–TM5–TM6, while the Gα subunit binds to the first intracellular loop (between TM1 and TM2) and the carboxyterminal domain. *Abbreviations*: N-1, amino-terminal residue; C-413, carboxy-terminal residue; extra, extracellular side; intra, intracellular side. *Source*: From Ref. 16.

which causes dissociation from the complex leaving the βγ-subunits as undissociable heterodimer. Both the Gα as well as the Gβγ subunits can inhibit or activate a variety of intracellular effectors including ion channels, phospholipases, adenylyl cyclase (AC) isoforms, phosphoinositide-3 kinase (PI3K), mitogen-activated protein kinase (MAPK), and others. The downstream signaling pathways involve sequential protein phosphorylation cascades ultimately affecting targets in the cytoplasm or operating via transcriptional factors affecting the gene expression profile (Fig. 2 and Table 1). A second group of enzymes, the protein phosphatases, are responsible for dephosphorylation and termination of the signaling. Many signaling components contain multiple phosphorylation sites and phosphorylation may either stimulate or inhibit signaling depending on their specific localization on the protein. All intracellular signaling pathways are interconnected and form a robust network with considerable redundancy (for review, see ref. 18). A decrease in the stimulating agent (circulating hormones, or exogenously administered drugs) does not terminate receptor signaling at a clearly defined time point. Rapid signal termination is induced by desensitization of the agonist-activated receptor through specific phosphorylation (homologous desensitization) by a G-protein-coupled receptor kinase (GRK). Desensitization may also be achieved by phosphorylation via a specific serine/threonine-kinase in the absence of agonist occupancy. This heterologous desensitization is regulated by the signaling of another receptor via an intermediary second messenger that stimulates a particular serine/threonine-kinase like protein kinase-A (PKA) or protein kinase-C (PKC) (18,44). Desensitization may or may not be followed by internalization of the GPCR, which subsequently is either degraded or recycled back to a functional membrane receptor. The accepted paradigm for signaling of GPCRs holds that a receptor functions as a single unit (monomer), inde-

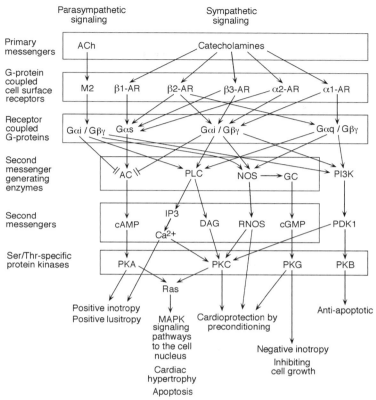

FIGURE 2 Simplified scheme of sympathetic and parasympathetic signaling cascades of GPCRs down to the level of cellular responses. Note the intimate cross-talk between the various signaling pathways. Lines with blunted ends (=) indicate inhibition. *Abbreviations*: AC, adenylyl cyclase; Ach, acetylcholine; AR, adrenergic receptor; cAMP, cyclic adenosine monophosphate; cGMP, cyclic guanosine monophosphate; DAG, diacylglycerol; GC, guanylyl cyclase; Gas, Gai, Gaq, Gbg, G-protein signaling components; IP3, inositol trisphosphate; M2, muscarinic acetylcholine receptor; MAPK, mitogen-activated protein kinase; NOS, nitric oxide synthase; PDK1, PI3K-dependent kinase; PI3K, phosphoinositide-3 kinase; PKA, PKB, PKC, PKG, target-specific serine/threonine protein kinases; PLC, phospholipase-C; Ras, small monomeric GTPase; RNOS, reactive nitric oxide species. *Source*: From Ref. 16.

pendently capable of coupling to a particular G-protein complex. However, recent reports on homo- and heterodimerization between GPCR subtypes suggest an additional receptor complexity that could account for previously unexplained pharmacological diversity (18,45,46). For instance, β_2-adrenergic receptors form homodimers that seem to be the agonist-induced active receptor species. Heterodimerization between β_1-receptors and β_2-receptors prevents agonist-induced internalization of β_2-receptors. Another interesting finding is that α_{1D}-receptors accumulate intracellularly and become only surface membrane targeted in smooth muscle cells when α_{1B}-receptors are coexpressed forming heterodimers with the α_{1D} species (47). Furthermore, functional interaction between β-receptors and angiotensin-II (AngII) type-1 receptor (AT$_1$) signaling described by in vitro and in

TABLE 1 Main Adrenergic Receptor Subtype Signaling Pathways and Functions in Nervous, Cardiac, and Vascular Tissues

Adrenergic receptor subtype	Main signaling pathways (compare Fig. 2)	Effects on nervous and cardiac tissue	Effects on vascular tissue
β_1	Gs–AC–cAMP–PKA	Positive effects on heart rate, inotropy, lusitropy, metabolism, growth, myocyte toxicity	
β_2	Gs–AC–cAMP–PKA, Gi-inhibiting AC, Gi–PLC–DAG–PKC, and G$\beta\gamma$–PI3K–PDK1–PKB	Positive effects on inotropy, lusitropy, metabolism, growth, myocyte survival Presynaptic stimulation of NA release	Relaxation of vascular smooth muscle cells
β_3	Gi-inhibiting AC, Gi–PLC–DAG–PKC, and Gi–NOS–NO–GC–cGMP–PKG	Negative inotropy and myocyte survival	
α_{1A}	Gq–PLC–IP3–Ca^{2+}	Positive effects on heart rate, inotropy, and growth in myocytes	Vasoconstriction
α_{1B}	Gq–PLC–IP3–Ca^{2+}		
α_{1D}	Gq–PLC–IP3–Ca^{2+}	Contraction of smooth muscle cells	Vasoconstriction
α_{2A}	Gi-inhibiting AC,	Presynaptically reduces sympathetic outflow	Lowers blood pressure
α_{2B}	Gi-inubiting AC and also G-stimulating AC	Postsynaptically counteracts the effects of α_{2A}	Vasoconstriction in the periphery
α_{2C}	Gi-inhibiting AC	Presynaptically reduces sympathetic outflow Postsynaptically lowers cAMP	Lowers blood pressure Participation in vasoconstriction after exposure to cold temperatures

Abbreviations: AC, adenylyl cyclase; cAMP, cyclic adenosine monophosphate; cGMP, cyclic guanosine monophosphate; DAG, diacylglycerol; Gs, Gi, Gq, G$\beta\gamma$ G-protein signaling components; GC, guanylyl cyclase; IP3, inositol trisphosphate; NO, nitric oxide; NOS, NO synthase; PDK1, PI3K-dependent kinase; PI3K, phosphoinositide-3 kinase; PKA, PKB, PKC, PKG, target-specific serine/threonine protein kinases; PLC, phospholipase-C.
Source: From Ref. 16.

vivo experiments reveals that β-blockers and AT$_1$ blockers each may gain dual control over these two signaling pathways (48). Because one of the receptors in the complex has to be free of antagonist in order to permit efficient coupling and signaling of the ligand-activated receptor, it may have a role in stabilizing the interaction of the activated receptor with its cognate G-protein. Thus, each antagonist not only blocks its own receptor but also the signaling of the reciprocal receptor by a transinhibition mechanism. These examples demonstrate the functional significance of GPCR dimerization, but this may just be the tip of the iceberg (for reviews, see refs. 49,50).

Different types of Gα-proteins stimulate (Gαs) or inhibit (Gαi) adenylyl cyclase, which generates the second messenger cAMP (Fig. 2) (18,30,39). cAMP activates PKA, which is responsible for an increase in intracellular Ca^{2+}, positive inotropy (enhanced contractile force), and accelerated lusitropy (hastened relaxation). Enhanced lusitropy is tightly coupled to positive inotropy in order to accommodate a faster heart rate by increasing the efficiency of the Ca^{2+}-pump of the sarcoplasmic reticulun (SR). β_1-Receptors exclusively couple to Gαs, whereas β_2-ARs may signal via Gαs, Gαi, and the Gβγ dimer. The diversity of signaling by β_2-receptors has been demonstrated in rodent and human hearts (51). The signaling of the Gαi complex is able to follow several different routes: (*i*) Gαi may activate phospholipase-C (PLC) resulting in generation of the two second messengers inositol trisphosphate (IP3) and diacylglycerol (DAG). DAG activates PKC, whereas IP3 releases Ca^{2+} from the SR. (*ii*) Gαi from the β_3-adrenergic receptor may stimulate endogenous myocardial nitric oxide (NO) synthase producing NO, which stimulates the guanylyl cyclase producing cyclic guanosine monophosphate (cGMP), which in turn activates protein kinase-G (PKG). This signaling pathway results in negative inotropy and cytoprotection. (*iii*) The Gβγ dimer from the β_2-receptor may initiate another cytoprotective signaling cascade involving phosphoinositide-3 kinase (PI3K), PI3K-dependent kinase-1 (PDK1), and protein kinase-B (PKB, also called Akt). This leads to increased expression of the antiapoptotic protein Bcl-2 and inhibition of proapoptotic factors such as caspase-9 and Fas-ligand (death factor) expression. The α_1-adrenergic receptor subtypes all signal via the Gαq–PLC–IP3–Ca^{2+} pathway increasing cytoplasmic Ca^{2+}, whereas the α_2-receptor subtypes inhibit AC by the Gαi component, thus lowering intracellular Ca^{2+}.

In general, the type-2 adrenergic receptors (α_2 and β_2) are found at the prejunctional site in the central and peripheral sympathetic nervous system, where activation of the α_2-receptor inhibits, and activation of β_2-receptor enhances norepinephrine release (Fig. 3 and Table 1). Presynaptically localized α_{2A} and α_{2C}-receptor subtypes are important in lowering sympathetic tone in the central nervous system as well as in decreasing norepinephrine release in cardiac sympathetic nerve terminals (31,34,52). In most effector cells such as cardiomyocytes, endothelial, or smooth muscle cells, type-2 adrenergic receptors are also present postsynaptically together with α_1, β_1, and β_3 receptors. Acute changes in myocardial function are, however, almost exclusively governed by the β-receptor signaling pathways. A functionally relevant contribution of α_1-receptors appears unlikely in humans under normal conditions. However, in

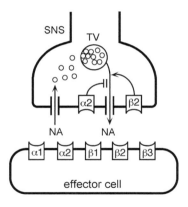

FIGURE 3 Schematic representation of adrenergic synaptic transmission in the central and peripheral nervous system as well as at the site of target tissues. The effector cells may comprise cardiomyocytes, smooth muscle cells, or endothelial cells. Line with blunted end (=) indicates inhibition. *Abbreviations*: SNS, sympathetic nervous system; TV, transmitter vesicle; NA, norepinephrine. *Source*: From Ref. 16.

heart failure, β-adrenergic receptors are desensitized and downregulated ($\beta_1 > \beta_2$), whereas the total amount of the α_1-adrenergic receptor subtypes remains constant or may be even upregulated. Under these conditions, the α_1-receptor-mediated inotropy may prove important (30,33,52,53). Although all three types of α_1-adrenergic receptor are expressed in the heart, the α_{1A} is the dominant subtype. Evidence from both in vitro and in vivo studies show that the α_{1A}-adrenergic receptor is the main subtype (around 90%) responsible for the sympathetic regulation of vascular tone and blood pressure (54,55). Some α_{1B}- and α_{1D}-adrenergic receptors can be found in different parts of the vascular system, but little is known about their specific function. No direct α_2-adrenergic receptor-mediated effects are discernible on the myocardium. Also, the negative inotropic effect of β_3-adrenergic receptor signaling mentioned above appears negligible under normal conditions (5,56). However, in the failing heart where β_3-adrenergic receptors are upregulated with concomitant downregulation of β_1-receptors, this negative inotropic effect may precipitate the deterioration of cardiac function. The heart rate is directly linked to β-adrenergic receptor signaling via the Gαs component which raises cAMP levels. Specific pacemaker channels reside in the sino-atrial node controlling heart rate and rhythm (57–59). These voltage-gated cation channels open during hyperpolarization following the action potential and allow sodium ions to enter the cell. This results in slow depolarization of the membrane until it reaches threshold level and elicits a new action potential. Stimulation of the pacemaker channels by sympathetic activity does not depend on phosphorylation but is induced by binding of cAMP to the channel protein. In contrast, stimulation of muscarinic acetylcholine receptors reduces cAMP levels via Gαi-mediated inhibition of adenylyl cyclase, so lowering the heart rate (Fig. 2). The presynaptic inhibitory α_2-adrenergic receptors are the main site of action for the nonsubtype-specific α_2-adrenergic receptor agonists clonidine and dexmedetomidine for the treatment of hypertension and postoperative pain. Some transitory peripheral vasoconstriction may be observed due to the postsynaptic α_{2B}-adrenergic receptor subtype (60,61). β-Adrenergic receptor blockers used as antihypertensive drugs may reduce sympathetic drive by dampening the signaling activity of presynaptic β_2-adrenergic receptors, whereas their cardioprotective effects are predominantly mediated at the peripheral postsynaptic receptor level by decreasing β_1- and β_2-receptor signaling in cardiomyocytes.

SYMPATHO-MODULATORY THERAPEUTIC STRATEGIES IN CURRENT CLINICAL PRACTICE
Cardioprotection by Systemic Medication

β-Adrenergic Receptor Antagonists
Basic Mechanisms and Cardiovascular Effects
Although some effects of β-adrenergic antagonists may be caused by central actions (62,63), the principal effect of these agents is at the end organ receptor level where they reduce β-adrenergic receptor signaling. This is fundamentally different from most of the α_2 agonists. Important mechanisms responsible for β-antagonist-mediated perioperative cardioprotection are (5):

1. Blunting of stress-induced increases in heart rate optimizing myocardial oxygen balance and stabilizing atherosclerotic plaques.
2. Improved Ca^{2+} handling and bioenergetics shifting ATP-production from oxidation of free fatty acid to less oxygen-consuming glucose oxidation.

3. Prevention of target protein hyperphosphorylation leading to decreased receptor desensitization and diastolic Ca^{2+} leakage by the ryanodine receptor.
4. Inhibition of β_1-adrenergic receptor-mediated cytotoxicity (altered gene expression, mechanical unloading, apoptosis, necrosis).
5. Antiarrhythmic effects.

In contrast to α_2 agonists, the untoward peripheral effects of β-adrenergic antagonists can be offset by counterregulatory production of endogenous catecholamines, explaining the good tolerability of this class of drugs (1,14,64,65). On the other hand, direct receptor blockade may be more cytoprotective under supramaximal autonomic stimulation (flat part of the sigmoid dose–response curve) than simply lowering catecholamine levels as observed with α_2 agonist treatment. Finally, selective inhibition of β_1-adrenergic receptor-mediated toxic effects leaves the beneficial effects of moderate β_2-adrenergic receptor stimulation unaffected and thus may further improve hemodynamic tolerance (5). Notably, β_1-adrenergic receptor antagonism enhances the inotropic response to β_2-adrenergic receptor stimulation (66). β_1-Adrenergic receptor blockade may increase postischemic and pharmacological coronary flow velocity reserve (67). Although many ancillary properties of individual β-antagonists are thought to be linked to clinical effectiveness and tolerability (68), their significance in perioperative medicine needs to be elucidated. The selection of a specific agent on the basis of individual drug profiles may be advantageous in specific clinical situations (Table 2). As with clonidine, β-antagonists improve the baroreflex sensitivity in elderly hypertensive patients, thus stabilizing blood pressure (69).

Clinical Aspects and Considerations

The evidence for the effectiveness of β-adrenergic antagonists in reducing perioperative cardiac events has been extensively reviewed (70). On the basis of the clinical evidence of mainly two well-designed randomized clinical trials (1,65), the perioperative use of β-antagonists is included in and supported by the updated (2002) Guidelines on Perioperative Evaluation of Patients Undergoing Noncardiac Surgery of the American Heart Association (AHA) (71). Mangano et al. (65) showed in a cohort of elderly male patients who had or were at risk of coronary artery disease undergoing major surgery (predominantly abdominal and vascular) that perioperative atenolol administration decreased long-term overall mortality by 55% and cardiac mortality by 65%. Comparing bisoprolol with standard care, Poldermans et al. (1) demonstrated a 10-fold reduction in the 30-day perioperative incidence of cardiac death and nonfatal myocardial infarction in patients with positive dobutamine stress echocardiography undergoing vascular surgery. Although these randomized clinical studies have been extensively criticized on a number of grounds (72), β-blockers represent the most effective treatment modality to prevent perioperative cardiac complications. According to the AHA guidelines, all patients on chronic β-blocker treatment, or who have definite coronary artery disease undergoing major vascular surgery, should be treated with perioperative β-blockade (Class I evidence for β-adrenergic antagonists). Other indications for the preventive use of perioperative β-blockers are less well supported by current evidence and need further clarification in randomized clinical studies. In an editorial accompanying an article by London et al. (72) on the physiologic foundations and clinical controversies of perioperative β-blocker treatment, Kertai et al. (73) recommended the widespread use of perioperative β-antagonist treatment in all surgical patients with only a single risk factor as well as the long-term continuation of such a treatment after

TABLE 2 β-Adrenergic Antagonists and Ancillary Properties

Drug	Selectivity ratio of β_1/β_2	Membrane-stabilizing activity	Intrinsic sympatho-mimetic activity	Lipid solubility	Clearance	Special
Propranolol	2.1	+	−	+++	Hepatic	Inverse agonist
Metoprolol	74	−	−	+	Hepatic stereo-selective	Inverse agonist β-AR↑
Atenolol	75	−	−	−	Renal	−
Esmolol	70	−	−	−	Erythrocyte esterase	−
Bisoprolol	119	−	−	(+)	Hepatic/renal	−
Celiprolol	~300	−	β2+		Hepatic/renal	β_2 agonist
Nebivolol	293	−	−	+	Hepatic	NO-release bronchodi lation
Carvedilol	7.2	−	β_1+(?)	+	Hepatic, stereo-selective	Antioxidant antiadhesive α_1-antagonist β-AR↓
Bucindolol	1.4	−	+(?)	+	Hepatic	α_1-antagonist

Abbreviations: NO, nitric oxide; +, effect present; − effect absent; ?, still under debate.
Source: From Ref. 15.

surgery. We would stress, however, that such high-impact recommendations should be based on more solid facts, namely randomized controlled trials. Some perioperative β-blocker studies have showed disappointing results without clear benefits [POBBLE Trial (74) and the Danish DIPOM⁺ (not yet published but presented as abstract at the 77th Annual Meeting of the American Heart Association)]. These recommendations should not be allowed to hinder future research in this important area and render the conduct of randomized controlled trials of perioperative β-blockade treatment impossible because of unjustified ethical objections and misconceptions about the currently available data.

Patients on chronic β-blocker treatment may need substantial perioperative supplementation. The currently recommended use of atenolol, bisoprolol, and metoprolol is cheap and safe if cautiously titrated (75). Whenever bradycardia occurs, it is important to discern whether discontinuation of treatment is really necessary. Although titration of β-adrenergic antagonists to individual ischemic thresholds using noninvasive stress tests appears rational, particularly with respect to side effects (12), it is hardly applicable in the clinical setting. (It would be too expensive and there are many patients with preexisting ST segment changes or left-bundle branch block that would preclude titration.) Also, the artificial conditions of noninvasive stress tests do not entirely simulate real perioperative conditions with significant changes in coagulation and cytokine release. β-Blocker therapy paradoxically decreases the ischemic threshold, and a heart rate of 90 beats per minute or even lower may represent a relative tachycardia (76). β-Blockers should be initiated as early as possible before surgery and maintained for at least one week (one month in vascular patients) after surgery, and tapered before discontinuation to avoid adrenergic withdrawal response. Administration of β-blockers should not be used instead of preoperative risk stratification and invasive interventions where unequivocally indicated (77). Alpha and beta adrenergic responses may be altered by downregulation and desensitization in sepsis, burns, cirrhosis, hemorrhagic shock, and cardiopulmonary bypass (78). Polymorphic metabolism of β-adrenergic antagonists may significantly affect clinical responsiveness. Accordingly, poor metabolizers with different variants of CYP23D6 (cytochrome P450 isoform) may have increased plasma levels of metoprolol (79). This is not the case for bisoprolol, which is independent of any genetic polymorphism of oxidation (80). Genetic background also appears to be responsible for observed variability in efficiency of β-adrenergic antagonist treatment in black and Asian patients (24). Finally, β-antagonists are of questionable value in heart failure patients with atrial fibrillation (81). Thus, it can be speculated that their perioperative administration in cardiac risk patients with atrial fibrillation might be of minimal or no advantage. Coronary artery disease represents a severe inflammatory process affecting the whole coronary tree ("pancoronaritis"). The territory of perioperative myocardial infarction is related only in 50% to the culprit coronary lesion or the site of the most critical coronary stenosis (82). Preoperative invasive interventions such as angioplasty or coronary surgery may therefore not replace but at most complement the protection afforded by perioperative β-blocker treatment. Coronary artery revascularization before elective vascular surgery does not significantly alter the long-term outcome in patients with stable cardiac symptoms (83). Whether the protection offered by perioperative β-blockade can be enhanced by additional administration of statins must be evaluated in future randomized controlled trials (84–86). Clinical studies of β-blockade in nonsurgical settings support the concept that bisoprolol might be more protective than atenolol. Perioperative β-blockade treatment should be used in accordance with available data obtained from perioperative randomized controlled trials.

Reluctant Use of Perioperative β-Blockers

Most anesthesiologists are aware of the promising results from recent perioperative β-adrenergic antagonist trials (87). However, many are reluctant to implement perioperative β-blockade their daily clinical practice. VanDenKerkhof et al. (87) conducted a questionnaire-based survey of members of the Canadian Anesthesiologists' Society with an overall response rate of 54%. Ninety-five percent of the responders were aware of the perioperative β-blocker literature, and 93% even agreed that β-blockers could be beneficial in patients with known coronary artery disease undergoing noncardiac surgery. In sharp contrast to this, however, was the fact that only 57% used prophylactic administration of β-blockers in these patients on a regular basis, and only 34% continued therapy beyond the early postoperative period. Only 9% of these anesthesiologists reported to have institutional guidelines for perioperative β-blocker use. Similar findings were obtained by London et al. (88) in an e-mail-based survey including anesthesiologists, surgeons, and cardiologists from 62 Veterans Affairs Medical Centers. Response rates in this study ranged from 40% to 60% depending on the specialty. Ninety-two percent of the responders agreed in that perioperative β-blockade could be effective in decreasing adverse short-term outcomes. However, only 60% thought that this would be the case for long-term adverse outcomes. Eighty-seven percent supported β-adrenergic antagonist use in patients with known coronary artery disease, but only 72% in patients with risk factors alone. There was a large range of opinions regarding the efficacy of perioperative β-blockade in various surgical settings as well as the proper timing of this therapy. In this study again, only 13% of the responders reported having institutional guidelines for perioperative β-blocker use. In both studies, methodological biases are likely to have affected the results. Nonresponders may have even less knowledge about the clinical use and possible benefits of perioperative β-blockade, and therefore tend to administer this treatment even less frequently. The frequency of withheld but indicated perioperative administration of β-blockers may substantially exceed the estimations by the authors of these surveys. Several causes may account for this. Controversy continues surrounding perioperative β-blockade (87,88), and many anesthesiologists advocate awaiting the results of larger-scale trials. Other concerns include possible side effects, unclear responsibilities for perioperative patient care, and lack of time. Taken together, these surveys confirm the results of previous studies, where perioperative β-blockade was established in only 30% to 40% of eligible patients despite the absence of clear contraindications (89,90).

Clinical and Economic Benefits from Perioperative β-Blockade

Lindenauer et al. (91) conducted a retrospective study of perioperative β-blockade in patients who developed postoperative myocardial infarction. Ninety-seven percent of the 72 patients with postoperative myocardial infarction were retrospectively identified as being at increased risk for cardiac complications. Eighty-one percent of these were ideal candidates for perioperative β-blockade (established indications present but no contraindication) but only 52% of these infarct patients received perioperative β-blockers. Another important finding of this study is the fact that patients, who developed postoperative myocardial infarction despite perioperative β-blockade, exhibited a markedly lower in-hospital mortality. This clearly supports the concept that β-blockade exerts cardioprotective effects in even highest risk patients with severe coronary artery disease by decreasing infarct size and related cardiovascular complications. The authors concluded that approximately 40% of the perioperative myocardial infarcts in this study could have been prevented by perioperative β-blockade.

In a retrospective cohort study, Schmidt et al. (89) tried to estimate the potential benefit of perioperative β-blockade on cardiac morbidity and mortality if existing practice guidelines were strictly applied. All adult patients treated over a one month period at a 550-bed community-based teaching hospital who were undergoing major noncardiac surgery but had no additional surgical procedures during the same hospitalization were studied. Of the 158 patients, 67 (42.4%) were "ideal" candidates for perioperative β-blocker treatment (established indications present but no contraindications). However, only 25 (37%) of these received a β-blocker during the perioperative period. By extrapolating these results, the authors calculated that between 560 and 801 untreated patients per year might have had benefited from perioperative β-blockade. The authors also calculated that in the hospital studied between 62 and 89 lives would be saved annually (at an overall cost of up to $40,210 for treatment with β-blockers) if β-blockers were strictly used in all eligible patients. This would result in yearly saving of additional costs related to cardiovascular complications in the range of between $318,000 and $463,000. Albeit retrospective in nature and based on simplified assumptions, this study provides new information on the clinical and financial impact of guideline-based administration of perioperative β-blockade.

Fleisher et al. (92) assessed the cost effectiveness of different strategies of perioperative β-blockade (among others Poldermans' and Mangano's schemes of administration) in elective aortic surgery patients using a "computer-based decision analytical model" including outcomes, their probabilities, and the costs of both treatment and outcome. One additional perioperative death was associated with additional health care costs of $21,909, whereas an additional perioperative myocardial infarct raised the costs by $15,000. Net hospital savings of $500 per patient were calculated if an oral β-blocker was used for a minimum of seven days in these patients. Importantly, all different strategies/protocols of perioperative β-blocker use were similarly effective. A strict administration of the life-saving perioperative β-blockade may have enormous clinical and economic benefits.

α_2-Adrenoreceptor Agonists (α_2-Adrenergic Receptor Agonists)
Basic Mechanisms and Cardiovascular Effects
α_2 agonists exert their cardioprotective effects predominantly by attenuation of catecholamine release and thus inhibition of stress-induced tachycardia. The hypotensive effect of this class of drugs is due to a lowering of central sympathetic tone via activation of α_2 adrenergic receptors and the pharmacologically less well-defined imidazoline1 receptors. This is consistent with the notion that clonidine is ineffective in controlling increased blood pressure in hypertensive tetraplegic patients (93). In contrast, bradycardic effects are elicited by vagomimetic effects, and are preserved in tetraplegic patients (94). Apart from their hemodynamic effects, α_2 agonists may induce analgesia (particularly in sympathetically maintained pain), anxiolysis, and sedation (95,96). Postjunctional α_{2B}-adrenergic receptors mediate a short-term hypertensive response via stimulation of L-type Ca^{2+} channels in smooth muscle cells of resistance vessels. Recently, etomidate was found to activate α_{2B}-adrenergic receptors thereby eliciting its well-known stabilizing cardiovascular effect (61). Prejunctional α_{2A}-adrenergic receptors have antiadrenergic effects, and postjunctional α_{2A}-adrenergic receptors have anesthetic effects via inhibition of L-type Ca^{2+} channels in neurons localized in the locus coeruleus and nucleus reticularis lateralis. Decreased ganglionic transmission and a concomitant increase of the counterregulatory vagal tone can further enhance the central effects of α_2 agonists (97). Interestingly, the antiarrhythmic effects of α_2 agonists are completely mediated via the vagal nerve, as antiarrhythmic effects are totally abolished by vagotomy (98). One of the potential advantages of central inhibition of sympathetic tone over peripheral receptor blockade is that the release of cotransmitters such as neuropeptide-Y, a major contributor to coronary vascular resistance, is equally suppressed. On the other hand, these neurotransmitters may exert trophic effects on cardiomyocytes. All α_2 agonists interact with imidazoline receptors due to their imidazole ring. Although the novel α_2 agonist moxonidine was developed to interact preferentially with imidazoline binding sites, it requires the α_2-adrenergic receptor to lower blood pressure because no hypotensive effects in response to moxonidine were observed in α_2-adrenergic receptor knockout mice (99). Similar to β-adrenergic receptors, α-adrenergic receptors can be up- or downregulated (78). However, their regulation and the subsequent physiological consequences have been poorly explored. Unfortunately, there are no subtype-selective agonists clinically available. At present, the most commonly used α_2 agonists are clonidine and dexmedetomidine. Their relative receptor specificities as compared to other α_2-As are listed in Table 3.

Clinical Aspects and Considerations
A recent meta-analysis on the efficacy of clonidine for the prevention of perioperative myocardial ischemia that included seven studies concluded that clonidine reduces cardiac ischemic events in patients with known or at risk of coronary artery disease

TABLE 3 α_2 Agonists and Specific Properties

Drug	Selectivity ratio of α_2/α_1	Selectivity ratio of $\alpha_2/I1^*$	Plasma half-life	Lipid solubility	Clearance	Special
Clonidine	40	16	9 hr	+	Hepatic/ renal	Sedative, analgesic, antishivering, antisialagogue, muscle relaxant
Mivazerol	400	215	4 hr	+	Hepatic/ renal	
Dexmede- tomidine	1600	30	2 hr	+	Hepatic/ renal	
Moxonidine	/	70	2 hr	+	Hepatic/ renal	

Abbreviations: +, effect present; I1*, centrally located imidazoline receptor-1; /, not known.
Source: From Ref. 15.

without increasing the incidence of bradycardia (8). Interestingly, this meta-analysis found a reduction in myocardial ischemia by clonidine in cardiac and noncardiac surgery, but only in the oral (mostly preoperative), but not the intravenous administration group. Mortality associated with myocardial ischemia was not evaluated because of the expected low number of myocardial infarctions and cardiac deaths. Another recent meta-analysis including studies with all α_2 agonists claims a lower cardiac morbidity in high-risk patients undergoing vascular and major surgery (100). Clonidine was found to decrease anesthetic-induced impairment of the baroreflex responses and thus to attenuate blood pressure lability (smaller hemodynamic fluctuations around a lower basal blood pressure) (101). Perioperative mivazerol has been reported to decrease perioperative ischemic events, and recently to decrease cardiac death (9.5% vs. 14% in placebo, $p=0.02$), but not myocardial infarction, in patients with coronary artery disease undergoing vascular surgery (11). However, this was a subgroup analysis and there was no effect of mivazerol on the incidence of all-cause deaths, cardiac deaths, or myocardial infarctions in the whole cohort of study patients undergoing all types of surgery. However, apart from their cardiovascular effects, α_2 agonists may exert indirect beneficial cardiac effects by their nonceiling analgesic, antishivering, and sedative effects (5). Sudden discontinuation should be avoided because of a serious withdrawal syndrome. Theoretically, α_2 agonists can jeopardize coronary flow reserve as intracoronary application of the α_2-antagonist yohimbine was shown to attenuate inhibition of coronary flow in patients undergoing coronary culprit lesion stenting (102). Conversely, α-adrenergic vasoconstriction reduces systolic retrograde coronary blood flow maintaining sufficient perfusion in subendocardial myocardium during adrenergic stimulation (103). Bradycardia as a side effect should be primarily treated with atropine, but higher doses of clonidine can markedly blunt the effect of atropine (104). Conversely, clonidine may significantly potentiate the pressor effects of catecholamines (105). At higher concentrations, α_2-As may promote coagulation (106). Collectively, there is currently less evidence for α_2-As than β-blockers for the prevention of perioperative cardiac complications. Although detrimental cardiac effects were reported after long-term use of α_2-As in heart failure patients, the short-term use of α_2 agonists at moderate doses in perioperative medicine can be advocated (thrombotic complications may be possible with high doses). Nonetheless, more selective modulation of α_2-adrenergic receptors would be highly desirable.

Cardioprotection by Regional Anesthesia
General Comments
Approximately one-third of patients undergo regional anesthesia for surgery. The anesthetic/analgesic power of epidural anesthesia has been illustrated recently by reports on coronary artery bypass grafting in awake patients under epidural anesthesia (107). In general, regional anesthesia more effectively decreases the neurohumoral response to surgery than general anesthesia, particularly with respect to the release of adrenal cortical and medullary hormones. Although some meta-analyses claim regional anesthesia and analgesia to be superior to general anesthesia with respect to cardiovascular and other outcome measures (deep vein thrombosis, pulmonary embolism, transfusion requirements, pneumonia and other infections, respiratory failure, renal failure, stroke) (7,9,108), most large-scale randomized trials have demonstrated that the choice of anesthesia does not influence cardiac morbidity and mortality (109–112). Hence, the currently available clinical data indicate that factors other than anesthetic technique are more important for cardiac outcome in even high-risk patients. However, uncertainty about the ultimate net benefits of regional anesthesia compared with general anesthesia will continue.

Spinal Anesthesia
Basic Aspects
Blockade of sympathetic nerves (T1–L2) and cardiac accelerator nerves (T1–Th5) can lead to sudden profound physiological changes during spinal anesthesia. The rapid distribution of the local anesthetic in the subarachnoidal space results in the blockade of all fibers of the anterior and posterior spinal roots including the sympathetic afferent and efferent fibers. Spinal cord penetration of the local anesthetic may also be responsible for specific anesthetic effects. The short diffusion path to small diameter B- and C-fibers makes them specifically susceptible to local anesthetic action. Much more than in epidural anesthesia and analgesia, the degree of sympathetic denervation is often unpredictable and quite extensive, albeit for a relatively limited time. The level of sympathetic blockade exceeds that of the sensory block, usually by two dermatomes, but sometimes by more than six dermatomes. The level of the block depends on age and position of the patient. Levels above T1 not only decrease venous return and thereby slow heart rate, but also abolish completely the sympathetic cardiac drive. Hypotension in spinal anesthesia is predominantly due to the marked fall in venous return followed by a decrease in cardiac output (20%) and stroke volume (25%). Systemic vascular resistance remains nearly unaffected (5%), as there is only little arteriolar dilation. In contrast to general anesthesia, no downregulation of lymphocyte β-adrenergic receptors was observed after cesarean section when performed under spinal anesthesia. The beneficial effects on β-adrenergic receptor preservation, stress response, and hemodynamics were also recently shown in patients undergoing coronary artery bypass grafting with a high spinal anesthesia as an adjunct to general anesthesia (113).

Clinical Aspects and Considerations
The incidence of cardiac arrest during spinal anesthesia is significant (1:10,000) and is thought to be mainly due to sympatho-vagal imbalance (114). Risk factors for cardiac

arrest under spinal (and epidural) anesthesia are: male gender, heart rate < 60 bpm, ASA Physical Status-I (i.e., healthy individuals!), β-blockade, age under 50 years, and sensory blockade above T6 (114,115). Marked hypotension may occur in 30% of patients and bradycardia in 15%. Prehydration, slow injection of the local anesthetic, and unilateral block may help to decrease adverse hemodynamic effects (116). Incremental continuous spinal anesthesia may provoke significantly less hypotensive episodes and ischemic cardiac events than bolus injection (117). Cardiovascular side effects may occur at all times during spinal anesthesia and even develop hours after surgery (118). The sympathetic denervation achieved by spinal anesthesia is fairly unpredictable, rather transient (except for continuous spinal anesthesia), and associated with a remarkably high incidence of hemodynamic instability and cardiac arrest.

Epidural Anesthesia and Analgesia
Basic Aspects
The dorsal and ventral roots are the primary sites of action in epidural anesthesia. However, local anesthetics can also cross the dura and penetrate the spinal cord. In general, sensory anesthesia is established prior to a sympathetic blockade, which is sufficient to induce systemic hypotension. Changes in blood pressure, heart rate, and cardiac output reflect the level of the blockade, but are in general less pronounced than in spinal anesthesia. With blocks below T5, there is rarely hypotension as compensatory vasoconstriction in unblocked segments occurs. In other words, the vasodilation below the level of sympathetic blockade is usually compensated for by vasoconstriction above the level of blockade, such that the decrease in blood pressure is relatively mild. Blockade above the level of T5 may affect cardiac fibers and no compensatory vasoconstriction may occur leading to marked hypotension, particularly in hypovolemic patients (119). Blockade up to T10 increases lower limb blood flow, but does not change coronary blood flow, provided there is no decrease in blood pressure (120). High levels of block (above T5) cause a decrease in coronary blood flow by up to 50% and an increase in coronary vascular resistance. However, as myocardial work is concomitantly decreased to a greater degree resulting in decreased heart rate and contractility, no adverse effects may be seen. Hypotension in lumbar epidural anesthesia may have the opposite effect on cardiac oxygen balance. Compensatory reflex activity in unblocked thoracic sympathetic segments may decrease coronary blood supply and provoke wall motion abnormalities (121). Hypotension in lumbar epidural anesthesia (T6–T12) may be therefore more critical in susceptible patients. Conversely, lumbar and thoracic epidural anesthesia have been reported to decrease left ventricular loading and improve global and regional ventricular function in patients with coronary artery disease. Thoracic epidural anesthesia also increases the diameter of stenotic coronary arteries (122). As with β-adrenergic antagonist treatment, there is a redistribution of myocardial blood from the epicardium to the endocardium blood flow in thoracic epidural anesthesia (123). The use of thoracic epidural anesthesia decreases ST segment changes and infarct size after coronary artery occlusion and may improve postischemic functional recovery (less stunning) (124).

Clinical Aspects
Thoracic epidural anesthesia has been reported to be effective in humans with myocardial ischemia refractory to conventional medical treatment, indicating that under specific conditions thoracic epidural anesthesia may be superior to antianginal medication (107). In patients with multivessel ischemic heart disease, thoracic epidural anesthesia normalized blood flow response to sympathetic stimulation.

Although some studies suggest that the use of epidural anesthesia with or without general anesthesia could improve perioperative cardiac outcome, there is currently little evidence from large-scale randomized controlled trials to support this view. Disappointingly, a large multicenter, randomized, unblinded study with 973 patients was unable to detect decreased 30-day mortality in patients undergoing abdominal surgery with combined epidural (thoracic or lumbar) and general anesthesia plus postoperative epidural analgesia versus general anesthesia alone (111). These findings reiterate the observations made by other investigators (125,126). However, postoperative epidural analgesia was found to significantly improve pulmonary outcome in a recent meta-analysis (108). Pulmonary dysfunction, stroke, acute renal failure, and acute confusion were also less frequently observed in patients undergoing CABG surgery when receiving postoperative thoracic epidural analgesia (127). In contrast to clonidine or dexmedetomidine, by inhibiting sympathetic spinal reflexes, thoracic epidural anesthesia can prevent bowel dysfunction after abdominal surgery and improve gastrointestinal recovery. High thoracic epidural anesthesia can also be used safely in patients with bronchial hyperreactivity (128). Although it has not been directly compared with respect to cardioprotection, lumbar epidural anesthesia does not appear to offer the same degree of protection. Serious complications including postdural puncture headache, neurologic injury, and epidural hematoma (<1:100,000) with paraplegia may be lower at the thoracic level. Overall, thoracic epidural anesthesia is a unique treatment modality combining effective pain relief with antiadrenergic properties. It also has the theoretical advantage of a lower cardiac complication rate in high-risk patients undergoing major surgery (129).

Combining Sympatho-modulatory Cardioprotective Strategies

Different antiadrenergic therapies affect the autonomic nervous system by different mechanisms and accordingly have different effects on hemodynamics (Table 4). The question arises of whether these treatment modalities should be combined to optimize cardiac protection. Some combinations such as β-adrenergic antagonists or α_2 agonists with regional anesthesia are occasionally used, but have not been

TABLE 4 Differential Hemodynamic Effects of Individual, Acutely Established Sympatho-modulatory Therapies

Parameter	Treatment				
	β-AA	α_2-A	LEA	TEA	SA
HR	⇓	⇓	⇓/⇔	⇓	⇓
BP	⇓	(⇑)/⇓	⇓	⇓	⇓
SVR	(⇑)	⇓	⇓	(⇔)	(⇔)
Afterload	⇓	⇓	⇓	(⇔)	(⇔)
LVEDP	⇑	⇑	⇓	⇓	⇓
CO	⇓	⇓	⇑	⇓	⇓
CVR	⇔	⇔	⇔/(⇑)	(⇓)	⇔/(⇑)
VO$_2$ myocardium	⇓	⇓	(⇑)	⇓	(⇑)
Arrhythmia	⇓	(⇓)	⇔	⇓	⇔

Abbreviations: β-AA, β-adrenergic antagonist; α-A, α agonist; BP, blood pressure; CO, cardiac output; CVR, coronary vascular resistance; HR, heart rate; LEA, lumbar epidural anesthesia; LVEDP, left ventricular end-diastolic pressure; SA, spinal anesthesia; SVR, systemic vascular resistance; TEA, thoracic epidural anesthesia; VO$_2$ myocardium, myocardial oxygen consumption; ⇓, decreased; ⇑,increased; ⇔, unchanged; ( ), variable.
Source: From Ref. 15.

prospectively evaluated with respect to cardiac outcome and adverse effects. There is sparse clinical and experimental data on efficacy and side effects of combined antiadrenergic treatments. A comparison between the effects of thoracic epidural anesthesia and β-adrenergic antagonists on hemodynamic parameters in conscious rats with acute myocardial infarction yielded intriguing findings (122). Thoracic epidural anesthesia decreased left ventricular end-diastolic pressure, and systemic vascular resistance remained unaffected; metoprolol in contrast increased both parameters. Heart rate and cardiac output were similarly decreased with both treatment regimens. Importantly, induction of thoracic epidural anesthesia during maximal metoprolol treatment did not cause any further hemodynamic changes (particularly no further decline in blood pressure). Similarly, in a clinical study evaluating the effect of thoracic epidural anesthesia (T1–T12) on cardiovascular function in patients with coronary artery disease receiving β-adrenergic antagonists, no further cardiac depression (decrease in blood pressure and heart rate) occurred (130). From this, it can be speculated that the favorable hemodynamic effects of thoracic epidural anesthesia may be synergistic with the cardioprotective effects of β-blockers. Good hemodynamic tolerance of β-blockers combined with epidural anesthesia was reported perioperatively in some clinical studies with small numbers of patients (1,13,131). Intrathecal and oral clonidine prolongs regional anesthesia and analgesia but increases the incidence of hypotension and bradycardia (60). Correcting epidural anesthesia-induced hypotension may provoke transient myocardial ischemia (121). Although the incidence of bradycardia and hypotension may be significantly increased with the combination of regional anesthetic techniques and β-blockers or α_2 agonists, there may be a net reduction in ischemic events and short- as well as long-term cardiovascular complications. However, this hypothesis must be evaluated in future randomized clinical trials. Combing β-blockers with α_2 agonists appears to be less useful except for α_2 agonists administered by the intrathecal or epidural route. An increased incidence of bradycardia and hypotension has previously been reported for mivazerol and dexmedetomidine administered alone (132,133), which may be worsened by coadministration with β-blockers. The combination of β-blockers and α_2 agonists is further complicated by the following additional observations. Coadministration of clonidine and sotalol annihilates the hypotensive effects and rather increases blood pressure, whereas propranolol and atenolol potentiate the hypotensive and bradycardic effects of clonidine in hypertensive patients (134). Notably, atenolol even more profoundly reduces blood pressure than the nonselective propranolol. Administration of prazosin (selective for α_1-adrenergic receptors) to clonidine further reduces blood pressure, but does not affect heart rate. Although clonidine is able to antagonize β-blocker-withdrawal, β-blockers may be dangerous in treating α_2 agonist withdrawal due to the pressure-raising effect of β-adrenergic antagonists during clonidine withdrawal. Overall, there is currently no evidence to support combining antiadrenergic treatments in perioperative medicine except for combining regional anesthetic techniques with β-blockers or intrathecally administered α_2 agonists. Owing to its simplicity, safety, and profound impact on basic physiological mechanisms in the heart, β-blockade remains the first choice for prevention of perioperative adverse cardiac events.

GENETIC MODULATION OF ADRENERGIC ACTIVITY:
THE NEW AGE OF HUMAN GENOMICS
Adrenergic Genetics and Genomics

Patient responses to β-blockers are often quite variable. This variability may have potent genetic determinants residing in the receptor proteins or in components of their downstream signaling cascades. Genetic heterogeneity not only constitutes the basis of the cardiovascular phenotype but also determines the course of progression of cardiovascular diseases (16,18). In contrast to rare mutations (<1%), polymorphisms are defined as having an allelic incidence of over 1%. Most polymorphisms (around 90%) concern one single base exchange within the genomic nucleotide sequence ("single nucleotide polymorphism" or SNP, pronounced "SNIP"). The human genome harbors about 10 million SNPs, or roughly one SNP per 300 bases (the total genome length comprises around 3 billion bases). The residual 10% of polymorphisms mostly represent insertions or deletions (indels) of nucleotide sequences with variable length. Owing to partial degeneration of the nucleotide code determining the amino acids in proteins (more than one nucleotide triplets coding for one amino acid), a particular SNP in a protein coding region (exon) may cause a change in amino acid sequence (nonsynonymous polymorphism) or may have no effect at all (synonymous polymorphism). In turn, a change in the amino acid sequence may have no consequence, or it may affect the protein function (uncontrollable loss of function or gain of function). A change of function potentially modifies the individual's responses to disease, environment (bacteria, viruses, toxins, chemicals), and therapy. SNPs in the noncoding regions (introns) often remain silent but, nevertheless, can also have distinct effects as well (see β_2-adrenergic receptor in following section). SNPs not causing a particular disease themselves may serve as a marker for disease loci on chromosomes, and thus help identifying the disease. Nonsynonymous polymorphisms have been found in seven of the nine adrenergic receptor subtypes (Table 5) (16,43,135). The effects of the individual polymorphisms are experimentally studied by heterologous expression of receptor gene constructs in cell systems in vitro as well as in transgenic animal models in vivo. Clinical findings, which correlate with experimental characteristics, have been described for a number of these polymorphisms (16,135–138). For some polymorphisms, however, clinical observations are not compatible with experimental findings, or appear even to be contradictory. A few examples are given to illustrate the link between clinical and experimental observations (see following section). Even where clinical and experimental findings appear contradictory, a detailed analysis of the effects of combinations of several polymorphisms occurring in one single gene, or distributed over more than one gene, may yield a mechanistic explanation for clinical observations. This arises when several allelic polymorphisms (some disease-related and some not) in series are inherited en bloc (136,139,140). Such co-inherited sets of polymorphisms are called haplotypes. A measure for the stability of co-inheritance of two given SNPs is their "linkage disequilibrium" (LD). In principle, the more distant two SNPs are located from one another, the more likely they become separated by chromosome recombination, i.e., they have a low LD. On the other side, more closely localized SNPs have a larger LD.

Stable haplotypes are generated by chromosome shuffling through repeated recombinations over many interbreeding generations (141). Today's extant haplotypes have been preserved over thousands of generations, and have thus survived hundreds and thousands of years. Relatively small numbers of all possible haplotypic SNP combinations have survived, whereas those harboring lethal disease traits

TABLE 5 Nonsynonymous Polymorphisms of Adrenergic Receptors

Receptor	Amino-acid position	Alleles coding for amino acids		Caucasians (%)	African Americans (%)	In vitro functional effects from studies on cell expression systems	Pathophysiological effects from human studies
		Major	Minor				
β1	49, near N-term	Ser	Gly	15	13	Gly49 enhances agonist-promoted down regulation	Gly49 allele is associated with improved survival
	389, in Gs-coupling domain	Arg	Gly	27	42	Arg389 strongly stimulates AC, Gly389 impairs Gs-coupling	Arg389 risk for heart failure only in combination with α_{2C} Del322–325
β2	16, near N-term	Gly	Arg	39	50	Gly16 enhances agonist-promoted downregulation	Gly16 segregates with hyper-tension (see text for discussion)
	27, near N-term	Gln	Glu	43	27	Glu27 resistant to agonist-promoted down regulation	Glu27 segregates with hyper-tension (see text for discussion)
	164, in the fourth transmembrane domain	Thr	Ile	2–5	2–5	Ile164 impairs coupling to the stimulatory Gs-protein	Heterozygous Ile164 entails rapid progression of heart failure with significant decrease of survival

β_3	64, end of first transmembrane domain	Trp	Arg	10	?	Arg64 possibly displays lower G-protein coupling	Arg64 may be involved in obesity and type-2 diabetes, relevance for the heart not well established
α_{1A}	492, near C-term	Cys	Arg	46	70	Similar pharmacological and functional characteristics	Similar prevalence of each polymorphic allele in various diseases
α_{2A}	251, in the third intracellular loop	Asn	Lys	0.4	5	Lys251, a rare polymorphism, enhanced Gi-coupling-function	Centrally mediated hypotension
α_{2B}	301–303, Glu–Glu–Glu	No deletion	Deletion	31	12	Only partially phosphorylatable, resistant to desensitization	Increased vasoconstriction, risk for coronary events when homozygous
α_{2C}	322–325, Gly–Ala–Gly–Pro	No deletion	Deletion	4	38	Control of basal NE release, impaired Gi-coupling	Risk for idiopathic and ischemic cardiomyopathies (homozygous)

Abbreviations: AC, adenylyl cyclase; Ala, alanine; Arg, arginine; Asn, asparagine; C-term, carboxyl-terminal residue; Cys, cysteine; Gln, glutamine; Glu, glutamic acid; Gly, glycine; Gs, Gi, G-protein signaling components; Ile, isoleucine; Lys, lysine; N-term, amino-terminal residue; NE, norepinephrine; Pro, proline; Ser, serine; Thr, threonine; Trp, tryptophan.
Source: From Ref. 16.

must have been eliminated (see β_2-adrenergic receptor in following section). The International HapMap Consortium prepares a catalogue (HapMap) of common haplotypes containing specified SNPs and other genetic variants as markers, which enables the genome-wide search for disease-related mutations (141). The HapMap covers samples from populations with ancestry from parts of Africa, Asia, and Europe. This strategy will allow for individual genetic characterization by screening some 300,000 to 600,000 SNPs, which is far fewer than the 10 million common SNPs in the human genome.

Clinically Relevant Polymorphisms

Correspondence exists between experimental and clinical observations for the 301–303 deletion of the postsynaptic α_{2B}-adrenergic receptor (Table 5). Impaired phosphorylation due to the loss of three glutamine residues from the third intracellular loop results in an increased resistance against desensitization. The enhanced signaling reinforces peripheral vasoconstriction (counteracting the vasodilatatory effect of the presynaptic α_{2A}-adrenergic receptor) producing an increased risk for coronary episodes, especially in the case of homozygotes (43,142). The resistance of α_{2B}-adrenergic receptor to desensibilization only becomes manifest during acute bouts of increased sympathetic tone, and is not associated with essential hypertension.

The 322–325 deletion (loss of four amino acid residues from the third intracellular loop) in the presynaptic α_{2C}-adrenergic receptor reduces its coupling to the Gi-protein resulting in increased activity of the adenylyl cyclase (increased release of norepinephrine in presynaptic nerve endings) with its cardiotoxic profile akin to the stimulation pattern of β_1-adrenergic receptor (43,136). Homozygotes are at a significant risk for early onset and progression of heart failure. The variable penetrance of the α_{2C}-deletion in heart failure and its 38% presence in Afro-Americans versus only 4% in Caucasian Americans (Table 5) suggested that haplotype variance could be implicated as well. Indeed, 20 polymorphisms were found in a multiethnic population, encompassing the promoter in the 5'-untranslated region (UTR), the coding sequence, and a stretch in the 3'-UTR downstream of the gene. These polymorphisms occur in 24 distinct haplotypes with complex organization and as yet ill-defined functions. Whole-gene transfection studies in human neuronal cells indicate that expression-specific haplotypes may amplify, attenuate, or dominate the cardiomyopathic effect attributed to the α_{2C}-deletion (136). Further studies are required for characterization of specific haplotype functions. Combination with the α_{2C} 322–325 deletion of arginine at position 389 in the β_1-adrenergic receptor greatly increases the heart failure risk (see here below).

In the β_1-adrenergic receptor common coding polymorphisms occur in amino acid positions 49 and 389 (43,137). The β_1-Glycine49 (instead of serine) receptor displays enhanced agonist-promoted downregulation in vitro because its interaction with the stimulatory Gs-protein is weakened, and, consequently has proved to be a protective genotype (Table 5). The β_1-Arginine389 polymorphism exhibits enhanced function (enhanced coupling to the Gs-protein) compared to β_1-Glycine389, and thus may influence heart failure progression. However, a robust relationship between haplotypes consisting of the polymorphic combination at positions 49 and 389 renders genotype interpretations more difficult (43). The gene–gene interaction between the β_1-Arginine389 and the α_{2C} 322–325 deletion alleles results from synergistic actions of the two variants leading to an enhanced risk for heart failure with an odds ratio of around 10 (43).

The β_2-adrenergic receptor has three clinically relevant sites of variation, at amino acids 16, 27, and 164 (Table 5) (16,43). The isoleucine164 variant displays marked dysfunction in heterozygous subjects. Experimentally, it is characterized by reduced coupling to the Gs-protein resulting in reduced activity of adenylyl cyclase. In the healthy myocardium, β_2-adrenergic receptors account for 20% to 30% of all β-adrenergic receptors (18). In failing hearts where the β_1-adrenergic receptors are significantly downregulated with not much change in the β_2-receptor content, the impaired β_2-isoleucine164 contributes to systolic dysfunction, reduced cardioprotection, and thus precipitates development of overt heart failure (43,143). Homozygosity for β_2-isoleucine164 has never been found. These findings are indicative of the β_2-adrenergic receptors playing a decisive role not only in the vascular smooth muscle, but also in the myocardium (18).

As the β_2-adrenergic receptor polymorphisms at positions glycine16arginine and glutamine27glutamate have less pronounced effects than that of threonine164isoleucine (Table 5), the correspondence between experimental and clinical findings is more difficult to establish (43,137,138). Here we encounter a case where, at first sight, experimental and clinical observations appear contradictory. Both positions, 16 and 27, contribute to cardiac function as well as to the long-term development of essential hypertension. At position 16, glycine imparts enhanced agonist-promoted downregulation, regardless of whether glutamine or glutamate occupies position 27 (144). Although the arginine16–glutamate27 combination displays less downregulation in vitro, this particular combination either never occurs or is very uncommon in humans. Therefore, position 16 seems to control the downregulation phenotype of the genotype combinations observed in humans. If the β_2-adrenergic receptor is beneficial in heart failure, the arginine16 variant would be the favorable genotype because it undergoes less downregulation than glycine16. Correspondingly, glycine instead of arginine at position 16 is associated with higher blood pressure and risk of heart disease. However, analysis of haplotype occurrence for the β_2-adrenergic receptor modifies this simplified picture (43,140,145). A mechanistic explanation of the observations in the clinical setting may be the strict co-inheritance of distinct alleles, each of which has characteristic effects on its own, but in combination produce a new phenotype.

Eight of 13 SNPs are located in the promoter region upstream of the start codon (nucleotide triplet ATG), whereas the reminder five SNPs reside in the first half of the β_2-adrenergic receptor coding gene. This 5'-UTR comprises several putative *cis*-acting regulatory elements including a short stretch with an open reading frame coding for an expression regulating peptide (ERP) of 19 amino acids. One polymorphism concerns the last amino acid residue of ERP, changing it from cysteine (homozygous in 30%) to arginine (homozygous in 13%), with the remainder being heterozygous. Thus, the allele frequency is 0.63 for cysteine and 0.37 for arginine in a Caucasian population without acute or chronic heart disease. Expression of β_2-adrenergic receptor in a cell culture system is almost half that with the arginine-containing ERP compared with the cysteine-containing ERP. In a subject carrying the β_2-glycine16 variant favoring receptor downregulation, this effect may be offset by receptor upregulation in combination with the cysteine-containing ERP, or else, may be aggravated by receptor downregulation in combination with the arginine-containing ERP. Both these combinations occur among the most common β_2-adrenergic receptor haplotypes with varying frequencies in different ethnic groups (16,43). Interestingly, out of the 8192 possible haplotypic allele combinations with the 13 SNPs mentioned above, only 12 are found in humans, with four being common, and the remainder eight being rare. Thus, over 8000 possible β_2-adrenergic receptor haplotypes must be incompatible with life and have been removed.

What Can We Learn from Adrenergic Genomics?

A recent survey of several studies on β-blocker treatment of heart failure (including V-HeFT1, V-HeFT2, SOLVD, US-Carv, BEST, MERIT-HF) indicates that the Afro-Americans exhibit on average a blood pressure over 60% higher than non-Afro-Americans (146). On the other hand, non-Afro-Americans suffered over 90% more often from coronary artery disease than the Afro-Americans. Nevertheless, with regard to all mortality, both ethnic groups similarly benefited from the treatment with β-adrenergic antagonists or ACE inhibitors, even though in the Afro-American patients the blood pressure reduction was less. In the BEST study, bucindolol significantly increased mortality among Afro-Americans, whereas a tendency of mortality reduction was apparent among the non-Afro-Americans at termination of the study after two years. As discussed recently, in view of the genotypic variability, we advocate clinical studies with genotyped individuals (16). Large population studies without knowledge of the genetic context may fail to identify most effective treatment modalities. Pharmacogenetic testing has so far mainly focused on pharmacokinetic mechanisms involving the large families of drug metabolizing enzymes (146). However, pharmacodynamic mechanisms appear now to account for most of the cardiovascular variations in response to drug therapy. The technical feasibility of a genome-wide search for relevant polymorphisms at affordable costs will help to individualize drug therapy for maximizing efficacy and limiting toxicity in the future.

CONCLUSIONS

Insight into complex sympathetic regulatory mechanisms may allow not only better therapeutic approaches in perioperative medicine, but may also help to explain unwanted or unexpected side effects of pharmacological modulators of adrenergic receptor activity. Relevant properties include adrenergic receptor signaling via different types of G-proteins, homologous and heterologous desensitization of adrenergic receptors, homo- and heterodimerization of adrenergic receptor subtypes, and the downstream signaling network connected to various different adrenergically modulated cellular functions. Adrenergic signaling relies, in principle, on two intracellular signaling modes: (*i*) reversible binding of Ca^{2+} ions to specific protein sites and (*ii*) protein phosphorylation cascades. Both signaling modes follow distinct pathways, which are intimately interlinked.

Selective stimulation of adrenergic receptor subtypes may exert beneficial or detrimental effects on the myocardium. Fine-tuning of complex adrenergic signaling may provide maximum cardioprotection. α_2 agonists nonselectively decrease sympathetic tone, whereas β_1-adrenergic agonists may be more selective. Unfortunately, no subtype-selective α_2 agonists are clinically available. Regional anesthetic techniques combine effective pain relief with inhibitory but rather unpredictable effects on sympathetic nerve activity. Administration of β_1-adrenergic agonists has been proven to be most effective in preventing perioperative adverse cardiac effects. However, there is currently no "sun and center" in the present armamentarium of perioperative sympatho-modulatory treatments. Identification of patients with critical polymorphisms of adrenergic receptors associated with adverse outcome as part of the perioperative risk management may directly improve patient management by allowing directed pharmacological interventions. Importantly, pharmacodynamic mechanisms now appear to account for most of the cardiovascular variations in response to drug therapy. Only a detailed understanding of the complex adrenergic signaling and intracellular Ca^{2+} handling as well as of the existing genetic polymorphisms will lead to novel more effective therapeutic strategies in perioperative medicine.

CURRENT DEVELOPMENTS IN PERIOPERATIVE BETA-BLOCKER RESEARCH (NOTE ADDED IN PROOF)

Three recent placebo-controlled trials (POBBLE, DIPOM, MaVS), one with high-risk vascular surgical patients, could not confirm the initial promising results calling into question whether the previous findings can be generalized to the vast majority of surgical patients (147,148,149). One large retrospective study even suggests that perioperative beta-blockade may be detrimental in patients at lower risk (150). Although not all of these new findings have been implemented into current practice guidelines, the updated version of the AHA guidelines now recommends perioperative beta-blocker therapy with Class I evidence exclusively for the following two conditions a) chronic (intercurrent) beta-blocker use and b) patients undergoing vascular surgery with positive (evoked ischemia) preoperative stress testing (151).

To date, no perioperative beta-blocker trial has addressed the role of adrenergic receptor polymorphisms on outcome or treatment effect. This important question will be addressed by the SWISS Beta-Blocker in Spinal Anesthesia (BBSA) study, the results of which will be soon available. In vitro studies of isoproterenol stimulation showed that Arg389 β_1-adrenergic receptors produce higher levels of cAMP because of enhanced G-protein coupling compared with Gly389 receptors ("gain-of-function" polymorphism). This is consistent with clinical studies showing increased prevalence of hypertension and myocardial infarct in Arg389 homozygotes. On the other side, if ischemic heart disease is established, individuals carrying the Arg389 receptor may have a better prognosis. Using a transgenic mouse model with cardiac-specific overexpression of the Gly389 or Arg389 containing β_1-adrenergic receptors, Akhtar et al. (152) showed that the Arg389 variant is linked to improved protection against myocardial ischemia/reperfusion due to adaptive signaling mechanisms. Arg389 carriers are also more likely to benefit from beta-blocker therapy. In the Beta-Blocker Evaluation of Survival Trial (BEST) study, Arg389 homozygotes treated with bucindolol had the largest benefit in mortality reduction (-38%), while Gly389 carriers had virtually no clinical benefit from bucindolol therapy compared to placebo (153). These findings imply that pre-selected patients being homozygous for the Arg389 would profit greatly from perioperative beta-blockade. On the other side, the benefits observed in some studies could have resulted from an uneven distribution of genotypes. Even large-scale trials (154) might be unable to ultimately decide whether perioperative beta-blockade is beneficial or not, unless detailed pharmacogenomic characterization of the study population will be performed (155). In support of this idea is the recent experience from the BEST trial with more than 1000 patients enrolled. Bucindolol therapy was only advantageous in the Arg389 variant and related to the degree of antagonized adrenergic activity and not—as previously speculated—by protection against excessive sympatholysis.

REFERENCES

1. Poldermans D, Boersma E, Bax JJ, et al. The effect of bisoprolol on perioperative mortality and myocardial infarction in high-risk patients undergoing vascular surgery. Dutch Echocardiographic Cardiac Risk Evaluation Applying Stress Echocardiography Study Group. N Engl J Med 1999; 341:1789–1794.
2. NCEPOD. Extremes of Age. The 1999 Report of the National Confidential Enquiry into Perioperative Deaths: The National Confidential Enquiry into Perioperative Deaths, 1999.
3. NCEPOD. Then and Now: The 2000 Report of the National Confidential Enquiry into Postoperative Deaths: The National Confidential Enquiry into Postoperative Deaths, 2001.
4. Ebert TJ. Is gaining control of the autonomic nervous system important to our specialty? Anesthesiology 1999; 90:651–653.
5. Zaugg M, Schaub MC, Pasch T, Spahn DR. Modulation of beta-adrenergic receptor subtype activities in perioperative medicine: mechanisms and sites of action. Br J Anaesth 2002; 88:101–123.
6. Zaugg M, Tagliente T, Lucchinetti E, et al. Beneficial effects from beta-adrenergic blockade in elderly patients undergoing noncardiac surgery. Anesthesiology 1999; 91:1674–1686.
7. Beattie WS, Badner NH, Choi P. Epidural analgesia reduces postoperative myocardial infarction: a meta-analysis. Anesth Analg 2001; 93:853–858.
8. Nishina K, Mikawa K, Uesugi T, et al. Efficacy of clonidine for prevention of perioperative myocardial ischemia: a critical appraisal and meta-analysis of the literature. Anesthesiology 2002; 96:323–329.
9. Rodgers A, Walker N, Schug S, et al. Reduction of postoperative mortality and morbidity with epidural or spinal anaesthesia: results from overview of randomised trials. Br Med J 2000; 321:1493.
10. Mamode N, Scott RN, McLaughlin SC, et al. Perioperative myocardial infarction in peripheral vascular surgery. Br Med J 1996; 312(7043):1396–1397.
11. Oliver MF, Goldman L, Julian DG, Holme I. Effect of mivazerol on perioperative cardiac complications during non-cardiac surgery in patients with coronary heart disease: the European Mivazerol Trial (EMIT). Anesthesiology 1999; 91:951–961.
12. Raby KE, Brull SJ, Timimi F, et al. The effect of heart rate control on myocardial ischemia among high-risk patients after vascular surgery. Anesth Analg 1999; 88:477–482.
13. Urban MK, Markowitz SM, Gordon MA, et al. Postoperative prophylactic administration of beta-adrenergic blockers in patients at risk for myocardial ischemia. Anesth Analg 2000; 90:1257–1261.
14. Zaugg M, Tagliente T, Lucchinetti E, et al. Beneficial effects from beta-adrenergic blockade in elderly patients undergoing noncardiac surgery. Anesthesiology 1999; 91:1674–1686.
15. Zaugg M, Schulz C, Wacker J, Schaub MC. Sympatho-modulatory therapies in perioperative medicine. Br J Anaesth 2004; 93:53–62.
16. Zaugg M, Schaub MC. Genetic modulation of adrenergic activity in the heart and vasculature: implications for perioperative medicine. Anesthesiology 2005; 102:429–446.
17. Zaugg M, Schaub MC, Foex P. Myocardial injury and its prevention in the perioperative setting. Br J Anaesth 2004; 93:21–33.
18. Zaugg M, Schaub MC. Cellular mechanisms in sympatho-modulation of the heart. Br J Anaesth 2004; 93:34–52.
19. Gaffney TE, Braunwald E. Importance of the adrenergic nervous system in the support of circulatory function in patients with congestive heart failure. Am J Med 1963; 34:320–324.
20. Bristow M. Antiadrenergic therapy of chronic heart failure: surprises and new opportunities. Circulation 2003; 107:1100–1102.
21. Bristow MR. Beta-adrenergic receptor blockade in chronic heart failure. Circulation 2000; 101:558–569.
22. Coats AJ. Heart Failure 99—the MOXCON story. Int J Cardiol 1999; 71:109–111.
23. Sabbah HN, Stanley WC, Sharov VG, et al. Effects of dopamine beta-hydroxylase inhibition with nepicastat on the progression of left ventricular dysfunction and remodeling in dogs with chronic heart failure. Circulation 2000; 102:1990–1995.

24. A trial of the beta-blocker bucindolol in patients with advanced chronic heart failure. N Engl J Med 2001; 344:1659–1667.

25. Amar D, Fleisher M, Pantuck CB, et al. Persistent alterations of the autonomic nervous system after noncardiac surgery. Anesthesiology 1998; 89:30–42.

26. Ziegeler S, Tsusaki BE, Collard CD. Influence of genotype on perioperative risk and outcome. Anesthesiology 2003; 99:212–219.

27. Schillinger W, Fiolet JW, Schlotthauer K, Hasenfuss G. Relevance of Na^+–Ca^{2+} exchange in heart failure. Cardiovasc Res 2003; 57:921–933.

28. Booth JV, Ward EE, Colgan KC, et al. Metoprolol and coronary artery bypass grafting surgery: does intraoperative metoprolol attenuate acute beta-adrenergic receptor desensitization during cardiac surgery? Anesth Analg 2004; 98:1224–1231.

29. Booth JV, Spahn DR, McRae RL, et al. Esmolol improves left ventricular function via enhanced beta-adrenergic receptor signaling in a canine model of coronary revascularization. Anesthesiology 2002; 97:162–169.

30. Brodde OE, Michel MC. Adrenergic and muscarinic receptors in the human heart. Pharmacol Rev 1999; 51:651–690.

31. Gavras I, Manolis AJ, Gavras H. The alpha2-adrenergic receptors in hypertension and heart failure: experimental and clinical studies. J Hypertens 2001; 19:2115–2124.

32. Koshimizu TA, Tanoue A, Hirasawa A, et al. Recent advances in alpha1-adrenoceptor pharmacology. Pharmacol Ther 2003; 98:235–244.

33. Michelotti GA, Price DT, Schwinn DA. Alpha 1-adrenergic receptor regulation: basic science and clinical implications. Pharmacol Ther 2000; 88:281–309.

34. Philipp M, Brede M, Hein L. Physiological significance of alpha(2)-adrenergic receptor subtype diversity: one receptor is not enough. Am J Physiol Regul Integr Comp Physiol 2002; 283:R287–R295.

35. Post SR, Hammond HK, Insel PA. Beta-adrenergic receptors and receptor signaling in heart failure. Annu Rev Pharmacol Toxicol 1999; 39:343–360.

36. Bers DM. Cardiac excitation-contraction coupling. Nature 2002; 415:198–205.

37. Neves SR, Ram PT, Iyengar R. G protein pathways. Science 2002; 296:1636–1639.

38. Oldenburg O, Qin Q, Krieg T, et al. Bradykinin induces mitochondrial ROS generation via NO, cGMP, PKG, and mitoKATP channel opening and leads to cardioprotection. Am J Physiol Heart Circ Physiol 2004; 286:H468–H476.

39. Rockman HA, Koch WJ, Lefkowitz RJ. Seven-transmembrane-spanning receptors and heart function. Nature 2002; 415:206–212.

40. Zaugg M, Schaub MC. Signaling and cellular mechanisms in cardiac protection by ischemic and pharmacological preconditioning. J Muscle Res Cell Motil 2003; 24:219–249.

41. Freddolino PL, Kalani MY, Vaidehi N, et al. Predicted 3D structure for the human beta 2 adrenergic receptor and its binding site for agonists and antagonists. Proc Natl Acad Sci USA 2004; 101:2736–2741.

42. Gouldson PR, Kidley NJ, Bywater RP, et al. Toward the active conformations of rhodopsin and the beta2-adrenergic receptor. Proteins 2004; 56:67–84.

43. Small KM, McGraw DW, Liggett SB. Pharmacology and physiology of human adrenergic receptor polymorphisms. Annu Rev Pharmacol Toxicol 2003; 43:381–411.

44. Bunemann M, Lee KB, Pals-Rylaarsdam R, et al. Desensitization of G-protein-coupled receptors in the cardiovascular system. Annu Rev Physiol 1999; 61:169–192.

45. Lavoie C, Mercier JF, Salahpour A, et al. Beta 1/beta 2-adrenergic receptor heterodimerization regulates beta 2-adrenergic receptor internalization and ERK signaling efficacy. J Biol Chem 2002; 277:35402–35410.

46. Angers S, Salahpour A, Bouvier M. Dimerization: an emerging concept for G protein-coupled receptor ontogeny and function. Annu Rev Pharmacol Toxicol 2002; 42:409–435.

47. Hague C, Uberti MA, Chen Z, et al. Cell surface expression of alpha1D-adrenergic receptors is controlled by heterodimerization with alpha1B-adrenergic receptors. J Biol Chem 2004; 279:15541–15549.

48. Barki-Harrington L, Luttrell LM, Rockman HA. Dual inhibition of beta-adrenergic and angiotensin II receptors by a single antagonist: a functional role for receptor–receptor interaction in vivo. Circulation 2003; 108:1611–1618.

49. Werry TD, Wilkinson GF, Willars GB. Mechanisms of cross-talk between G-protein-coupled receptors resulting in enhanced release of intracellular Ca^{2+}. Biochem J 2003; 374:281–296.
50. Breitwieser GE. G protein-coupled receptor oligomerization: implications for G protein activation and cell signaling. Circ Res 2004; 94:17–27.
51. Kilts JD, Gerhardt MA, Richardson MD, et al. Beta(2)-adrenergic and several other G protein-coupled receptors in human atrial membranes activate both G(s) and G(i). Circ Res 2000; 87:705–709.
52. Riemann B, Schafers M, Law MP, et al. Radioligands for imaging myocardial alpha- and beta-adrenoceptors. Nuklearmedizin 2003; 42:4–9.
53. Turnbull L, McCloskey DT, O'Connell TD, et al. Alpha 1-adrenergic receptor responses in alpha 1AB-AR knockout mouse hearts suggest the presence of alpha 1D-AR. Am J Physiol Heart Circ Physiol 2003; 284:H1104–H1109.
54. Piascik MT, Hrometz SL, Edelmann SE, et al. Immunocytochemical localization of the alpha-1B adrenergic receptor and the contribution of this and the other subtypes to vascular smooth muscle contraction: analysis with selective ligands and antisense oligonucleotides. J Pharmacol Exp Ther 1997; 283:854–868.
55. Price DT, Lefkowitz RJ, Caron MG, et al. Localization of mRNA for three distinct alpha 1-adrenergic receptor subtypes in human tissues: implications for human alpha-adrenergic physiology. Mol Pharmacol 1994; 45:171–175.
56. Tavernier G, Toumaniantz G, Erfanian M, et al. Beta3-adrenergic stimulation produces a decrease of cardiac contractility ex vivo in mice overexpressing the human beta3-adrenergic receptor. Cardiovasc Res 2003; 59:288–296.
57. Kaupp UB, Seifert R. Molecular diversity of pacemaker ion channels. Annu Rev Physiol 2001; 63:235–257.
58. Moosmang S, Stieber J, Zong X, et al. Cellular expression and functional characterization of four hyperpolarization-activated pacemaker channels in cardiac and neuronal tissues. Eur J Biochem 2001; 268:1646–1652.
59. Biel M, Ludwig A, Zong X, Hofmann F. Hyperpolarization-activated cation channels: a multi-gene family. Rev Physiol Biochem Pharmacol 1999; 136:165–181.
60. Dobrydnjov I, Axelsson K, Samarutel J, Holmstrom B. Postoperative pain relief following intrathecal bupivacaine combined with intrathecal or oral clonidine. Acta Anaesthesiol Scand 2002; 46:806–814.
61. Paris A, Philipp M, Tonner PH, et al. Activation of alpha 2B-adrenoceptors mediates the cardiovascular effects of etomidate. Anesthesiology 2003; 99:889–895.
62. Shyong EQ, Lucchinetti E, Tagliente TM, et al. Interleukin balance and early recovery from anesthesia in elderly surgical patients exposed to beta-adrenergic antagonism. J Clin Anesth 2003; 15:170–178.
63. Zaugg M, Tagliente T, Silverstein JH, Lucchinetti E. Atenolol may not modify anesthetic depth indicators in elderly patients—a second look at the data. Can J Anaesth 2003; 50:638–642.
64. Gottlieb SS, Fisher ML, Kjekshus J, et al. Tolerability of beta-blocker initiation and titration in the Metoprolol CR/XL Randomized Intervention Trial in Congestive Heart Failure (MERIT-HF). Circulation 2002; 105:1182–1188.
65. Mangano DT, Layug EL, Wallace A, Tateo I. Effect of atenolol on mortality and cardiovascular morbidity after noncardiac surgery. Multicenter Study of Perioperative Ischemia Research Group. N Engl J Med 1996; 335:1713–1720.
66. Hall JA, Kaumann AJ, Brown MJ. Selective beta 1-adrenoceptor blockade enhances positive inotropic responses to endogenous catecholamines mediated through beta 2-adrenoceptors in human atrial myocardium. Circ Res 1990; 66:1610–1623.
67. Billinger M, Seiler C, Fleisch M, et al. Do beta-adrenergic blocking agents increase coronary flow reserve? J Am Coll Cardiol 2001; 38:1866–1871.
68. Soriano JB, Hoes AW, Meems L, Grobbee DE. Increased survival with beta-blockers: importance of ancillary properties. Prog Cardiovasc Dis 1997; 39:445–456.
69. Cleophas TJ, Grabowsky I, Niemeyer MG, et al. Paradoxical pressor effects of beta-blockers in standing elderly patients with mild hypertension: a beneficial side effect. Circulation 2002; 105:1669–1671.
70. Auerbach AD, Goldman L. Beta-blockers and reduction of cardiac events in noncardiac surgery: scientific review. J Am Med Assoc 2002; 287:1435–1444.

71. Eagle K-A, Berger P-B, Calkins H, et al. ACC/AHA guideline update for perioperative cardiovascular evaluation for noncardiac surgery—executive summary: a report of the American College of Cardiology/American Heart Association Task Force on Practice Guidelines (Committee to Update the 1996 Guidelines on Perioperative Cardiovascular Evaluation for Noncardiac Surgery). J Am Coll Cardiol 2002; 39(3):542–553.

72. London MJ, Zaugg M, Schaub MC, Spahn DR. Perioperative beta-adrenergic receptor blockade: physiologic foundations and clinical controversies. Anesthesiology 2004; 100:170–175.

73. Kertai MD, Bax JJ, Klein J, Poldermans D. Is there any reason to withhold beta blockers from high-risk patients with coronary artery disease during surgery? Anesthesiology 2004; 100:4–7.

74. Brady AR, Gibbs JS, Greenhalgh RM, et al. Perioperative beta-blockade (POBBLE) for patients undergoing infrarenal vascular surgery: results of a randomized double-blind controlled trial. J Vasc Surg 2005; 41:602–609.

75. Salpeter SR, Ormiston TM, Salpeter EE. Cardioselective beta-blockers in patients with reactive airway disease: a meta-analysis. Ann Intern Med 2002; 137:715–725.

76. Tzivoni D, Medina A, David D, et al. Effect of metoprolol in reducing myocardial ischemic threshold during exercise and during daily activity. Am J Cardiol 1998; 81:775–777.

77. Fleisher LA, Eagle KA, Shaffer T, Anderson GF. Perioperative- and long-term mortality rates after major vascular surgery: the relationship to preoperative testing in the medicare population. Anesth Analg 1999; 89(4):849–855.

78. Smiley RM, Kwatra MM, Schwinn DA. New developments in cardiovascular adrenergic receptor pharmacology: molecular mechanisms and clinical relevance. J Cardiothorac Vasc Anesth 1998; 12:80–95.

79. Jonkers RE, Koopmans RP, Portier EJ, van Boxtel CJ. Debrisoquine phenotype and the pharmacokinetics and beta-2 receptor pharmacodynamics of metoprolol and its enantiomers. J Pharmacol Exp Ther 1991; 256:959–966.

80. Leopold G. Balanced pharmacokinetics and metabolism of bisoprolol. J Cardiovasc Pharmacol 1986; 8 (suppl 11):S16–S20.

81. Fung JW, Chan SK, Yeung LY, Sanderson JE. Is beta-blockade useful in heart failure patients with atrial fibrillation? An analysis of data from two previously completed prospective trials. Eur J Heart Fail 2002; 4:489–494.

82. Dawood MM, Gutpa DK, Southern J, et al. Pathology of fatal perioperative myocardial infarction: implications regarding pathophysiology and prevention. Int J Cardiol 1996; 57:37–44.

83. McFalls EO, Ward HB, Moritz TE, et al. Coronary–artery revascularization before elective major vascular surgery. N Engl J Med 2004; 351:2795–2804.

84. Poldermans D, Bax JJ, Kertai MD, et al. Statins are associated with a reduced incidence of perioperative mortality in patients undergoing major noncardiac vascular surgery. Circulation 2003; 107:1848–1851.

85. Durazzo AE, Machado FS, Ikeoka DT, et al. Reduction in cardiovascular events after vascular surgery with atorvastatin: a randomized trial. J Vasc Surg 2004; 39:967–975.

86. Ali IS, Buth KJ. Preoperative statin use and in-hospital outcomes following heart surgery in patients with unstable angina. Eur J Cardiothorac Surg 2005; 27:1051–1056.

87. VanDenKerkhof EG, Milne B, Parlow JL. Knowledge and practice regarding prophylactic perioperative beta blockade in patients undergoing noncardiac surgery: a survey of Canadian anesthesiologists. Anesth Analg 2003; 96:1558–1565.

88. London MJ, Itani KM, Perrino AC Jr, et al. Perioperative beta-blockade: a survey of physician attitudes in the Department of Veterans Affairs. J Cardiothorac Vasc Anesth 2004; 18:14–24.

89. Schmidt M, Lindenauer PK, Fitzgerald JL, Benjamin EM. Forecasting the impact of a clinical practice guideline for perioperative beta-blockers to reduce cardiovascular morbidity and mortality. Arch Intern Med 2002; 162:63–69.

90. Boersma E, Poldermans D, Bax JJ, et al. Predictors of cardiac events after major vascular surgery: role of clinical characteristics, dobutamine echocardiography, and beta-blocker therapy. J Am Med Assoc 2001; 285:1865–1873.

91. Lindenauer PK, Fitzgerald J, Hoople N, Benjamin EM. The potential preventability of postoperative myocardial infarction: underuse of perioperative beta-adrenergic blockade. Arch Intern Med 2004; 164:762–766.
92. Fleisher LA, Corbett W, Berry C, Poldermans D. Cost-effectiveness of differing perioperative beta-blockade strategies in vascular surgery patients. J Cardiothorac Vasc Anesth 2004; 18:7–13.
93. Mathias CJ, Reid JL, Wing LM, et al. Antihypertensive effects of clonidine in tetraplegic subjects devoid of central sympathetic control. Clin Sci (Lond) 1979; 57 (suppl 5):425S–428S.
94. Reid JL, Tangri KK, Wing LM. The central hypotensive action of clonidine and propranolol in animals and man. Prog Brain Res 1977; 47:369–383.
95. Khan ZP, Ferguson CN, Jones RM. Alpha-2 and imidazoline receptor agonists: their pharmacology and therapeutic role. Anaesthesia 1999; 54:146–165.
96. Kamibayashi T, Maze M. Clinical uses of alpha2-adrenergic agonists. Anesthesiology 2000; 93:1345–1349.
97. McCallum JB, Boban N, Hogan Q, et al. The mechanism of alpha2-adrenergic inhibition of sympathetic ganglionic transmission. Anesth Analg 1998; 87:503–510.
98. Hayashi Y, Maze M. Drugs affecting adrenoceptors: alpha2-agonists. In: Bowdle TA, Horita A, Kharasch ED, eds. The Pharmacologic Basis of Anaesthesiology. New York: Churchill Livingstone, 1994:602–623.
99. Tan CM, Wilson MH, MacMillan LB, et al. Heterozygous alpha 2A-adrenergic receptor mice unveil unique therapeutic benefits of partial agonists. Proc Natl Acad Sci USA 2002; 99:12471–12476.
100. Wijeysundera DN, Naik JS, Beattie WS. Alpha-2 adrenergic agonists to prevent perioperative cardiovascular complications: a meta-analysis. Am J Med 2003; 114:742–752.
101. Parlow JL, Begou G, Sagnard P, et al. Cardiac baroreflex during the postoperative period in patients with hypertension: effect of clonidine. Anesthesiology 1999; 90:681–692.
102. Gregorini L, Marco J, Farah B, et al. Effects of selective alpha1- and alpha2-adrenergic blockade on coronary flow reserve after coronary stenting. Circulation 2002; 106: 2901–2907.
103. Morita K, Mori H, Tsujioka K, et al. Alpha-adrenergic vasoconstriction reduces systolic retrograde coronary blood flow. Am J Physiol 1997; 273:H2746–H2755.
104. Nishikawa T, Dohi S. Oral clonidine blunts the heart rate response to intravenous atropine in humans. Anesthesiology 1991; 75:217–222.
105. Nishikawa T, Kimura T, Taguchi N, Dohi S. Oral clonidine preanesthetic medication augments the pressor responses to intravenous ephedrine in awake or anesthetized patients. Anesthesiology 1991; 74:705–710.
106. Theodorou AE, Mistry H, Davies SL, et al. Platelet alpha 2-adrenoceptor binding and function during the menstrual cycle. J Psychiatr Res 1987; 21:163–169.
107. Aybek T, Kessler P, Dogan S, et al. Awake coronary artery bypass grafting: utopia or reality? Ann Thorac Surg 2003; 75:1165–1170.
108. Ballantyne JC, Carr DB, deFerranti S, et al. The comparative effects of postoperative analgesic therapies on pulmonary outcome: cumulative meta-analyses of randomized, controlled trials. Anesth Analg 1998; 86:598–612.
109. Rigg JR, Jamrozik K, Myles PS, et al. Epidural anaesthesia and analgesia and outcome of major surgery: a randomised trial. Lancet 2002; 359:1276–1282.
110. Peyton PJ, Myles PS, Silbert BS, et al. Perioperative epidural analgesia and outcome after major abdominal surgery in high-risk patients. Anesth Analg 2003; 96:548–554.
111. Park WY, Thompson JS, Lee KK. Effect of epidural anesthesia and analgesia on perioperative outcome: a randomized, controlled Veterans Affairs cooperative study. Ann Surg 2001; 234:560–569.
112. Norris EJ, Beattie C, Perler BA, et al. Double-masked randomized trial comparing alternate combinations of intraoperative anesthesia and postoperative analgesia in abdominal aortic surgery. Anesthesiology 2001; 95:1054–1067.
113. Lee TW, Grocott HP, Schwinn D, Jacobsohn E. High spinal anesthesia for cardiac surgery: effects on beta-adrenergic receptor function, stress response, and hemodynamics. Anesthesiology 2003; 98:499–510.

114. Carpenter RL, Caplan RA, Brown DL, et al. Incidence and risk factors for side effects of spinal anesthesia. Anesthesiology 1992; 76:906–916.
115. Pollard JB. Cardiac arrest during spinal anesthesia: common mechanisms and strategies for prevention. Anesth Analg 2001; 92:252–256.
116. Liu SS, McDonald SB. Current issues in spinal anesthesia. Anesthesiology 2001; 94:888–906.
117. Favarel-Garrigues JF, Sztark F, Petitjean ME, et al. Hemodynamic effects of spinal anesthesia in the elderly: single dose versus titration through a catheter. Anesth Analg 1996; 82:312–316.
118. Ponhold H, Vicenzi MN. Incidence of bradycardia during recovery from spinal anaesthesia: influence of patient position. Br J Anaesth 1998; 81:723–726.
119. Bonica JJ, Kennedy WF, Akamatsu TJ, Gerbershagen HU. Circulatory effects of peridural block. 3. Effects of acute blood loss. Anesthesiology 1972; 36:219–227.
120. Sivarajan M, Amory DW, Lindbloom LE. Systemic and regional blood flow during epidural anesthesia without epinephrine in the rhesus monkey. Anesthesiology 1976; 45:300–310.
121. Saada M, Duval AM, Bonnet F, et al. Abnormalities in myocardial segmental wall motion during lumbar epidural anesthesia. Anesthesiology 1989; 71:26–32.
122. Blomberg S, Ricksten SE. Effects of thoracic epidural anesthesia on central hemodynamics compared to cardiac beta adrenoceptor blockade in conscious rats with acute myocardial infarction. Acta Anesthesiol Scand 1990; 34:1–7.
123. Klassen GA, Bramwell RS, Bromage PR, Zborowska-Sluis DT. Effect of acute sympathectomy by epidural anesthesia on the canine coronary circulation. Anesthesiology 1980; 52:8–15.
124. Meissner A, Rolf N, Van Aken H. Thoracic epidural anesthesia and the patient with heart disease: benefits, risks, and controversies. Anesth Analg 1997; 85:517–528.
125. Urwin SC, Parker MJ, Griffiths R. General versus regional anaesthesia for hip fracture surgery: a meta-analysis of randomized trials. Br J Anaesth 2000; 84:450–455.
126. O'Hara DA, Duff A, Berlin JA, et al. The effect of anesthetic technique on postoperative outcomes in hip fracture repair. Anesthesiology 2000; 92:947–957.
127. Scott NB, Turfrey DJ, Ray DA, et al. A prospective randomized study of the potential benefits of thoracic epidural anesthesia and analgesia in patients undergoing coronary artery bypass grafting. Anesth Analg 2001; 93:528–535.
128. Groeben H. Effects of high thoracic epidural anesthesia and local anesthetics on bronchial hyperreactivity. J Clin Monit Comput 2000; 16:457–463.
129. Loick HM, Schmidt C, Van Aken H, et al. High thoracic epidural anesthesia, but not clonidine, attenuates the perioperative stress response via sympatholysis and reduces the release of troponin T in patients undergoing coronary artery bypass grafting. Anesth Analg 1999; 88:701–709.
130. Stenseth R, Berg EM, Bjella L, et al. The influence of thoracic epidural analgesia alone and in combination with general anesthesia on cardiovascular function and myocardial metabolism in patients receiving beta-adrenergic blockers. Anesth Analg 1993; 77: 463–468.
131. Poldermans D, Boersma E, Bax JJ, et al. Bisoprolol reduces cardiac death and myocardial infarction in high-risk patients as long as 2 years after successful major vascular surgery. Eur Heart J 2001; 22:1353–1358.
132. Perioperative sympatholysis: beneficial effects of the alpha 2-adrenoceptor agonist mivazerol on hemodynamic stability and myocardial ischemia. McSPI—Europe Research Group. Anesthesiology 1997; 86:346–363.
133. Talke P, Li J, Jain U, et al. Effects of perioperative dexmedetomidine infusion in patients undergoing vascular surgery. The Study of Perioperative Ischemia Research Group. Anesthesiology 1995; 82:620–633.
134. Lilja M, Jounela AJ, Juustila H, Mattila MJ. Interaction of clonidine and beta-blockers. Acta Med Scand 1980; 207:173–176.
135. Mialet Perez J, Rathz DA, Petrashevskaya NN, et al. Beta 1-adrenergic receptor polymorphisms confer differential function and predisposition to heart failure. Nat Med 2003; 9:1300–1305.

136. Small KM, Mialet-Perez J, Seman CA, et al. Polymorphisms of cardiac presynaptic alpha2C adrenergic receptors: diverse intragenic variability with haplotype-specific functional effects. Proc Natl Acad Sci USA 2004; 101:13020–13025.

137. Forleo C, Resta N, Sorrentino S, et al. Association of beta-adrenergic receptor polymorphisms and progression to heart failure in patients with idiopathic dilated cardiomyopathy. Am J Med 2004; 117:451–458.

138. Kaye DM, Smirk B, Finch S, et al. Interaction between cardiac sympathetic drive and heart rate in heart failure: modulation by adrenergic receptor genotype. J Am Coll Cardiol 2004; 44:2008–2015.

139. Carlson CS, Eberle MA, Kruglyak L, Nickerson DA. Mapping complex disease loci in whole-genome association studies. Nature 2004; 429:446–452.

140. Drysdale CM, McGraw DW, Stack CB, et al. Complex promoter and coding region beta 2-adrenergic haplotypes alter receptor expression and predict in vivo responsiveness. Proc Natl Acad Sci USA 2000; 97:10483–10488.

141. The International HapMap Project. Nature 2003; 426:789–796.

142. Snapir A, Heinonen P, Tuomainen TP, et al. An insertion/deletion polymorphism in the alpha2B-adrenergic receptor gene is a novel genetic risk factor for acute coronary events. J Am Coll Cardiol 2001; 37:1516–1522.

143. Brodde OE, Buscher R, Tellkamp R, et al. Blunted cardiac responses to receptor activation in subjects with Thr164Ile beta(2)-adrenoceptors. Circulation 2001; 103:1048–1050.

144. Liggett SB. Polymorphisms of beta-adrenergic receptors in heart failure. Am J Med 2004; 117:525–527.

145. McGraw DW, Forbes SL, Kramer LA, Liggett SB. Polymorphisms of the 5' leader cistron of the human beta2-adrenergic receptor regulate receptor expression. J Clin Invest 1998; 102:1927–1932.

146. Schwartz GL, Turner ST. Pharmacogenetics of antihypertensive drug responses. Am J Pharmacogenomics 2004; 4:151–160.

147. Brady AR, Gibbs JS, Greenhalgh RM, Powell JT, Sydes MR. Perioperative beta-blockade (POBBLE) for patients undergoing infrarenal vascular surgery: results of a randomized double-blind controlled trial. J Vasc Surg 2005; 41:602–609.

148. Yang H, Raymer K, Butler R, Parlow J, Roberts R. The effects of perioperative beta-blockade: results of the Metoprolol after Vascular Surgery (MaVS) study, a randomized controlled trial. Am Heart J 2006; 152:983–990.

149. Juul AB, Wetterslev J, Gluud C, Kofoed-Enevoldsen A, Jensen G, Callesen T, Norgaard P, Fruergaard K, Bestle M, Vedelsdal R, Miran A, Jacobsen J, Roed J, Mortensen MB, Jorgensen L, Jorgensen J, Rovsing ML, Petersen PL, Pott F, Haas M, Albret R, Nielsen LL, Johansson G, Stjernholm P, Molgaard Y, Foss NB, Elkjaer J, Dehlie B, Boysen K, Zaric D, Munksgaard A, Madsen JB, Oberg B, Khanykin B, Blemmer T, Yndgaard S, Perko G, Wang LP, Winkel P, Hilden J, Jensen P, Salas N. Effect of perioperative beta blockade in patients with diabetes undergoing major non-cardiac surgery: randomised placebo controlled, blinded multicentre trial. BMJ 2006; 332:1482.

150. Lindenauer PK, Pekow P, Wang K, Mamidi DK, Gutierrez B, Benjamin EM. Perioperative beta-blocker therapy and mortality after major noncardiac surgery. N Engl J Med 2005; 353:349–361.

151. Fleisher LA, Beckman JA, Brown KA, Calkins H, Chaikof E, Fleischmann KE, Freeman WK, Froehlich JB, Kasper EK, Kersten JR, Riegel B, Robb JF, Smith SC, Jr., Jacobs AK, Adams CD, Anderson JL, Antman EM, Faxon DP, Fuster V, Halperin JL, Hiratzka LF, Hunt SA, Lytle BW, Nishimura R, Page RL. ACC/AHA 2006 guideline update on perioperative cardiovascular evaluation for noncardiac surgery: focused update on perioperative beta-blocker therapy: a report of the American College of Cardiology/American Heart Association Task Force on Practice Guidelines (Writing Committee to Update the 2002 Guidelines on Perioperative Cardiovascular Evaluation for Noncardiac Surgery): developed in collaboration with the American Society of Echocardiography, American Society of Nuclear Cardiology, Heart Rhythm Society, Society of Cardiovascular Anesthesiologists, Society for Cardiovascular Angiography and Interventions, and Society for Vascular Medicine and Biology. Circulation 2006; 113:2662–2674.

152. Akhter SA, D'Souza KM, Petrashevskaya NN, Mialet-Perez J, Liggett SB. Myocardial beta1-adrenergic receptor polymorphisms affect functional recovery after ischemic injury. Am J Physiol Heart Circ Physiol 2006; 290:H1427–H1432.

153. Liggett SB, Mialet-Perez J, Thaneemit-Chen S, Weber SA, Greene SM, Hodne D, Nelson B, Morrison J, Domanski MJ, Wagoner LE, Abraham WT, Anderson JL, Carlquist JF, Krause-Steinrauf HJ, Lazzeroni LC, Port JD, Lavori PW, Bristow MR. A polymorphism within a conserved beta1-adrenergic receptor motif alters cardiac function and beta-blocker response in human heart failure. Proc Natl Acad Sci 2006; 103:11288–11293.

154. Devereaux PJ, Yang H, Guyatt GH, Leslie K, Villar JC, Monteri VM, Choi P, Giles JW, Yusuf S. Rationale, design, and organization of the PeriOperative ISchemic Evaluation (POISE) trial: a randomized controlled trial of metoprolol versus placebo in patients undergoing noncardiac surgery. Am Heart J 2006; 152:223–230.

155. Zaugg M, Schaub MC. Genetic modulation of adrenergic activity in the heart and vasculature: implications for perioperative medicine. Anesthesiology 2005; 102:429–446.

Intraoperative Management of the Patient with Ischemic Heart Disease

J. Berridge

Department of Anesthesia and Critical Care, The General Infirmary at Leeds, Leeds, U.K.

THE PROBLEM

Coronary heart disease is common. It is responsible for over 110,000 deaths in the United Kingdom each year (1). There are 1.4 million people with angina in the United Kingdom. It is inevitable that many patients who present for major surgery will have a history of ischemic heart disease. In addition to patients with overt ischemic heart disease is a significant population of surgical patients who have occult coronary artery disease. This is perhaps best exemplified by the asymptomatic diabetic patient, who is at high risk of adverse perioperative cardiovascular events such as death, myocardial infarction (MI), or episodes of severe heart failure following elective surgery. There are many scoring systems for identifying those at high risk of perioperative MI (2–4). Table 1 has a simplified system divided into factors that greatly increase the risk, factors that moderately increase the risk, and factors that slightly increase the risk. The only factor that has been associated with a reduction in risk is having a success of coronary artery bypass grafting within the previous six years. A particular problem is that of surgery soon after intracoronary stenting, particularly when a drug-eluting stent has been used. These stents reduce restenosis rates, but delays endothelium coverage making the stent extremely vulnerable to thrombosis if antiplatelet therapy is interrupted for major surgery. A recent study suggests that elective surgery should be delayed for at least three months after stenting and some people opine the delay should be 12 months (5). It should be remembered that three or more moderate risk factors in the same patient equate to a high risk of adverse perioperative cardiovascular events or death. For example, a 75-year-old diabetic patient undergoing a hemicolectomy is a high-risk patient even if there are no symptoms of cardiovascular disease and the ECG is normal.

Clinical risk factors are easily identified when the patient is assessed preoperatively, so it should be possible to detect patients at particular risk and put in place systems to reduce the perioperative cardiovascular risk. This chapter is not concerned with the place of perioperative medication such as aspirin, statins, β-blockers, or α_2-adrenergic agonists in reducing risk as these are discussed elsewhere; we will examine the influence of anesthetic technique, perioperative monitoring, and hemodynamic manipulation on outcome in the patient with ischemic heart disease undergoing surgery. We will also attempt to provide some guidance as to what to do when the patient develops myocardial ischemia or infarction during or immediately after surgery.

INFLUENCE OF ANESTHETIC TECHNIQUE

The literature concerning the association between anesthetic technique and cardiovascular morbidity and mortality is surprisingly limited. Slogoff and Keats

TABLE 1   Risk Factors for Perioperative MI

High risk	Moderate risk	Slight risk	Decreased risk
MI within 6 wk	Age greater than 70	Previous MI	Coronary artery bypass
Coronary stenting within 3 mo (bare metal)	Emergency surgery	Grade I–II hypertension without end organ	graft within 6 yr
	Thoracic or abdominal surgery	damage	
Coronary stenting within 1 yr (drug eluting)	Type II diabetic over 50 yr old	Class I angina (treated)	
		Class I heart failure (treated)	
	Type I diabetic for greater than 10 yr	Asymptomatic abnormal ECG	
Grade III or IV angina	MI between 6 wk and 3 mo	Previous coronary stent	
Grade III or IV heart failure	Coronary stent after 3 mo (bare metal) or 1 yr (drug eluting)		
Added heart sounds or elevated JVP			
	Class II angina		
Severe aortic stenosis (gradient greater than 50 mmHg)	Class II heart failure		
	Moderate aortic stenosis (gradient 25–50)		
	Grade III hypertension		
	Grade II hypertension with end organ damage		
	Rhythm other than sinus		

Abbreviations: MI, myocardial infarction; ECG, electrocardiogram.

(6) demonstrated that one anesthetist out of a group of nine cardiac anesthetists had excess mortality after coronary artery surgery despite using broadly similar anesthetic drugs to his colleagues. The fault appeared to be that he (anesthetist number 7) failed to control heart rate before bypass and his patients suffered more perioperative ischemia. The implication of this study is that the conduct of the anesthetic is more important than the drugs used to produce anesthesia. However, it is increasingly clear from work done in cardiac surgery that volatile anesthesia has a protective role in patients suffering from myocardial ischemia. There are now a number of studies that show the benefit from volatile anesthesia compared with total intravenous techniques in patients undergoing coronary artery revascularization. In one study from Antwerp conducted in patients undergoing coronary artery surgery on bypass, patients were randomized to one of four anesthetic regimens: propofol, midazolam, sevoflurane, or desflurane. The two groups who received a volatile, anesthetic agent spent less time on the intensive care unit, less time in hospital stay, and a smaller troponin rise (7). A multicenter study conducted in Italy showed a similar effect in patients having off-pump coronary surgery when desflurane was compared to propofol (8). The cardioprotective mechanism of action of volatile agents is thought to be due to opening of mitochondrial adenosine triphosphate sensitive potassium ion channel (K_{ATP}) (9). There are data to suggest that δ-opioid receptor stimulation also leads to K_{ATP} channel activation (10,11) with evidence of preconditioning in animal models (12) and isolated human myocytes (13). One study has demonstrated echocardiographic evidence of better

preserved cardiac function in patients given morphine than in patients given fentanyl in patients having coronary artery bypass surgery (14). Although such studies give an indication as to what may or not be beneficial for the heart that is prone to ischemia, there has been surprisingly little similar work in patients undergoing noncardiac surgery. Such work as has been done is in relation to the potential for isoflurane to induce myocardial ischemia. Early reports suggested that isoflurane may induce ischemia by coronary vasodilatation resulting in a steal phenomenon. It is now thought that if tachycardia and hypotension are avoided, the use of isoflurane is not associated with increased myocardial ischemia (15). Indeed, when used in conjunction with insulin to maintain normoglycemia in diabetics undergoing coronary artery surgery, isoflurane was associated with better outcomes and a lower troponin rise when compared to intravenous anesthesia (16). Isoflurane and sevoflurane have a similar incidence of myocardial ischemia when used in high-risk patients (17,18).

REGIONAL ANESTHESIA

Regional anesthesia is superficially an attractive option for the management of patients with ischemic heart disease. The hypothesis is that reducing the stress of surgery reduces the demand on the heart by reducing heart rate and the metabolic response. The results of clinical studies are disappointing. A study comparing spinal anesthesia with general anesthesia in the management of transurethral prostatectomy showed no difference in ST segment changes (19). A study that examined myocardial ischemia in elderly patients showed a reduced ischemic burden in those who had an incremental spinal via spinal catheter when compared to one-off spinal anesthetic and general anesthesia (20). Two papers have come to differing conclusions with one from Canada suggesting that regional anesthesia may well reduce the incidence of adverse cardiovascular events in patients undergoing infrarenal aortic aneurysm surgery (21). The other group from Australasia failed to demonstrate any reduction in cardiovascular morbidity or death between high-risk patients given an epidural or those who had general anesthesia alone (22). Other papers suggest that well-conducted regional anesthesia may reduce the incidence of perioperative ischemia; this is by no means proven (23,24).

GLYCEMIC CONTROL

There has been an upsurge in interest in glycemic control in the critically ill patients after van den Berghe's group demonstrated reduced mortality in longer stay patients after predominantly cardiac surgery who were subjected to tight glycemic control (25). The concept of improved perioperative outcome in patient subject to tight glycemic control is given added plausibility by the results of the original Dextrose Insulin and Glucose in the Management of Acute Myocardial Infarction (DIGAMI) study. This showed a prolonged mortality benefit in patients intensively treated with insulin after acute MI (26). However, to date, the only studies showing perioperative benefit are in diabetic patients undergoing cardiac surgery. One cohort study showed that a switch from subcutaneous intermittent insulin to intravenous insulin was associated with better glycemic control and lower mortality (27). A randomized controlled trial that compared intravenous insulin and tighter glucose control to subcutaneous insulin with poorer glycemic control demonstrated a mortality benefit at two years (28). Interestingly, a paper from Italy suggests that cessation of gliben-clamide and conversion to insulin with tight glycemic control is essential if isoflu-rane is to have a cardioprotective effect in patients undergoing coronary artery surgery (16). This is consistent with the fact that sulfonylureas block the opening of the K_{ATP} channel by volatile anesthetic agents.

There is effectively no outcome data on glycemic control regimens during sur-gery in nondiabetics. Nor is there any good evidence on the benefits of periopera-tive glycemic control in diabetics undergoing noncardiac surgery. However, it would appear sensible to attempt to try and achieve physiological blood glucose levels in patients undergoing surgery. Although untested in noncardiac surgery, avoidance of sulfonylureas and conversion to insulin the night before surgery is likely to be a sensible policy. This may improve outcome by allowing volatile agents to exert their anesthetic preconditioning effect.

TEMPERATURE

Hypothermia has a complex effect on the heart. Cooling of the heart is used for its cardioprotective properties during cardiac surgery. However, one paper from Helsinki suggests that modest hypothermia after elective surgery leads to a large increase in ischemia related to noradrenaline release (29). It would seem prudent to attempt to maintain normothermia in high-risk patients.

PERIOPERATIVE OPTIMIZATION AND MONITORING

There have been a number of studies in which intensive cardiovascular monitoring and controlled manipulation of the cardiovascular system have improved outcome in high-risk patients undergoing major surgery. Rao et al. (30) studied pulmonary artery catheterization and tight management of early ischemia in patients with an extremely high risk of MI and showed a marked reduction in death and rate of MI. However, because the study used historical controls, this evidence of the effect of intense monitoring and hemodynamic control should be viewed skeptically. Boyd et al. (31) demonstrated an 85% reduction in mortality with preoperative resuscita-tion with fluids and dopexamine to a target cardiac index and oxygen delivery com-pared to intensive monitoring alone. Wilson et al. (32) studied a similar regime but randomized patients to receive targeted fluid loading and either adrenaline or dopex-amine or routine care. They demonstrated with a significant reduction in mortality in both treatment groups and a reduction in morbidity in the dopexamine group. Both studies have been criticized because it is perceived that the control groups received inferior care postoperatively. That criticism is only partially valid as the control patients received the normal standard of care given to such patients at that time in their respective hospitals. At the very least, the results suggest that improving the car-diovascular physiology as far as possible in patients will improve outcome.

Patients with ischemic heart disease do better with tight heart rate control dur-ing their care (33). It would appear to be consistent with the findings on periopera-tive β-blockade. A recent paper suggests that atenolol is superior to metoprolol due to its longer duration of action (34). This paper supports the assertion that it is not the use of β-blockers itself that is effective, but the heart rate control.

Electrocardiographic (ECG) monitoring for intraoperative ischemia is the only commonly used useful continuous monitor. In order to capture periopera-tive ischemia, a five-lead system with automatic ST segment analysis should be used. In expert hands, transesophageal echocardiography is the most sensitive monitor of significant ischemia. However, due to the need for a skilled operator dedicated to examining the images, it is not practical outside the setting of cardiac surgery in many parts of the world. It remains, however, a powerful tool for diagnosis in complex cases and should be considered in patients who are not responding to simple management. It should also be remembered that an immediate postoperative 12-lead ECG is a useful screening tool in patients having vascular surgery as an abnormal ECG at that time is a pointer to patients at higher risk of adverse events (35).

In patients who have had evidence of intraoperative (or early postoperative) myocardial ischemia, it is important to perform timely cardiac enzyme assays. In patients who have had surgery, a simple creatine kinase level is of limited value due to skeletal muscle damage. The modern mainstay of diagnosis is cardiac troponin levels. It must be remembered that the troponin level needs to be measured at least six hours after the insult. The usefulness of the troponin lies in its ability to stratify the risk of further adverse cardiac events. It is useful in diagnosing MI, and has particular value in directing the management of in patients with perioperative ischemia but without ST-elevation MI.

MANAGEMENT OF INTRAOPERATIVE ISCHEMIA

When there is evidence of intraoperative ischemia, management is in three parts:

1. Immediate hemodynamic management,
2. Early antithrombotic management, and
3. Late definitive management.

IMMEDIATE HEMODYNAMIC MANAGEMENT

When there is evidence of intraoperative myocardial ischemia from the ECG, pulmonary arterial pressures, or echocardiography, the first line of treatment is heart rate control and normalization of the blood pressure. This may require volume resuscitation or red cell transfusion in the hypovolemic, bleeding patient. It may require increased analgesia or anesthesia. Esmolol has been shown to be effective in acute heart rate control in at-risk patients where tachycardia, which may be relative rather than absolute, is the precipitating cause (36). Hypotension should be treated with adequate volume resuscitation and then vasoconstrictors in small titrated doses with such drugs as phenylephrine and metaraminol. In certain patients who are on long-acting angiotensin system inhibitors, terlipressin may be needed to treat refractory hypotension (37). Hypertension should be initially managed by ensuring effective analgesia and anesthesia, but thereafter initial therapy should be intravenous nitrate followed by β-blockade. It is unusual during surgery to need to do more than this but if other agents are needed clonidine may well have a role. A recent paper suggests that clonidine in patients undergoing carotid endarterectomy reduces postoperative hypertension and neurological sequelae, and this is in addition to its established anti-ischemic properties (38).

Patients with aortic stenosis are also at increased risk of adverse myocardial events, principally due to myocardial ischemia. These patients are distinct from those with coronary artery disease in that they get subendocardial ischemia when there is a fall in perfusion pressure. It is essential to maintain the patient's normal

TABLE 2   Features of Patients at High Risk of Further Adverse Events Postoperatively Following an Episode of Perioperative Ischemia

ECG changes	Biochemical factors	Symptoms
Persistent tachycardia New ST or T-wave changes	Elevated troponin levels	Continuing chest pain Heart failure

diastolic blood pressure during surgery. In essence, it does not matter how this is done as long as the anesthesia is well controlled. It is important that ST segment changes in these patients are not managed by the administration of nitrates until coronary perfusion has been restored with vasoconstrictors. If this is done, then the outcomes in such patients can be as good as age-matched controls (39).

EARLY ANTITHROMBOTIC MANAGEMENT

ST segment changes under anesthesia should be regarded as manifestations of an acute coronary syndrome and managed as such. The use of antithrombotic treatments should be dictated by the nature of the surgery, the risk of bleeding, and the severity of the cardiac dysfunction. There are no published studies to suggest that any one strategy is better than any other. What can be supported is the routine use of aspirin (300 mg) in patients who have no contraindications. This should be given on the basis of ECG changes alone. In patients who develop an ST elevation MI, thrombolysis or primary angioplasty should be considered where there is severe cardiac dysfunction or the surgery has not been intracranial, abdominal, or thoracic. It should be remembered that primary angioplasty involves aggressive antiplatelet therapy that may well need managing with platelet transfusion if bleeding is severe.

Other interventions that should be considered are: high-dose enoxaparin, intravenous heparin, clopidogrel, and high-dose statin therapy.

LATE DEFINITIVE MANAGEMENT

Patients should have their risk stratified and managed according to standard cardiological practices. Patients at high risk of further adverse events are summarized in Table 2.

Such patients require urgent assessment by a cardiologist. Patients may need angiography or stress testing later depending on symptoms. What is certain is that all patients who have evidence of perioperative ischemia need full secondary prevention. This will include β-blockade, angiotensin system antagonists, aspirin, and statin therapy.

CONCLUSIONS

The management of patients at risk of intraoperative ischemia begins preoperatively and such patients should receive all their routine cardioprotective medications which may include β-blockers, statins, and aspirin. It may be sensible to consider using volatile anesthesia instead of total intravenous anesthesia in patients requiring general anesthesia. Regional anesthesia is at worst as safe in these patients as general anesthesia alone and may bring benefits in postoperative analgesia and respiratory impairment. It would seem sensible to maintain tight glycemic control particularly in diabetics who should be converted to insulin therapy prior to surgery if they are on oral hypoglycemic drugs. The ECG should be monitored closely and any hemodynamic disturbance corrected paying particular attention to heart rate control. This can be effective in the management of moderate-to-severe aortic stenosis as well. An early postoperative 12-lead ECG is of value for predicting future adverse events.

In the event of intraoperative myocardial ischemia, give aspirin as early as possible unless the patient is undergoing intracranial surgery. ST-segment elevation myocardial infarction (STEMI) should be managed conventionally with thrombolysis or PTCA unless there are overwhelming risks of hemorrhage. Cardiological management in acute coronary syndromes other than STEMI should be guided by the postoperative ECG, symptoms, and troponin levels. Give aggressive secondary prevention to all patients who develop perioperative ischemia.

REFERENCES

1. Coronary Heart Disease. Department of Health. United Kingdom. www.dh.gov.uk/PolicyAndGuidance/HealthAndSocialCareTopics/CoronaryHeartDisease/fs/en.
2. Lee TH, Marcantonio ER, Mangione CM, et al. Derivation and prospective validation of a simple index for prediction of cardiac risk of major noncardiac surgery. Circulation 1999; 100:1043–1049.
3. Eagle KA, Berger PB, Calkins H, et al. ACC/AHA Guideline Update for Perioperative Cardiovascular Evaluation for Noncardiac Surgery—Executive Summary. A Report of the American College of Cardiology/American Heart Association Task Force on Practice Guidelines (Committee to Update the 1996 Guidelines on Perioperative Cardiovascular Evaluation for Noncardiac Surgery). Anesth Analg 2002; 94:1052–1064.
4. Hlatky MA, Boineau RE, Higginbotham MB, et al. A brief self-administered questionnaire to determine functional capacity (the Duke Activity Status Index). Am J Cardiol 1989; 64:651–654.
5. Vicenzi MN, Meislitzer T, Heitzinger B, Halaj M, Fleisher LA, Metzler H. Coronary artery stenting and non-cardiac surgery—a prospective outcome study. Br J Anaesth 2006; 96:686–693.
6. Slogoff S, Keats AS. Does perioperative myocardial ischemia lead to postoperative myocardial infarction? Anesthesiology 1985; 62:107–114.
7. De Hert SG, Van der Linden PJ, Cromheecke S, et al. Choice of primary anesthetic regimen can influence intensive care unit length of stay after coronary surgery with cardiopulmonary bypass. Anesthesiology 2004; 101:9–20.
8. Guarracino F, Landoni G, Tritapepe L, et al. Myocardial damage prevented by volatile anesthetics: a multicenter randomized controlled study. J Cardiothorac Vasc Anesth 2006; 20:477–483.
9. Zaugg M, Lucchinetti E, Uecker M, Pasch T, Schaub MC. Anaesthetics and cardiac preconditioning. Part I. Signalling and cytoprotective mechanisms. Br J Anaesth 2003; 91:551–565.
10. Schultz JEJ, Hsu AK, Gross GJ. Ischemic preconditioning and morphine-induced cardioprotection involve the delta-opioid receptor in the intact rat heart. J Mol Cell Cardiol 1997; 29:2187–2195.
11. Schultz JEJ, Hsu AK, Gross GJ. Ischemic preconditioning in the intact rat heart is mediated by δ_1 but not μ or κ opioid receptors. Circulation 1998; 97:1282–1289.
12. Schultz JE-J, Hsu AK, Nagase H, Gross GJ. TAN-67, a delta 1-opioid receptor agonist, reduces infarct size via activation of Gi/o proteins and KATP channels. Am J Physiol Heart Circ Physiol 1998; 274:H909–H914.
13. Bell SP, Sack MN, Patel A, Opie LH, Yellon DM. Delta opioid receptor stimulation mimics ischemic preconditioning in human heart muscle. J Am Coll Cardiol 2000; 36:2296–2302.

14. Murphy GS, Szokol JW, Marymont JH, Avram MJ, Vender JS. Opioids and cardioprotection: the impact of morphine and fentanyl on recovery of ventricular function after cardiopulmonary bypass. J Cardiothorac Vasc Anesth 2006; 20:493–502.

15. Agnew NM, Pennefather SH, Russell GN. Isoflurane and coronary heart disease. Anaesthesia 2002; 57:338–347.

16. Forlani S, Tomai F, De Paulis R, et al. Preoperative shift from glibenclamide to insulin is cardioprotective in diabetic patients undergoing coronary artery bypass surgery. J Cardiovasc Surg (Torino) 2004; 45:117–122.

17. Rooke GA, Ebert TJ, Muzi M, Kharasch ED. The hemodynamic and renal effects of sevoflurane and isoflurane in patients with coronary artery disease and chronic hypertension. Anesth Analg 1996; 82:1159–1165.

18. Ebert TJ, Kharasch ED, Rooke GA, Shroff A, Muzi M. Myocardial ischemia and adverse cardiac outcomes in cardiac patients undergoing non-cardiac surgery with sevoflurane and isoflurane. Anesth Analg 1997; 85:993–999.

19. Edwards ND, Callaghan LC, White T, Reilly CS. Perioperative myocardial ischaemia in patients undergoing transurethral surgery: a pilot study comparing general with spinal anaesthesia. Br J Anaesth 1995; 74:368–372.

20. Juelsgaard P, Sand NP, Felsby S, et al. Perioperative myocardial ischaemia in patients undergoing surgery for fractured hip randomized to incremental spinal, single-dose spinal or general anaesthesia. Eur J Anaesthesiol 1998; 15:656–663.

21. Beattie WS, Badner NH, Choi P. Epidural analgesia reduces postoperative myocardial infarction: a meta-analysis. Anesth Analg 2001; 93:853–858.

22. Peyton PJ, Myles PS, Silbert BS, Rigg JA, Jamrozik K, Parsons R. Perioperative epidural analgesia and outcome after major abdominal surgery in high-risk patients. Anesth Analg 2003; 96:548–554.

23. Matot I, Oppenheim-Eden A, Ratrot R, et al. Preoperative cardiac events in elderly patients with hip fracture randomized to epidural or conventional analgesia. Anesthesiology 2003; 98:156–163.

24. Scheini H, Virtanen T, Kentala E, et al. Epidural infusion of bupivacaine and fentanyl reduces perioperative myocardial ischaemia in elderly patients with hip fracture—a randomized controlled trial. Acta Anesthesiol Scand 2000; 44:1061–1070.

25. van den Berghe G, Wouters P, Weekers F, et al. Intensive insulin therapy in the critically ill patients. N Engl J Med 2001; 345:1359–1367.

26. Malmberg K. Prospective randomised study of intensive insulin treatment on long term survival after acute myocardial infarction in patients with diabetes mellitus. DIGAMI (Diabetes Mellitus, Insulin Glucose Infusion in Acute Myocardial Infarction) Study Group. Br Med J 1997; 314:1512–1515.

27. Lazar HL, Chipkin S, Fitzgerald CA, Bao Y, Cabral H, Apstein CA. Tight glycemic control in diabetic coronary artery bypass graft patients improves perioperative outcomes and decreases recurrent ischemic events. Circulation 2004; 109:1497–1502.

28. Furnary AP, Gao G, Grunkemeier GL. Continuous insulin infusion reduces mortality in patients with diabetes undergoing coronary artery bypass grafting. J Thorac Cardiovasc Surg 2003; 125:1007–1021.

29. Backlund M, Lepantalo M, Toivonen L, et al. Factors associated with post-operative myocardial ischaemia in elderly patients undergoing major non-cardiac surgery. Eur J Anaesthesiol 1999; 16:826–833.

30. Rao TLK, Jacobs KH, El-Etr AA. Reinfarction following anesthesia in patients with myocardial infarction. Anesthesiology 1983; 59:499–505.

31. Boyd O, Grounds RM, Bennett ED. A randomized clinical trial of the effect of deliberate perioperative increase of oxygen delivery on mortality in high-risk surgical patients. J Am Med Assoc 1993; 270:2699–2707.

32. Wilson J, Woods I, Fawcett J, et al. Reducing the risk of major elective surgery: randomised controlled trial of preoperative optimisation of oxygen delivery. Br Med J 1999; 318:1099–1103.

33. Raby KE, Brull SJ, Timimi F, et al. The effect of heart rate control on myocardial ischemia among high-risk patients after vascular surgery. Anesth Analg 1999; 88:477–482.

34. Redelmeier D, Scales D, Kopp A. Beta blockers for elective surgery in elderly patients: population based, retrospective cohort study. Br Med J 2005; 331:932.
35. Bottiger BW, Motsch J, Teschendorf P, et al. Postoperative 12-lead ECG predicts perioperative myocardial ischaemia associated with myocardial cell damage. Anaesthesia 2004; 59:1083–1090.
36. Harwood TN, Butterworth J, Prielipp RC, et al. The safety and effectiveness of esmolol in the perioperative period in patients undergoing abdominal aortic surgery. J Cardiothorac Vasc Anesth 1999; 13:555–561.
37. Eyraud D, Brabant S, Nathalie D, et al. Treatment of intraoperative refractory hypotension with terlipressin in patients chronically treated with an antagonist of the renin–angiotensin system. Anesth Analg 1999; 88:980–984.
38. Schneemilch CE, Bachmann H, Ulrich A, Elwert R, Halloul Z, Hachenberg T. Clonidine decreases stress response in patients undergoing carotid endarterectomy under regional anesthesia: a prospective, randomized, double-blinded, placebo-controlled study. Anesth Analg 2006; 103:297–302.
39. Raymer K, Yang H. Patients with aortic stenosis: cardiac complications in non-cardiac surgery. Can J Anaesth 1998; 45:855–859.

9 Diagnosis of Perioperative Ischemia and Infarction

George D. Lappas and Mark Stafford-Smith
Department of Cardiothoracic Anesthesiology, Duke University Medical Center, Durham, North Carolina, U.S.A.

INTRODUCTION

As the population ages, and patients presenting for surgery are increasingly elderly with numerous comorbidities, perioperative management is becoming ever more challenging. Some of the most serious comorbidities involve the cardiovascular system, and cardiovascular disease is an extremely important contributor to risk. Perioperative myocardial ischemia or infarction has major implications for overall surgical outcome. A clear understanding of the armamentarium of approaches available to anticipate or recognize these serious complications is key to successful anesthetic management.

Mortality rates for patients with coronary artery disease correlate with the number of significantly narrowed vessels and are highest for those with disease of the left main coronary artery. These same factors correlate with risk of myocardial infarction (MI) and death in the perioperative period, making the preoperative recognition of coronary artery disease a particularly relevant aspect of the overall strategy to minimize cardiovascular complications.

Technology to diagnose perioperative ischemia and infarction is evolving. Previously, the stethoscope, the standard electrocardiogram (ECG), and clinical acumen were the primary tools that guided the clinician. Although these tools remain useful, improved understanding of the electrophysiology of the heart and computerized processing of the ECG have contributed to, and in some cases exceeded, physician interpretation skills, improving the ability of the clinician to identify myocardial ischemic episodes. In addition, risk factor algorithms and newer investigations such as stress testing, echocardiography, nuclear imaging, and even magnetic resonance imaging are now available and being used in ways that help the clinician predict myocardial ischemia.

Laboratory advances are also contributing to our understanding of the biochemistry of myocardial ischemia, injury, and infarction and are facilitating the development of novel markers with utility as predictors of the occurrence and significance of ischemic events. In the future, advances in genomic research may allow for even earlier identification of at-risk individuals so that preventative strategies and interventions can be implemented long before ischemia or infarction occurs.

In the operating room, several ischemia-detection strategies exist, including computerized monitoring for ST segment changes, pulmonary artery (PA) pressure wave form monitoring, and transesophageal echocardiography (TEE) to detect regional wall motion abnormalities (RWMAs). Controversy exists as to the most valuable of these tools. During the postoperative period, when patients are still at significant risk for myocardial ischemic events, many of the modalities listed above can also be helpful.

The aim of this chapter is to review the knowledge and tools available, and their value in predicting or diagnosing ischemic myocardial disease.

BACKGROUND
Myocardial Ischemia, Infarction, and Hibernation

Myocardial ischemia occurs when there is an imbalance between myocardial oxygen supply and demand. This is commonly due to fixed coronary artery obstructions (e.g., atherosclerotic stenoses), but can also be due to the inability of coronary vessels to dynamically adapt to increased demand for blood flow. Stated another way, ischemia may be due to inadequate supply of oxygenated blood (*supply ischemia*) or excessive demand (*demand ischemia*).

MI occurs when unrelieved ischemia leads to cell death. As energy requirements, metabolic activity, and oxygen extraction are greatest in the subendocardium, this region is the most susceptible region to ischemic injury and necrosis (1).

Supply Ischemia

Reduction in coronary arterial blood flow in the setting of unchanging oxygen requirements, for example, due to vasospasm or other causes of acute coronary obstruction (e.g., thrombus), results in supply ischemia. This phenomenon, termed "low-flow" ischemia, is characterized by both oxygen deprivation and insufficient removal of metabolites *and is the cause of MI and most episodes of unstable angina*. The Gregg effect refers to the normal improvement in left ventricular systolic performance seen with increased coronary blood flow and perfusion pressure; similarly, the Salisbury effect refers to the related reduction in left ventricular diastolic distensibility. In the setting of supply ischemia, both the Gregg effect and the Salisbury effect are reversed, as left ventricular systolic and diastolic functions are impaired due to a buildup of metabolites that reduces the calcium sensitivity of myofilaments. Supply ischemia can also occur in the setting of normal coronary arteries; hypoxia resulting from anemia, carbon monoxide poisoning, low oxygen tension (FiO_2), hemoglobinopathies, cyanotic heart disease, or cor pulmonale have the effect of reducing oxygen delivery without impairing coronary artery blood flow.

Demand Ischemia

In the presence of chronic coronary atherosclerosis, there is fixed coronary blood flow. During stress or exercise, tachycardia leads to an increase in myocardial oxygen consumption. As the coronary blood flow is fixed, there is insufficient increase in coronary blood flow to meet metabolic demand, producing demand ischemia. This phenomenon can be termed "high-flow" ischemia and is *responsible for most episodes of chronic stable angina*.

Usually, supply and demand ischemia coexist. In the extreme case, if oxygen supply remains inadequate to meet metabolic demands, a destructive cascade ensues that leads to myocardial injury and ultimately cell necrosis.

Consequences of Ischemia

Cardiac myocytes have very low oxygen stores and rely on a continuous supply of oxygenated blood for aerobic metabolism. Within seconds of coronary occlusion, myocardial oxygen tension falls and left ventricular dysfunction occurs, related to alterations in intracellular calcium handling. Other adverse consequences of ischemia include decreased myocardial compliance, leading to increased resistance to ventricular filling, elevated ventricular filling pressures, and ultimately pulmonary congestion.

Compensatory coronary artery mechanisms aimed at preserving myocardial perfusion are activated during myocardial ischemia; paracrine responses include local release of vasodilator substances and dilation of affected vessels. Subendocardial ischemia reduces ventricular contractile force, ultimately stretching and paradoxically elongating the myocardium during systole. As the myocardium elongates with each subsequent contraction, the cellular transmembrane potential decreases and ischemic electrocardiographic abnormalities appear.

Stunning and Hibernation

As our understanding of the pathophysiology of ischemic myocytes becomes clearer, new entities such as myocardial stunning and hibernation have been described. Myocardial stunning occurs when a brief episode of critical ischemia causes prolonged myocardial dysfunction. This mechanism contributes to the global myocardial dysfunction seen after cardiopulmonary bypass with aortic cross-clamping. Although both stunning and infarction result in extended periods of impaired contractility, cell death does not occur with stunning, and gradual return of contractile activity occurs. Myocardial stunning limited to a single coronary artery manifests clinically through persistent regional myocardial dysfunction, without chest pain, or ECG, and regional perfusion abnormalities (2). After an MI, myocardial stunning in the tissue surrounding the necrotic myocardium may significantly contribute to the overall impairment of contractile function.

Myocardial hibernation occurs when chronically reduced coronary blood flow leads to impaired resting left ventricular function. The important feature of hibernating myocardium is that contractile function, even in akinetic (noncontracting) myocardial segments, can sometimes regain function after revascularization. The term "hibernation" is appropriate because this is thought to be an adaptive mechanism whereby reducing myocardial contractility reduces oxygen consumption in the affected tissue (3).

Both stunning and hibernation are important clinical concepts because not only must these dynamic phenomena be kept in mind when interpreting the results of myocardial function tests, but they offer the potential for pharmacotherapies and revascularization procedures to improve left ventricular function, which may be an important consideration prior to a high-risk surgical procedure. The contrasting features of ischemia, stunning, and hibernation are summarized in Table 1.

TABLE 1 Clinical Features of Myocardial Ischemia, Infarction, and Stunning/Hibernation

	Coronary blood flow	Myocardial contractile impairment
Normal	Normal	Unimpaired
Ischemia	Reduced	Transient
Infarction	Absent	Permanent
Stunning	Normal	Restored after a period of time
Hibernation	Reduced	Restored after revascularization

Source: From Ref. 4.

Perioperative Ischemia

In addition to the comorbidities that a patient brings with them, and the specific characteristics of a particular surgical procedure, there are numerous added myocardial challenges that characterize the perioperative period. Prior to surgery, patients are often emotionally stressed, a condition that may be associated with tachycardia and increased myocardial oxygen demand. In addition, during surgery, stress hormone release in response to surgical stimulation includes a number of vasoactive substances, such as epinephrine and norepinephrine. Other conditions that may further add to myocardial demands and are common to the perioperative period include intravascular volume depletion, ongoing blood loss, and even aspects of general anesthesia. In the postoperative period, patients may be anemic and volume-depleted, and oxygen supply may be further diminished by intrapulmonary shunting (atelectasis) and poor respiratory effort due to pain. Furthermore, postoperative pain promotes ongoing stress hormone release. Patients are often hypothermic after surgery, leading to shivering that can increase myocardial oxygen utilization by as much as 400%.

At any point during the perioperative period when these contributors to increased myocardial demand exceed reserve, then ischemia or infarction will result. It is not surprising that during the postoperative period, especially in the first 72 hours, the patient is at significant risk for myocardial ischemia and infarction.

The incidence of myocardial ischemia varies with the type of surgery, comorbid conditions, and intraoperative control of hemodynamic variables. The greatest incidence of perioperative ischemia occurs with vascular surgical procedures.

A recent review (5) provides a summary of the current knowledge on perioperative myocardial ischemia and includes recent data for over 2400 patients undergoing both vascular and nonvascular surgery. In this study, the overall incidence of perioperative myocardial ischemia, infarction, and death were 7.3%, 3.9%, and 1%, respectively.

LABORATORY DIAGNOSIS OF MYOCARDIAL INFARCTION

During the acute phase of an evolving MI, as the integrity of the cell membrane is compromised and myocytes become necrotic, intracellular macromolecules diffuse into the cardiac interstitium and subsequently appear in circulating blood (6). Increases in the concentration of serum "cardiac markers" have been the standard method for detection of MI over the last 30 years. The chronology and kinetics of the various markers depend on their location in the myocyte, their molecular weight, and their mechanism of clearance from the circulation (Fig. 1). Creatinine phosphokinase-MB (CK-MB) fraction was previously the preferred marker available to indicate myocardial necrosis. Today, the cardiac troponins have been accepted as a standard serologic test of myocardial cell death. As evidence continues to accumulate indicating that early detection of MI has the potential to significantly alter therapy and the short- and long-term outcome of this condition, there is a continuing search for markers that will allow for earlier diagnosis and intervention.

Creatine Kinase

Creatine kinase (CK) is an enzyme found in large quantities in cardiac and skeletal muscle. Increases in serum CK are detectable within three to eight hours with a peak at 12 to 24 hours after MI. However, due to the widespread distribution of this

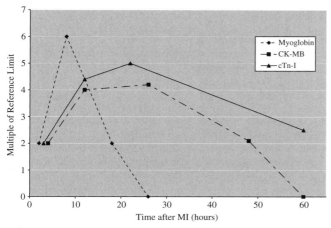

FIGURE 1 The time course of biomarker appearance after MI. After an MI, elevations in myoglobin peak within four hours, followed by cardiac troponin-I and CK-MB. Myoglobin levels return to baseline within 30 hours. Troponin levels peak within 24 hours and will remain elevated for several days. CK-MB levels peak latest, usually after 24 hours, and return to baseline within 72 hours. *Abbreviations*: cTn-I, cardiac troponin-I; MI, myocardial infarction; CK-MB, creatinine phosphokinase-MB.

enzyme throughout the body, the clinical utility of total CK levels as a marker of MI is limited. Currently, determination of the total CK is rarely used as more than a screening test for MI.

CK exists as three distinct isoenzymes (MM, BB, and MB) that are differentially distributed throughout the body and can be characterized by electrophoresis. Both MM and MB isoenzymes are present in cardiac muscle. The CK-MB isoenzyme represents the most "cardiac-specific" variant of the CK enzyme. Notably, skeletal muscle contains principally MM but also contains a small amount of the MB isozyme (1–3%). In contrast, brain and kidney contain predominantly the BB isoenzyme.

As myocardial cells are by far the largest source of CK-MB, the appearance of CK-MB in the serum is highly suggestive of MI. Circulating levels of CK-MB characteristically peak 12 to 24 hours after myocardial cell injury and normalize within two to three days. Although an elevated CK-MB level is strongly associated with MI and poor prognosis, curiously the peak level does not correlate well with infarct size, regardless of the magnitude of elevation (7,8). Interestingly, CK-MB elevations are common following percutaneous intervention procedures (20–30%) and coronary artery bypass surgery (greater than 90%) and their magnitude strongly predicts adverse outcome (9,10).

A more sophisticated analysis of CK-MB elevation is possible that can help in determining the timing of a myocardial ischemic event. This methodology relies on the observation that, within hours of release into the circulation, serum enzymes cleave the terminal amino acids from all CK isoforms. Electrophoresis can identify patterns of CK-MM and CK-MB degradation and provide a "fingerprint" for determining the timing of an MI. In patients with equivocal evidence for MI, isoform analysis may provide the clinician with valuable diagnostic information (11,12).

Problems exist with CK and CK-MB as markers of MI. As small quantities of CK-MB exist in skeletal muscle, measurements of CK and CK-MB at a single point in time are not reliable; the temporal rise and fall of these enzymes in serially obtained blood samples is more useful. For example, skeletal muscle release of CK-MB (i.e., from strenuous exercise) generally remains elevated for a longer time than myocardial release of CK-MB. Cardiac-specific troponins I and T can distinguish skeletal from cardiac muscle damage and, therefore, have replaced CK-MB as the preferred biomarker for diagnosing MI.

Troponins

The troponin (Tn) protein complex consists of three subunits that regulate the calcium-mediated contractile process of striated muscle. Although both cardiac and skeletal muscle contain TnT and TnI, the myocardial and skeletal muscle forms of these proteins are encoded by different genes with differing amino acid sequences. It has been possible to produce subtype-specific antibodies for the cardiac isoforms (cTnT and cTnI) that can be used for quantitative assays in the detection of MI. cTnT and cTnI are normally present at very low levels in the peripheral circulation but typically increase more than six times above the upper limit of normal during MI.

A specific pattern of troponin elevation in the circulation is characteristic following myocardial injury; there is a biphasic rise that corresponds to early leakage of free cytoplasmic troponin and later prolonged release from cell necrosis. Within three hours of the onset of ischemia, circulating levels of both cTnT and cTnI rise above reference levels, slightly preceding changes in CK-MB levels; troponin elevations persist for up to 7 to 10 days after MI. The sensitivity of TnT approaches 50% within three to four hours, 75% at six hours, and almost 100% at 12 hours after onset of symptoms. Positive troponin levels during an acute coronary event are strongly associated with adverse outcome, whereas a negative test predicts low risk (13). Preoperative and postoperative elevations of troponin levels are also predictive of short- and long-term adverse outcome following coronary artery bypass surgery (14,15).

Myoglobin

Myoglobin is a low-molecular-weight heme protein released into the circulation from injured myocardial cells. This protein is not specific, however, to myocardial cells. Nevertheless, it can be detected within a few (1–2) hours after the onset of infarction, and peak levels of serum myoglobin are reached within one to four hours (11). Although high levels of myoglobin are not useful to "rule in" for a diagnosis of MI, low myoglobin levels have a 100% negative predictive value (i.e., absence of myoglobin is useful to "rule out" a patient for MI) (16). Serial determinations of serum myoglobin improve prediction of MI; for example, a doubling of serum myoglobin within two hours of presentation is 95% sensitive and specific for the diagnosis of MI (16). Unfortunately, many problems exist that make it unlikely that myoglobin can be improved as an early test to diagnose MI. Myoglobin from myocardium is not distinguishable from skeletal muscle myoglobin, and levels are elevated in patients with renal failure because of reduced clearance.

B-Type (Brain) Natriuretic Peptide

B-type natriuretic peptide (BNP) has been identified as a serum marker in the diagnosis of MI (17–20). In addition to its usefulness in diagnosis, BNP levels may offer prognostic information in patients with an MI. BNP is released from ventricular muscle in response to increased wall tension, and has become a diagnostic tool for congestive heart failure. BNP levels increase after MI and unstable angina; however, the magnitude of BNP rise in patients with MI is lower than commonly seen with heart failure, falling in the range seen with other conditions such as left ventricular hypertrophy, asymptomatic left ventricular dysfunction, pulmonary embolus, and cor pulmonale. Elevated BNP levels are therefore suggestive of ischemia or infarction, but are not sufficient to diagnose MI (17). However, the prognostic information offered by BNP levels in the setting of an MI creates a very valuable asset in a myocardial ischemia biomarker panel. BNP is useful in predicting those at risk for developing heart failure and increased mortality risk; it should be noted that a low BNP value does not ensure a benign clinical course and cannot detect those patients at high risk for reinfarction (19).

GENETIC BASIS OF CORONARY ARTERY DISEASE

It has long been known that heredity contributes to coronary artery disease. Premature heart attacks tend to "run in families" with individuals experiencing their first MI well before the age of 40, while males tend to develop heart disease earlier than females. Extreme but rare examples of vulnerability to coronary artery disease have already been attributed to variation in a single gene; for example, 90% of patients with type III hyperlipoproteinemia (familial dysbetalipoproteinemia) are homozygous for the uncommon apolipoprotein ε2 allele. However, subtle variations in many genes are suspected to contribute to the majority of risk for atherosclerotic heart disease, making this disorder fit the definition of a common complex genetic disease.

In two studies, genetic fingerprints were found that are relevant to the pathophysiology of atherosclerosis (21,22). In a study of postoperative vascular surgery patients, platelet polymorphisms were shown to be independently associated with postoperative myocardial ischemia even after accounting for comorbidities and surgical risk factors (23).

As we gain further insight into the human genome, it may be possible to quantify genetic predisposition for coronary artery disease prior to surgery. Beyond preoperative evaluation, identification of susceptibility genes at the preoperative visit could also provide a time for counseling and personalized drug approaches to influence the long-term outcomes of surgical procedures (24).

PREOPERATIVE DETECTION OF MYOCARDIAL ISCHEMIA/INFARCTION
History and Physical Examination

A focused history and physical examination is the cornerstone of preoperative diagnosis of myocardial ischemia or infarction. The history should identify past cardiac problems and symptoms such as angina, recent or past MI, heart failure, and symptomatic arrhythmias. The preoperative interview should include specific questions about chest pain or discomfort, palpitations, shortness of breath, and details of any exercise threshold that elicits these symptoms.

A simple evaluation of exercise tolerance is to gauge how many flights of stairs an individual can climb before rest is required. One way of comparing exercise tolerance for different activities is how much energy expenditure they require in comparison to that consumed at rest. The average human consumes, at rest, 1 cal kg/hr and 3.5 mL oxygen/kg/min; the term one "metabolic equivalent" or MET has been coined to describe the metabolic demand of rest. Thus, an activity that consumes 6 METs is six times more demanding than rest. Although METs have typically been used as a unit measure to describe the exercise level achieved during a treadmill stress test, METs are also useful to compare the demands of daily activities. For example, the Duke Activity Status Index (25), a commonly used assessment of the activities of daily living, uses MET units to rate daily activities by their energy requirements (Table 2). In general, activities rating 3 to 6 METs are of moderate intensity, whereas more than 6 METs are of vigorous or high intensity.

Several classification systems have been developed to grade the severity of cardiac symptoms, for example, the Canadian Cardiovascular Society Functional Classification of Angina Pectoris (Table 3). Similar grading systems can be used to describe activity limitations related to congestive heart failure symptoms.

Angina, the uncomfortable feeling that occurs with myocardial oxygen supply/demand imbalance, may not be recognized as important by the patient and may be described as a pressure, heaviness, or pain, typically with exertion, that is usually substernal but may radiate to the arm, neck, jaw, or back. Patients may have a painless "angina-equivalent" such as acute shortness of breath that is particularly important to recognize as it may reflect severe coronary artery disease with global myocardial impairment. The interview should also include questions about risk factors for coronary artery disease. The presence of comorbidities such as cerebrovascular or peripheral vascular disease, hypertension, hypercholesterolemia, diabetes, renal disease, chronic pulmonary disease, and of high-risk behaviors such as smoking may support a diagnosis of myocardial ischemic symptoms.

The physical examination need not be exhaustive. Nevertheless, several physical signs are of value in the assessment of cardiovascular status. General appearance including cyanosis, dyspnea, and obesity are useful. Auscultation of the heart may reveal a murmur or a third heart sound indicative of left ventricular failure.

TABLE 2 Energy Requirements of Common Daily Activities

Activity level	Activity	METs
	Lying quietly	1.0
	Taking out trash	3.0
	Vacuuming	3.5
	Climbing stairs (two flights)	4.0
	Gardening (no lifting)	4.4
	Mowing lawn (push mower)	4.5
Mild		
	Golf (with cart)	2.5
	Walking (2 mph)	2.5
Moderate		
	Walking (3 mph)	3.3
	Cycling	3.5
	Golf (without cart)	4.4
	Walking (4 mph)	4.5
Vigorous		
	Chopping wood	4.9
	Tennis (doubles)	5.0
	Cycling (moderately)	5.7
	Swimming	7.0
	Walking (5 mph)	8.0
	Jogging (10-min mile)	10.2

Abbreviation: METs, metabolic equivalents (see text for definition).
Source: From Ref. 26.

TABLE 3 Canadian Cardiovascular Society Functional Classification of Angina Pectoris

Class	Definition	Specific activity scale[a]
I	Ordinary physical activity (e.g., walking and climbing stairs) does not cause angina; angina occurs with strenuous, rapid, or prolonged exertion at work or recreation	Some vigorous activities will cause angina
II	Slight limitation of ordinary activity; angina occurs on walking or climbing stairs rapidly; walking uphill; walking or stair climbing after meals, in cold, in wind, or under emotional stress; or only during the few hours after awakening; when walking greater than two blocks on level ground; or when climbing more than one flight of stairs at a normal pace and in normal conditions	Some moderate activities will cause angina
III	Marked limitation of ordinary physical activity; angina occurs on walking one to two blocks on level ground or climbing one flight of stairs at a normal pace in normal conditions	Some mild activities will cause angina
IV	Inability to perform any physical activity without discomfort; anginal symptoms may be present at rest	Inability to perform activities without angina developing; angina may develop at rest

[a]See Table 2 for MET equivalents.
Source: From Ref. 27.

Auscultation of the neck over the carotid arteries for bruits may reveal cerebrovascular disease. Determination of jugular venous pressure and lung auscultation may suggest the presence of heart failure. Examination of the extremities may reveal edema, bruits, or abnormal pulses; evidence of vascular disease should heighten suspicion of occult coronary artery disease.

Findings from the history and physical examination may support a presumptive diagnosis of congestive heart failure, arrhythmia, or significant coronary artery disease, or reassure the physician that none of these conditions are likely. Commonly, clinical examination cannot confirm the status of the coronary arteries, but evidence that occult coronary artery disease cannot be ruled out may justify further investigations. The first test ordered should be a 12-lead ECG.

Electrocardiography

The ECG was first described by Einthoven in 1902 (28) and represents a graphic display of the electrical activity of the heart as recorded by a galvanometer attached to leads on the body surface. Examination of the 12-lead ECG is a sensitive test to detect myocardial ischemia.

Lead Placement

The heart acts as a volume conductor allowing the surface ECG to be measured at any point in the body. By convention, *standard electrodes* are placed on the left and

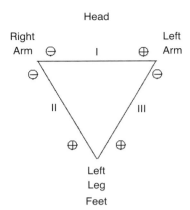

FIGURE 2   Einthoven's triangle. *Source*: From Ref. 28.

right arms, and the left leg, and *the standard leads* measure potential differences between these electrodes; as these leads measure the potential differences between pairs of electrodes, they are also known as *bipolar leads*. The standard leads that form Einthoven's Triangle are designated leads I, II, and III; I is from the right to the left arm, II is from the right arm to the left leg, and III is from the left arm to the left leg (Fig. 2).

Other electrode placement strategies have been developed that can provide a detailed picture of the electrical activity of the heart. For example, the most familiar ECG system uses nine electrodes to achieve 12 different leads or views of the heart (the 12-lead ECG). Key to developing the additional leads for the 12-lead ECG was the development of the concept of the *central terminal* by Wilson in the early 1930s. The central terminal is the potential derived from the average of potentials at the three standard electrodes. Wilson suggested that the central terminal could be considered a "neutral" potential to which other potentials could be compared from any electrode placement; leads measuring potential differences between the central terminal and an electrode are also known as *unipolar leads*. The central terminal was used to describe three additional limb leads, V_R, V_L, and V_F, by using the standard electrodes as unipolar leads. In 1942, Goldberger noted that the signal strength of these standard unipolar leads could be augmented by 50% by omitting the central terminal and comparing the combined potential of two limb leads with the third, for example, the combined potential of the left and right arms to the left leg. These three new *augmented* unipolar leads (aV_R, aV_L, and aV_F) were incorporated into the 12-lead ECG; aV_R is from the combined left arm and right leg to the right arm, aV_L is from the combined right arm and left leg to the left arm, and aV_F is from the combined left and right arms to the left leg. To complete the 12 ECG views of the heart, in addition to the six limb leads (I, II, III, aV_R, aV_L, and aV_F), a standardized group of unipolar precordial leads were developed that compare electrodes placed on the chest wall with the central terminal. The six precordial electrodes (V_1, V_2, V_3, V_4, V_5, and V_6) are placed in a row between the right sternal border at the fourth intercostal space and the left midaxillary line at the fifth intercostal space (Fig. 3). Numerous other ECG lead placement strategies exist, each with their own merits and shortcomings (Fig. 4).

Description and analysis of ECG waveforms are well described elsewhere and have become a refined specialty, particularly with regard to the characteristics of the

Chest Lead Placement

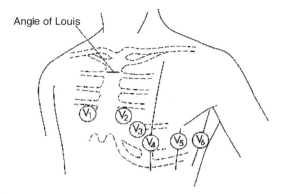

Angle of Louis

FIGURE 3 Precordial ECG lead placement. *Source*: From Ref. 29.

ST segment and T-waves, which can yield important information about myocardial ischemia and infarction.

Repolarization (ST-T Wave) Abnormalities

The normal ECG reflects electrical activity related to the mechanical activity of the heart. Standard ECG characteristics include the P-wave that represents atrial contraction, the QRS complex that represents ventricular contraction, and the ST-T wave that reflects ventricular repolarization (Fig. 5). As the ventricles repolarize, the ST segment is normally a flat neutral line (i.e., isoelectric) in all leads; this is because all myocardial cells repolarize approximately simultaneously. Changes in the ST segment related to myocardial ischemia are well characterized (Fig. 6). An early ECG sign of myocardial ischemia is a change of the ST segment from flat to sloping and/or a deflection of the ST segment from the baseline. This is due to the change in the repolarization potentials of ischemic and infarcted myocardial cells, relative to normal cells. In the early 1950s, Rakita et al. (32) demonstrated that within 60 seconds of coronary artery occlusion, ST segment elevation could be seen on the ECG. The electrophysiologic basis for this observation has been described as altered resting membrane potentials (33).

Acute ischemia can reduce the resting membrane potential of the cardiac myocyte and shorten the duration of the action potential. As a result, a voltage gradient develops between normal and ischemic myocytes, causing abnormal current flow between the normal and ischemic areas. On the ECG, these currents are represented by upward or downward sloping of the ST segment and perturbations of the T-wave. ST segment abnormalities are the earliest and most consistent ECG finding during acute myocardial ischemia (34).

ECG criteria for ischemia were initially established for patients undergoing treadmill stress tests (31). However, in the awake, nonstressed, or even anesthetized patient, the same criteria can be used to establish a diagnosis of myocardial ischemia. These criteria include horizontal or downsloping of the ST segment greater than 1 mm (0.1 mV) and elevation of the ST segment greater than 1 mm.

ST segment and T-wave abnormalities are thus considered key ECG criteria for diagnosis of acute coronary ischemia and infarction. Up to 85% of coronary care unit patients with isolated ST segment elevation are subsequently shown to have suffered

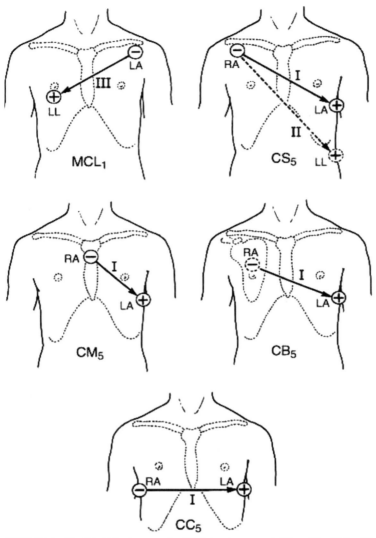

FIGURE 4 Modified bipolar standard limb lead system: MCL_1, CS_5, CM_5, CB_5, CC_5. *Source*: From Ref. 30.

an MI (35–37); if both Q-waves and ST segment elevation are present, this number increases to 94% (37). In contrast, ST segment depression usually indicates subendocardial ischemia. If these abnormalities are new, persistent, and marked, the likelihood of MI increases.

The location of regional myocardial ischemia can be inferred by the distribution of ST segment abnormalities among the ECG leads. For example, ST segment elevation in leads II, III, and aV_F is typical of inferior ischemia in the distribution of the right coronary artery, whereas ST elevation in leads I and aV_R is characteristic of lateral wall ischemia and circumflex artery ischemia. Finally, ST changes in the

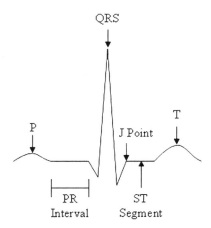

FIGURE 5 Nomenclature describing the deflections of the normal ECG.

precordial leads V_{1-6} are typical of anterior and antero-septal ischemia in the distribution of the left anterior descending artery.

The ST segment is not a perfect tool for diagnosing ischemic myocardial events. ST segment elevation can occur in the absence of ischemia, as with nonspecific "early repolarization" abnormalities, left ventricular hypertrophy, and pericarditis. Conversely, a significant percentage of patients with MI present with initially normal ECGs (36).

T-waves represent myocardial repolarization and may also reflect acute myocardial ischemia. Isolated T-wave inversion is present in the ECG of 10% of patients admitted to coronary care units (38), and 22% of these individuals will subsequently be confirmed to have acute myocardial ischemia. T-wave changes may reflect prior myocardial damage or left ventricular strain. Nevertheless, Pope et al. (36) found that 39% of coronary care patients with inverted T-waves of at least 1 mm or greater had suffered an MI.

Ambulatory Electrocardiography

Ambulatory electrocardiography, also called Holter monitoring after Norman J. Holter, the engineer who invented the procedure, is a method that can be used to record ECG signals for long periods in the outpatient setting. Holter monitors are cassette or digital recorders that monitor two or three ECG leads, usually leads V_1, V_5, and a modified aVF. The patients are encouraged to keep an event diary, and monitors are equipped with event buttons to identify episodes, such as chest pain or dyspnea, for later correlation with ECG findings. In addition to detection of ECG-ST segment abnormalities during an episode, the ambulatory ECG monitor can record arrhythmias caused by or responsible for ischemic episodes (Fig. 7).

The Holter monitoring system does have limitations. For example, horizontal or downsloping ST segment depression may result from body position, hyperventilation, or cardiac drugs (40,41). The role of ambulatory ECG in the preoperative diagnosis of myocardial ischemia is not yet completely defined; however, it has shown some value as a prognostic guide. For example, Stern et al. (42) found that the ambulatory ECG had a sensitivity of 91% and a specificity of 78% in documenting coronary artery disease confirmed later by angiography. The absence of ST segment shifts

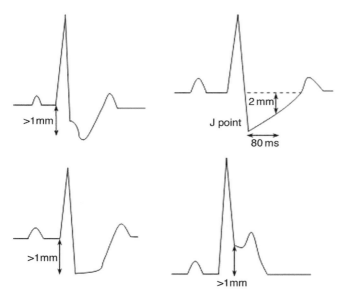

FIGURE 6 ECG criteria for myocardial ischemia consist of 1 mm or more of J-point depression with downsloping or horizontal ST segments; slowly upsloping ST segment depression, defined as 2 mm of ST depression measured 80 milliseconds from the J point; and ST segment elevation. *Abbreviation:* ECG, electrocardiogram. *Source:* From Ref. 31.

on ambulatory monitoring predicts a low risk of cardiac complications in patients undergoing noncardiac surgery.

Stress Testing

The basis of stress testing is that stress, as generated by exercise or various pharmacologic agents, can increase myocardial oxygen demand and precipitate myocardial ischemia that will manifest with ECG ST segment abnormalities. Stress testing is useful in assessing preoperative risk. Although mild disease may not be detected, a strongly positive test is highly predictive of significant underlying coronary atherosclerosis that requires further investigation and possibly intervention (e.g., angioplasty).

Treadmill exercise testing is a standard investigation for the diagnosis of coronary artery disease. The test involves having the patient exercise in a graded fashion (Table 4) (44) so that blood pressure and heart rate rise. As myocardial oxygen demand increases, myocardial ischemia may result and be manifest by repolarization (ST T-wave) abnormalities. The treadmill test is stopped when the patient is unable to continue exercising, either due to fatigue, angina, diagnostic ST segment changes, arrhythmias, or when heart rate reaches 85% to 90% of a predicted, age-related maximum.

Abnormalities of the ST segment are most sensitive for the ECG detection of myocardial ischemia. During acute subendocardial ischemia, the electrical forces responsible for the ST segment are directed towards the inner layers of the heart causing ST depression. With transmural ischemia, the forces are directed outwards

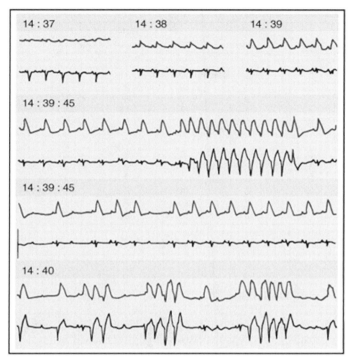

FIGURE 7 A sample ambulatory ECG Holter monitor recording in a patient with atypical angina. The top channel reflects an inferior lead, and the bottom channel records an anterior lead. Note progressive ST segment elevation in the inferior lead, eventually resembling a monophasic action potential. Bursts of nonsustained ventricular tachycardia result. Then, sinus slowing and Wenckebach atrioventricular (AV) block occur from a vasodepressor reflex response elicited by ischemia of the inferior myocardial wall or possibly caused by ischemia of the sinus and AV nodes. In the bottom tracing, both AV block and ventricular arrhythmias are apparent. Numbers indicate time (e.g., 2:37 P.M.). *Abbreviation*: ECG, electrocardiogram. *Source*: From Ref. 39.

towards the epicardium, and ST segment elevation results. In patients without myocardial ischemia, the ST segment is flat or horizontal. With increasing ischemia, there is downsloping of the ST segment that leads, eventually, to inversion of the T-wave. As the ischemia becomes greater still, multiple leads are involved, and the patient may experience angina.

Significant ST segment evidence of myocardial ischemia by stress testing criteria requires J-point depression greater than 1 mm (0.1 mV) relative to the isoelectric PQ interval (Fig. 6). Furthermore, the ST depression must persist for at least 80 milliseconds after the J point in at least three consecutive beats. ST segment elevation during exercise testing is only considered abnormal in non-Q-wave leads. Importantly, exercise-induced ST segment depression does not localize the site of myocardial ischemia, nor does it necessarily provide clues as to the coronary artery involved. For example, it is not uncommon for patients with isolated right coronary distribution disease to exhibit exercise-induced ST segment changes in anterior leads that are related to the left main coronary artery distribution.

TABLE 4 Sample Exercise Protocols

Protocol	Stage	Duration (min)	Grade	Rate (mph)	METs
Modified Bruce protocol	1	3	0	2	3
	2	3	10	2	5
	3	3	12	3	7
	4	3	14	3	10
	5	3	16	4	13
Naughton protocol	0	2	0	2	2
	1	2	4	2	3
	2	2	7	2	4
	3	2	11	2	5
	4	2	14	2	6
	5	2	18	2	7

Abbreviations: METs, metabolic equivalents; mph, miles per hour.
Source: From Ref. 43.

Myocardial Perfusion Imaging Modalities

When a patient demonstrates a "positive" stress test, modalities to assess myocardial perfusion can be useful to confirm and better characterize the existence of vulnerable myocardium. Specifically, myocardial perfusion imaging is used as a test for evaluating the adequacy of blood flow to various regions of the myocardium. Because of its noninvasive nature, myocardial perfusion imaging is often used in preference to coronary angiography to detect coronary artery disease. Perfusion analysis, which measures the adequacy of blood flow, is a functional test that is fundamentally different from assessing the patency of coronary arteries, done during coronary angiography. Interestingly, for this reason, correlation between coronary angiography and perfusion is not always exact. For example, although a coronary artery may be occluded, perfusion to the related myocardium may be normal if sufficient collateral vessels have developed. Current technologies used in the clinical evaluation of myocardial perfusion include single-photon emission computed tomography (SPECT), and less commonly positron emission tomography (PET) or contrast echocardiography.

Single-Photon Emission Computerized Tomography

SPECT imaging of myocardial perfusion is currently the most commonly performed nuclear cardiology study. It is based on the premise that increased regional blood flow will result in increased delivery of a tracer to the myocardium. If a suitable labeled tracer is extracted and retained only by viable myocytes and can be imaged, then absence of the tracer can be used to identify abnormalities in myocardial perfusion.

The tracer is usually an isotope that emits radiation that can be detected by a gamma camera; data are converted to represent the magnitude and location of signal. SPECT imaging creates multiple tomograms that form a digital display representing radiotracer distribution throughout the myocardium (Fig. 8). The long axis of the left ventricle and tomographic images in three standard planes are derived. Short-axis images, representing "donut-like" slices of the heart cut perpendicular to the long axis of the heart, are displayed beginning toward the apex and moving toward the base.

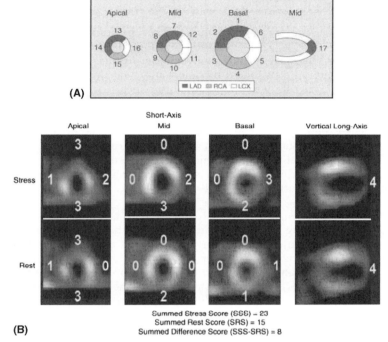

(A)

(B)

Summed Stress Score (SSS) = 23
Summed Rest Score (SRS) = 15
Summed Difference Score (SSS-SRS) = 8

FIGURE 8 (**A**) The 17-segment model. (**B**) Segmented scoring of a patient whose stress and rest SPECT perfusion images show an apical fixed defect, extending into the inferoapical and anteroapical walls. There is evidence of reversible defects in the interior and lateral walls. As described in the text, the summed stress score (SSS), summed rest score (SRS), and the summed difference score (SDS) representing the extent of ischemia are shown. *Abbreviations*: SPECT, single-photon emission computed tomography; LAD, left anterior descending; LCX, left circumflex; RCA, right coronary artery. *Source*: From Ref. 45.

The radiotracer most often used in SPECT is thallium-201. It is a monovalent cation with biological properties similar to those of potassium. In addition, as potassium is virtually absent in scar tissue but found in high concentrations in the intracellular fluid of viable myocytes, thallium-201 is a good choice to view viable myocardium. Thallium-201, therefore, can "differentiate" normal and ischemic from scarred myocardium (46).

Thallium-201 testing can be performed under stress or resting conditions. During stress, thallium-201 is less taken up by threatened myocardium than by well-perfused myocardium. Reversible perfusion defects disappear upon reimaging at rest and are highly suggestive of ischemic myocardium. Similarly, thallium injected at rest may identify defects that demonstrate "reversibility" from the initial images to delayed redistribution images (at three to four hours), reflecting viable myocardium that is hypoperfused even at rest. When a scarred or infarcted region of myocardium is present, thallium defects persist over time and are termed "irreversible" or "fixed" defects.

SPECT images are analyzed using visual and computer-aided techniques. A score is assigned to represent perfusion for each of the standard 17 (47) segments of the myocardium (Figs. 8 and 9). Perfusion in each segment is graded on a scale of 0 (normal perfusion) to 4 (very severe perfusion defect), and these are summed at rest and during stress. The SSS and the SRS are subtracted from one another. The result, the SDS, represents the extent and severity of stress-induced ischemia.

ECG-gated SPECT imaging takes this modality one step further. With this technique, myocardial performance is evaluated by determining ejection fraction and identifying regional left ventricular wall motion abnormalities. The details of the technique are beyond the scope of this chapter but are well discussed elsewhere (48). The combination of left ventricular function with perfusion data provides added prognostic information. Gated SPECT imaging has also been an important advance in differentiating attenuation artifact from infarct. For example, regions with persistent low counts that show normal motion and thickening represent soft-tissue artifacts rather than scar. Thus, gated SPECT has improved the specificity of perfusion imaging for ruling out coronary artery disease (49–51).

Echocardiography

Imaging of the left ventricle using ultrasound can provide real-time two- and even three-dimensional images of the contracting myocardium. In addition, Doppler echocardiography can characterize flow patterns across heart valves and tissue movement that reveals important information about myocardial performance. Echocardiographic characteristics of contracting myocardium include systolic, ventricular wall thickening, and inward motion of the endocardium.

When myocardial ischemia occurs, energy-dependent systolic and diastolic changes can be recognized in the echocardiography images. An area of myocardium that visibly fails to contract to the same degree as surrounding myocardium is termed "hypokinetic." With ischemia, myocardial thickening during systole also decreases, and there is reduced inward motion of the endocardium. As ischemia becomes more pronounced, the ventricular region may fail to contract or thicken altogether, leading to an "akinetic" area. Severe ischemia, infarction, or scarring of the myocardium may result in a sufficiently weakened ventricular region that a ballooning or outward movement, termed "dyskinesis," may occur during systole. These changes in ventricular contraction patterns are called RWMA. Depending on the location of the ventricular segment, and with knowledge of coronary anatomy, speculation about restricted blood flow to a myocardial region can be made based on the location of a RWMA. RWMA description has been standardized to a 17-segment model of the left ventricle (Figs. 9 and 10) (47).

An ischemic heart demonstrates impaired ventricular relaxation during diastole. Diastolic abnormalities precede systolic dysfunction at the onset of myocardial ischemia. Using pulsed-wave Doppler technology, blood flow velocity across the mitral valve can provide diastolic evidence of ischemia. The normal patterns include two waves: the E-wave, which corresponds to early passive ventricular filling, and the A-wave, which represents filling from atrial contraction (Fig. 11). The relative size of E and A waves (E/A ratio) reflects the relative speed of blood flow across the mitral valve during these times and can be used to characterize diastolic function of the ventricle. The normal E/A ratio of 0.75 to 1.5 reflects a relatively minor role for atrial contraction in overall stroke volume; the A-wave is often smaller than the E-wave. In contrast, diastolic mitral blood flow in the setting of ischemia meets a "stiffer" ventricle that fails to relax, and atrial contraction becomes more important for ventricular

Left Ventricular Segmentation

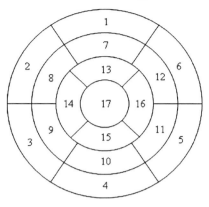

1. Basal Anterior
2. Basal Anteroseptal
3. Basal Inferoseptal
4. Basal Inferior
5. Basal Inferolateral
6. Basal Anterolateral
7. Mid Anterior
8. Mid Anteroseptal
9. Mid Inferoseptal
10. Mid Inferior
11. Mid Inferolateral
12. Mid Anterolateral
13. Apical Anterior
14. Apical Septal
15. Apical Inferior
16. Apical Lateral
17. Apex

FIGURE 9 Left ventricular segmentation. *Source*: From Ref. 52.

filling; consequently, the A-wave becomes more prominent, and the E/A ratio is reduced. With worsening ischemia and more severe diastolic dysfunction, more blood remains in the atrium after atrial contraction; eventually, the buildup results in higher atrial pressures. Once atrial pressures are sufficiently high, the contribution of passive filling to blood flow across the mitral valve once again becomes the predominant wave (53–55). The increased E/A ratio now represents a restrictive physiology (Fig. 12).

Coupling real-time myocardial imaging with stress testing has developed into the field of stress echocardiography. This testing can be performed with treadmill, upright or supine bicycle exercise, or by using pharmacological stressors such as dobutamine or dipyridamole. Transthoracic images are acquired at rest as a baseline. The patient is then stressed according to the standard protocols, and another set of images are acquired for comparison with the baseline images. Note is made of new RWMA, which would signify an inducible ischemic segment or new-onset diastolic dysfunction.

Although the stress echocardiogram is a relatively straightforward, noninvasive test, there is considerable variability in the literature about the sensitivity for detection of coronary artery disease. Nevertheless, as a risk stratification tool, stress echo has been shown to be valuable. For example, in one study that included 1500 patients, a normal stress echocardiography study was associated with 0.9% per year rate of cardiac event rate (57). There is no evidence, however, that resting transthoracic or TEE adds appreciably to the information provided by routine clinical and electrocardiographic data for predicting adverse outcomes (58).

Contrast Echocardiography

Myocardial contrast echocardiography is a relatively new field that shows great promise for providing information about myocardial perfusion from contrast-enhanced echocardiograms. Its use is still being studied and a substantial amount of technical skill and expertise as well as specialized imaging equipment are required for its appropriate utilization (59,60). Currently, perfluorocarbon-based agents that form

REGIONAL WALL SEGMENTS

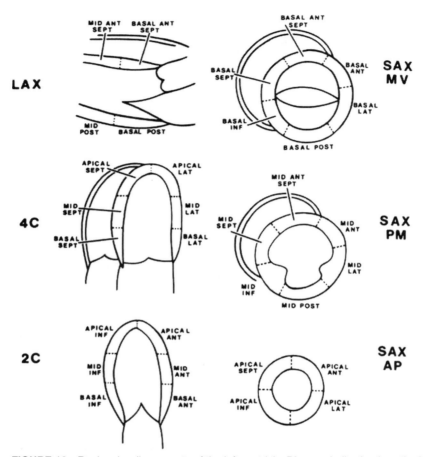

FIGURE 10 Regional wall segments of the left ventricle. Diagram indicating how the left ventricle can be divided into segments for two-dimensional transthoracic echocardiography. One can identify these segments in a series of longitudinal (LAX, 4C, 2C) or short-axis views (SAM MV, SAX PM, SAX AP). The longitudinal and short-axis views overlap and complement each other. *Abbreviations*: LAX, long axis; 4C, 4-chamber; 2C, 2-chamber; SAX MV, short-axis mitral valve; SAX PM, short-axis midpapillary muscle; SAX AP, short-axis apex. *Source*: From Ref. 47.

tiny microspheres when agitated and injected into the circulation are used. The microspheres are echodense, and act as contrast agents that can reveal differences in regional myocardial perfusion. The appearance of contrast in the myocardium parallels the distribution of actual myocardial blood flow.

The basis of contrast echocardiography is straightforward; the absence of contrast suggests the absence of significant blood flow, whereas its presence suggests normal capillary flow. Intermediate levels of contrast appearance indicate delayed capillary flow and suggest the presence of underlying obstructive coronary artery disease (61). In clinical studies, total absence of contrast in the myocardium has been correlated with

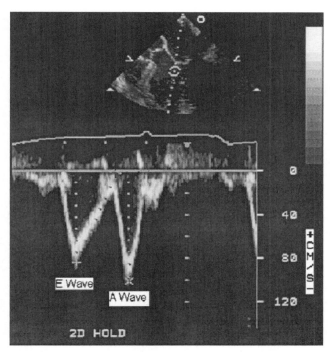

FIGURE 11 Normal E (early diastolic) and A (atrial contraction) waves by pulsed-wave Doppler across the mitral valve. In this case, the E velocity is 84 cm/s and A velocity is 104 cm/s. Therefore, the E/A ratio is 0.84.

the presence of MI. Preserved capillary flow as demonstrated by myocardial contrast echocardiography is also an accurate predictor of myocardial viability (62).

In addition, using specialized echocardiography transducers, it is possible to directly visualize the proximal portions of the left main and right coronary arteries and detect areas of atherosclerotic involvement and calcification. Detection of calcification

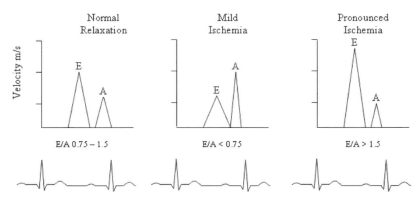

FIGURE 12 Normal and abnormal ischemic diastolic transmitral valve left ventricular filling patterns recorded using pulsed-wave Doppler echocardiography. *Source*: From Ref. 56.

within the proximal left anterior descending artery appears to be a reliable marker for significant obstructive coronary artery disease (63). It is also possible to use pulsed-wave Doppler in the coronary artery lumen and to determine a pulsatility index and quantify phasic flow (63,64).

Detection of contrast within the myocardium requires imaging algorithms that rely on analysis of sequential pulses. Limitations of this technique include a substantial learning curve, the requirement for highly specialized imaging platforms, and the tendency for more distal structures to be shadowed and thus mimic absence of perfusion (51).

Radionuclide Ventriculography

Similar to echocardiography, radionuclide ventriculography (RVG) quantitates right- and left-ventricular contractile functions, as well as diastolic function. Technetium-99m-labeled red blood cells are used to produce images that are acquired by "first-pass" or "equilibrium gated" techniques. Qualitative inspection of equilibrium studies allows assessment of: (*i*) global function, including assessment of left ventricular ejection fraction, (*ii*) the size of heart chambers, and (*iii*) regional wall motion.

Early reports of exercise RVG to detect coronary artery obstructions included predominantly patients with extensive disease resulting in high sensitivity. As the test has been more widely applied to healthier populations, reported sensitivity values have been lower. The sensitivity of this test can be improved by inducing stress by pharmacologic means. The response of left ventricular ejection fraction to exercise as determined by RVG is a powerful prognostic indicator, even though it is a relatively insensitive marker for coronary artery disease (65). For example, an ejection fraction of less than 50% by RVG is strongly associated with increased risk of postoperative congestive heart failure in patients undergoing open abdominal aortic aneurysm repair (66). RWMA detected by RVG during exercise is a sensitive marker for obstructive coronary artery disease. However, limitations of this technique include limited views of the inferior wall, and RWMAs are insensitive for disease of the right coronary artery (67).

In general, RVG is not commonly used for coronary artery disease detection, as sensitivity and specificity are modest, and visual image analysis of RWMAs is challenging.

Positron Emission Tomography

Positron emission tomography, or PET scanning, is a sophisticated imaging modality that uses positron-emitting isotopes of elements, such as carbon, nitrogen, oxygen, and fluorine. Incorporating such elements allows interrogation of physiologically relevant processes in normal and diseased states (68). Cardiac PET radiotracers fall within two broad categories: those that evaluate myocardial perfusion and those that evaluate myocardial metabolism. Emission data are displayed as tomograms in the horizontal and vertical long-axis and short-axis views (69). These data can then be used to derive myocardial perfusion and metabolic data in milliliters of blood per gram per minute for blood flow and moles per gram per minute for metabolism (Fig. 13).

PET agents that assess myocardial perfusion can be used in place of the SPECT agents to assess myocardial perfusion imaging under resting and stress conditions. In addition, because it is possible to obtain quantitative perfusion data, PET can be used to assess coronary flow reserve as a measure of coronary stenosis. However, PET is considerably more expensive than SPECT, and a cost-effective

Stress

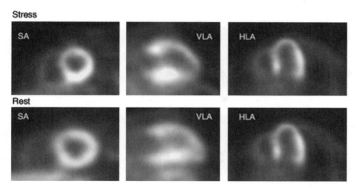

FIGURE 13 Sample PET image of a patient with chest pain. Rest and stress myocardial perfusion imaging with PET using ^{13}N-ammonia in a 47-year-old man complaining of exertional chest pain. The selected images of stress and rest myocardial perfusion in short axis (SA), vertical long axis (VLA), and horizontal long axis (HLA) demonstrate a large area of moderate reduction in tracer uptake in the mid and distal anterior wall and apex at peak exercise stress with normal myocardial perfusion at rest. *Abbreviation*: PET, positron emission tomography. *Source*: From Ref. 68.

analysis to justify the use of PET will be essential in justifying the use of this technology in place of SPECT. Currently, PET is used as a modality to image myocardial perfusion only when other, established imaging modalities are indeterminate or inconclusive (68).

Coronary Angiography
Over the past several decades, the evaluation of myocardial ischemia and infarction has relied increasingly on coronary angiography, and this procedure is now the "gold standard" in characterizing the contribution of coronary artery disease to myocardial ischemia and infarction. The procedure requires cannulation of a peripheral artery (usually the femoral artery) and insertion of shaped catheters into the aorta that are directed into the coronary ostia. Injection of radiolucent dye into the left and right coronary arteries follows. During injection, fluoroscopy is used to obtain orthogonal images as the dye courses through the coronary arteries. This provides clinicians with multiple views to visualize the major coronary arteries and their branches (Fig. 14).

Coronary stenosis is a decrease in the diameter of the coronary artery. It appears as a narrowing in the diameter of the contrast flow. Coronary stenoses of greater than 70% are considered significant (i.e., the ones most likely to produce angina). Complete coronary occlusion can also be detected using this technique.

Magnetic Resonance Imaging
Cardiovascular magnetic resonance (CMR) imaging is becoming an increasingly popular, clinically useful tool for the noninvasive evaluation of ischemic heart disease. CMR can assess cardiac size, function, myocardial perfusion, valvular morphology, and coronary artery anatomy. This modality offers high spatial and contrast resolution with a large, unrestricted field of view. It may also be superior to other modalities which are limited by the need for iodinated contrast, ionizing radiation, blurring from respiratory motion, or the inability to image the entire heart because of limited acoustic windows. With regard to patient safety, nonionizing modalities

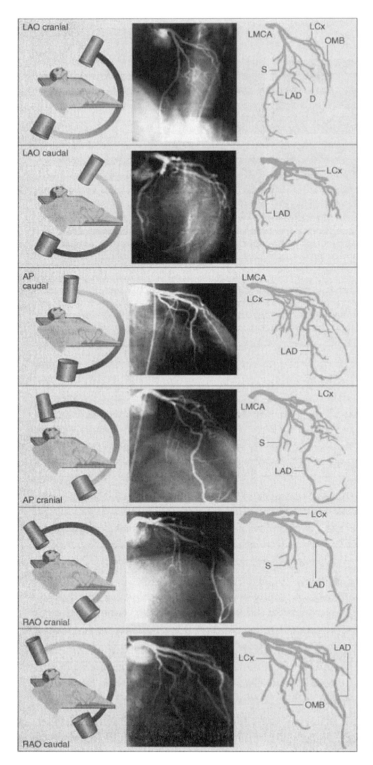

FIGURE 14

such as CMR or echocardiography may be preferred in the future. Unfortunately, CMR is complex and nonportable as compared to echocardiography. CMR provides superior image quality but is significantly more expensive than echocardiography.

The physics behind CMR are complex and beyond the scope of this chapter. The reader is referred to an excellent review for further details (70). Briefly, the frequency of radiowave absorption depends on the strength of the external magnetic field. Hydrogen nuclei behave like magnets and align to an external magnetic field. Thus, a tissue can be excited by a pulse of radiowave causing all the excited hydrogen nuclei to rotate away from the direction of the main magnetic field axis. Once the excitation pulse is finished, the net magnetization decays to its former position (relaxation), and energy is transmitted as a radio signal. The signal is then captured by a receiver antenna. Additional magnetic fields in various spatial planes are rapidly switched on and off, and a magnetic resonance image is constructed that represents a spatially resolved map of radio signals.

The three-dimensional image that is generated is useful for quantifying the volumes and mass of the ventricles. In addition, CMR is valuable to assess regional contractile function, such as quantification of wall motion and thickening of the left and right ventricles. To detect myocardial ischemia, a bolus of contrast is infused, and the sequential progression of contrast through the right ventricle, lungs, left ventricle, and myocardium is imaged. In myocardium that is vulnerable to ischemia, there is delayed and diminished myocardial enhancement in the presence of pharmacologic stress but normal enhancement at rest (Fig. 15). Additionally, the characteristic gradient of contrast from subepicardium towards the darker subendocardium within the perfusion defect aids in differentiation from artifact.

Recently, CMR has been applied to angiography with some encouraging results. Coronary MR angiography has high sensitivity and specificity for the evaluation of proximal coronary artery anomalies. The sensitivity and negative predictive values for detection of clinically significant (less than 50%) disease of the left main coronary artery or three-vessel disease is 100% (72,73). Unfortunately, the applicability of coronary MR angiography for the evaluation of more distal coronary arteries is limited by poor visualization of these structures. However, there is significant interest in the further development of coronary MR angiography as a potential technology to replace cardiac catheterization for the complete evaluation of coronary lumen stenosis.

MI can be detected with high resolution using a protocol known as "late gadolinium-enhancement CMR." The element gadolinium acts predominantly as an extracellular contrast agent. In areas of infarction, due to the expanded extracellular

---

FIGURE 14 (*Previous page*) Sample left coronary angiography. Angiographic views of the left coronary artery. The positions of the X-ray tube and image intensifier are shown for each of the commonly used angiographic views. The left anterior oblique (LAO cranial) shows the ostium and distal portion of the left main coronary artery (LMCA), the middle and distal portions of the left anterior descending artery (LAD), septal perforators (S), diagonal branches (D), and the proximal left circumflex (LCx) and superior obtuse marginal branch (OMB). The left anterior oblique (LAO caudal) shows the proximal LMCA and the proximal segments of the LAD and LCx. The anteroposterior projection (AP caudal) shows the distal LMCA and proximal segments of the LAD and LCx. The anteroposterior projection (AP cranial) also shows the midportion of the LAD and its septal (S) branches. The right anterior oblique projection (RAO cranial) shows the course of the LAD and its septal (S) and diagonal branches. The right anterior oblique projection (RAO caudal) shows the LCx and obtuse marginal branches (OMB). *Source*: From Ref. 51.

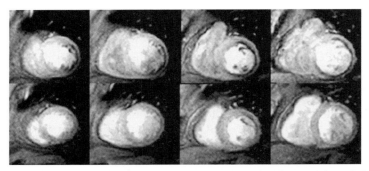

FIGURE 15   Cardiac magnetic resonance imaging perfusion defect. Selected short-axis views obtained during pharmacologic stress (*top row*) and during resting conditions (*bottom row*). The apex of the heart is to the viewer's left with successive images to the right more toward the base. These images illustrate perfusion defects as evidenced by diminished enhancement in the subendocardial zone of the lateral wall and extending into the anterior wall and inferior wall toward the base of the heart. *Source*: From Ref. 71.

compartment, there is increased distribution of gadolinium. Therefore, CMR gadolinium signals are strong in areas of infarction relative to normal myocardium; this is the reverse of SPECT, PET, and contrast CMR myocardial perfusion imaging, where infarction manifests as an absence of signal. Gadolinium-enhancement CMR is useful in the identification of both Q-wave and non-Q-wave MIs (74).

INTRAOPERATIVE DETECTION OF MYOCARDIAL ISCHEMIA AND INFARCTION

During surgery, as the patient typically cannot report symptoms and physical examination is limited, diagnosis of ischemia and infarction must rely on other modalities. Computer ST segment ECG analysis, invasive pressure monitoring, and intraoperative TEE all identify changes in myocardial performance that manifest during the development of ischemia and infarction. The value of these tools will be reviewed below.

Intraoperative Electrocardiographic Analysis

According to the 2004 ASA guidelines, all patients receiving anesthesia require continuous ECG monitoring throughout a procedure. In addition to providing information about the heart rate and rhythm, as previously discussed, the ECG can be useful in the detection of myocardial ischemia. However, operating room use of the ECG to diagnose episodes of ischemia is limited by the continuous observation required; brief abnormalities and subtle trends are particularly likely to be missed in the hectic surgical setting.

The usefulness of automated ST segment ECG monitoring to increase the efficiency of intraoperative ischemia detection is well established (75). Operating room monitoring systems with integrated ST segment analysis technology are now widely available. Although monitors differ in the ST segment analysis algorithms they employ, the basic principles across systems are similar; a baseline ST segment position is "learned" from a baseline or "template" ECG complex. Repeated sampling and comparison of subsequent ST segment positions to the baseline provides a graphic representation of ST segment changes over time that can be used to detect myocardial ischemia. To estimate the ST segment position from an ECG complex, the computer algorithm identifies the isoelectric point, at a predefined duration prior to the onset of the QRS (e.g., 40 milliseconds), and the ST segment, at a predefined time after the offset of the QRS (e.g., 60 milliseconds). It is significant that, although this technology has been embraced, no randomized clinical trials have assessed whether the addition of computerized ST segment ischemia monitoring improves patient outcomes. One intraoperative study of an ST segment monitoring system in cardiac surgery patients concluded that awareness for ischemic changes was heightened among the participating anesthesiologists, and therapeutic interventions were more rapidly instituted, possibly leading to improved outcome (76).

London et al. (77) addressed the question of which ECG leads are the most likely to identify intraoperative ischemic episodes by using continuous 12-lead ECG monitoring of 105 patients with known or suspected coronary artery disease undergoing noncardiac surgery. Of the 51 ischemic episodes that were recorded (ST segment depression or elevation greater than 1 mm), 45 involved ST depression alone, and the remainder involved both ST depression and elevation. Sensitivity for ST segment deviation was greatest in V5 and V4. These authors also noted that lead II, while superior for detection of atrial arrhythmias, was insensitive for detection of ischemia (Fig. 16). Combining leads V4 and V5 increased sensitivity to 90%, while the standard clinical combination, II and V5, was only 80% sensitive. Sensitivity increased to 96% by combining II, V4, and V5. The further addition of V2 and V3 (five leads) increased sensitivity to 100%. This study suggested that the use of II, V4, and V5 is the optimal arrangement for most clinical needs. Similar conclusions came from a second study involving 66 ischemic episodes during 185 vascular surgeries (78).

Pulmonary Artery Catheters
PA catheters are balloon-tipped, percutaneously inserted catheters that are used to measure pressures in the PA. Balloon inflation causes the tip to be carried into small branch

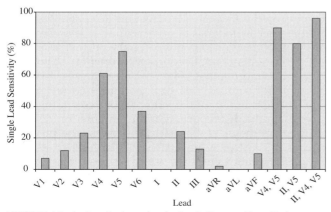

FIGURE 16 Ischemia detection by lead. *Source*: From Ref. 77.

vessels where it occludes the vessel; a "static" column of blood is formed between the tip of the catheter and the left atrium. Therefore, the pressure determined at the tip of the catheter reflects left atrial pressure (79). One of the early consequences of myocardial ischemia is diastolic dysfunction, which causes mean left atrial pressure to rise. Sometimes myocardial ischemia will precipitate mitral valve regurgitation. Both these hemodynamic changes may be reflected by abnormalities in the PA occlusion pressure waveform. Thus, a sudden rise in the PA occlusion pressure may reflect ischemia, and the PA catheter is generally accepted as a monitor of myocardial ischemia (80).

In general, the waveform that is transduced from the tip of the PA catheter when the balloon is occluding the pulmonary vasculature is analogous to the left atrial pressure waveform. That is, distinct a, c, and v waves can be identified, with the corresponding x and y descents. The a-wave pressure is elevated in any condition that increases the resistance to left ventricular filling as may occur with diastolic dysfunction or systolic failure. The v-wave may be increased in ischemic mitral insufficiency due to regurgitation of blood into the left atrium during ventricular systole. Following MI, papillary muscle rupture may lead to giant v-waves due to acute mitral insufficiency. However, it is important to note that no study had shown that routine PA pressure monitoring is superior to ECG monitoring in detecting intraoperative myocardial ischemia. Nevertheless, PA catheter use is prevalent among anesthesiologists for the management of high-risk vascular and cardiac surgery patients.

Intraoperative Transesophageal Echocardiography
Normal left and right ventricular contractions, including myocardial wall thickening and inward motion, are easily visualized using intraoperative TEE and are disturbed by ischemia and infarction. TEE evidence of ventricular impairment manifests visually through reduced or absent inward motion or even paradoxical outward bulging of the affected ventricular wall on the TEE image. Diastolic ventricular function also demonstrates typical changes that can be documented with TEE during episodes of ischemia. Finally, when ischemic myocardium affects the integrity of valvular apparatus, TEE diagnosis of ischemic regurgitation using color Doppler flow imaging may herald myocardial ischemia (e.g., ischemic mitral regurgitation). A characteristic sequence of events occurs in the development of ischemia (Fig. 17); diastolic dysfunction precedes systolic RWMAs and ECG changes then become manifest. Abnormalities specific to areas of myocardium that accompany ischemia are indications of the adequacy of regional coronary perfusion, and in this regard TEE can be informative not only about contractile function, but also in predicting culprit coronary vessel abnormalities (Fig. 18). For example, RWMAs involving the left ventricular anterior septum, free wall, and apex correlate with abnormal perfusion in the typical distribution of the left anterior descending coronary artery. Furthermore, a lesion in the distal portion of the left anterior descending coronary artery may only affect the apex. Similarly, disease in the posterior descending coronary artery causes RWMAs in the left ventricular inferior septum, posterior and inferior free wall. Circumflex coronary artery lesions often produce RWMAs of the lateral and posterior left ventricular walls, a particularly useful observation in this region that is often "silent" electrocardiographically. Proximal right coronary artery disease causes RWMAs in the right ventricular free wall.

More subtle patterns of RWMAs may occur with lesions in the branches of the three primary coronary arteries. Isolated disease in a diagonal branch of the left

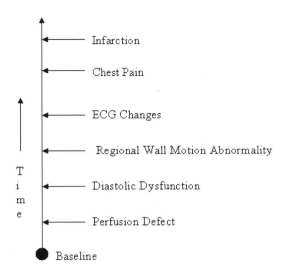

FIGURE 17 Temporal sequence of events during an episode of myocardial ischemia. After the initial insult (perfusion defect) diastolic dysfunction occurs first followed by RWMAs, ECG changes, and clinical signs. *Abbreviations*: RWMA, regional wall motion abnormality; ECG, electrocardiogram. *Source*: From Ref. 81.

anterior descending artery or obtuse marginal branch of the circumflex artery typically causes abnormalities of the anterolateral wall of the left ventricle. Notably, variations in coronary anatomy can cause different RWMAs from the same arterial lesion. For example, coronary artery "dominance" is variable among patients; "left dominant" individuals provide blood flow to the posterior descending artery from the left circumflex artery, conversely, "right dominant" patients provide flow from the right coronary artery; therefore, RWMAs resulting from a proximal obstruction of the right coronary artery would be different in patients with left or right dominant coronary circulations. Interpretation of RWMAs becomes even more complex in individuals with patent coronary bypass grafts to locations on diseased native vessels. Although RWMAs are most clearly visible on the left ventricle, they can also be seen in the right ventricle; in both ventricles, an increase in afterload can exaggerate existing RWMAs. One of the limitations of TEE as a diagnostic tool for myocardial ischemia is the need for significant image acquisition and interpretation skill. Consequently, extensive training in acquisition and interpretation of TEE images, and certification exams, have become an important part of training in the subspecialty of cardiac anesthesia. In addition to the significant personnel resources required to perform TEE, the technology is expensive, and concerns have been raised regarding the potential for TEE to distract anesthesia providers from routine patient care.

Occasionally, intraoperative diagnosis of myocardial ischemia may be aided by epicardial or transthoracic echocardiography imaging, although TEE typically provides superior image quality than those images obtained via chest wall echo. In the TEE midesophageal position, a "four-chamber" view of the heart can be obtained in the zero degree imaging plane, with excellent views of the inferior wall and septum possible; rotating the probe plane to 60° results in the "two-chamber" view, with visualization of the anterior and inferior walls; rotation to 120° results in a "long-axis" left ventricular view, that images the anterior septum and posterior wall. By advancing the TEE probe into the stomach, transgastric "short-axis" views of the LV and RV can be obtained.

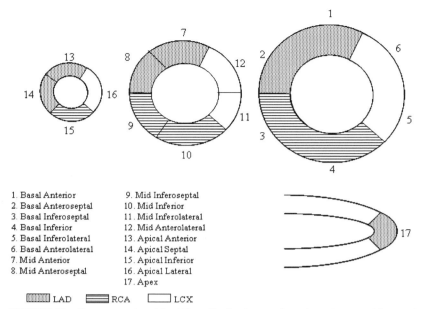

1. Basal Anterior
2. Basal Anteroseptal
3. Basal Inferoseptal
4. Basal Inferior
5. Basal Inferolateral
6. Basal Anterolateral
7. Mid Anterior
8. Mid Anteroseptal

9. Mid Inferoseptal
10. Mid Inferior
11. Mid Inferolateral
12. Mid Anterolateral
13. Apical Anterior
14. Apical Septal
15. Apical Inferior
16. Apical Lateral
17. Apex

LAD   RCA   LCX

FIGURE 18   Coronary artery blood flow distribution as viewed on short- and long-axis TEE views of the left ventricle. *Abbreviations*: LAD, left anterior descending coronary artery; RCA, right coronary artery, LCX, left circumflex coronary artery; TEE, transesophageal echocardiography. *Source*: From Ref. 52.

Comparison of Various Modalities

The relative value of available intraoperative ischemia-detection techniques has gained some attention. In 1989, Leung et al. (82) compared the prognostic significance of TEE-detected RWMAs with ECG and hemodynamic measurements such as blood pressure (BP) and PA pressure. In their study of 50 CABG patients, they found that TEE was superior to ECG (20% vs. 7%) in detecting ischemia. In the postbypass period, and in the first four hours in the ICU, TEE was again found to be superior to ECG and pressure monitoring in detecting myocardial ischemia. These authors also found that after separation from cardiopulmonary bypass, TEE-detected ischemia was predictive of outcome; six of 18 patients with postbypass TEE ischemia had adverse outcomes versus zero of 32 without TEE ischemia ($P=0.001$). Finally, the authors found that 73% of the ischemic episodes detected by TEE were not associated with acute change (±20% of control) in heart rate, BP, or PA pressure.

In another study, Smith et al. (83) studied 50 patients undergoing major vascular or coronary artery bypass graft. Of the patients studied, 48% developed RWMAs compared to only 12% that developed ST segment changes. They also found that RWMAs preceded ST segment changes in 21 of 24 patients. All three patients that experienced an intraoperative MI had persistent intraoperative RWMAs, whereas only one patient had ST segment changes. They too concluded that TEE was superior to electrocardiography for the intraoperative detection of myocardial ischemia. Furthermore, they found that when new RWMA persisted to the conclusion of surgery, MI was likely to have occurred.

POSTOPERATIVE DETECTION OF MYOCARDIAL ISCHEMIA/INFARCTION

Many issues regarding the pathophysiology of acute cardiac events remain unresolved, including whether postoperative MI is most often an acute thrombotic process as a consequence of coronary artery plaque rupture, or due to the cumulative burden on the myocardium of the stress and inflammatory responses to surgery, increased thrombogenicity, and high concentrations of circulating tissue factor (84,85). The postoperative period, particularly the second and third postoperative days, are the most common times for perioperative MI to occur.

Most of the techniques described above are suitable as methods to detect myocardial ischemia and infarction throughout the perioperative period. However, the challenge in diagnosing postoperative myocardial ischemia is that patients have the residual consequences of recent surgery. During the early postoperative period, most patients are poor historians; some have a clouded sensorium that may be contributed to by sedative and analgesic medications, whereas others simply have difficulty differentiating the symptoms of recovery from the symptoms of myocardial ischemia. Therefore, the presentation of MI is anything but typical in the postoperative patient. A clinical history of chest pain, shortness of breath, or other similar complaints may

TABLE 5 Detection of MI after Cardiac Surgery

	Symptoms
Early (less than 24-hr post-op)	Not reliable due to residual anesthetic effects and analgesics
Late (greater than 24-hr post-op)	Potentially reliable but may be confused with incisional pain and pleuritic pain from chest tubes, pericarditis
ECG	
New, persistent Q-waves	Most reliable diagnostic finding, but only if the Q-waves persist on serial EGGs over several days
Evolutionary ST-T changes	Supportive data favoring the diagnosis or MI only if a typical evolutionary pattern is observed; because of the effects of cardiopulmonary bypass, hypothermia, postoperative pericarditis, mediastinal chest tubes, and medications (e.g., digitalis), a variety of nonspecific ST-T wave abnormalities may be seen and should not be relied on for diagnosing perioperative MI
Myocardial-specific enzymes	
Total CK	Elevated total CK levels postoperatively may arise from multiple sources, including skeletal muscle in the thorax and calf, as well as myocardium
CK-MB	Myocardial-specific CK may be released from ischemia occurring during cardiopulmonary bypass, as well as myocardial and aortic incisions made intraoperatively (e.g., right atrium for cannulation of the cavae); because of the nearly universal release of CK-MB, a diagnosis of MI should not be made unless CK-MB is significantly elevated (e.g., greater than 30 units/L)
Echocardiogram	An RWMA is a helpful finding, particularly if it can be shown to be a new finding by comparison with a perioperative study; paradoxical motion of the high anterior portion of the interventricular septum is a common finding postoperatively in the absence of MI and should not be taken as the sole evidence of new perioperative myocardial necrosis

Abbreviations: post-op, postoperative; ECG, electrocardiogram; MI, myocardial infarction; CK, creatine kinase; RWMA, regional wall motion abnormality; CK-mB, myocardial isoform of creatine kinase.
Source: From Ref. 86.

lead the clinician to suspect the presence of myocardial ischemia. A new physical finding such as a murmur or pulmonary edema may also be suggestive, but most commonly, ECG findings identify postoperative myocardial ischemia and infarction; new and persistent Q-waves, especially those accompanied by ST-T wave abnormalities are the most helpful criteria.

Bedside echocardiograms (transthoracic or transesophageal) can contribute to establishing the diagnosis of a perioperative MI by detecting new RWMAs in cases where ECG or serum marker measurements are equivocal. New echocardiograms are particularly helpful when a preoperative study is available for comparison.

Detection of myocardial ischemia and infarction after cardiac surgery can be especially difficult, because postoperatively nonspecific ST-T wave ECG abnormalities and elevated CK are ubiquitous consequences of the surgery that make diagnosis difficult (Table 5).

If the patient is at high risk for myocardial ischemia, a 12-lead ECG should be obtained immediately after surgery and daily for two to three days postoperatively, while measurement of total CK and CK-MB should be made every eight hours for the first 24 to 36 hours if perioperative MI is suspected (51).

SUMMARY

It has been estimated that up to 30% of patients who present for surgical procedures suffer from myocardial ischemia. The clinician has an impressive armamentarium of tests available to identify the myocardium at risk during the perioperative period, and numerous interventions to treat myocardial ischemia. Although these tools have improved risk stratification and recognition of perioperative myocardial ischemia and infarction, these serious problems continue to be distressingly common, and are strongly associated with postoperative mortality. Research continues to characterize the most effective ways to cost-efficiently predict and prevent myocardial ischemia and infarction during the perioperative period.

REFERENCES

1. Bogaert J, Maes A, Van de Werf F, et al. Functional recovery of subepicardial myocardial tissue in transmural myocardial infarction after successful reperfusion: an important contribution to the improvement of regional and global left ventricular function. Circulation 1999; 99:36–43.
2. Bolli R, Marban E. Molecular and cellular mechanisms of myocardial stunning. Physiol Rev 1999; 79:609–634.
3. Elsasser A, Schlepper M, Klovekorn WP, et al. Hibernating myocardium: an incomplete adaptation to ischemia. Circulation 1997; 96:2920–2931.
4. Opie LH. Heart Physiology: From Cell to Circulation. 4th ed. Philadelphia: Lippincott Williams & Wilkins, 2004.
5. Landesberg G. Monitoring for myocardial ischemia. Best Pract Res Clin Anaesthesiol 2005; 19:77–95.
6. Antman EM. Decision making with cardiac troponin tests. N Engl J Med 2002; 346: 2079–2082.
7. Apple FS. Tissue specificity of cardiac troponin I, cardiac troponin T and creatine kinase-MB. Clin Chim Acta 1999; 284:151–159.
8. Gibson CM, Murphy SA, Marble SJ, et al. Relationship of creatine kinase-myocardial band release to thrombolysis in myocardial infarction perfusion grade after intracoronary stent placement: an ESPRIT substudy. Am Heart J 2002; 143:106–110.

9. Kong TQ, Davidson CJ, Meyers SN, Tauke JT, Parker MA, Bonow RO. Prognostic implication of creatine kinase elevation following elective coronary artery interventions. J Am Med Assoc 1997; 277:461–466.

10. Brener SJ, Lytle BW, Schneider JP, Ellis SG, Topol EJ. Association between CK-MB elevation after percutaneous or surgical revascularization and three-year mortality. J Am Coll Cardiol 2002; 40:1961–1967.

11. Apple FS. Creatine kinase isoforms and myoglobin: early detection of myocardial infarction and reperfusion. Coron Artery Dis 1999; 10:75–79.

12. Wu AH, Apple FS, Gibler WB, Jesse RL, Warshaw MM, Valdes R Jr. National Academy of Clinical Biochemistry Standards of Laboratory Practice: recommendations for the use of cardiac markers in coronary artery diseases. Clin Chem 1999; 45:1104–1121.

13. Hamm CW, Goldmann BU, Heeschen C, Kreymann G, Berger J, Meinertz T. Emergency room triage of patients with acute chest pain by means of rapid testing for cardiac troponin T or troponin I. N Engl J Med 1997; 337:1648–1653.

14. Thielmann M, Massoudy P, Neuhauser M, et al. Risk stratification with cardiac troponin I in patients undergoing elective coronary artery bypass surgery. Eur J Cardiothorac Surg 2005; 27:861–869.

15. Kathiresan S, Servoss SJ, Newell JB, et al. Cardiac troponin T elevation after coronary artery bypass grafting is associated with increased one-year mortality. Am J Cardiol 2004; 94:879–881.

16. Gibler WB, Gibler CD, Weinshenker E, et al. Myoglobin as an early indicator of acute myocardial infarction. Ann Emerg Med 1987; 16:851–856.

17. de Lemos JA, Morrow DA. Combining natriuretic peptides and necrosis markers in the assessment of acute coronary syndromes. Rev Cardiovasc Med 2003; 4(suppl 4):S37–S46.

18. de Lemos JA, Morrow DA, Bentley JH, et al. The prognostic value of B-type natriuretic peptide in patients with acute coronary syndromes. N Engl J Med 2001; 345:1014–1021.

19. Harrison A, Amundson S. Evaluation and management of the acutely dyspneic patient: the role of biomarkers. Am J Emerg Med 2005; 23:371–378.

20. Morrow DA, de Lemos JA, Sabatine MS, et al. Evaluation of B-type natriuretic peptide for risk assessment in unstable angina/non-ST-elevation myocardial infarction: B-type natriuretic peptide and prognosis in TACTICS-TIMI 18. J Am Coll Cardiol 2003; 41:1264–1272.

21. Shimokata K, Yamada Y, Kondo T, et al. Association of gene polymorphisms with coronary artery disease in individuals with or without nonfamilial hypercholesterolemia. Atherosclerosis 2004; 172:167–173.

22. Yamada Y, Izawa H, Ichihara S, et al. Prediction of the risk of myocardial infarction from polymorphisms in candidate genes. N Engl J Med 2002; 347:1916–1923.

23. Faraday N, Martinez EA, Scharpf RB, et al. Platelet gene polymorphisms and cardiac risk assessment in vascular surgical patients. Anesthesiology 2004; 101:1291–1297.

24. Topol EJ. The genomic basis of myocardial infarction. J Am Coll Cardiol 2005; 46:1456–1465.

25. Hlatky MA, Boineau RE, Higginbotham MB, et al. A brief self-administered questionnaire to determine functional capacity (the Duke Activity Status Index). Am J Cardiol 1989; 64:651–654.

26. Pasternak RC. Comprehensive rehabilitation of patients with cardiovascular disease. In: Zipes DP, Libby P, Bonow RO, Braunwald E, eds. Braunwald's Heart Disease: A Textbook of Cardiovascular Medicine. 7th ed. Philadelphia: Elsevier/Saunders, 2005 (chapter 43).

27. Goldman L, Hashimoto B, Cook EF, Loscalzo A. Comparative reproducibility and validity of systems for assessing cardiovascular functional class: advantages of a new specific activity scale. Circulation 1981; 64:1227–1234.

28. Einthoven W. Galvanometrische registratie van het menschilijk electrocardiogram. In: Rosenstein SS, ed. Herinneringsbundel. Leiden: Eduard Ijdo, 1902:101–107.

29. Goldberger AL. Clinical Electrocardiography: A Simplified Approach. 6th ed. St. Louis: Mosby, 1999.

30. Griffin RM, Kaplan JA. ECG lead systems. In: Thys DM, Kaplan JA, eds. The ECG in Anesthesia and Critical Care. New York: Churchill Livingstone, 1987:267 (chapter 2).

31. Goldschlager N. Use of the treadmill test in the diagnosis of coronary artery disease in patients with chest pain. Ann Intern Med 1982; 97:383–388.

32. Rakita L, Borduas JL, Rothman S, Prinzmetal M. Studies on the mechanism of ventricular activity. XII. Early changes in the RS-T segment and QRS complex following acute coronary artery occlusion: experimental study and clinical applications. Am Heart J 1954; 48:351–372.
33. Prinzmetal M, Toyoshima H, Ekmekci A, Mizuno Y, Nagaya T. Myocardial ischemia: nature of ischemic electrocardiographic patterns in the mammalian ventricles as determined by intracellular electrographic and metabolic changes. Am J Cardiol 1961; 8:493–503.
34. Zimetbaum PJ, Josephson ME. Use of the electrocardiogram in acute myocardial infarction. N Engl J Med 2003; 348:933–940.
35. Fesmire FM, Percy RF, Wears RL, MacMath TL. Initial ECG in Q wave and non-Q wave myocardial infarction. Ann Emerg Med 1989; 18:741–746.
36. Pope JH, Ruthazer R, Beshansky JR, Griffith JL, Selker HP. Clinical features of emergency department patients presenting with symptoms suggestive of acute cardiac ischemia: a multicenter study. J Thromb Thrombolysis 1998; 6:63–74.
37. Rude RE, Poole WK, Muller JE, et al. Electrocardiographic and clinical criteria for recognition of acute myocardial infarction based on analysis of 3,697 patients. Am J Cardiol 1983; 52:936–942.
38. Granborg J, Grande P, Pedersen A. Diagnostic and prognostic implications of transient isolated negative T waves in suspected acute myocardial infarction. Am J Cardiol 1986; 57:203–207.
39. Miller JM, Zipes DP. Diagnosis of cardiac arrhythmias. In: Zipes DP, Libby P, Bonow RO, Braunwald E, eds. Braunwald's Heart Disease: A Textbook of Cardiovascular Medicine. 7th ed. Philadelphia: Elsevier/Saunders; 2005 (chapter 29).
40. McKenna WJ, Chetty S, Oakley CM, Goodwin JF. Arrhythmia in hypertrophic cardiomyopathy: exercise and 48 hour ambulatory electrocardiographic assessment with and without beta adrenergic blocking therapy. Am J Cardiol 1980; 45:1–5.
41. Kennedy HL, Wiens RD. Ambulatory (Holter) electrocardiography and myocardial ischemia. Am Heart J 1989; 117:164–176.
42. Stern S, Tzivoni D, Stern Z. Diagnostic accuracy of ambulatory ECG monitoring in ischemic heart disease. Circulation 1975; 52:1045–1049.
43. Braunwald E, Goldman L, eds. Primary Cardiology. 2nd ed. Philadelphia: Saunders, 2003.
44. Goldman L, Ausiello DA. Cecil Textbook of Medicine. 22nd ed. Philadelphia, PA: Saunders, 2004.
45. Udelson JE, Dilsizian V, Bonow RO. Nuclear cardiology. In: Zipes DP, Libby P, Bonow RO, Braunwald E, eds. Braunwald's Heart Disease: A Textbook of Cardiovascular Medicine. 7th ed. Philadelphia: Elsevier Saunders, 2005 (chapter 13).
46. Dilsizian V, Narula J, Braunwald E. Atlas of Nuclear Cardiology. Philadelphia: Current Medicine, 2003.
47. Cerqueira MD, Weissman NJ, Dilsizian V, et al. Standardized myocardial segmentation and nomenclature for tomographic imaging of the heart: a statement for healthcare professionals from the Cardiac Imaging Committee of the Council on Clinical Cardiology of the American Heart Association. Circulation 2002; 105:539–542.
48. Germano G, Berman D. Clinical Gated Cardiac SPECT. Armonk, NY: Futura Publishing, 1999.
49. Taillefer R, DePuey EG, Udelson JE, Beller GA, Latour Y, Reeves F. Comparative diagnostic accuracy of Tl-201 and Tc-99m sestamibi SPECT imaging (perfusion and ECG-gated SPECT) in detecting coronary artery disease in women. J Am Coll Cardiol 1997; 29:69–77.
50. Crean A, Dutka D, Coulden R. Cardiac imaging using nuclear medicine and positron emission tomography. Radiol Clin North Am 2004; 42:619–634.
51. Popma JJ. Coronary angiography and intravascular ultrasound imaging. In: Zipes DP, Libby P, Bonow RO, Braunwald E, eds. Braunwald's Heart Disease: A Textbook of Cardiovascular Medicine. 7th ed. Philadelphia: Elsevier/Saunders; 2005:2183 (chapter 18).
52. American Society of Nuclear Cardiology. Imaging guidelines for nuclear cardiology procedures, part 2. J Nucl Cardiol 1999; 6:G47–G84.
53. Khouri SJ, Maly GT, Suh DD, Walsh TE. A practical approach to the echocardiographic evaluation of diastolic function. J Am Soc Echocardiogr 2004; 17:290–297.
54. Moller JE, Egstrup K, Kober L, Poulsen SH, Nyvad O, Torp-Pedersen C. Prognostic importance of systolic and diastolic function after acute myocardial infarction. Am Heart J 2003; 145:147–153.

55. Moller JE, Sondergaard E, Poulsen SH, Egstrup K. Pseudonormal and restrictive filling patterns predict left ventricular dilation and cardiac death after a first myocardial infarction: a serial color M-mode Doppler echocardiographic study. J Am Coll Cardiol 2000; 36:1841–1846.
56. Redfield MM, Jacobsen SJ, Burnett JC Jr, Mahoney DW, Bailey KR, Rodeheffer RJ. Burden of systolic and diastolic ventricular dysfunction in the community: appreciating the scope of the heart failure epidemic. J Am Med Assoc 2003; 289:194–202.
57. Yao SS, Qureshi E, Sherrid MV, Chaudhry FA. Practical applications in stress echocardiography: risk stratification and prognosis in patients with known or suspected ischemic heart disease. J Am Coll Cardiol 2003; 42:1084–1090.
58. Mangano DT, Goldman L. Preoperative assessment of patients with known or suspected coronary disease. N Engl J Med 1995; 333:1750–1756.
59. Senior R, Villanueva F, Vannan MA. Myocardial contrast echocardiography in acute coronary syndromes. Cardiol Clin 2004; 22:253–267.
60. Ward RP, Mor-Avi V, Lang RM. Assessment of left ventricular function with contrast echocardiography. Cardiol Clin 2004; 22:211–219.
61. Tong KL, Wei K. Myocardial contrast echocardiography in the detection of coronary stenosis. Cardiol Clin 2004; 22:233–251.
62. Balcells E, Powers ER, Lepper W, et al. Detection of myocardial viability by contrast echocardiography in acute infarction predicts recovery of resting function and contractile reserve. J Am Coll Cardiol 2003; 41:827–833.
63. Gradus-Pizlo I, Sawada SG, Wright D, Segar DS, Feigenbaum H. Detection of subclinical coronary atherosclerosis using two-dimensional, high-resolution transthoracic echocardiography. J Am Coll Cardiol 2001; 37:1422–1429.
64. Watanabe N, Akasaka T, Yamaura Y, et al. Noninvasive detection of total occlusion of the left anterior descending coronary artery with transthoracic Doppler echocardiography. J Am Coll Cardiol 2001; 38:1328–1332.
65. Klocke FJ, Baird MG, Lorell BH, et al. ACC/AHA/ASNC guidelines for the clinical use of cardiac radionuclide imaging—executive summary: A Report of the American College of Cardiology/American Heart Association Task Force on Practice Guidelines (ACC/AHA/ASNC Committee to Revise the 1995 Guidelines for the Clinical Use of Cardiac Radionuclide Imaging). Circulation 2003; 108:1404–1418.
66. Baron JF, Mundler O, Bertrand M, et al. Dipyridamole-thallium scintigraphy and gated radionuclide angiography to assess cardiac risk before abdominal aortic surgery. N Engl J Med 1994; 330:663–669.
67. Borer JS. Measurement of Ventricular Volume and Function. St. Louis: Mosby, 1999.
68. Takalkar A, Mavi A, Alavi A, Araujo L. PET in cardiology. Radiol Clin North Am 2005; 43:107–119.
69. Bacharach SL, Bax JJ, Case J, et al. PET myocardial glucose metabolism and perfusion imaging. Part 1. Guidelines for data acquisition and patient preparation. J Nucl Cardiol 2003; 10:543–556.
70. Manning WJ PD. Cardiovascular Magnetic Resonance. Philadelphia: Churchill Livingstone, 2002.
71. Dembo LG, Shifrin RY, Wolff SD. MR imaging in ischemic heart disease. Radiol Clin North Am 2004; 42:651–673.
72. Kim WY, Danias PG, Stuber M, et al. Coronary magnetic resonance angiography for the detection of coronary stenoses. N Engl J Med 2001; 345:1863–1869.
73. Dirksen MS, Lamb HJ, Doornbos J, Bax JJ, Jukema JW, de Roos A. Coronary magnetic resonance angiography: technical developments and clinical applications. J Cardiovasc Magn Reson 2003; 5:365–386.
74. Wu E, Judd RM, Vargas JD, Klocke FJ, Bonow RO, Kim RJ. Visualisation of presence, location, and transmural extent of healed Q-wave and non-Q-wave myocardial infarction. Lancet 2001; 357:21–28.
75. Kotrly KJ, Kotter GS, Mortara D, Kampine JP. Intraoperative detection of myocardial ischemia with an ST segment trend monitoring system. Anesth Analg 1984; 63:343–345.
76. Kotter GS, Kotrly KJ, Kalbfleisch JH, Vucins EJ, Kampine JP. Myocardial ischemia during cardiovascular surgery as detected by an ST segment trend monitoring system. J Cardiothorac Anesth 1987; 1:190–199.

77. London MJ, Hollenberg M, Wong MG, et al. Intraoperative myocardial ischemia: localization by continuous 12-lead electrocardiography. Anesthesiology 1988; 69:232–241.
78. Landesberg G, Mosseri M, Wolf Y, Vesselov Y, Weissman C. Perioperative myocardial ischemia and infarction: identification by continuous 12-lead electrocardiogram with online ST-segment monitoring. Anesthesiology 2002; 96:264–270.
79. Lappas D, Lell WA, Gabel JC, Civetta JM, Lowenstein E. Indirect measurement of left-atrial pressure in surgical patients—pulmonary-capillary wedge and pulmonary-artery diastolic pressures compared with left-atrial pressure. Anesthesiology 1973; 38:394–397.
80. Sandham JD, Hull RD, Brant RF, et al. A randomized, controlled trial of the use of pulmonary–artery catheters in high-risk surgical patients. N Engl J Med 2003; 348:5–14.
81. Otto CM. Textbook of Clinical Echocardiography. 3rd ed. Philadelphia: Elsevier/Saunders, 2004.
82. Leung JM, O'Kelly B, Browner WS, Tubau J, Hollenberg M, Mangano DT. Prognostic importance of postbypass regional wall-motion abnormalities in patients undergoing coronary artery bypass graft surgery. SPI Research Group. Anesthesiology 1989; 71:16–25.
83. Smith JS, Cahalan MK, Benefiel DJ, et al. Intraoperative detection of myocardial ischemia in high-risk patients: electrocardiography versus two-dimensional transesophageal echocardiography. Circulation 1985; 72:1015–1021.
84. Landesberg G. The pathophysiology of perioperative myocardial infarction: facts and perspectives. J Cardiothorac Vasc Anesth 2003; 17:90–100.
85. Le Manach Y, Perel A, Coriat P, Godet G, Bertrand M, Riou B. Early and delayed myocardial infarction after abdominal aortic surgery. Anesthesiology 2005; 102:885–891.
86. Adams DH, Filsoufi F, Antman EM. Medical management of the patient undergoing cardiac surgery. In: Zipes DP, Libby P, Bonow RO, Braunwald E, eds. Braunwald's Heart Disease: A Textbook of Cardiovascular Medicine. Philadelphia: Elsevier Saunders, 2005 (chapter 76).

Management of Perioperative Ischemia and Infarction

Micha Dorsch and Jim McLenachan

Yorkshire Heart Centre, The General Infirmary at Leeds, Leeds, U.K.

INTRODUCTION

Despite all efforts at prevention, perioperative myocardial ischemia and myocardial infarction (MI) remain a problem. Conservative estimates suggest that 2% of adults at the age of 50 or older undergoing elective noncardiac surgery have a major perioperative cardiac event (1). The risk is thought to be even higher in patients undergoing urgent or emergency surgery (2). The diagnosis of perioperative ischemia and infarction is not straightforward. Even in the nonoperative setting about 20% of MI presents with symptoms other than chest pain (3). In the operative setting, the majority of ischemic events occur in the first three days after surgery (4,5) when many patients are either on analgesics, or even still intubated and sedated. Therefore, only a small minority of patients present with the typical symptom of chest pain. In the worst-case scenario this means that the diagnosis of MI is completely missed, while in other cases a significant delay in establishing the correct diagnosis is likely (6). The challenges in correctly diagnosing perioperative MI have been discussed in a previous chapter and will not be reiterated at this stage.

PATHOPHYSIOLOGY OF ISCHEMIA AND INFARCTION

Myocardial ischemia implies an imbalance between myocardial oxygen demand and myocardial oxygen supply. Most frequently this is caused by atheromatous narrowing of the coronary arteries leading to a reduction in supply. This will usually produce ST-segment depression on the resting electrocardiogram (ECG). At other times, ischemia can occur because of increased demand. In the operative setting, an increase in heart rate, or the development of atrial fibrillation with a rapid ventricular rate, may lead to ischemic pain and ECG changes in the absence of any dynamic changes in the coronary arteries. Similarly, hypovolemia or anemia may induce ischemic pain and ECG changes in the absence of fresh pathology in the coronary arteries.

MI implies death of myocardial cells and is usually caused by reduced supply due to complete obstruction of a coronary artery. Classically, this will be accompanied by ST-segment elevation on the ECG. In many cases, patients with ST-segment depression will later be shown to have suffered a MI based on the results of troponin or creatinine kinase Mb (CKMB) measurements. These results are useful to make a retrospective diagnosis and to help plan further investigation or treatment, but are usually not available to plan immediate treatment. The 12-lead ECG, therefore, is the key investigation in deciding how to manage the patient. Patients with ST-segment elevation require immediate treatment aimed at re-opening the occluded coronary vessel; this can be done either pharmacologically (by i.v. thrombolysis) or mechanically [by coronary angioplasty (percutaneous coronary intervention or PCI)].

Patients with ST-segment depression may ultimately require coronary revascularization [PCI or coronary artery bypass graft (CABG)], but should be treated medically in the first instance.

DEFINITIONS

The development of newer, more sensitive markers of myocardial injury have made a new nomenclature necessary; this has caused some confusion among health care professionals. Figure 1 gives an overview. Patients presenting with symptoms suggestive of acute ischemia can be given a diagnosis of acute coronary syndrome (ACS). Depending on whether the first ECG shows ST-segment elevation or not, patients can be divided into those with ST-segment elevation MI (STEMI) or non-ST–segment elevation ACS. Patients without ST-elevation on the initial ECG can experience a non-ST–segment elevation MI (NSTEMI), if markers of myocardial injury (troponin, CK etc.) are later detected in the blood. If not, a diagnosis of unstable angina (UA) is made, if it is felt that the patient's symptoms were due to myocardial ischemia.

As the pathogenesis and clinical presentation of UA and NSTEMI are very similar and the conditions cannot be differentiated at presentation, it seems sensible to discuss the management of these conditions together. This is now common practice in the cardiology literature and this concept has been adapted by the relevant advisory committees who have published different guidelines for the management of STEMI and NSTEMI (7,8).

ASSESSMENT OF RISK

The above considerations on different forms of MI highlight the fact that UA and MI are not one or two distinct diseases, but a continuum of problems that can last from a short, self-limiting episode of myocardial ischemia without any cell damage to a large full thickness infarct with subsequent severe impairment of left ventricular function. It is obvious that these two extremes will not only carry very different prognosis, but also pose completely different challenges to the physician treating the respective patients. To optimize an individual patient's treatment the physician will

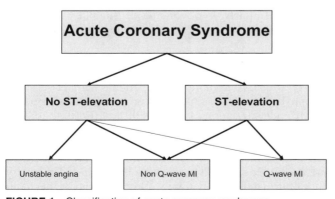

FIGURE 1   Classification of acute coronary syndromes.

need to have a very clear idea about his patient's risk of having further events and/or death. This has been an area of much debate in the cardiology community in recent years. A number of risk models have been developed. Currently the most widely accepted risk stratifying tool is the TIMI-risk score. The TIMI risk score for NSTEMI and UA was developed using the unfractionated heparin cohort of the TIMI-11B Trial (9,10). TIMI 11b was a multicenter randomized controlled clinical trial comparing the low-molecular weight heparin enoxaparin with unfractionated heparin in the management of ACS. It has subsequently been validated in additional trials and in one registry (11–13). It evaluated the composite endpoint of death, MI, and severe ischemia requiring revascularization within 14 days. Seven variables were used in the model:

1. age above 65 years
2. three or more coronary risk factors
3. known coronary stenosis of 50% or more
4. ST-segment deviation at presentation
5. two or more anginal events within the previous 24 hours
6. use of aspirin within the previous seven days
7. elevated cardiac markers.

Patients score one for each risk factor with a maximum total score of seven. Table 1 gives risk of the composite endpoint and individual endpoints. The same group also developed a risk score for STEMI that can be calculated from clinical variables available at the time of admission to hospital (14). The model was derived from a population of nearly 15,000 patients with STEMI who were recruited into the InTime II trial, a thrombolytic trial comparing the newer fibrinolytic agent lanoteplase to accelerated alteplase (15). The model was validated in the TIMI9 trial cohort (16). This score predicts mortality at 30 days. The variables are shown in Table 2. Table 3 shows the odds of death by 30 days depending on the risk score.

There are no risk prediction models specifically for MI occurring in the perioperative period. Given the generally worse outcome for perioperative ischemia/infarction when compared to events in the nonoperative setting, and the fact that risk scores derived from a clinical trial population almost always underestimate the risk when applied to a real life population, it seems likely that the risks quoted above are minimum risks.

TABLE 1 TIMI Risk Score for Non-ST–Segment Elevation Myocardial Infarction (MI)/Unstable Angina

Number of risk factors	Death (%)	MI (%)	Revascularization (%)	Composite (%)
0/1	1.2	2.3	1.2	4.7
2	1.0	2.1	6.0	8.3
3	1.7	3.7	9.5	13.2
4	2.5	5.0	12.2	19.9
5	5.6	8.5	14.3	26.2
6/7	6.5	15.8	20.9	40.9

Note: Percent risk of death, MI, need for urgent revascularization, and the composite depending on the number of risk factors (age ≥ 65 years; ≥ 3 risk factors; known coronary stenosis ≥ 50%; ST-segment deviation at presentation; ≥ 2 anginal events within the previous 24 hours; use of aspirin within the previous seven days; elevated cardiac markers).
Abbreviation: TIMI, thrombolysis in myocardial infarction.
Source: From Ref. 10.

TABLE 2 Factors Included in the TIMI Risk Score for STEMI

Age 65–74 yr	2 points
Age 75	3 points
Diabetes, hypertension, or angina	1 point
Systolic BP < 100 mmHg	3 points
HR > 100	2 points
Killip class II–IV	2 points
Weight < 67 kg	1 point
Anterior STEMI or LBBB	1 point
Time to treatment > 4 hr	1 point
Risk score = total	(0–14)

Abbreviations: BP, blood pressure; HR, heart rate; LBBB, left bundle branch block; MI, myocardial infarction; STEMI, ST-segment elevation MI; TIMI, thrombolysis in myocardial infarction.
Source: From Ref. 14.

GENERAL MEASURES IN THE MANAGEMENT OF ISCHEMIA OR INFARCTION

Once a diagnosis of perioperative ischemia has been made or is at least suspected, some general principles of the acute management of ischemia in the nonoperative setting should be followed.

Bed rest is advised while ischemia is ongoing. Adequate oxygenation will improve myocardial ischemia. Therefore, continuous measurement of oxygen saturation should be initiated. Supplemental oxygen should definitely be given if the oxygen saturation declines to less than 90%. Although it is common practice, there is no evidence available to support the routine administration of oxygen to all patients with acute myocardial ischemia in the absence of respiratory distress or arterial hypoxemia (8).

In the nonoperative setting, pain and distress are treated with intravenous morphine or diamorphine, usually given together with an antiemetic. The usefulness of this treatment has not been assessed in randomized clinical trials. However, morphine is a potent vasodilator and reduces heart rate through increased vagal tone. Its analgesic and anxiolytic effects will decrease blood pressure. All these mechanisms will reduce myocardial oxygen demand thereby alleviating myocardial ischemia.

TABLE 3 TIMI Risk Score for ST-Segment Elevation Myocardial Infarction (Odds of Death by 30 Days Depending on Risk Score)

Risk score	Odds of death by 30 days (95% CI)
0	0.1 (0.1–0.2)
1	0.3 (0.2–0.3)
2	0.4 (0.3–0.5)
3	0.7 (0.6–0.9)
4	1.2 (1.0–1.5)
5	2.2 (1.9–2.6)
6	3.0 (2.5–3.6)
7	4.8 (3.8–6.1)
8	5.8 (4.2–7.8)
>8	8.8 (6.3–12)

Note: The risk score is derived from the clinical variables described in Table 2.
Abbreviation: CI, confidence interval.
Source: From Ref. 14.

Given the high mortality and morbidity associated with myocardial ischemia and infarction in the perioperative period, the patient should be managed in some form of high dependency area with an adequate nursing to patient ratio and facilities for continuous 12-lead ECG monitoring. Whether this is an intensive care unit, a surgical, or medical high dependency unit, or a coronary care unit will depend on local factors and the individual needs of a specific patient. Continuous ECG monitoring will allow detection of ventricular fibrillation, which is the major preventable cause of death in the early period of myocardial ischemia and infarction. If continuous 12-lead ECG monitoring is not available, repeat 12-lead ECGs will also detect ST-segment shift as a sign of ongoing or recurrent ischemia.

In the perioperative setting, it can be very difficult to work out whether hypotension is the cause or the consequence of ischemia. The possibility that hypotension caused by surgical bleeding has precipitated myocardial ischemia should be considered. Hypotension due to neuroaxial blockade can also cause reduced coronary blood flow and myocardial ischemia, particularly in the context of preexisting coronary artery disease (CAD). Myocardial oxygen delivery may also be compromised by arterial hypoxemia due to pneumonia, atelectasis, and pneumothorax all of which may complicate surgery.

Although most episodes of perioperative ischemia or infarction occur in the postoperative period, some events occur during surgery. If this is the case the operating surgeon should be informed and a joint decision should be taken whether or not to stop the operation. Clearly this will have to be an individualized decision taking into account the nature and urgency of the operation, the stage of the procedure when ischemia occurs, the severity of ischemia/infarction, and its response to initial treatment.

BALANCING RISKS

Many of the pharmacological treatment strategies for myocardial ischemia involve the use of potent antiplatelet and antithrombotic drugs. These increase the risk of hemorrhagic complications. This is increasingly being recognized as a problem in the management of ACS in the nonoperative setting and bleeding complications are now frequently a part of composite endpoints in modern clinical trials. It is obvious that the potential for these drugs causing harm is even greater in the perioperative setting. When making decisions on pharmacotherapy for patients with perioperative ischemia and infarction one needs to consider at least the following three factors:

1. Whether or not to use an antithrombotic or antiplatelet drug in a given patient will depend on details and bleeding risks of the operation. In specific types of surgery where bleeding complications could have devastating consequences, such as intracranial surgery, eye surgery, or spinal cord surgery, particular caution is required.
2. The severity of the ischemia, its response to initial therapy, the time interval between surgery and the onset of ischemia, the angiographic findings and the planned management strategy (medical, PCI, CABG) will influence the use of antithrombotic and antiplatelet therapy.
3. Finally different antiplatelet and antithrombotic therapies have different associated bleeding risks. The most severe bleeding complications are usually seen with thrombolytic and fibrinolytic agents such as streptokinase and tissue plasminogen activator (t-PA). Given the fact that primary PCI has been shown

to be a superior management strategy for patients with STEMI, it is the author's view that thrombolysis should not be used in perioperative STEMI and all efforts should be made to treat/transfer the respective patients to an experienced PCI-center in a timely fashion.

The bleeding risks associated with antiplatelet agents are significantly smaller. Burger et al. (17) analyzed the data available for aspirin. The authors reviewed 41 studies on perioperative aspirin related bleeding risk. Their conclusion was that while aspirin increased the rate of bleeding complications by a factor of 1.5, it did not lead to a higher level of the severity of bleeding complications except in intracranial surgery.

The data for other antiplatelet agents in the perioperative setting is extremely limited. Clopidogrel was assessed in the CURE trial (18). The risk of perioperative bleeding was increased for patients who underwent CABG within the first five days after clopidogrel was discontinued. However, in a small randomized trial of 150 patients undergoing carotid endarterectomy there was no increase in bleeding complications or blood transfusions in the clopidogrel group when compared to placebo (19).

Data is even more limited on glycoprotein (GP) IIb/IIIa receptor antagonists. Currently, we do not routinely recommend the use of these agents for patients who suffer a perioperative episode of MI or ischemia, particularly if noninterventional management of the patient is planned. If it is planned to take the patient to the catheter laboratory, decision making is more difficult and will have to take into account the nature and time of the operation, the severity, duration and time of ischemia, the angiographic findings, and the availability of alternative agents, such as Bivalirudin.

The bleeding risks associated with the use of heparin (including low-molecular weight heparins) is higher than that with most antiplatelet agents (up to 7% major bleeding in one trial in the nonoperative setting). There is also the suggestion of an even higher bleeding risk with the low-molecular weight heparins (20,21). In practice, decision making is relatively easy for patients undergoing PCI, where heparin (or Bivalirudin) is considered absolutely necessary to perform the procedure safely. If a conservative approach is chosen and a decision to give heparin was taken, we would recommend using unfractionated heparin, because it has a shorter half-life and it can be more reliably reversed with protamin.

Given the complexities as discussed above we strongly believe that therapy should be individualized for each case on the basis of close discussion between the surgical, anesthetic, and cardiology teams.

IMPORTANCE OF THE ECG IN GUIDING TREATMENT

Despite the many advances in noninvasive and invasive cardiac investigations, the 12-lead ECG remains the most important single investigation in the management of acute ischemia or infarction. It is imperative, therefore, that a good quality 12-lead ECG be performed and correctly interpreted, as quickly as possible. If the ECG fulfills the standard criteria for STEMI (Table 4), then the patient should be considered for immediate reperfusion therapy. This could be achieved either by coronary angioplasty (PCI) or by the systemic administration of thrombolysis. If the 12-lead ECG does not fulfill the criteria for immediate PCI or thrombolysis, then they should be managed as for ischemia/NSTEMI. This group, however, should be monitored closely with frequent

TABLE 4　Standard Criteria for Initiation of Reperfusion Therapy

ST-segment elevation > 0. 1 mV in at least 2 inferior leads (II, III, avF)
ST-segment elevation > 0. 2 mV in at least 2 contiguous anterior leads (V2–V6)
New left bundle branch block

further ECGs because the ECG may evolve into an ST-segment elevation pattern, which may then require reperfusion therapy. It is important to realize that blood tests (CK, CKMB, troponin etc.) have no part to play in the acute setting. These tests are useful for making a retrospective diagnosis, and for risk stratification, but are generally not available at a time to influence immediate decisions about angioplasty, thrombolysis, and other aspects of drug treatment.

MANAGEMENT OF STEMI

Management of STEMI is one of the few real emergencies in medicine. Numerous observational studies and clinical trials have proven beyond doubt that both mortality and long-term morbidity increase with increasing time delay between the onset of symptoms and reperfusion of the infarct related territory (22–24). General measures of management have been discussed in a previous chapter and should be put into place. Administration of 300 mg of aspirin should be done as soon as possible. A decision on a revascularization strategy, preferably primary PCI, should be made early and the logistics of how it can be delivered, should be explored immediately.

PCI for STEMI

Primary PCI is now the gold standard treatment for STEMI and should be considered in all patients. Since its inception in 1977, angioplasty has made enormous strides and is now the most commonly used revascularization strategy. Initial problems with acute vessel closure were largely solved with the advent of stenting. More recently the development of drug eluting stents has reduced the problem of in-stent-restenosis, which now allows interventional cardiologists to take on more complex lesions and disease in smaller vessels. Initially designed as a treatment of stable angina, PCI has now found its role as an important management tool for ACS.

Primary PCI has been tested as a treatment strategy for STEMI in a large number of small randomized controlled trials. These have been summarized in a recent meta-analysis (25). In this study, 7739 thrombolytic eligible patients from 23 trials have been analyzed. Primary PCI was associated with a reduction in the combined endpoint of death, nonfatal infarction and stroke from 14% to 8%. Moreover, when the endpoints were analyzed individually, there was a statistically significant reduction in all of these including mortality on its own. More recently, two studies (PRAGUE-2 and DANAMI-2) have extended these findings from patients directly admitted to angioplasty centers to those who needed transport from a local hospital to an interventional center (26–28).

The superiority of primary PCI when compared to thrombolytic therapy critically depends on whether or not the intervention can be provided in a timely fashion.

Nallamothu and Bates (29) used data from Keeley's (25) meta-analysis and were able to show that the benefit from primary PCI as compared to thrombolytic therapy is lost when the PCI related time delay (compared to thrombolyis) is 95 minutes or more. Consequently the relevant American Heart Association/American College of Cardiology (AHA/ACC) guidelines recommend primary PCI as the preferred treatment strategy for STEMI provided it can be delivered with a door-to-balloon time of less than 90 minutes and a call-to-balloon time of less than 120 minutes (7). Many hospitals around the world are currently developing the logistics of care-pathways to achieve these targets for patients suffering an acute STEMI in the nonoperative setting. These existing pathways should be used for the optimal management of patients with a perioperative STEMI, as this high-risk group of patients with significant bleeding risk would particularly benefit from primary PCI.

Thrombolysis

If PCI is not available within a period of 90 to 120 minutes, consideration should be given to intravenous thrombolysis. Clearly, this will involve balancing the risk to the patient of not treating the MI against the risk of bleeding. Recent surgery and risk of bleeding were standard exclusion criteria in all of the major thrombolytic studies. There are, therefore, no data about the relative risks of thrombolysis and MI in the perioperative setting. In normal clinical practice, the superiority of thrombolysis compared to placebo has been well established in a number of randomized controlled trials. In ISIS-2,17,187 patients with STEMI were randomized to streptokinase versus placebo (30). Five-week mortality was reduced from 12% to 9.2% ($p < 0.001$). There was an excess of cerebral hemorrhage (0.1% vs. 0.0%) and bleeds requiring transfusion (0.5% vs. 0.2%) in the treatment group. These findings were confirmed in the GISSI-1 study (31).

Further studies such as GUSTO-I have evaluated other thrombolytic strategies and have proven the superiority of t-PA over streptokinase (32). Newer agents, such as tenectaplase, may have slightly improved efficacy but do not confer any reduction of the bleeding risk.

Adjunctive Drug Treatment for STEMI

Aspirin in STEMI

Aspirin 300 mg should be given orally, immediately to all conscious STEMI patients. The single most important trial in this context is probably ISIS-2 (30). Seventeen thousand one hundred and eighty seven patients admitted with suspected acute MI were randomized in a two-by-two factorial design to one month of aspirin and 1.5 MU of streptokinase versus placebo. At five weeks aspirin use on its own was associated with a 23% relative risk reduction in vascular death when compared to placebo.

The optimal dose of aspirin therapy has been a matter of intense discussions over recent years. The Antiplatelet Trialists Collaboration concluded in their meta-analysis that there was no appreciable evidence that a higher-dose aspirin was more effective than medium-dose aspirin in preventing vascular events (33). Consequently, the ACC/AHA Guidelines recommend an initial dose of 162–325 mg aspirin followed by 75–160 mg daily.

Aspirin is usually given in its oral form. In the perioperative period this might be a problem when there could be problems with oral intake and/or absorption. If this was the case a rectal formulation (same dose) is available. Intravenous aspirin is not available in the United Kingdom.

Clopidogrel in STEMI

Clopidogrel is a thienopyridine adenosine diphosphate antagonist, which irreversibly inhibits platelet aggregation and is a more potent inhibitor of platelet activation than aspirin.

A recent large-scale trial (COMMIT) assessed clopidogrel in addition to standard therapy (including aspirin and thrombolysis) in 45,852 patients with acute MI. The composite primary endpoint of death, reinfarction and stroke was significantly reduced from 10.1% to 9.2%. There was also a significant reduction in mortality. No excess risk of bleeding was observed (34). Current clinical practice is to give clopidogrel in a loading dose of either 300 mg or 600 mg followed by 75 mg daily to all STEMI patients whether being treated with primary PCI or with thrombolysis. For patients undergoing primary PCI, dual antiplatelet therapy with clopidogrel and aspirin for one year is standard treatment.

GP IIb/IIIa Antagonists in STEMI

GP IIb/IIIa receptor is abundant on the platelet surface and is involved in the final and obligatory pathway for platelet aggregation. Two different types of GP IIb/IIIa antagonists with characteristic pharmacokinetic and pharmacodynamic properties have been developed. Abciximab, a monoclonal antibody, has a short half-life, but binds irreversibly to the receptor. The action of abciximab, therefore, can only be overcome when the platelets are replenished. The small molecule IIb/IIIa inhibitors Eptifibatide and Tirofiban are peptides; they have a plasma half-life of two to three hours. Platelet function returns to normal four to eight hours after discontinuation of the drug. Two large studies have shown the benefits of abciximab in patients with ST-segment elevation MI (ADMIRAL and CADILLAC). In the ADMIRAL study, 300 patients were randomized to either abciximab or placebo prior to PCI. The active treatment reduced the composite endpoint of death, reinfarction, or revascularization at 30 days and at six months (35). In the CADILLAC study, 2082 patients with acute MI were randomized in a two-by-two factorial design to undergo PTCA alone, PTCA plus abciximab therapy, stenting alone or stenting plus abciximab. A composite endpoint of death, reinfarction, stroke, and ischemia driven target vessel revascularization (repeat PCI or CABG) was analyzed at six months. It had occurred in 20% of patients with PTCA alone, 16.5% after PTCA plus abciximab, 11.5% after stenting, and 10.2% after stenting plus abciximab. All these differences were driven by target vessel revascularization (36). Based on this and other small studies, the ACC/AHA guidelines concluded that IIb/IIIa inhibitor treatment should be started treatment as early as possible before primary PCI.

Heparins in STEMI

This group of drugs includes unfractionated heparin and various low-molecular weight heparins. Heparin activates antithrombin, a proteoloytic enzyme that inactivates thrombin and factors IXa and Xa. Therefore, it prevents thrombus formation but does not lyse existing thrombi.

The need for heparin in STEMI depends on the reperfusion strategy chosen. For primary PCI it is common practice to use weight-adjusted boluses of 70–100U/kg heparin. Again this information is not directly derived from trials in primary PCI but from general observations in angioplasty (37)

The nonspecific fibrinolytic agents such as streptokinase produce a systemic coagulapathy and the need for systemic anticoagulation is doubtful. This question has been addressed in ISIS-3 and GISSI-2 and no significant reduction in 30-day mortality could be demonstrated when subcutaneous heparin was used together with nonspecific thrombolytic agents (38,39).

Heparin is routinely used after treatment of STEMI with fibrin-specific thrombolytic agents. This is mainly based on angiographic studies that have shown that intravenous heparin in conjunction with alteplase led to higher rates of infarct related artery perfusion (7).

The role of low-molecular weight heparins for patients with STEMI remains unclear. In ASSENT-3 unfractionated heparin was compared to enoxaparin as adjunctive therapy to tenecteplase. The composite endpoint of 30-day mortality, in-hospital reinfarction, and in-hospital recurrent ischemia was reduced with enoxaparin treatment. However, there was a tendency toward more bleeding complications including intracranial hemorrhage in the enoxaparin group (40).

Given the concerns about a possibly increased bleeding risk with low-molecular weight heparins, it seems sensible to use unfractionated heparin in the context of perioperative STEMI. This has the advantage that the drug is more quickly eliminated after discontinuation of the infusion and that the effects of unfractionated heparin can be reversed with protamine in the case of life threatening bleeding.

Other Anti-thrombin Agents in STEMI

Bivlirudin is a thrombin inhibitor, which has been tested in several studies, mostly involving non-STEMI patients. Bivalirudin is currently being compared with unfractionated heparin and a IIb/IIIa inhibitor in a large study of STEMI patients being treated with primary PCI (HORIZONS study). Currently, however, there is no evidence to favor bivalirudin over the combination of heparin and abciximab in the treatment of ST-segment elevation MI.

Beta-Blockers in STEMI

Beta-blockers competitively inhibit the effects of catecholamines on beta-adrenoreceptors in the cell wall. These agents have a negative chronotropic and a negative inotropic effect resulting in decreased oxygen demand of the myocardium. A large number of trials have been performed assessing the short- and long-term benefits of beta-blockers after MI. In a meta-analysis of these trials, Freemantle et al. (41) found a 23% reduction in the odds of death in long-term trials. This equates to a number needed to treat for two years to avoid one death of 42. Benefits have been demonstrated for patients with and without concomitant therapy, both early and late after STEMI (7). Prompt administration of oral beta-blockers has received a class I recommendation by the relevant ACC/AHA guidelines (7). The use of very early and intravenous beta-blockade has been a matter of debate over the years. The most recent ACC/AHA guidelines gave a class IIa recommendation for intravenous beta-blockers. Since publication of these guidelines the results of the Clopidogrel and Metoprolol in MI trial have been made available (42). In this Chinese Megatrial 45,852 patients admitted to 1250 hospitals were randomly allocated to intravenous followed by oral Metoprolol or matching placebo. Neither total mortality nor the composite endpoint of death, reinfarction, or cardiac arrest was significantly reduced by the active treatment. Current clinical practice is not to give intravenous beta-blockers, but to give most MI patients an oral beta-blocker provided they have no preexisting contraindications and have no evidence of heart block, shock, or pulmonary edema.

Calcium Antagonists in STEMI

These drugs inhibit both myocardial and vascular smooth muscle contraction by reducing cell transmembrane inward calcium flux. The nondihydropyridine drugs Verapamil and Diltiazem also depress sinus and AV-node function. This group of drugs was intensively studied in various randomized controlled trials in the nonoperative setting.

There is no clear evidence to support the use of any type of calcium antagonist after MI The ACC/AHA guidelines for STEMI conclude that Diltiazem or Verapamil could be considered in patients who have an absolute contraindication to beta-blockers for relief of ongoing ischemia or to control the ventricular rate in atrial flutter of fibrillation (7).

Nitrates in STEMI

Nitrates are endothelium-independent vasodilators that reduce myocardial oxygen consumption and increase myocardial oxygen delivery. In the acute setting glyceryl trinitrate (GTN) is the preferred nitrate given its rapid onset of action. Nitrates might be useful as an initial measure when vasospasm is thought to be the cause of the ST-segment elevation. Routine use of a nitrate infusion is probably not necessary for patients suffering from a STEMI (43,44). However, nitrate infusions have a role for the management of hypertension and pulmonary edema in the context of STEMI and this has been endorsed by the relevant practice guidelines (7,45). Nitrates should be avoided in right ventricular infarction and hypotension.

Angiotensin Converting Enzyme Inhibitors in STEMI

In the context of acute MI, angiotensin converting enzyme (ACE)-inhibitors have been assessed in the AIRE, GISSI-3, ISIS-4, and other smaller studies. These have proven the benefit of ACE-inhibition with a variety of different agents after MI (43,44,46). Patients with anterior MI, evidence of pulmonary edema or an ejection fraction of less than 40% have been shown to benefit most from treatment with an ACE-inhibitor. Treatment should begin with a low dose of an ACE-inhibitor (such as Ramipril 1.25 mg b.d.) within 24 hours of an acute event, provided the renal function is normal and the systolic blood pressure is greater than 100 mmHg.

Statins in STEMI

As with ACE-inhibitors, the main benefits of this class of drugs are in secondary prevention. Recently studies have compared high versus low dose statin therapy and have shown some benefit with the more aggressive approach (47). In general, therefore, all patients with cardiac ischemia or infarction should be started on a high dose statin as soon as is feasible.

MANAGEMENT OF NON-ST-SEGMENT ELEVATION MI/UA

As discussed previously, patients presenting with myocardial ischemia and ST-segment depression form a single group at the time of presentation. It is only when the results of cardiac marker tests, such a troponin or CK, are available several hours later, that these patients can be categorized into non-ST-segment elevation MI (with elevated markers) or UA (without elevated markers). These patients will generally have significant CAD and the majority will require revascularization, either by coronary angioplasty (PCI) or by coronary artery surgery (CABG). However, revascularization is usually not required immediately, unlike the situation with the

STEMI patient. In most NSTEMI/UA patients, the ischemia will settle with appropriate medical treatment (plaque passivation) allowing planned angiography and revascularization within 24 to 48 hours.

Drug Treatment of NSTEMI /UA
Nitrates
Nitrates are available as spray, sublingual tablet, and as an intravenous formulation. The usual starting dose is $10\,\mu g/min$, which can be rapidly titrated up to a usual ceiling dose of $200\,\mu g/min$. Dose escalation is often limited by the development of hypotension. Tolerance to its hemodynamic effects usually develops after 24 hours.

Both in the operative and in the nonoperative setting nitrates are often considered as first line treatment for acute myocardial ischemia. Curiously, the effects of nitrates on symptoms in the acute setting have never been evaluated in large-scale clinical trials. Whether or not the use of nitrates has an effect on mortality has been an issue of some debate. Yusuf et al. (48) published an overview of small randomized trials suggesting a 35% reduction in mortality. This hypothesis was then formally tested in ISIS-4 and GISSI-3 and no statistically significant mortality benefit could be demonstrated (43,44). However, clinical experience suggests that intravenous nitrates are useful in this setting and their use has been endorsed by the AHA/ACC guidelines for UA and NSTEMI, where a class Ic recommendation has been given (8).

Aspirin in UA and NSTEMI
There is good evidence supporting the use of aspirin for patients with UA (49). One thousand two hundred and sixty six men with UA were randomized to 325 mg aspirin versus placebo for 12 weeks. There was an impressive 51% relative risk reduction (5.1% absolute risk reduction) in the combined endpoint of death and MI at 12 weeks. The Antiplatelet Trialists Collaboration (33) quoted an absolute risk reduction in vascular events of 5% in patients with UA.

Clopidogrel in UA and NSTEMI
Clopidogrel has been studied as an adjunct to aspirin therapy in ACS patients in the CURE-study (18). Twelve thousand five hundred and sixty two patients with UA were randomized to clopidogrel (300 mg loading dose followed by 75 mg daily). Patients were followed up for 3 to 12 months. There was a statistically significant 20% relative risk reduction (absolute risk reduction: 2.2%) for the primary composite endpoint of cardiovascular death, MI, or stroke. These salutary effects have to be weighed up against the increased bleeding risks of dual antiplatelet therapy. In CURE the risk of major bleeding was increased from 2.7% in the placebo group to 3.7% in the clopidogrel group. There was also a nonsignificant trend for an increase in life threatening bleeding. Currently, in the nonoperative setting, it is our practice to give clopidogrel to all patients who are scheduled to undergo PCI and to those who are admitted with a marker or ECG-positive ACS.

Heparin in UA and NSTEMI
Several small randomized controlled trials have tried to analyze whether intravenous heparin reduces the frequency of MI and death in patients admitted with UA (50–52). All of these trials lacked the power to answer this question. Braunwald et al. (8)

examined the available evidence and found that treatment with intravenous heparin reduced the absolute risk of death or MI at one week from 5.5% to 2.6% ($p < 0.018$).

LMWH have been assessed in clinical trials of patients with UA. In the FRISC study, patients admitted with UA or non-Q–wave MI were randomized to Dalteparin (120 IU/kg bodyweight, b.i.d.) versus placebo for six days. The primary endpoint of death or MI at six days was reduced from 4.8% to 1.8%. This benefit persisted at 40 days (21).

Two trials (FRIC and FRAX.I.S.) compared intravenous heparin to low-molecular weight heparins (dalteparin and nadroparin) and were unable to demonstrate any statistically significant difference between the treatment groups (53,54). As there was a trend toward harm with the low-molecular weight heparins in these trials dalteparin and nadroparin are now rarely used in clinical praxis. Two further trials (TIMI 11b and ESSENCE) compared Enoxaparin to intravenous heparin and showed small but statistically significant reductions in early events with the low-molecular weight heparins (9,20).

It is not possible to explain the differences between different low-molecular weight heparins from the available data. Most institutions have switched to using LMWH, usually Enoxaparin for at least 48 hours as part of the medical management of NSTEMI/UA.

GP IIb/IIIa Inhibitors in UA and NSTEMI

These agents have been shown to reduce adverse events, particularly MI, in ACS patients undergoing PCI. For abciximab, this has been demonstrated in the EPIC, EPILOGUE and EPISTENT studies (55–57). Subgroup analysis suggests that patients who are troponin positive and diabetic patients tend to benefit most.

The small molecules Tirofiban and Eptifibatide were assessed in the PRISM, PRISM-PLUS, and PURSUIT trials (58–60). These trials showed a modest reduction in early combined ischemic endpoints in the active treatment group.

The only published head-to-head comparison between different GP IIb/IIIa receptor antagonists is the TARGET trial (61). In this study of 5308 patients scheduled to undergo elective or urgent PCI, abciximab was significantly better than tirofiban in preventing the combined endpoint of death or MI.

While the benefit of GP IIb/IIIa receptor antagonists, particularily abciximab, is well documented during PCI, the results of the trials in primarily medically treated patients are less clear. Boersma et al. (62) performed a meta-analysis of all major randomized clinical trials involving 31,402 patients with ACS who were not routinely scheduled to undergo coronary revascularization. The composite endpoint of death or MI at 30 days was reduced from 11.8% to 10.8% (relative risk reduction: 9%). Major bleeding complications were seen in 2.4% of the GP IIb/IIIa receptor antagonists group and 1.4% of the placebo group ($p < 0.0001$). However, the observed benefit was confined to those patients, who (although not scheduled for routine coronary revascularization) underwent PCI or CABG within the next 30 days. This simply reinforces the modern view that there are two stages to the management of NSTEMI/UA, namely medical treatment ("plaque passivation") and revascularization, usually by PCI but occasionally by CABG.

Bivalirudin in UA and NSTEMI

Bivalirudin is part of a class known as direct thrombin inhibitors. Hirudin is the prototype and has been studied against unfractionated heparin in the GUSTO-IIb and

TIMI 9B and OASIS trials (16,63,64). So far superiority over intravenous heparin has not been demonstrated and there seems to be an excess of bleeding complications in the hirudin group. Currently the only indication for hirudin could be patients with heparin-induced thrombocytopenia.

Bivalirudin is a synthetic analog of hirudin that has recently gained some interest as an alternative to intravenous heparin and abciximab in PCI. In the REPLACE-2 trial 6010 patients undergoing elective or low risk emergency PCI were randomized to either bivalirudin with provisional GP IIb/IIIa inhibition or heparin with planned GP IIb/IIIa inhibition (65). The trial was designed as a noninferiority trial. There was no difference in the composite endpoint of death, MI, and urgent repeat revascularization at 30 days between the two treatment groups. However, in-hospital major bleeding rates were significantly reduced by bivalirudin (2.4% vs. 4.1%; $p < 0.001$).

The ACUITY-trial has at the time of writing only been published in abstract format (66). Thirteen thousand eight hundred and nineteen patients with moderate-to high-risk ACS were included. The trial design was rather complex involving various treatment arms and randomization steps. The main result seems to be that bivalirudin monotherapy significantly reduces bleeding complications, when compared to a combination of heparin and 2b3a-inhibitor without increasing the incidence of ischemic complications. It seems likely that the use of bivalirudin might well increase in the future, particularly in patients who are supposed to have a high bleeding risk, such as those with perioperative ischemia and infarction.

Beta-Blockers in UA and NSTEMI

Although there is some evidence to support the prophylactic use of beta-blockers in patients at high risk of a perioperative event, there are no randomized controlled trials supporting the use of beta-blockers as a treatment for perioperative myocardial ischemia. Even in the nonoperative setting there were only small and uncontrolled studies. A meta-analysis of double-blind, randomized trials showed a 13% reduction of the risk of progression to acute MI (67). Based on our pathophysiologic considerations and the trial data on CAD in the nonoperative setting we recommend the use of oral (for low risk) and intravenous beta-blockade in the case of ongoing chest pain and inability to take/absorb oral medication first.

True asthma and AV-node disease (degree AV-block with PR > 0.24 ms; all forms of higher degree AV-block) remain absolute contraindications to the use of beta-blockers. In patients with chronic obstructive pulmonary disease (COPD) a small dose of a beta-1–specific drug (such as metoprolol 25 mg or bisoprolol 1.25 mg) can be tried cautiously, particularly if the patient is felt to be at high risk (recurrent pain; biomarker positivity; dynamic ECG changes).

Calcium-Antagonists in UA and NSTEMI

These agents have a limited role in the acute management of acute ischemia. In general, verapamil or diltiazem can be considered for patients who have contraindications to or cannot tolerate beta-blockade. However, given their negative inotropic effect, these agents should be avoided if the patient is in pulmonary edema or has severely impaired left ventricular function.

Statins

There is a wealth of data to support the use of 3-hydroxy-3-methylglutaryl coenzyme A (HMG-CoA)–reductase inhibitors or statins in primary and secondary prevention of CAD (68–70). More recently studies have compared high versus low dose statin therapy and have shown some benefit with the more aggressive approach (47). It is our current practice to start every patient who presents to us with any form of an ACS (UA, NSTEMI, STEMI) on a statin such as simvastatin 40 mg once daily or atorvastatin 40 mg once daily.

PCI for UA/NSTEMI

Most patients who develop UA/NSTEMI should be considered for coronary angiography with a revascularization either by PCI (around 80%) or coronary bypass surgery (around 20%). This policy is based on the results of recent clinical trials (FRISC 2, TACTICS-TIMI 18, RITA 3) comparing an early invasive strategy to a conservative approach in this group of patients. These trials have consistently shown a reduction in death, recurrent MI, and refractory angina, both early and late after the initial event (71–74).

How can this information be applied to patients who have a perioperative episode of NSTEMI or UA? Subgroup analysis has demonstrated that the highest risk patients are those who have most to gain from an early invasive approach (74,75). As outlined above patients with a perioperative event are at high risk per se and would therefore qualify for an early invasive approach. The potential benefits of this approach have to be balanced against potential bleeding complications. High risk patients undergoing acute PCI are usually treated with a cocktail of aspirin, clopidogrel, heparin, and frequently abciximab. In TACTICS-TIMI 18 the rate of major bleeding was 1.9% in the invasive group and 1.3% in the conservative group. The respective figures for all bleeding episodes were 5.5% in the invasive group and 3.3% in the conservative group (72). These figures demonstrate that although the bleeding risk with an interventional strategy is somewhat higher, even the conservative strategy with prolonged duration of antithrombotic and antiplatelet drug therapy is not without its associated bleeding complications.

MANAGEMENT OF HEART FAILURE ASSOCIATED WITH ACUTE ISCHEMIA OR INFARCTION

Heart failure in patients with an ACS is a serious complication associated with a one-year mortality of between 40% to 60% in patients with cardiogenic shock (76). In about 75% of patients heart failure is due extensive LV dysfunction (7). Other important causes include mechanical complications of MI such as acute severe mitral regurgitation, ventricular septal rupture, and subacute free-wall rupture with tamponade. These conditions need to be actively ruled out and early echocardiography is recommended. Heart failure can present as pulmonary edema or low output state/cardiogenic shock. Principles of treatment are similar and discussed below. Figure 2 summarizes our recommended treatment strategy.

Oxygenation

Oxygen supplementation to achieve arterial saturation greater than 90% is a class Ic recommendation of the AHA/ACC-guidelines for the management of pulmonary congestion in the context of STEMI (7). Oxygen can be delivered by simple facemasks, but more recently noninvasive ventilation with continuous positive airway pressure (CPAP) and noninvasive positive pressure ventilation (NPPV) has gained considerable interest. Several small randomized trials have been performed comparing noninvasive ventilation with standard therapy and CPAP with biphasic positive

Management of Acute Heart Failure in ACS

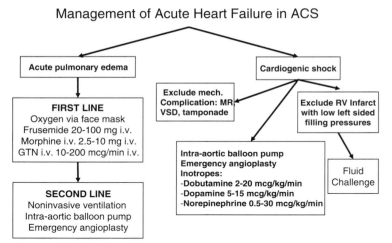

FIGURE 2   Treatment strategies for acute pulmonary edema and cardiogenic shock.
Abbreviations: ACS, acute coronary syndrome; i.v., intravenous; MR, mitral regurgitation; RV, right ventricular; VSD, ventricular septal defect.

airways pressure (BIPAP). Peter et al. (77) performed a meta-analysis of all trials assessing noninvasive ventilation in acute cardiogenic pulmonary edema. This confirmed a definite mortality reduction with CPAP versus standard therapy (relative risk 0.59, 95% CI 0.38–0.90, $p=0.015$). For NPPV a trend toward reduced mortality was seen. The need for invasive ventilation was significantly reduced with both forms of noninvasive ventilation. It is our current practice to treat all patients with pulmonary edema who do not quickly settle on standard therapy (oxygen via face mask, diamorphine, diuretics) with CPAP.

Optimization of Filling Pressures

Left ventricular filling pressures may rise rapidly in ACS due to acute systolic or diastolic dysfunction. This causes rapid redistribution of fluid from the intravascular space to the lung interstitium and alveoli. The diagnosis can generally be made by lung auscultation and chest X-ray. Immediate management consists of adequate oxygenation as described above and preload reduction. This can usually be achieved with a combination of opiates (morphine sulfate 2.5–10 mg i.v.), diuretics (furosemide 20–100 mg i.v.) and nitrates (GTN 10–200µ g i.v.). These measures have received class Ic recommendation by the joint ACC/AHA guidelines (7). All the drugs described have a tendency to lower blood pressure. This is usually well tolerated, as the physiological response to pulmonary edema is sympathetic stimulation causing a rise in blood pressure. In the presence of pulmonary edema, a systolic pressure of less than 100 mmHg indicates cardiogenic shock with pulmonary edema. In this situation nitrates should not be given and inotropic support may be required.

Sometimes patients with acute MI present with hypotension and no evidence of pulmonary edema. In this situation it is important to rule out right ventricular infarction. The diagnosis can be suspected by performing an ECG looking at the right ventricular leads. It can be confirmed by invasive hemodynamic monitoring with a pulmonary artery catheter and is characterized by low left sided filling pressures and elevated right atrial pressures. The adequate treatment consists of prompt expansion of intravascular volume with normal saline.

Inotropes

When arterial hypotension fails to respond to fluid challenge inotropic and vaso-pressor agents need to be considered. Unfortunately, there are no large-scale randomized controlled trials to support the use of these agents. The rationale for their use is mainly clinical observations and pathophysiologic principles.

Incautious use of inotropes in cardiogenic shock may, via various mechanisms (tachycardia, coronary artery constriction), trigger further myocardial ischemia and necrosis resulting in even lower blood pressure. Therefore, our preferred initial strategy in patients with cardiogenic shock in the context of acute myocardial ischemia is the insertion of an intra-aortic balloon pump and emergency PCI.

Intra-aortic Balloon Pump

The intra-aortic balloon pump (IABP) improves diastolic coronary blood flow and reduces myocardial work. It might, therefore, be a useful device in patients with acute MI who are in cardiogenic shock or who have ongoing or recurrent ischemic

TABLE 5 Suggested Management of Perioperative Myocardial Ischemia and Infarction

General measures

Bed rest
Oxygen therapy
High dependency area (continuous ECG monitoring
   or repeat 12-lead ECGs)
Involve cardiology team early
Exclude noncoronary causes of ischemia
   (hypovolemia, hypoxemia)

Immediate management	
Unstable angina/N-STEMI	STEMI
Aspirin 300 mg p.o./p.r.	Aspirin 300 mg p.o./p.r.
Sublingual/i.v. nitrates	Try sublingual GTN
Morphine sulfate 2–10 mg i.v.	Morphine sulfate 2–10 mg i.v.
β-Blockade (metoprolol 50–100 mg p.o., atenolol 2.5–10 mg i.v.)	Discuss feasibility primary PCI
Consider unfractionated or low-molecular weight-heparin[a]	
Consider clopidogrel 300 mg p.o.[a]	
Consider GP IIb/IIIa[a]	
Consider early revascularization	

Long-term management

Cardiac rehabilitation program
Aspirin 75 mg for life
Clopidogrel 75 mg for 1 yr
Beta-blocker (metoprolol 50–100 mg b.d.; bisoprolol 5–10 mg o.d.)
Statin (simvastatin 40 mg p.o. once, atorvastatin 20 mg p.o. once)
ACE inhibitor (ramipril 2.5–5 mg b.d., perindopril 4–8 mg p.o. once)

[a]Benefit of treatment must be assessed against increased bleeding risk
Abbreviations: ACE, angiotensin converting enzyme; ECG, electrocardiogram; GP, glycoprotein; GTN, glyceryl trinitrate; MI, myocardial infarction; NSTEMI, non-ST–segment elevation MI; PCI, percutaneous coronary intervention; STEMI, ST-segment elevation MI.

discomfort. It is important to understand that IABP usually are a bridge to a more definite treatment such as revascularization or a way to buy some time (stunned myocardium). In this context, the use of IABP has been endorsed by the relevant ACC/AHA guidelines (7). Currently there is no trial evidence to support the use of IABP in acute MI. Its use is solely based on pathophysiologic principles and clinical observations.

SUMMARY

Managing patients who suffer perioperative MI or ischemia is a clinical challenge. This is not helped by the fact that there is very little in the way of evidence to guide the physician treating this vulnerable group of patients. It is our approach to use the evidence available from ACS in the nonoperative setting and modify it according to the demands of the perioperative setting. This also means that individualized decisions need to be made that take into account the severity of the ischemia, its response to initial therapy, the type of surgery that has been performed, and the time interval between surgery and the onset of ischemia. Optimal individual decisions can only be made on the basis of close discussion between the surgical, anesthetic, and cardiology teams. Table 5 summarizes the outline of a possible management strategy for perioperative MI or ischemia.

REFERENCES

1. Lee TH, Marcantonio ER, Mangione CM, et al. Derivation and prospective validation of a simple index for prediction of cardiac risk of major noncardiac surgery. Circulation 1999; 100(10):1043–1049.
2. Kumar R, McKinney WP, Raj G, et al. Adverse cardiac events after surgery: assessing risk in veteran population. J Gen Intern Med 2001; 16(8):507–518.
3. Dorsch MF, Lawrance RA, Sapsford RJ, et al. Poor prognosis of patients presenting with symptomatic MI but without chest pain. Heart 2001; 86(5):494–498.
4. Badner NH, Knill RL, Brown JE, et al. MI after noncardiac surgery. Anesthesiology 1998; 88(3):572–578.
5. Fleischmann KE, Goldman L, Young B, et al. Association between cardiac and noncardiac complications in patients undergoing noncardiac surgery: outcomes and effects on length of stay. Am J Med 2003; 115(7):580–581.
6. Devereaux PJ, Goldman L, Yusuf S, et al. Surveillance and prevention of major perioperative ischemic cardiac events in patients undergoing noncardiac surgery: a review. CMAJ 2005; 173(7):779–788.
7. Antman EM, Anbe DT, Armstrong PW, et al. ACC/AHA guidelines for the management of patients with ST-elevation MI: a report of the American College of Cardiology/American Heart Association task force on practice guidelines. J Am Coll Cardiol 2004; 44(3):E1–E211.
8. Braunwald E, Antman EM, Beasley JW, et al. ACC/AHA guidelines for the management of patients with unstable angina and non-ST–segment elevation MI: a report of the American College of Cardiology/American Heart Association task force on practice guidelines. J Am Coll Cardiol 2000; 36:970–1062.
9. Antman EM, McCabe CH, Gurfinkel EP, et al. Enoxaparin prevents death and cardiac ischemic events in unstable angina/non-Q–wave MI: results of the Thrombolysis in MI (TIMI) 11B trial. Circulation 1999; 100:1593–1601.
10. Antman EM, Cohen M, Bernink PJLM, et al. The TIMI risk score for unstable angina/non-ST elevation MI. JAMA 2000; 284(7):835–842.
11. Morrow DA, Antman EM, Snapinn SM, et al. An integrated clinical approach to predicting the benefit of tirofiban in non-ST elevation acute coronary syndromes. Application of the TIMI risk score for UA/NSTEMI in PRISM-PLUS. Eur Heart J 2000; 23(3):187–191.

12. Budaj A, Yusuf S, Mehta SR, et al. Benefit of Clopidogrel in patients with acute coronary syndromes without ST-segment elevation in various risk groups. Circulation 2002; 106(13):1622–1626.
13. Scirica BM, Cannon CP, Antman EM, et al. Validation of the thrombolysis in MI risk score for unstable angina pectoris and non-ST-elevation MI in the TIMI III registry. Am J Cardiol 2002; 90(3):303–305.
14. Morrow DA, Antman EM, Charlesworth A, et al. TIMI risk score for ST-elevation MI: a convenient, bedside, clinical score for risk assessment at presentation: an intravenous nPA for treatment of infarcting myocardium early II trial substudy. Circulation. 2000; 102(17):2031–2037.
15. InTime II Investigators. Intravenous NPA for the treatment of infarcting myocardium early; in TIME-II, a double-blind comparison of a single-bolus lanoteplase vs. accelerated alteplase for the treatment of patients with acute MI. Eur Heart J 2000; 21:2005–2013.
16. Antmann EM. Hirudin in acute MI. Thrombolysis and thrombin inhibition in MI (TIMI) 9B trial. Circulation. 1996; 94(5):911–921.
17. Burger W, Chemnitius JM, Kneissl GD, et al. Low-dose aspirin for secondary cardiovascular prevention—cardiovascular risk after its perioperative withdrawal versus bleeding risks with its continuation—review and meta-analysis. J Intern Med 2005; 257(5):399–414.
18. Clopidogrel in Unstable Angina to Prevent recurrent Events Trial Investigators. Effects of clopidogrel in addition to aspirin in patients with acute coronary syndromes without ST-segment elevation. N Engl J Med 2001; 345:494–502.
19. Payne DA, Jones CI, Hayes PD, et al. Beneficial effects of clopidogrel combined with aspirin in reducing cerebral emboli in patients undergoing carotid endarterectomy. Circulation 2004; 109(12):1442–1444.
20. Cohen M, Demers C, Gurfinkel EP, et al. A comparison of low-molecular weight heparin with unfractionated heparin for unstable coronary artery disease. N Engl J Med 1997; 337:447–452.
21. FRISC Study group. Low-molecular-weight heparin during instability in coronary artery disease. Lancet 1996; 347(9001):561–568.
22. Cannon CP, Gibson CM, Lambrew CT, et al. Relationship of symptom-onset-to-balloon time and door-to-balloon time with mortality in patients undergoing angioplasty for acute MI. JAMA 2000; 283(22):2491–2497
23. Goldberg RJ, Mooradd M, Gurwitz JH, et al. Impact of time to treatment with tissue plasminogen activator on morbidity and mortality following acute MI (the Second National Registry of MI). Am J Cardiol 1998; 82:259–264.
24. Berger PB, Ellis SG, Holmes DR, et al. Relationship between delay in performing direct coronary angioplasty and early clinical outcome in patients with acute MI: results from the Global Use of Strategies to Open Occluded Arteries in Acute Coronary Syndromes (GUSTO-IIb) trial. Circulation 1999; 100:14–20.
25. Keeley EC, Boura JA, Grines CL. Primary angioplasty versus intravenous thrombolytic therapy for acute MI: a quantitative review of 23 randomised trials. Lancet 2003; 361(9351):13–20.
26. Widimsky P, Groch L, Zelizko M, et al. Multicentre randomised trial comparingtransport to primary angioplasty vs immediate thrombolysis vs combined strategy for patients with acute MI presenting to a community hospital without a catheterisation laboratory. The PRAGUE study. Eur Heart J 2000; 21(10):823–831.
27. Widimsky P, Budesinsky T, Vorac D, et al. Long distance transport for primary angioplasty vs immediate thrombolysis in acute MI. Final results of the randomized national multicentre trial–PRAGUE-2. Eur Heart J 2003; 24(1):94–104.
28. Andersen HR, Nielsen TT, Rasmusen K, et al. A comparison of coronary angioplasty with fibrinolytic therapy in acute MI. N Engl J Med 2003; 349(8):733–742.
29. Nallamothu BK, Bates ER. Percutaneous coronary intervention versus fibrinolytic therapy in acute MI: is timing (almost) everything? Am J Cardiol 2003; 92(7):824–826
30. ISIS-2 Collaborative Group. Randomised trial of intravenous streptokinase, oral aspirin, both, or neither among 17187 cases of suspected acute MI: ISIS2. Lancet 1988; ii:349–360.
31. GISSI-1 Study Group. Effectiveness of intravenous thrombolytic treatment in acute MI. Lancet 1986; I:397–402.
32. GUSTO 1 Investigators. An international randomised trial comparing four thrombolytic strategies for acute MI. N Engl J Med 1993; 329:673–682.

33. Antiplatelet Trialists' Collaboration. Collaborative overview of randomised trials of antiplatelet therapy I: prevention of death, MI, and stroke by prolonged antiplatelet therapy in various categories of patients. 1994; 308:81–106.

34. Chen ZM, Jiang LX, Chen YP, et al. Addition of clopidogrel to aspirin in 45,852 patients with acute MI: randomized placebo-controlled trial. Lancet 2005; 366(9497):1607–1621.

35. Montalescot G, Barragan P, Wittenberg O, et al. Platelet glycoprotein IIb/IIIa inhibition with coronary stenting for acute MI. N Engl J Med 2001; 344:1895–1903.

36. Stone GW, Grines CL, Cox DA. Comparison of angioplasty with stenting, with or without abciximab, in acute MI. N Engl J Med 2002; 346(13):957–966.

37. Narrins CR, Hillegass WB, Nelson CL, et al. Relation between activated clotting time during angioplasty and abrupt closure. Circulation. 1996; 93(4):667–671.

38. GISSI-2 Study Group. GISSI-2: a factorial randomised trial of alteplase versus streptokinase and heparin versus no heparin among 12490 patients with acute MI. Lancet 1990; 336:65–71.

39. ISIS-3 Collaborative Group. ISIS-3: a randomised comparison of streptokinase vs tissue plasminogen activator vs. antistreplase and of aspirin plus heparin vs aspirin alone among 41,299 cases of suspected acute MI. Lancet 1992; 339:753–770.

40. Wallentin L, Goldstein P, Armstrong PW, et al. Efficacy and safety of tenecteplase in combination with the low-molecular weight heparin enoxaparin or unfractionated heparin in the prehospital setting: the Assessment of the Safety and Efficacy of a New Thrombolytic Regimen (ASSENT)-3 Plus randomised trial in acute MI. Circulation 2003; 108(2):135–142.

41. Freemantle N, Cleland J, Young P, et al. Beta blockade after MI: systematic review and meta regression analysis. BMJ 1999; 318(7200):1730–1737.

42. Chen ZM, Pan HC, Chen YP, et al. Early intravenous then oral metoprolol in 45,852 patients with acute MI: randomized placebo-controlled trial. Lancet 2005; 366(9497):1622–1632.

43. ISIS-4 Collaborative Group. ISIS-4: a randmised factorial trial assessing early oral captopril, oral mononitrate, and intravenous magnesium sulphate in 58,050 patients with suspected acute MI. Lancet; 1995; 345:669–685.

44. GISSI-3 Study Group. GISSI-3: effects of lisinopril and transdermal glyceryl trinitrate singly and together on 6-week mortality and ventricular function after MI. Lancet 1994; 343:1115–1122.

45. Van de Werf F, Ardissino D, Betriu A, et al. Management of acute MI in patients presenting with ST-segment elevation. The Task Force on the Management of Acute MI of the European Society of Cardiology. Eur Heart J 2003; 24(1):28–66.

46. The Acute Infarction Ramipril Efficacy (AIRE) Study Investigators. Effect of ramipril on mortality and morbidity of survivors of acute MI with clinical evidence of heart failure. Lancet 1993; 342:821–828.

47. Cannon CP, Braunwald E, McCabe CH, et al. Intensive versus moderate lipid lowering with statins after acute coronary syndromes. N Engl J Med 2004; 350(15):1495–1504.

48. Yusuf S, Collins R, MacMahon S, et al. Effect of intravenous nitrates on mortality in acute MI: an overview of the randomized trials. Lancet 1988; 1(8594):1088–1092.

49. Lewis HD, Davis JW, Archibald DG, et al. Protective effects of aspirin against acute MI and death in men with unstable angina. Results of a Veterans Administration Cooperative Study N Engl J Med 1983; 309(7):396–403.

50. Theroux P, Ouimet H, McCans J, et al. Aspirin, heparin, or both to treat acute unstable angina. N Engl J Med 1988; 319(17):1105–1111.

51. RISC Group. Risk of MI and death during treatment with low dose aspirin and intravenous heparin in men with unstable coronary artery disease. Lancet 1990; 636(8719):827–830.

52. Cohen M, Adams PC, Parry G, et al. Combination antithrombotic therapy in unstable rest angina and non-Q-wave infarction in nonprior aspirin users. Primary end points analysis from the ATACS trial. Circulation 1994; 89(1):81–88.

53. Klein W, Buchwald A, Hillis SE, et al. Comparison of low-molecular-weight heparin with unfractionated heparin acutely and with placebo for 6 weeks in the management of unstable coronary artery disease. Fragmin in unstable coronary artery disease study (FRIC). Circulation 1997; 96(1):61–68.

54. FRAX.I.S. Study group. Comparison of two treatment durations (6 and 14 days) of a low molecular weight heparin with a 6-day treatment of unfractionated heparin in the initial management of unstable angina or non-Q-wave MI. Eur Heart J 1999; 20(21):1553–1562.

55. EPIC Investigators. Use of a monoclonal antibody directed against the platelet glycoprotein IIb/IIIa receptor in high risk coronary angioplasty. The EPIC Investigation. N Engl J Med 1994; 330(14):956–961.
56. EPILOG Investigators. Platelet glycoprotein IIb/IIIa receptor blockade and low-dose heparin during percutaneous coronary revascularization. N Engl J Med 1997; 336(24): 1689–1696.
57. EPISTENT Investigators. Randomized placebo-controlled and balloon-angioplasty-controlled trial to assess safety of coronary stenting with use of platelet glycoproteinIIb/IIIa blockade. The EPISTENT Investigators. Evaluation of platelet IIb/IIIa inhibitor for stenting. Lancet 1998; 352(9122):87–92.
58. PRISM Investigators. A comparison of aspirin plus tirofiban with aspirin plus heparin for unstable angina. N Engl J Med 1998; 338:1498–1505.
59. PRISM-PLUS Investigators. Inhibition of the platelet glycoprotein IIb/IIIa receptor with Tirofiban in unstable angina and Non-Q-wave MI. N Engl J Med 1998; 338: 1488–1497.
60. PURSUIT Investigators. Inhibition of platelet glycoprotein IIb/IIIa with eptifibatide in patients with acute coronary syndromes. N Engl J Med 1998; 339:436–443.
61. Topol EJ, Moliterno DJ, Herrmann HC, et al. Comparison of two platelet glycoprotein IIb/IIIa inhibitors, tirofiban and abciximab, for the prevention of ischemic events with percutaneous coronary revascularisation. N Engl J Med 2001; 344:1888–1894.
62. Boersma E, Harrington RA, Moliterno DJ, et al. Platelet glycoprotein IIb/IIIa inhibitors in acute coronary syndromes: a meta-analysis of all major randomised clinical trials. Lancet 2002; 359(9302):189–198.
63. GUSTO IIb Investigators. A comparison of recombinant hirudin with heparin for the treatment of acute coronary syndrome. N Engl J Med 1996; 335:775–782.
64. OASIS-2 Investigators. Effects of recombinant hirudin (lepirudin) compared with heparin on death, MI, refractory angina, and revascularisation procedures in patients with acute myocardial ischemia without ST elevation. A randomised trial. Lancet 1999; 353(9151): 429–438.
65. Lincoff AM, Bittl JA, Harrington RA, et al. Bivalirudin and provisional glycoprotein IIb/IIIa blockade compared with heparin and planned glycoprotein IIb/IIIa blockade during percutaneous coronary intervention: REPLACE-2 randomised trial. JAMA 2003; 289(13):853–863.
66. Stone GW. ACUITY trial results. Late Breaking Clinical Trials. ACC, 2006.
67. Yusuf S, Wittes J, Friedman L. Overview of results of randomized clinical trials in heart disease. I. Treatments following MI. JAMA 1988a; 260(14):2088–2093.
68. Sacks FM, Pfeffer MA, Moye L, et al. The effect of pravastatin on coronary events after MI in patients with average cholesterol levels. N Engl J Med 1996; 335:1001–1009.
69. Scandinavian Simvastatin Survival Study Group. Randomized trial of cholesterol lowering in 4444 patients with coronary heart disease: the Scandinavian Simvastatin Survival Study (4S). Lancet 1994; 344(8934):1383–1389.
70. Shepherd J, Cobbe SM, Ford I, et al. Prevention of coronary heart disease with pravastatin in men with hypercholesterolaemia. N Engl J Med 1995; 333:1301–1307.
71. Wallentin L, Lagerqvist B, Husted S, et al. Outcome at 1 year after an invasive compared with a non-invasive strategy in unstable coronary-artery disease: the FRISC II invasive randomised trial. Lancet 2000; 356(9223):9–16.
72. Cannon CP, Weintraub WS, Demopoulos LA, et al. Comparison of early invasive and conservative strategies in patients with unstable coronary syndromes treated with the glycoprotein IIb/IIIa inhibitor Tirofiban. N Engl J Med 2001; 344:1879–1887.
73. Fox KA, Poole-Wilson PA, Henderson RA, et al. Interventional versus conservative treatment for patients with unstable angina or non-ST-elevation MI: the British Heart Foundation RITA 3 randomised trial. Lancet 2002; 360(9335):743–751.
74. Fox KA, Poole-Wilson PA, Clayton TC, et al. 5-year outcome of an interventional strategy in non-ST-elevation acute coronary syndrome: the British Heart Foundation RITA 3 randomised trial. Lancet 2005; 366(9489):914–920.
75. Braunwald E, Antman EM, Beasley JW, et al. ACC/AHA 2002 guideline update for the management of patients with unstable angina and non-ST-segment elevation MI—summary

article: a report of the American College of Cardiology/American Heart Association task force on practice guidelines. J Am Coll Cardiol 2002; 40:1366–1374.

76. Hochman JS, Sleeper LA, White HD, et al. One year survival following early revascularisation for cardiogenic shock. JAMA. 2001, 285:190-192.

77. Peter JV, Moran JL, Philipps-Hughes J, et al. Effect of non-invasive positive pressure ventilation (NIPPV) on mortality in patients with acute cardiogenic pulmonary oedema: a meta-analysis. Lancet 2006; 367(9517):1155–1163.

78. Fleischmann KE, Goldman L, Young B, et al. Association between cardiac and noncardiac complications in patients undergoing noncardiac surgery: outcomes and effects on length of stay. Am J Med 2003; 115(7):580–581.GUSTO IV-ACS randomised trial. Lancet 2001; 357(9272):1915–1924.

11 Arrhythmias and the Surgical Patient

Andrew D. McGavigan and Andrew C. Rankin
Department of Cardiology, Glasgow Royal Infirmary, Glasgow, U.K.

INTRODUCTION

Rhythm disturbances are common in the general population. Indeed, atrial fibrillation (AF), the most widespread arrhythmia, has an overall prevalence of 1%, rising with age, affecting nearly 10% of those aged over 80 years (1–3). Another 0.2% to 0.8% of people have experienced an episode of supraventricular tachycardia (SVT) at some point in their lives (4,5) and 3% of the population have had a myocardial infarction in the past (6), providing a potential substrate for ventricular arrhythmias.

Given the frequency of rhythm disturbances in the general population, it is not surprising that arrhythmias impact on routine surgical and anesthetic practice. In this chapter, we will discuss the epidemiology, mechanisms, diagnosis, treatment, and prophylaxis of arrhythmias commonly encountered in the perioperative setting.

EPIDEMIOLOGY
Incidence

The Multicenter Study of General Anesthesia reported an incidence of any disturbance of heart rate in 70.3% of 17,201 patients undergoing anesthesia for a variety of surgical interventions (7). However, the majority of these were transient tachycardia or bradycardia of sinus origin. Only 10.9% of patients had events classified as arrhythmias and less than 1% of the patient population had an adverse outcome due to a rhythm disturbance. This study illustrates why the reported incidence of perioperative rhythm disturbances displays such large variation within the literature. The incidence of arrhythmias is largely a function of the definition of an arrhythmic event, the method of assessment, and the type of surgery performed.

For example, a study by Amar et al. (8) demonstrated that ventricular tachyarrhythmias can be detected in 15% of patients in the few days following noncardiac thoracic surgery. However, Topol et al. (9) reported an incidence of ventricular arrhythmias of less than 1% following cardiac surgery. This apparent disparity can be explained by the fact that Amar's study utilized continuous Holter monitoring and defined an arrhythmic event as three or more consecutive beats of ventricular tachycardia (VT), whereas Topol did not use continuous monitoring and reported only clinically significant arrhythmia [sustained VT or ventricular fibrillation (VF)] as the endpoint. Similar conflicting data are present for the reported incidence of atrial arrhythmias in the perioperative setting, ranging from 6.1% to 53% of patients depending on the population studied and clinical definition of arrhythmia (10–12). The epidemiology of specific dysrhythmias is discussed further later in this chapter.

Risk Factors

Regardless of the true incidence of perioperative arrhythmias, it is clear that there are factors which contribute to arrhythmogenesis. These include patient characteristics, the type of surgery, and the anesthetic process.

The most consistent risk factor for the development of any arrhythmia in the general population is older age, and this is mirrored in the perioperative setting. In the Multicenter Study of General Anesthesia, increasing age was associated with increased incidence of both atrial and ventricular arrhythmias (13). Indeed, the risk of atrial arrhythmia in those aged 50 years was around 0.5%, rising to 2% at age 70 and peaking at more than 10% in those over 80 years. This finding has been confirmed in numerous other studies (11,14–16). This is unsurprising as older people have an increased risk of structural heart disease, myocardial ischemia, and hypertension and are prone to the risks of polypharmacy, all of which are risk factors for arrhythmogenesis. Furthermore, aging itself leads to changes in electrical conduction and refractoriness which may predispose to arrhythmia production (17,18). Previous history of myocardial infarction, LV dysfunction, or arrhythmia also increase risk of perioperative events (9,13,19).

Arrhythmias are more common following cardiovascular and noncardiac thoracic surgery (13,19,20). This may be due to direct trauma to the myocardium or autonomic fibers (16,21). Indeed, alterations in autonomic balance may alter cardiac conduction properties, thereby predisposing to the creation of arrhythmias (21–23). Postoperative pain or ischemia may produce catecholamine surges which may be proarrhythmic.

Finally, the choice of anesthetic agent has a direct impact on the incidence of arrhythmias. It is beyond the scope of this chapter to provide a comprehensive review of the mode of action, electrophysiological effects, and interaction of all the intravenous and volatile agents and adjunctive therapies used in modern anesthetic practice. However, in general terms, most inhalation agents depress sinoatrial and atrioventricular (AV) nodal function (24,25), and alter conduction times across the His-Purkinje system and myocardium (26,27), due to their effects on cardiac ion channels (28). This may lead to bradycardia or produce dispersion of refractoriness, creating a potential environment for reentry and arrhythmogenesis. Local anesthetic and intravenous agents also have the potential to alter electrophysiological properties and may therefore be arrhythmogenic (29). However, the degree of proarrhythmia is not constant within the same class of agent. For example, in the Multicenter Study of General Anesthesia, the use of halothane was associated with a 8.6% incidence of severe ventricular arrhythmia compared to a 1.3% and 0.8% incidence with fentanyl and isoflurane, respectively (13). The more modern volatile agents may be less proarrhythmic (30).

Accurate preoperative assessment of the patient history and risk factors may help to predict those at risk of arrhythmias which, if anticipated, may allow a reduction in incidence or improve outcome through correction of preoperative electrolyte abnormalities, careful selection of anesthetic agent, and early diagnosis and treatment of perioperative rhythm disturbances.

MECHANISMS

One may consider that arrhythmias are due to the intersection of structural heart disease and transient changes to the electrophysiological milieu. This simplification is essentially correct as arrhythmogenesis depends on the interplay between substrate and triggers.

Substrate

Potential substrates can be present from birth, and others develop due to disease or to cardiac surgical or percutaneous intervention. The most common substrates are those which predispose to the formation of reentrant circuits. For example, AV bypass tracts (accessory pathways) provide an inherent potential substrate for SVT due to AV reentry, using the AV node as one limb of the circuit and the accessory pathway as the other (Fig. 1A). A similar reentrant mechanism can produce SVT in the presence of dual AV nodal physiology, where the two limbs of the circuit are contained within the AV node. An example of acquired substrate would be ventricular scarring due to previous myocardial infarction. This provides a potential reentrant circuit around a scar, predisposing to VT (Fig. 1B). Reentry is also the mechanism for both typical and atypical atrial flutter (often following cardiac surgery). Alterations in cardiac conduction time may predispose to reentry circuits and may be due to the anesthetic agent (13), but may reflect changes in plasma electrolytes (31), perioperative ischemia, and hypoxia (32).

However, reentry is not the sole mechanism for arrhythmogenesis. Other mechanisms include increased automaticity which is responsible for the majority of focal atrial tachycardia, inappropriate sinus tachycardia, and some focal forms of VT. Triggered activity underlies Torsade de Pointes and some forms of VT seen in structurally normal hearts. AF has features of all three mechanisms (33).

Triggers

Regardless of the precise mechanism, not everyone with a potential arrhythmic substrate develops an arrhythmia. Triggers are required to initiate and sometimes sustain arrhythmias and can be diverse in origin. Premature beats may trigger a reentrant arrhythmia, and may have an automatic or triggered mechanism. In addition, they may be due to direct mechanical stimulation of the heart by the surgeon. Similar mechanical irritation can be produced by the placement of central venous cannulae, which may produce transient or sustained rhythm disturbance. Stimulation of the adrenergic nervous system is also proarrhythmic, whether the stimulation is direct by inotropic agents or indirect through pain, urinary retention, or constipation (10,34). Often the substrate for arrhythmogenesis is not modifiable, making it important to keep in mind the potential factors which may predispose to a rhythm disturbance, which may be minimized or be completely avoidable (Table 1).

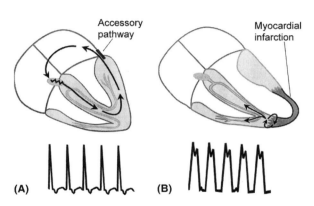

FIGURE 1 Reentrant arrhythmias. (**A**) The macro-reentrant circuit of AVRT includes an accessory pathway, the atria, the conducting system, and the ventricles. The tachycardia has a narrow QRS complex morphology. (**B**) The micro-reentrant circuit of scar-related VT involving the border zone of a myocardial infarction. The tachycardia has a broad QRS complex morphology. *Abbreviations*: AVRT, atrioventricular reentrant tachycardia; VT, ventricular tachycardia.

TABLE 1   Factors Contributing to Arrhythmogenesis

Type of surgery	Cardiac > thoracic > vascular > abdominal > others
Anesthetic agent	Halothane > fentanyl > isoflurane > sevoflurane
Mechanical cardiac irritation	Surgeon, central venous catheter, pacing wire, intercostals drains
Vagal stimulation	Laryngoscopy, endotracheal intubation, pain, nausea, and vomiting
Adrenergic stimulation	Awareness during anesthesia, pain, sympatho-mimetics, constipation, urinary retention
Metabolic derangement	Hyper/hypokalemia, hypomagnesemia, hypoxia, hypercapnia
Drugs	Withdrawal or newly instigated; all antiarrhythmic therapy, inotropes, drugs which prolong QT interval

DIAGNOSIS

Regardless of the mechanism, it is important to recognize the development of a perioperative arrhythmia and to diagnose it correctly, to allow quick, appropriate, and effective treatment. The importance of a 12-lead electrocardiogram (ECG) cannot be overemphasized, as reliance on a single ECG strip or electronic monitoring devices can lead to misdiagnosis. Similarly, it is important to record a preoperative baseline 12-lead ECG. Rate, regularity, QRS duration, axis and morphology, the relationship of P-wave to QRS and P-wave morphology are all important in the accurate classification of arrhythmias. Bradycardia and tachycardia are defined as less than 60 and greater than 100 beats per minute, respectively. Focusing on tachycardia, one of the simplest classifications is by QRS duration using 120 milliseconds to dichotomize tachyarrhythmias into narrow and broad complex tachycardia (Table 2). Intravenous adenosine causes transient AV nodal block which may be of therapeutic or diagnostic value, terminating tachycardias which are dependent on the AV node (Fig. 2) or revealing underlying atrial tachyarrhythmia, thus allowing assessment of atrial rate and P-wave morphology (35).

Narrow Complex Tachycardia

Narrow complex tachycardias with a QRS duration of <120 milliseconds are almost invariably supraventricular in origin, regardless of the precise mechanism. The most commonly encountered tachycardia in the perioperative setting is sinus tachycardia (13). This may be due to many factors including volume loss, infection, or pain, and treatment should be directed at the cause. In this setting, the ECG should show regular QRS activity (although sinus arrhythmia can produce some irregularity in P–P

TABLE 2   Narrow and Broad Complex Tachycardias

Narrow complex tachycardia	Sinus tachycardia
	Atrial fibrillation
	Atrial flutter
	Atrial tachycardia
	Supraventricular tachycardia
Broad complex tachycardia	All of the above in the presence of bundle branch block
	Ventricular tachycardia
	Preexcited AV reentrant tachycardia
	Preexcited AF

Abbreviation: AF, atrial fibrillation.

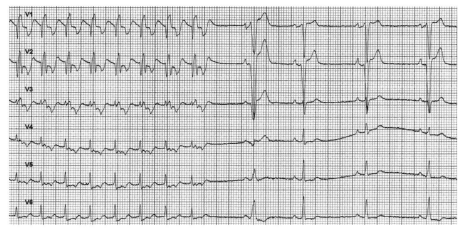

FIGURE 2 Termination of tachycardia (AVRT) following intravenous injection of adenosine (12 mg). The chest leads are shown, V1–V6. There is right bundle branch block during tachycardia. *Abbreviation*: AVRT, atrioventricular reentrant tachycardia.

and therefore R–R interval), with a P-wave preceding each QRS. The P-wave should be of identical morphology to previously documented baseline ECG and usually is positive in the inferior leads and biphasic in lead V1. An irregular rate with no apparent recurring pattern of R–R intervals accompanied by no discernable P-wave, or with evidence of highly variable and chaotic atrial activity, suggests AF.

If P-waves outnumber QRS complexes, then the likely diagnosis is atrial flutter or tachycardia with AV block. Typical flutter is due to a macro-reentrant circuit contained within the right atrium which passes through an isthmus between the inferior vena cava and the tricuspid annulus. It produces a characteristic "sawtooth" pattern of atrial activity, negative inferiorly, with no clear isoelectric interval between complexes (Fig. 3). Often 2:1 AV block is present, producing a ventricular rate around 150 beats per minute, and this mechanism should be considered in any

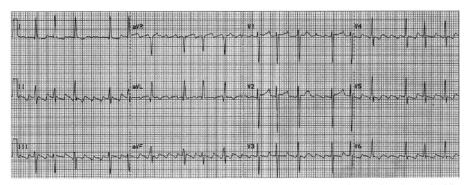

FIGURE 3 Atrial flutter with variable block. The AV conduction is mainly 2:1, but the typical "sawtooth" pattern of atrial flutter is apparent in the inferior leads when the block increases, e.g., after third QRS complex. *Abbreviation*: AV, atrioventricular.

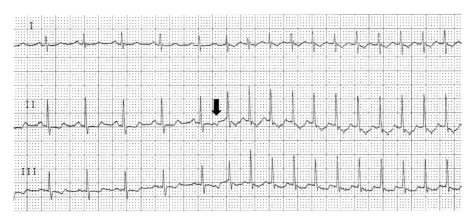

FIGURE 4 Onset of AVRT. After the fifth QRS, there is an atrial premature beat (*arrow*), which initiates the tachycardia. During the tachycardia, retrograde atrial activity, with inverted P-waves, can be seen following the QRS, in the ST segment. *Abbreviation*: AVRT, atrioventricular reentrant tachycardia.

tachycardia of this rate. Atypical and clockwise flutters produce different P-wave morphologies, but again have no clear isoelectric interval between complexes, which helps differentiate them from focal atrial tachycardias. Focal atrial tachycardia is usually of a slower rate than flutter, and P-wave morphology is dependent on the site of origin. They can usually be differentiated from sinus rhythm, although this may not be obvious on single- or dual-channel recordings, especially in the setting of one-to-one AV conduction. Focal tachycardias arising from the region of the sinus node can mimic sinus tachycardia, and careful comparison to the baseline ECG and the speed and mode of onset are helpful to distinguish between them. The response to intravenous adenosine may help establish the diagnosis by revealing the underlying atrial rate.

Atrioventricular reentrant tachycardia (AVRT) and AV nodal reentrant tachycardia (AVNRT) are often referred to as supraventricular tachycardias (SVTs). They are regular, narrow complex tachycardias, with no obvious P-wave activity or P-waves that immediately follow the QRS. The P-waves are typically negative in the inferior leads, reflecting retrograde ventriculoatrial conduction with atrial depolarization progressing in a superior direction (Fig. 4). Adenosine typically terminates SVT.

Broad Complex Tachycardia

All the above arrhythmias can produce a broad complex QRS morphology of a left or right bundle branch morphology in presence of His-Purkinje conduction delay (Fig. 5). This creates potential difficulty in differentiating a supraventricular arrhythmia with bundle branch block from VT. This is less problematic if the conduction delay is fixed, with left bundle branch block (LBBB) or right bundle branch block (RBBB) present on the baseline ECG, as the QRS morphology should be identical, or near-identical, to that in sinus rhythm. However, His-Purkinje delay or block can be dynamic, with aberrancy only developing at fast heart rates, producing a different morphology to baseline. In this case, it is often difficult to distinguish these arrhythmias from VT.

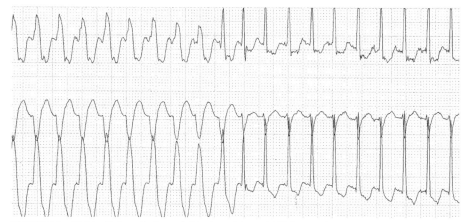

FIGURE 5 SVT with bundle branch block and broad QRS complexes, which changes to narrow complex tachycardia when the bundle branch block resolves. *Abbreviation*: SVT, supraventricular tachycardia.

Clues can be gleaned from the 12-lead ECG. Aberrancy should be typical of LBBB or RBBB, and the features of P-wave relation and morphology outlined above may help in the diagnosis. Clear evidence of AV dissociation, the presence of fusion and capture beats, and the absence of an RS pattern across all precordial leads (negative concordance) favor VT and there are many algorithms to aid in the diagnosis (36,37). Intravenous adenosine may help by unmasking the underlying atrial activity or terminating SVT (Fig. 2). The clinical setting should also be considered. For example, the development of a regular broad complex tachycardia in an elderly patient with previous myocardial infarction and LV dysfunction is likely to be VT, whereas a young patient with a structurally normal heart and a history of SVT is much more likely to have SVT with aberrancy. However, we would stress that one should err on the side of caution and, if in doubt, the arrhythmia should be assumed to be ventricular in origin.

SPECIFIC TACHYARRHYTHMIAS

Correct diagnosis of the cardiac arrhythmia is important because of the differences in the clinical significance, management options, and prognosis with specific tachyarrhythmias. Although some arrhythmias may be rare, such as preexcited AF or Torsades de Pointes, the recognition of them will contribute to optimal management.

Atrial Fibrillation
Preoperative Atrial Fibrillation
Given the frequency of AF in the general population, it is common for this arrhythmia to be present before surgical intervention. The diagnosis may have been made previously, and suitable risk stratification already been performed. The main treatment issues during the perioperative period are ensuring adequate rate control during and after the stresses of anesthesia and surgery, and whether anticoagulation should be temporarily discontinued. With regard to rate control, AV nodal blocking

agents such as β-blockers and calcium antagonists may have to be maintained, increased, or decreased during this period and should be guided by ventricular rate and hemodynamic status.

Asymptomatic AF may be diagnosed at the time of preoperative assessment, and become the subject of debate as whether to proceed with surgery. There are really little data to help guide strategy, but given the ubiquitous nature of AF within the community and the fact that <1% of patients with newly diagnosed AF will have an obvious discernible and potentially dangerous cause such as thyrotoxicosis, myocarditis, recent myocardial infarction, or pulmonary thromboembolus (38), it is reasonable to proceed with surgery, unless the patients were symptomatic or had evidence of an acute illness. This has to be taken in the context of patient characteristics, type and urgency of surgery, and degree of rate control. Echocardiography may help in selected cases, and coupled with clinical risk factors and duration of arrhythmia will guide the need for anticoagulation following surgery.

Peri- and Postoperative Atrial Fibrillation

Potentially more problematic is the development of new AF during the perioperative period. Polanczyk et al. (11) prospectively examined 4181 patients in sinus rhythm undergoing a variety of noncardiac surgical procedures and detected an incidence of supraventricular arrhythmias in 7.6% of patients, the majority of which occurred in the first three days following surgery. AF comprised the majority of these in the postoperative period. Perhaps unsurprisingly, predictors included older age, a history of arrhythmia, vascular and thoracic procedures, asthma, and LV dysfunction.

The effects of AF can range from a transient phenomenon producing minimal or no symptoms to prolonged arrhythmia producing significant hemodynamic compromise. The latter is most likely in those with structural heart disease where loss of atrial transport has profound effect on cardiac output and is often associated with an increased duration of hospital stay (11). Treatment of AF will be guided by the clinical situation. Factors such as electrolyte imbalance, hypoxia, and ischemia should be identified and corrected if possible. In the presence of severe hemodynamic compromise, electrical cardioversion should be undertaken. However, this is not to be recommended in the absence of hemodynamic instability, as only a minority of patients will remain in sinus rhythm following successful DC cardioversion in the immediate postoperative setting (39).

With regard to chemical cardioversion, there are few trials to support or refute this approach. A recent meta-analysis of amiodarone for cardioversion of recent-onset AF demonstrated spontaneous reversion rates at 6 and 24 hours of 43% and 56%, respectively, which increased to 56% and 82% with intravenous amiodarone (40). In the nonsurgical setting, reversion rates of up to 76% and 91% can be achieved with single doses of the class Ic drugs propafenone and flecainide, respectively (41), but this may not be applicable to the perioperative arena. It is important to remember that all these agents have the potential for proarrhythmia. There are also data that suggest that once AF has developed, pursuing sinus rhythm by either electrical or pharmacological means, provides no improvement in outcome when compared to a rate control strategy (42,43). Indeed, AF is usually self-limiting, with more than 90% of patients being in sinus rhythm six weeks following surgery (44). We would, therefore, reserve chemical cardioversion for those in whom continuation of AF may be deleterious in the immediate postoperative period. This may include those with LV dysfunction and hemodynamic instability.

Control of the ventricular rate is the key to treatment in the majority of patients who develop AF. Numerous drugs will slow AV nodal conduction and reduce ventricular rate. Digoxin is often ineffective in the hyperadrenergic state following surgery and is probably best avoided (38), except in those with cardiac failure. Other options include β-blockers and calcium channel blockers, the choice of which will be dictated by the clinical circumstances. For example, β-blockers may be first choice in those with ischemic heart disease, but contraindicated in asthmatics and cautioned in those with heart failure. Sometimes, a combination of drugs will be required to achieve adequate rate control, and any sudden changes in AV nodal blocking requirements should prompt a search for an underlying cause such as ischemia, hypovolemia, heart failure, etc. Once the patient is stabilized, further investigation, treatment, and follow-up, including the decision regarding anticoagulation, should be made in conjunction with the local cardiological service.

Prophylaxis of Atrial Fibrillation
Most of the data on the prevention of postoperative AF come from studies in cardiac surgical patients. Multiple drug regimes using various agents have been assessed with varying results (45). Both calcium antagonists and procainamide have been shown to decrease the incidence of supraventricular arrhythmias following cardiac surgery, but is unclear as to whether this translates into superior outcome, and results are not consistent (46–48).

Two meta-analyses have demonstrated the effectiveness of β-blocker therapy as prophylaxis (45,49), and have shown a reduction in duration of hospital stay. However, results are again not consistent across the trials. In the recent Beta-blocker Length of Stay trial, metoprolol showed no reduction in incidence of AF or length of stay (50). Newer agents such as carvedilol may be superior (51), as may sotalol (a β-blocker with class III antiarrhythmic action), especially in conjunction with magnesium (49,52,53). A recent meta-analysis of prophylactic magnesium administration alone showed a reduction in the incidence of postoperative AF from 28% to 18% in those undergoing cardiac surgery, but had no effect on length of stay (54).

The most robust data comes from the numerous trials of amiodarone as prophylaxis, and there appears to be consistent findings from these trials (49). The Amiodarone Reduction in Coronary Heart trial demonstrated a reduction in AF from 47% to 35% in those undergoing coronary heart surgery who were loaded intravenously with amiodarone for 24 to 48 hours before surgery (55). Superior results may be achieved with a more prolonged loading phase, with one trial showing a halving of incidence of AF from 53% to 25% in those orally loaded for one week prior to operation (56). Again, although trials have consistently demonstrated the efficacy of amiodarone in reducing the incidence of perioperative AF (57), it is less clear whether this translates into an improved outcome.

Given the relative lack of prospective large-scale trials in the noncardiac surgical setting, we would support current guidelines on this issue (38). β-Blockers as prophylaxis are recommended in those undergoing cardiac surgery. In the noncardiac patient, prophylactic sotalol or amiodarone is suggested if the patient is believed to be at high risk of perioperative AF.

Atrial Flutter and Tachycardia
Other atrial arrhythmias seen in the perioperative period include atrial flutter and atrial tachycardia, although they are not common in this setting. Risk factors for

typical flutter are similar to those for AF, and it is important to remember that antiar-rhythmic treatment for AF may allow the formation of a stable flutter circuit. Those with previous cardiac operations (with the exception of coronary bypass) may be at risk of atypical flutter circuits around areas of intra-atrial scarring. Pharmacological cardioversion of flutter is rarely successful and initial treatment should be aimed at control of the ventricular rate, although this is often more difficult to achieve than with AF. Often a combination of AV nodal blocking drugs (such as β-blocker and digoxin) is required. DC cardioversion should be considered in cases of atrial flutter associated with hemodynamic compromise and if the arrhythmia fails to revert. Other options include overdrive atrial pacing, although this should be reserved for selected cases, such as in the setting of postcardiac surgery.

Focal atrial tachycardia can be unifocal, with only one P-wave morphology evi-dent, or multifocal. These arrhythmias are often catecholamine sensitive, and can be precipitated by hyperadrenergic states or sympatho-mimetic agents. Other precipi-tants include electrolyte abnormalities and pulmonary disease, especially in the case of multifocal atrial tachycardia. Treatment should be expectant, with control of rate with AV nodal blocking agents if necessary and removal or correction of triggers such as pain or electrolyte imbalance. β-Blocker therapy is a reasonable first-line drug for rate control and some forms will terminate with intravenous adenosine.

Supraventricular Tachycardia

The reentrant arrhythmias AVRT and AVNRT comprise the remainder of the supraven-tricular arrhythmias. The incidence of SVT is less than that of AF but still occurs in up to 3% of patients undergoing general anesthesia (11). However, unlike AF, which often develops one to three days following surgery, SVT typically occurs during anesthesia, producing a narrow complex tachycardia with either no discernible atrial activation or evidence of retrograde atrial activation. In contrast to atrial tachycar-dia, there are no warm up or warm down phenomena; SVTs are characterized by a sudden onset, often preceded by a premature atrial or ventricular beat, and usually terminate abruptly.

Regardless of whether the AV reentrant circuit is confined to the AV node, or involves an accessory pathway, the AV node is an obligate part of the circuit. There-fore, blocking this should terminate the arrhythmia, making intravenous adenosine an effective treatment in the anesthetic room or theatre (35,58). If the atrial arrhyth-mia continues with AV block, the AV node is not part of the circuit and the diag-nosis is therefore not SVT. Adenosine may fail to terminate the arrhythmia or be contraindicated (e.g., bronchospasm), and other AV nodal blocking agents such as intravenous β-blockers or verapamil can be utilized. Adenosine may also cause AF which is usually nonsustained. SVTs are usually self-limiting, relatively easy to deal with, and tend not to recur in the postoperative period. Cardiological advice should be sought in those with recurrent paroxysms.

Ventricular Preexcitation and the Wolff–Parkinson–White Syndrome

Ventricular preexcitation, indicating conduction down an accessory pathway, pro-duces a short PR interval and delta waves on a 12-lead ECG (Fig. 6) and has preva-lence of 2.5 per 1000 population (59). The Wolff–Parkinson–White (WPW) syndrome is characterized by the presence of symptomatic arrhythmias in the presence of ven-tricular preexcitation on a resting electrocardiogram. The ECG features of preexcita-tion reflect simultaneous conduction from atria to ventricles over both the AV node

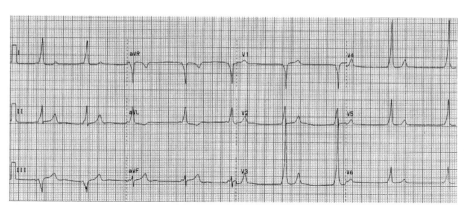

FIGURE 6   Ventricular pre-excitation in the ECG from a patient with WPW syndrome. The initial slurred upstroke of the QRS complex (delta wave) is due to early ventricular activation via an accessory pathway, resulting in a short PR interval. The pathway is *right-sided*, producing an "LBBB" morphology. *Abbreviations*: ECG, electrocardiogram; WPW, Wolff–Parkinson–White; LBBB, left bundle branch block.

and an accessory pathway. The degree of preexcitation is variable being dependent on heart rate, site of pathway, and speed of AV nodal and accessory pathway conduction. Therefore, the pattern of preexcitation may be variable from one ECG to another.

The typical arrhythmia associated with WPW is AVRT, one of the SVTs producing a regular narrow complex tachycardia. Antegrade AV conduction is via the AV node, with normal ventricular activation, and the accessory pathway acts as the retrograde limb of the circuit (Fig. 1A). More rarely, activation is in the opposite direction, with the accessory pathway as the antegrade limb and the AV node as the retrograde limb, producing a broad complex regular tachycardia. These tachycardias are managed in a similar way to other SVTs, as both have the AV node as an obligate part of the circuit. In patients with known WPW or who have preexcited SVTs, adenosine should be used with caution due to the incidence of conversion to AF which may be preexcited. Drugs which have an effect on both the pathway and the AV node, such as procainamide or flecainide, are alternatives. Preexcited AF is the potentially most serious arrhythmia in WPW syndrome. An accessory pathway may allow rapid activation of the ventricles during AF, which may degenerate into VF (60). The 12-lead ECG shows an irregular wide complex tachycardia with beat-to-beat variation of QRS width and morphology (Fig. 7). A class Ic antiarrhythmic drug or amiodarone should be given, or electrical cardioversion undertaken in the presence of hemodynamic instability or very fast ventricular rates.

Preexcitation may be found incidentally on a 12-lead ECG and is sometimes noted for the first time at anesthetic review. Its presence demonstrates antegrade conduction over the accessory pathway, but does not prove that it is capable of sustaining one of the arrhythmias outlined above. Indeed, the majority of people with preexcitation never have symptoms and it often disappears over time (59). However, preexcitation on the ECG should alert one to the presence of a potential substrate for arrhythmias, and a history suggestive of arrhythmia should be sought from the patient. In the absence of previous symptoms or documented rhythm disturbance, we would propose that surgery could proceed, with early treatment of arrhythmias

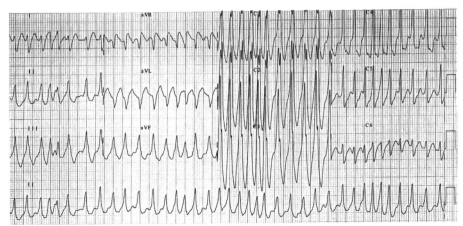

FIGURE 7   Preexcited AF, with rapid ventricular activation via an accessory pathway. The pathway is *left-sided*, producing an "RBBB" morphology. *Abbreviations*: AF, atrial fibrillation; RBBB, right bundle branch block.

if they were to develop. In the presence of symptoms, or documented preexcited AF, cardiological advice should be sought before surgery.

Ventricular Arrhythmias
Ventricular Ectopy and Nonsustained VT
Simple ventricular ectopy and nonsustained VT (defined as >3 beats but lasting <30 seconds) is common in the perioperative period, occurring in up to 15% of patients undergoing noncardiac thoracic surgery (8), and does not appear to be associated with an adverse outcome (8,19,61,62). Attempts to suppress ectopy do not improve outcome (63), and given the potential for proarrhythmia with this strategy in other settings (64), this approach cannot be supported, and no specific action is required other than supportive care. However, ventricular ectopy and nonsustained tachycardia should alert to the possibility of ischemia, electrolyte imbalance, acid–base disorders, or drug toxicity.

Sustained Monomorphic Ventricular Tachycardia and Ventricular Fibrillation
These factors may also be implicated in the genesis of sustained monomorphic VT, which is often a manifestation of underlying structural heart disease. The majority of patients with perioperative VT have impaired LV function (9,65), and cardiac ischemia is often implicated in its etiology. Fortunately, sustained VT or VF is rare in the perioperative setting, with a reported incidence of around 0.6% in a large unselected general surgical series (7) increasing to 1% in cardiac surgical series (9,65). However, mortality has been reported to be as high as 50% (9,65), and preoperative cardiological input may be of value in patients with a history of ventricular tachyarrhythmias. Perioperative β-blockade should be considered in high-risk patients undergoing noncardiac surgery, as this has been demonstrated to reduce mortality, although whether its primary effect is reduction in ischemic or arrhythmic death is not clear (66).

Acute treatment of VT is no different than in nonsurgical settings and includes DC cardioversion (usually in the presence of hemodynamic compromise), overdrive

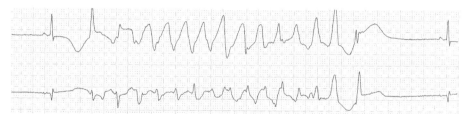

FIGURE 8 Torsades de Pointes, a polymorphic VT, associated with prolongation of the QT inter-val, which can be seen in the first beat, in sinus rhythm. Two monitor leads are shown. *Abbreviation*: VT, ventricular tachycardia.

ventricular pacing, and intravenous antiarrhythmic therapy such as lidocaine, sotalol, or amiodarone. Myocardial ischemia and electrolyte imbalance should be corrected if present. VF should of course be treated with immediate defibrillation.

Polymorphic Ventricular Tachycardia and Torsades de Pointes

Polymorphic VT is characterized by a wide complex tachycardia with continuously changing axis, and may be caused by acute myocardial ischemia. This should be actively sought and treated. Torsades de Pointes is polymorphic VT in the presence of QT prolongation (Fig. 8). Although long QT can be congenital, the vast majority are due to acquired disease or are drug induced (Table 3). Treatment should be aimed at the underlying cause and may involve correction of electrolyte abnormalities and withdrawal of drugs which prolong the QT interval (these may include drugs given to treat other arrhythmias). Intravenous magnesium sulfate, e.g., 8 mM $MgSO_4$ (4 mL of 50% solution) in 100 mL N-saline over 5 to 15 minutes, may be of benefit. Pacing or isoprenaline infusion may help with pause-dependent torsade. Cardiological input should be sought.

Perioperative Bradycardia

With the exception of some forms of cardiac surgery, the incidence of severe peri-operative bradycardia necessitating treatment is low at around 0.4%, although transient and clinically insignificant bradycardia occurs in 18.9% (7). This is often due to suppression of sinus node activity, causing a sinus bradycardia or junc-tional escape rhythm and is usually amenable to short-term pharmacological ther-apy (e.g., atropine, or β-agonists), but atrial pacing by either the transvenous or transesophageal route can be considered in resistant cases with hemodynamic compromise.

Transient AV block may be due to high vagal tone or effects of drugs, but sus-tained second- or third-degree AV block may require temporary pacing, transcuta-neously or by transvenous lead insertion, especially in the context of hemodynamic deterioration. Further management, including the issue of permanent pacing, should be discussed with the local cardiology service.

Patients with a history of high-grade AV block should also be discussed with cardiology preoperatively, and the procedure delayed if permanent pacemaker implantation is necessary. The prophylactic insertion of a temporary pacemaker is only indicated if surgery cannot be delayed. In the absence of AV block, asympto-matic bi- or tri-fascicular block is not an indication for pacemaker insertion (67).

TABLE 3 Causes of Long QT Interval

Congenital	Long QT syndromes Lange–Neilson syndrome Romano–Ward syndrome
Acquired	Electrolyte imbalance— hypokalemia, hypomagnesemia, hypocalcemia Myocardial ischemia Heart failure Myocarditis Severe bradycardia Intracerebral bleed Anorexia nervosa Anaphylaxis Hypothyroidism Hypothermia
Drug-induced	Antiarrhythmic drugs—class Ia and III Antibiotics—macrolides, ampicillin, trimethoprim-sulfamethoxazole Antifungals Antimalarials Antivirals Tricyclic antidepressants Antipsychotics Nonsedating antihistamines Steroids

CONCLUSIONS

Arrhythmia management in the perioperative setting poses significant challenges to the anesthetist and surgeon and is not limited to the immediate operative period. Management starts at the preoperative assessment and continues throughout the postoperative period. Early identification of patients at risk of arrhythmias, early diagnosis, and appropriate treatment of both the rhythm disturbance and potential triggers are necessary to optimize care in this high-risk group of patients.

REFERENCES

1. Kannel WB, Abbott RD, Davage DD, Mcnamara PM. Epidemiologic features of chronic atrial fibrillation: the Framingham study. N Engl J Med 1982; 306:1018–1022.
2. Furberg CD, Psaty BM, Manolio TA, et al. Prevalence of atrial fibrillation in elderly subjects. The Cardiovascular Health Study. Am J Cardiol 1994; 74:236–241.
3. Go AS, Hylek EM, Phillips KA, et al. Prevalence of diagnosed atrial fibrillation in adults. J Am Med Assoc 2001; 285(18):2370–2375.
4. Orejarena LA, Vidaillet H, Destefano F, et al. Paroxysmal supraventricular tachycardia in the general population. J Am Coll Cardiol 1998; 31:150–157.
5. US Department of Health and Human Services. Current Estimates from the National Health Interview Survey (1996). No. 99-1528. Centers for Disease Control Vital and Health Statistics, 1999.
6. Ghandi M. Clinical epidemiology of coronary heart disease in the UK. Br J Hosp Med 1997; 58:1–2.
7. Forrest JB, Cahalan MK, Rehder K, et al. Multicenter study of general anesthesia. II. Results. Anesthesiology 1990; 72:262–268.
8. Amar D, Zhang H, Roistacher N. The incidence and outcome of ventricular arrhythmias after noncardiac thoracic surgery. Anesth Analg 2002; 95:537–543.

9. Topol EJ, Lerman BB, Baughman KL, et al. De novo refractory ventricular tachyarrhythmias after coronary revascularization. Am J Cardiol 1986; 57:57–59.
10. Mathew JP, Parks R, Savino JS. Atrial fibrillation following coronary artery bypass graft surgery: predictors, outcomes, and resource utilization. Multicenter Study of Perioperative Ischemia Research Group. J Am Med Assoc 1996; 276:300–306.
11. Polanczyk CA, Goldman L, Marcantonio ER, et al. Supraventricular arrhythmia in patients having noncardiac surgery: clinical correlates and effect on length of stay. Ann Intern Med 1998; 129:279–285.
12. Stamou SC, Dangas G, Hill PC, et al. Atrial fibrillation after beating heart surgery. Am J Cardiol 2000; 86:64–67.
13. Forrest JB, Rehder K, Cahalan MK, Goldsmith CH. Multicenter study of general anesthesia. III. Predictors of severe perioperative adverse outcomes. Anesthesiology 1992; 76:3–15.
14. Amar D, Roistacher N, Burt M, et al. Clinical and echocardiographic correlates of symptomatic tachydysrhythmias after non-cardiac thoracic surgery. Chest 1995; 108:349–354.
15. Amar D, Zhang H, Leung HY, et al. Older age is the strongest predictor of postoperative atrial fibrillation. Anesthesiology 2002; 96:352–356.
16. Maisel WH, Rawn JD, Stevenson WG. Atrial fibrillation after cardiac surgery. Ann Intern Med 2001; 135:1061–1073.
17. Allessie MA, Boyden PA, Camm AJ, et al. Pathophysiology and prevention of atrial fibrillation. Circulation 2001; 103:769–777.
18. Kistler PM, Sanders P, Fynn SP, et al. Electrophysiologic and electroanatomic changes in the human atrium associated with age. J Am Coll Cardiol 2004; 44(1):109–116.
19. Mahla E, Rothman B, Rehak P, et al. Perioperative ventricular dysrhythmias in patients with structural heart disease undergoing noncardiac surgery. Anesth Analg 1998; 86(1):16–21.
20. Ommen SR, Odell JA, Stanton MS. Atrial arrhythmias after cardiothoracic surgery. N Engl J Med 1997; 336:1429–1434.
21. Cox JL. A perspective of postoperative atrial fibrillation in cardiac operations. Ann Thorac Surg 1993; 56:405–409.
22. Amar D, Zhang H, Miodownik S, Kadish AH. Competing autonomic mechanisms precede the onset of postoperative atrial fibrillation. J Am Coll Cardiol 2003; 42:1262–1268.
23. Mayr A, Knotzer H, Pajk W, et al. Risk factors associated with new onset tachyarrhythmias after cardiac surgery—a retrospective analysis. Act Anaesth Scand 2001; 45:543–549.
24. Bosjnak ZJ, Kampine JP. Effects of halothane, enflurane, and isoflurane on the SA node. Anesthesiology 1983; 58:314–321.
25. Atlee JL, Brownlee SW, Burstrom RE. Conscious state comparisons of the effects of inhalational anesthetics on specialised atrioventricular conduction times in dogs. Anesthesiology 1986; 64:703–710.
26. Atlee JL, Rusy BF, Kreul JF, Eby T. Supraventricular excitability in dogs during anesthesia with halothane and enflurane. Anesthesiology 1978; 49:407–418.
27. Turner LA, Bosnjak ZJ, Kampine JP. Electrophysiological effects of halothane on Purkinje fibers from normal and infarcted canine hearts. Anesthesiology 1987; 67:619–629.
28. Huneke R, Fassl J, Rossaint R, Luckhoff A. Effects of volatile anesthetics on cardiac ion channels. Act Anaesth Scand 2004; 48(5):547–561.
29. Atlee JL, Bosnjak ZJ. Mechanisms for cardiac dysrhythmia during anesthesia. Anesthesiology 1990; 72:347–374.
30. Novalija E, Hogan QH, Kulier AH, et al. Effects of desflurane, sevoflurane and halothane on post-infarction spontaneous dysrhythmias in dogs. Act Anaesth Scand 1998; 42(3):353–357.
31. Parra L, Fita G, Gomar C, et al. Plasma magnesium in patients submitted to cardiac surgery and its influence on perioperative morbidity. J Cardiovasc Surg 2001; 42(1):37–42.
32. Aranki SF, Shaw DP, Adams DH, et al. Predictors of atrial fibrillation after coronary artery surgery: current trends and impact on hospital resources. Circulation 1996; 94:390–397.
33. Wu TJ, Kerwin WF, Hwang C, et al. Atrial fibrillation: focal activity, re-entry, or both? Heart Rhythm 2004; 1(1):117–120.
34. Argalious M, Motta P, Khandwala F, et al. "Renal dose" dopamine is associated with the risk of new-onset atrial fibrillation after cardiac surgery. Crit Care Med 2005; 33(6):1447–1448.

35. Conti J, Belardinelli L, Curtis A. Usefulness of adenosine in diagnosis of tachyarrhythmias. Am J Cardiol 1995; 75:952–955.
36. Kindwall KE, Brown J, Josephsen ME. Electrocardiographic criteria for ventricular tachycardia in wide complex left bundle branch block morphology tachycardias. Am J Cardiol 1988; 61:1279–1283.
37. Brugada P, Brugada J, Mont L, et al. A new approach to the differential diagnosis of a regular tachycardia with a wide QRS complex. Circulation 1991; 83:1649–1659.
38. Fuster V, Ryden LE, Asinger RW, et al. ACC/AHA/ESC guidelines for the management of patients with atrial fibrillation: executive summary. A Report of the American College of Cardiology/American Heart Association Task Force on Practice Guidelines and The European Society of Cardiology Committee for Practice Guidelines and Policy Conferences (Committee to Develop Guidelines for the Management of Patients with Atrial Fibrillation). Circulation 2001; 104:2118–2150.
39. Mayr A, Ritsch N, Knotzer H, et al. Effectiveness of direct-current cardioversion for treatment of supraventricular tachyarrhythmias, in particular atrial fibrillation, in surgical intensive care patients. Crit Care Med 2003; 31:401–405.
40. Chevalier P, Durand-Dubief A, Burri H. Amiodarone versus placebo and class Ic drugs for cardioversion of recent-onset atrial fibrillation: a meta-analysis. J Am Coll Cardiol 2003; 41:255–262.
41. Suttorp MJ, Kingma JH, Jessurun ER, et al. The value of class Ic antiarrhythmic drugs for acute conversion of paroxysmal atrial fibrillation or flutter to sinus rhythm. J Am Coll Cardiol 1990; 16:1722–1727.
42. Lee JK, Klein GJ, Yee R, et al. Rate control versus conversion strategy in postoperative atrial fibrillation: a prospective, randomized pilot study. Am Heart J 2000; 140:871–877.
43 Soucier R, Silverman D, Abordo M, et al. Propafenone versus ibutilide for post operative atrial fibrillation following cardiac surgery: neither strategy improves outcomes compared to rate control alone. The PIPAF Study. Med Sci Monit 2003; 9:19–23.
44. Stebbins D, Igidbashian L, Goldman SM, et al. Clinical outcome of patients who develop atrial fibrillation after coronary artery bypass graft surgery. Pace 1995; 18:798.
45. Crystal E, Healey J, Connolly SJ. Atrial fibrillation after cardiac surgery: update on the evidence on the available prophylactic interventions. Card Electrophysiol Rev 2003; 7:189–192.
46. Malhotra R, Mishra M, Kler TS, et al. Cardioprotective effects of diltiazem infusion in the perioperative period. Eur J Cardiothorac Surg 1997; 12:420–427.
47. Gold MR, O'gara PT, Buckley MJ, et al. Efficacy and safety of procainamide in preventing arrhythmias after coronary artery bypass surgery. Am J Cardiol 1996; 78:975–979.
48. Wijeysundera DN, Beattie WS, Rao V, et al. Calcium antagonists reduce cardiovascular complications after cardiac surgery: a meta-analysis. J Am Coll Cardiol 2003; 41:1496–1505.
49. Crystal E, Connolly SJ, Sleik K. Interventions on prevention of postoperative atrial fibrillation in patients undergoing heart surgery: a meta-analysis. Circulation 2002; 106:75–80.
50. Crystal E, Thorpe KE, Connolly SJ, et al. Metoprolol prophylaxis against postoperative atrial fibrillation increases length of hospital stay in patients not on pre-operative β blockers: the β Blocker Length of Stay (BLOS) trial. Heart 2004; 90:941–942.
51. Merritt JC, Niebauer M, Tarakji K, et al. Comparison of effectiveness of carvedilol versus metoprolol or atenolol for atrial fibrillation appearing after coronary artery bypass grafting or cardiac valve operation. Am Heart J 2003; 92:735–736.
52. Forlani S, De Paulis R, De Nortaris S, et al. Combination of sotalol and magnesium prevents atrial fibrillation after coronary artery bypass grafting. Ann Thorac Surg 2002; 74:720–726.
53. Parikka H, Toivonen L, Heikkila L, et al. Comparison of sotalol and metoprolol in the prevention of atrial fibrillation after coronary artery bypass surgery. J Cardiovasc Pharmacol 1998; 31:67–73.
54. Miller S, Crystal E, Garfinkle M, et al. Effects of magnesium on atrial fibrillation after cardiac surgery: a meta-analysis. Heart 2005; 91(5):618–623.
55. Guarnieri T, Nolan S, Gottlieb SO, et al. Intravenous amiodarone for the prevention of atrial fibrillation after open heart surgery. the Amiodarone Reduction in Coronary Heart (ARCH) Trial. J Am Coll Cardiol 1999; 34:343–347.

56. Daoud EG, Strickberger SA, Man KC, et al. Preoperative amiodarone as prophylaxis against atrial fibrillation after heart surgery. N Engl J Med 1997; 337:1785–1791.
57. Stamou SC, Hill PC, Sample GA, et al. Prevention of atrial fibrillation after cardiac surgery—the significance of postoperative oral amiodarone. Chest 2001; 120:1936–1941.
58. Camm AJ, Garrat C. Adenosine and supraventricular tachycardia. N Engl J Med 1991; 325:1621–1629.
59. Krahn AD, Manfreda J, Tate RB, et al. The natural history of electrocardiographic preexcitation in men. The Manitoba Follow-up Study. Ann Intern Med 1992; 116(6):456–460.
60. Klein GJ, Bashore TM, Sellers TD, et al. Ventricular fibrillation in the Wolff–Parkinson–White syndrome. N Engl J Med 1979; 301:1080–1085.
61. Mangano DT, Browner WS, Hollenberg M, et al. Long-term cardiac prognosis following noncardiac surgery. J Am Med Assoc 1992; 268:233–239.
62. Smith RC, Leung JM, Keith FM, et al. Ventricular dysrhythmias in patients undergoing coronary artery bypass graft surgery: incidence, characteristics, and prognostic importance. Study of Perioperative Ischemia (SPI) Research Group. Am Heart J 1992; 123:73–81.
63. Johnson RG, Goldberger AL, Thurer RL, et al. Lidocaine prophylaxis in coronary revascularization patients: a randomized prospective. Ann Thorac Surg 1993; 55:1180–1184.
64. Echt DS, Liebson PR, Mitchell LB, et al. Mortality and morbidity in patients receiving encainide, flecainide, or placebo. The Cardiac Arrhythmia Suppression Trial. N Engl J Med 1991; 324(12):781–788.
65. Tam SK, Miller JM, Edmunds LH, et al. Unexpected, sustained ventricular tachyarrhythmia after cardiac operations. J Thorac Cardiovasc Surg 1991; 102:883–889.
66. Lindenauer PK, Pekow P, Wang K, et al. Perioperative beta-blocker therapy and mortality after major noncardiac surgery. N Engl J Med 2005; 353(4):412–414.
67. Gregaratos G, Abrams J, Epstein AE, et al. ACC/AHA/NASPE 2002 Guideline update for implantation of cardiac pacemakers and antiarrhythmia devices: summary article. A Report of the American College of Cardiology/American Heart Association Task Force on Practice Guidelines (ACC/AHA/NASPE Committee to Update the 1998 Pacemaker Guidelines). Circulation 2002; 106(16):2145–2161.

12

Heart Failure and the Surgical Patient

Karl Skarvan

Department of Anesthesia, University Hospital Basel,
Basel, Switzerland

INTRODUCTION

All diseases of the heart can evolve towards the stage of heart failure (HF). HF develops either insidiously or suddenly and encompasses a wide spectrum of clinical conditions, ranging from asymptomatic cardiac lesions to life-threatening pulmonary edema or cardiogenic shock. Heart disease can progress from asymptomatic to symptomatic, from gradual or acute decompensation to recompensation, and eventually to terminal or end-stage failure. However, the chance of an event-free survival varies considerably, depending on the nature of the disease. The etiology of heart disease has changed greatly in the course of last century; in Europe, at the beginning of twentieth century, rheumatic and infectious etiologies were responsible for 70% of all heart diseases (1). Today, coronary artery disease is not only responsible for 80% of all cardiac deaths, but also for most cases of HF (2,3). The prevalence of HF increases dramatically with increasing age. Because of prolonged life spans and efficacious therapies for coronary artery disease, the absolute numbers of people with HF in the community is increasing. Consequently, more patients suffering from HF are admitted to hospital and require anesthesia and surgery. In the past, anesthesiologists caring for patients with coronary artery disease focused mainly on perioperative myocardial ischemia and learned how to recognize, treat, and prevent it. Now anesthesiologists may meet patients who survived their infarctions and episodes of ischemia. When these patients present for surgery, they are carrying a new major risk, that of a failing heart.

This chapter reviews the present concepts of the clinical syndrome of HF in accordance with the published guidelines for management of chronic and acute HF (4–7). It also provides information that can be helpful in understanding the diverse problems that may arise when patients with chronic HF undergo surgery or when acute HF develops in the perioperative period.

DEFINITION

When defining HF, textbooks traditionally focus on the failure of the heart pump to meet the metabolic demands of the body. An example is the definition of HF proposed by Denolin more than 20 years ago: "the state of any heart disease in which, despite adequate ventricular filling, the heart's output is decreased or in which the heart is unable to pump blood at a rate adequate for satisfying the requirements of the tissues with function parameters remaining within normal limits" (8). Unfortunately, none of the classic definitions is quite satisfactory and certainly not helpful in clinical practice. A definition based on objective measurements and cut-off values for hemodynamic, imaging, or metabolic parameters does not exist either. A definition that is helpful in making the diagnosis of HF must be based on clinical judgment that in turn is supported by history, physical examination, and noninvasive or invasive investigations

(5). Accordingly, HF is present if (*i*) there are symptoms of HF and if (*ii*) there is objective evidence of cardiac dysfunction at rest. It is important that both criteria be fulfilled. Where the diagnosis is still in doubt (*iii*), the response to treatment directed towards HF should be taken into account (5). For practical purposes, it is useful to distinguish chronic HF from acute HF. However, many cases of acute HF represent an acute decompensation of preexisting chronic HF. Patients with HF either have abnormal or preserved left ventricular (LV) systolic function. If evidence of LV diastolic dysfunction is found in patients with HF and preserved LV systolic function, the HF is classified as diastolic HF. On the other hand, almost every patient with systolic dysfunction and systolic HF also has an impaired diastolic function. It is also important to distinguish between predominant LV failure and isolated right ventricular (RV) failure. Still in use are other terms such as forward and backward HFs. An extreme example of forward LV failure is cardiogenic shock; an example of LV backward failure is pulmonary edema. The widely used term "congestive HF" refers to the presence of venous hypertension and edema in either systemic or pulmonary circulation and, accordingly, designates decompensated HF. Finally, the terms asymptomatic, compensated, decompensated, and recompensated and end-stage HFs are used to describe the severity of HF and its changes over the course of time (6). The term perioperative or postoperative HF refers to acute HF that develops during the perioperative period. Acute HF is considered a major adverse outcome of anesthesia and surgery.

EPIDEMIOLOGY

The overall prevalence of symptomatic chronic HF varies between 0.4% and 3.6% according to the population studied and the methodology used. The true prevalence in adult European population is about 1.5%, doubles with each age decade, and may be as high as 3% to 5% in persons over the age of 75 years. The mean age of patients with HF is 74 to 76 years and there is a marked gender difference with higher prevalence of HF in men than in women (9–11). Because the population in Western countries is aging, the prevalence of HF is steadily increasing. At the age of 40, the lifetime risk for developing HF is 21% for men and 20% for women (12,13). The incidence of new cases of HF in adult population is estimated to range between two and three cases of HF per 1000 population per year and to increase more than fivefold in people over the age of 65 (10). Considering these figures, it is not surprising that HF consumes up to 2% of the annual health care budget (14). Most of the costs are due to frequent hospital admissions because of repeated decompensation of HF. In the United Kingdom, about 300,000 discharges or deaths per year because of HF are registered. This number corresponds to 800 patients treated in a middle-sized hospital each year (12).

HF usually evolves over a long period from underlying LV dysfunction. The prevalence of LV systolic dysfunction in the adult population has been reported to be 3%, rising to 4% to 6% in subjects over 65 years of age. Between one-half and two-thirds of these subjects are asymptomatic (12). The absence of symptoms in patients with LV dysfunction implies that their heart disease is neither diagnosed nor treated. Nevertheless, even asymptomatic LV dysfunction confers a significant five-year mortality of 5% (12). HF has a poor prognosis: approximately half of the patients with diagnosis of HF die within four years and more than half of those with severe form of HF will die within one year (5). The median survival can be as low as 1.7 and 3.2 years for men and women, respectively. Although clinical therapeutic studies documented a significant improvement in survival of HF, it is unlikely that this already reflects the situation in the entire population. It has been suggested that only one-half of patients with symptomatic HF receive appropriate therapy, including diuretics, ACE inhibitors, and beta-blockers (15). Consequently, there is still substantial potential for improvement.

ETIOLOGY

The leading cause of HF is chronic and acute coronary artery disease. The prevalence of coronary artery disease in patients with HF varies between 50% and 75% (5). Most patients have a history of myocardial infarction and evidence of either hibernation or reversible ischemia (12). Although hypertension is present in the majority of patients and represents an important risk factor for the development of HF, only 10% of HF cases are directly caused by hypertensive heart disease. As third rank cardiomyopathies (dilatative, restrictive, hypertrophic), followed by valvular and adult congenital heart disease, pericardial diseases, myocarditis, cardiotoxic drugs, alcohol, and thyreotoxocosis (10,16).

PATHOPHYSIOLOGY

Losses of contractile myocardium and long-lasting pressure or volume overload are the main causes of ventricular dysfunction, which in the course of time progresses towards overt HF. As the weakened or overloaded ventricle becomes unable to adequately empty during systole, end-systolic volume increases, whereas ejection fraction and stroke volume fall. The impaired ejection leads to a rise in end-diastolic pressure and volume and, according to the Frank-Starling law, the stroke volume is restored (17). However, systolic wall stress, an important determinant of myocardial oxygen demand, increases and triggers the development of *ventricular hypertrophy* (18). At the beginning, the hemodynamic function remains normal at rest, but during exercise the cardiac reserve becomes exhausted and cardiac output does not meet the metabolic needs of active tissues. The pump failure is sensed by the carotid and aortic baroceptors, which in turn initiate a neurohumoral chain reaction that subsequently affects all tissues and organs of the body, determines the course of the cardiac disease, and induces structural changes in the heart itself. The systems activated in response to the failing ventricular function are the *sympathetic, parasympathetic, renin–angiotensin–aldosterone system (RAAS), hypothalamo-neurohypophyseal*, and *immune* systems as well as *vascular endothelium* (19,20). The activation of the sympathetic system causes vasoconstriction and produces a positive chronotropic and inotropic response. Its activity is reflected by increased plasma levels of noradrenaline. The tachycardia of HF is also increased by the withdrawal of parasympathetic activity. The RAAS, with its end-products angiotensin II and aldosterone, is responsible for further vasoconstriction, water, and sodium retention and potassium loss. The release of antidiuretic hormone (ADH, vasopressin) contributes to increased water reabsorption and to peripheral vasoconstriction (21). An additional powerful vasoconstricting stimulus stems from the activated endothelium, which releases endothelin-1 (22). A consequence of this vasoconstriction is diminished perfusion of peripheral tissues and organs with the kidney as the prominent victim. At first, the kidney compensates for the decreased renal blood flow by increasing filtration fraction and maintaining glomerular filtration. With prolonged and severe reduction in renal flow, however, an ischemic renal failure can develop. The function and integrity of the liver and gut also suffer from the diminished oxygen delivery. Finally, skeletal muscle function is also impaired in chronic HF (23). Defective vasodilation in working muscles during exercise, structural changes, and low anaerobic threshold are probably responsible for chronic fatigue and exercise intolerance of patients with chronic HF. In addition, skeletal muscle weakness may be related to impaired peripheral glucose utilization caused by insulin resistance, which is also held responsible for cardiac cachexia (24).

The cardiovascular system possesses a system that is also activated in cachexia and opposes the vasoconstriction and fluid retention produced by the RAAS. This is the system of natriuretic peptides [atrial (ANP) and brain natriuretic peptides (BNP)], synthesized and released by cardiac myocytes, which promote vasodilation and diuresis. Adrenomedullin and dopamine, secreted from the adrenal gland, and prostacyclin released from the endothelium also have similar effects (21). Recently, evidence of activation of the immune system was found, manifest by increases in proinflammatory cytokines TNF-α, IL-1, and IL-6 (25). Although this neurohumoral response is initially beneficial and allows restoration of perfusion pressure and cardiac output, in the long-term it becomes deleterious and in the absence of appropriate therapy can lead to terminal multiorgan failure. The understanding of all these complex mechanisms is the basis of present therapeutic strategies for acute and chronic HF (26). In addition, the plasma levels of mediators of the neuroendocrine response are now used as markers of the HF and its severity (noradrenaline, natriuretic peptides).

From the very beginning of the process, the myocardium undergoes pronounced structural *remodeling* (27,28). The overloaded cardiac muscle becomes hypertrophic by parallel or in series multiplication of sarcomeres, whereas the lost myocytes are replaced by fibrotic tissue (scar). Myocardial tissue repair is significantly influenced by the paracrine and autocrine action of angiotensin II locally synthetized in the myocardium and responsible for progressive accumulation of fibrous tissue. Fibrosis takes place not only at the site of injury (reparative fibrosis) but also in the remote myocardium (reactive fibrosis). The local action of angiotensin II, in concert with endothelin-1 and fibrogenic peptide TGF-β1, is responsible for deleterious structural changes in the myocardium, going from hypertrophy to necrosis and apoptosis of the myocytes and to widespread fibrosis (29,30). The consequence of this remodeling process is the progressive increase in stiffness and decrease in contractility of the myocardium (28). The ACE inhibitors and the angiotensin receptor blockers are able to interrupt or reverse this local process (*reverse remodeling*) even if there is no systemic activation of the RAAS (30). Initially, an adequate LV hypertrophy can temporarily normalize LV wall stress and, to a large extent, the global LV function. In contrast, inadequate hypertrophy is associated with permanently elevated wall stress, increased myocardial oxygen demand, further *dilatation*, and progressive impairment in LV function. The increasing LV volume is associated with a conspicuous change of LV geometry from a conical to spherical form. This change in shape impairs the contractile function of myocardial fibers. The remodeling process of ischemic heart causes an apical and outward displacement of papillary muscles with consequences for the function of the mitral valve. The leaflets become increasingly tethered in the ventricle during systole and fail to oppose properly. In this form of mitral regurgitation, the mitral valve leaflets are normal and exhibit a restricted motion during systole (31). The condition is known as *functional mitral valve regurgitation* and is a common finding in patients with coronary artery disease, particularly in those with history of myocardial infarction (ischemic mitral regurgitation). The presence of moderate or severe ischemic regurgitation in patients with HF is associated with a large increase in the risk of HF and death (32).

Surgical trauma activates the same systems as the failing heart: the sympathoadrenergic system with increases in noradrenaline and adrenaline plasma levels, the RAAS, the adrenal cortex (cortisol), the pituitary gland (adrenocorticotropic hormone, growth hormone, vasopressin, ADH) and the endothelium (endothelin). The overall result of this orchestrated stress response is vasoconstriction, hypertension, tachycardia, renal conservation of sodium and water, and loss of potassium (33). During surgery, this stress response is attenuated by general and/or regional anesthesia, but in the postoperative period, it becomes unopposed and can have deleterious effects in patients with reduced cardiac reserve or limited myocardial oxygen supply.

CLINICAL CONSIDERATIONS
Diagnosis
As mentioned above, the ESC Guidelines require for the diagnosis of HF the presence of *signs* and *symptoms* of HF and objective evidence of cardiac dysfunction at rest. The classical symptoms of HF are *exertional dyspnea, orthopnea, paroxysmal nocturnal dyspnea, fatigue,* and *edema*. The sensitivity of these symptoms varies from 23% (edema) to 66% (dyspnea) and the specificity from 52% (dyspnea) to 81% orthopnea (34). The interobserver reproducibility of the characteristic signs of HF, including *peripheral edema, raised jugular venous pressure, third heart sound and pulmonary crepitations*, is generally poor. Moreover, the signs may be absent in a substantial proportion of patients (12). Thus, "asymptomatic" patients with LV dysfunction can easily elude the clinical diagnosis and preoperative risk stratification. The algorithm for the diagnosis of HF and LV dysfunction is presented in Figure 1. The objective proof of LV dysfunction should be based on four investigations: ECG, chest X ray, echocardiography, and BNP assay (5).

A normal ECG has a high negative predictive value, whereas the presence of precordial Q-waves and long QRS intervals is suggestive of an abnormal LV function (35). In addition, ECG is invaluable for assessment of heart rhythm and conduction abnormalities.

The *chest X ray* should be a part of every initial diagnostic work-up and evaluated for cardiac size and shape, cardiothoracic ratio, pulmonary venous congestion or edema, and pleural effusion. *Echocardiography* plays a key role in the diagnostic process (5,12). It provides information on systolic and diastolic function and size of LV and RV, regional wall motion, ventricle hypertrophy, valvular function, pericardium, and pulmonary artery pressure. The most important single measurement is the LV ejection fraction (EF). The EF is usually derived from measurements of end-diastolic and end-systolic volumes in two planes (4-chamber and 2-chamber view) by the modified Simpson's method (Fig. 2). In general, an LV EF of 40% or less is considered as abnormal and an LV EF of 30% or less indicates a severe LV dysfunction. On the other hand, LV EF of 50% or more indicates preserved LV systolic function (5,36). Interestingly, the degree of LV dysfunction expressed as LV EF does not correlate with the symptoms of HF or New York Heart Association (NYHA) class. Intraoperatively, most anesthesiologists use instead of LV EF the LVFAC (LV fractional area change) derived from the transgastric short axis view by means of transesophageal echocardiography. In agreement with the transthoracic LV EF, an FAC value of 50% or more is compatible with preserved systolic function. LV end-diastolic and end-systolic size (or volume), a restrictive LV filling pattern, and mitral regurgitation are all independent echocardiographic predictors of adverse

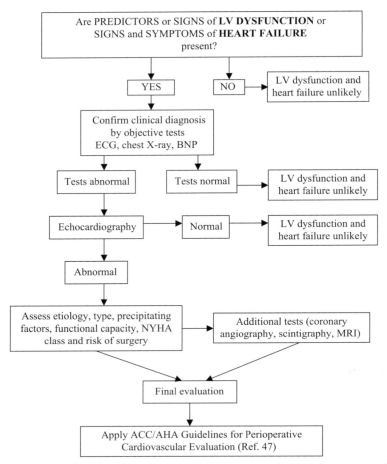

FIGURE 1   Algorithm for preoperative diagnosis of heart failure. *Source*: From Ref. 5.

outcome in chronic HF (37).When evaluating the ventricular size, one has to be aware that anesthesia and mechanical ventilation reduce the chamber dimensions and volumes (38).

Out of the family of natriuretic peptides, ANP and BNP are now available for use as biomarkers of HF (39). Although ANP is synthetized and stored in and released from the atrial myocardium, BNP is released from the ventricular myocardium. Synthesis takes place in cardiomyocytes and leads from the prepropeptides and propeptides NT-proANP and NT-proBNP to the active peptides ANP and BNP. The stimulus for the release of ANP and BNP is the stretching of the myocytes caused by increase of filling pressure and wall stress (40). BNP and NT-proBNP better reflect LV wall stress and dys-function and have therefore become the preferred and commercially widely available markers. The diagnostic value of BNP and NT-proBNP is identical. BNP/NT-proBNP levels increase slightly with increasing age and in LV hypertrophy, atrial fibrillation, RV failure, and renal failure. BNP or NT-proBNP is particularly useful for exclusion of LV dysfunction and HF in patients with equivocal symptoms and signs. The negative

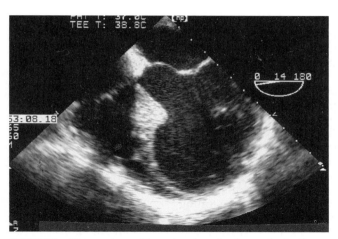

FIGURE 2   Mid-esophageal four-chamber view in a patient with coronary artery disease, history of anteroseptal myocardial infarction, and decompensated HF. The echocardiogram shows marked LV remodeling with extended scarring of the septum and the apex, eccentric hypertrophy of the vital myocardium, and general spherical dilatation. The LV EF measured in this and two-chamber view was 30%. The RV function was normal. *Abbreviations*: HF, heart failure; LV, left ventricular; EF, ejection fraction; RV, right ventricular.

predictive value of BNP/NT-proBNP has been reported to be as high as 98% (41,42). The use of BNP in differential diagnosis of acute dyspnea has resulted in shortening of hospital length of stay as well as in reduction of hospital costs (43). The high sensitivity of BNP/NT-proBNP already allows identification of asymptomatic NYHA class I patients with LV dysfunction who would benefit from therapy with ACE inhibitors. BNP/NT-proBNP levels correlate with the NYHA class and are useful for objective assessment of the severity of chronic HF. BNP/NT-proBNP is also a valuable and independent predictor of cardiac death and appears to be superior to other markers such as noradrenaline (44). Finally, preliminary results suggest that BNP/NT-proBNP may be useful in guiding the therapy of HF (45).

Functional Capacity
Aerobic capacity is the main determinant of functional status; it correlates with the severity of HF and predicts outcome. The information provided by patients on their ability to walk, climb stairs, etc., is the basis for the *NYHA classification*. Despite its subjective character, NYHA classification performs very well as predictor of cardiac death and adverse cardiac outcomes. In order to further improve the cardiac risk stratification, more objective measures of physical performance and functional capacity have been proposed (46). The ACC/ASA Guidelines for Preoperative Cardiac Risk Assessment (47) recommend the use of *metabolic equivalents* (1 MET = 3.5 mL O_2/kg/min). Limitation of aerobic capacity to less than 4 METs allows the patients only to walk slowly on level ground and is a predictor of increased perioperative and long-term cardiac risk. Another simple test is the *6-minute walk*. When patients are not able to cover a distance of more than 300 m, their functional status is poor and the risk is high (48,49). *Climbing two flights of stairs* demands more than 4 METs (approximately 5.5 METs) and if not possible, it is a predictor of perioperative complications (50). If true objective assessment of functional capacity is needed, e.g., before lung resection, lung or heart

transplantation, bicycle or treadmill *ergometry* has to be used (48). Ergometry allows measuring not only maximal tolerated *workload* but also *maximal oxygen consumption* (max VO_2 or peak VO_2) and various respiratory parameters such as oxygen pulse (VO_2/ heart rate). In patients with HF, a peak VO_2 cut-off value of less than $10 \, mL/kg/min$ is associated with high, and that of more than $18 \, mL/kg/min$ with low risk of death and complications (4). Patients with peak VO_2 of less than $10 \, mL/kg/min$ are usually considered as inoperable. Maximal VO_2 measured at the peak of exhaustive exercise, usually well beyond the anaerobic threshold, still depends on patient's cooperation. Therefore, new methods have been introduced that are patient-independent, involve submaximal bicycle exercise, and are better predictors than peak VO_2. The slope of the linear relation between ventilation (V_E), and CO_2 elimination (VCO_2) (V_E/VCO_2) reflects the abnormal increase in ventilation relative to gas exchange. In patients with HF, a value of the V_E/VCO_2 ratio greater than $34 \, 1/1$ was associated with a fivefold increase of cardiac death within six months of testing (51,52). An alternative method with a comparable predictive power is the determination of oxygen consumption at anaerobic threshold ($VO_2 \, AT$) (52). A $VO_2 \, AT$ value of less than $11 \, mL/kg/min$ increases the risk of cardiac death similar to V_E/VCO_2 ratio (51). For a favorable outcome of surgery, an AT of $14 \, mL/kg/min$ is deemed adequate (46).

Arrhythmias and Left Atrial Function
Abnormal cardiac rhythms are common in HF. They include supraventricular and ventricular arrhythmias as well as atrioventricular conduction abnormalities and are responsible for substantial morbidity, HF decompensation, and sudden death (53,54). The most common arrhythmia is *atrial fibrillation.* It is present in 10% to 50% of patients with HF and its incidence is proportional to the severity of HF (55). Atrial fibrillation occurring in HF can be regarded as an electromechanical failure of the left atrium (LA) caused by long-standing LV dysfunction. Normal LA function consists of *reservoir, conduit,* and *booster pump function* (56). In conditions associated with elevated resistance to LV filling, there is a compensatory increase in LA conduit and booster pump (atrial systolic function) function (Fig. 3). The redistribution of the LA function is visible in pulmonary veins as a marked increase in diastolic flow and reduction in systolic flow. In the presence of LV dysfunction or failure, the pressure in LA increases, leading to increase in LA wall stress, dilatation, hypertrophy, ischemia, and structural changes (fibrosis) of the LA wall. The latter becomes the electrophysiological substrate of atrial arrhythmias, which can be triggered in the perioperative period by increased sympathetic tone or further atrial distention by volume overload. The abnormalities of LA in patients with LV dysfunction or failure include increased LA volume, decreased passive and increased active emptying, and increased LA ejection force. Left atrial hypertrophy and enhanced booster pump function are able to compensate for impaired LV relaxation and increased LV stiffness (57) but this compensation is lost if the LA itself suffers from ischemia (58). The deterioration of LA systolic function or its complete loss due to atrial fibrillation or flutter is accompanied by marked impairment of LV filling. Left atrial systolic failure can be induced experimentally by fast atrial pacing or clinically by any supraventricular tachycardia, including atrial fibrillation or flutter (57). Decreased atrial function after prolonged period of atrial fibrillation with rapid ventricular rate is known as *atrial stunning* and requires a continuation of anticoagulation for several weeks to prevent stroke. The time required for recovery of atrial function is proportional to the duration of the arrhythmia (59,60). During this time, the LA will not be able to compensate for impairment of early filling in the event of an acute LV dysfunction.

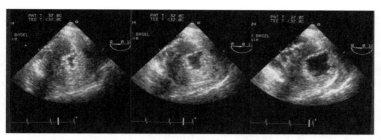

FIGURE 3 LV concentric remodeling and left atrial booster pump function. Three transgastric short-axis views in a female patient with coronary artery disease, hypertension, and acute pulmonary edema. Although the LV mass index is still within normal limits, the LV wall thickness and relative wall thickness are significantly increased (15 mm and 1.0, respectively). Doppler studies revealed an impaired relaxation pattern. *Left*: near-obliteration of the LV cavity at end-systole. *Middle*: passive filling of the LV prior to atrial contraction. *Right*: marked increase in LV volume at end-diastole after atrial contraction. *Abbreviation*: LV, left ventricular.

Interestingly, in healthy and spontaneously breathing subjects inhalational anesthetics impaired LA systolic function and reduced the atrial contribution to LV filling (61,62). Thus, LA plays a key role in the pathophysiology and clinical course of HF. The size and function of LA may be regarded as an integral reflection of LV diastolic function (63). Indeed, LA volume was found to be a predictor of poor outcome in a community-based population of elderly subjects (64).

Ventricular arrhythmias are common in patients with HF. Ventricular tachycardia and ventricular fibrillation have been identified as the main cause of *sudden death* of patients with HF; a few patients may also die suddenly because of bradyarrhythmias (heart block) or electromechanical dissociation. The risk of sudden death is increased ninefold in patients with HF, and sudden death is responsible for as many as half of all deaths from HF (65). In patients with coronary artery disease, ischemia, infarction, and myocardial scarring represent the electrophysiological substrate of ventricular arrhythmias and promote reentry. The mechanism of arrhythmia generation is usually different in nonischemic cardiomyopathy where macroentry via bundle branches or fascicles and focal automaticity is involved (66).

Diastolic Dysfunction and Diastolic Heart Failure

Diastolic function is primarily determined by active relaxation, elastic recoil, and the passive elastic properties of the myocardium. LV diastolic function is of critical importance for global LV function and overall cardiovascular performance (67). It is normal if the LV is able to fill during diastole to an end-diastolic volume compatible with adequate stroke volume and normal filling pressures. LV diastolic dysfunction refers to a condition of increased resistance of the LV to filling, associated with detectable abnormalities in LV diastolic function. There is substantial evidence that diastolic dysfunction can lead to chronic or acute HF (68). If patients with diastolic dysfunction undergo surgery, they are at risk of developing complications as the result of perioperative fluid and blood volume shifts. On the one hand, they may be less tolerant to blood loss, hypovolemia, and anemia; on the other hand, they may be particularly susceptible to volume overload. During exercise, postoperative sympatho-adrenergic stimulation, producing tachycardia and hypertension, can contribute to the manifestations of diastolic dysfunction. Thus, hemodynamic instability, impaired oxygenation, and acute

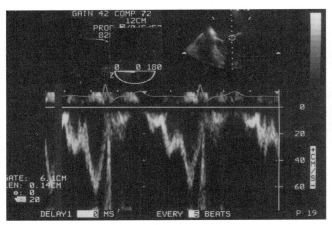

FIGURE 4 Transmitral blood flow velocity recorded by pulsed-wave Doppler in a patient with coronary artery disease, history of myocardial infarction, and poorly controlled hypertension. The flow pattern is characterized by low early filling velocity with prolonged deceleration time and high late diastolic velocity caused by atrial contraction. This flow pattern is compatible with impaired (slowed) LV relaxation. *Abbreviation*: LV, left ventricular.

pulmonary edema may all be consequences of impaired LV filling. In addition, volume overload in the presence of the diastolic dysfunction can distend the atria and precipitate atrial fibrillation with deleterious hemodynamic effects.

The criteria for diagnosis of LV diastolic dysfunction defined by European Study Group on Diastolic Heart Failure (69) include evidence of (*i*) slow isovolumic LV relaxation and/or (*ii*) slow early LV filling and/or (*iii*) reduced LV diastolic distensibility and/or (*iv*) increased LV chamber or myocardial muscle stiffness. The rate of isovolumic relaxation is measured by time constant τ of LV isovolumic pressure decay by means of left heart catheterization. Although the time constant τ is widely accepted as a reliable parameter of myocardial relaxation, it has been criticized because of its dependence on loading conditions (70). The parameters of LV distensibility and stiffness require construction of LV pressure/volume curve (71). In fact, the leftward and upward shift of the diastolic LV pressure/volume relation expressing the need for a higher filling pressure at any given end-diastolic volume is the only unequivocal proof of LV diastolic dysfunction. Although a reliable diagnosis of LV dysfunction requires left heart catheterization, in practice and in epidemiologic studies, noninvasive Doppler techniques are widely used (Fig. 4). However, the Doppler-derived information on diastolic dysfunction is subject to serious limitations. The Doppler parameters are measures of LV filling dynamics and, therefore, are affected by a variety of factors apart from intrinsic diastolic properties. Doppler parameters are highly load-dependent and their abnormalities mostly result from elevated LV filing pressure. Thus, they cannot provide reliable information on intrinsic diastolic properties or chamber stiffness (71). There is a high prevalence of Doppler-derived diastolic abnormalities in the community and, consequently, in the population of patients undergoing surgery as well (72). Applying the criteria of the European Study Group, abnormalities in Doppler parameters were found in 11% of a large population sample. Including only patients treated with diuretics or with left atrial enlargement (as evidence of dysfunction) resulted in a prevalence of 3.1% (73). In a recently studied population aged 45 years or older, the overall prevalence of diastolic dysfunction was 21%, with 6.6% having a clinically relevant moderate and 0.7% having a severe dysfunction. Interestingly, less than half of the patients with moderate or severe diastolic dysfunction had symptomatic chronic HF (74). The prevalence of diastolic dysfunction is higher in men than in women and increases with age: it was shown to be less than 3% in individuals younger than 35 years but to be present in 15.8% of those older than 65 years (73). This age dependency may be explained by increasing prevalence of predictors of diastolic dysfunction with age. The predictors are arterial hypertension, LV hypertrophy, coronary artery disease, obesity, renal disease, and diabetes mellitus (73,74). The prevalence data have been recently challenged because of the limitations on which they are based. Indeed, a 16-fold difference in the prevalence of diastolic dysfunction and poor concordance between the commonly used Doppler measures of LV diastolic function were recently reported (75). It is likely that the epidemiologic studies based on Doppler measurements substantially overestimate the prevalence of diastolic dysfunction (70). Despite the controversy regarding the relation of Doppler parameters to intrinsic diastolic properties, diastolic dysfunction, diagnosed by Doppler in a large population sample, is a predictor of all-cause mortality, independent of gender, age, and LV EF (74–76). In 11% to 15% of patients older than 65 years and no clinical evidence of heart disease but with Doppler evidence of LV diastolic dysfunction, a symptomatic HF developed within five years of the Doppler study (36). In addition, Doppler indices were helpful in intraoperative management of patients undergoing open heart surgery, predicting need for fluids or difficult weaning from cardiopulmonary bypass (77,78).

Many now agree that *diastolic HF* is a heterogenous entity and can be caused not only by true diastolic dysfunction, but also by subtle systolic dysfunction, renal failure or excessive arterial stiffening, and reduced aortic distensibility (79). However, a recent study found no evidence of abnormal systolic performance, function, and contractility in patients with diastolic HF (80). Although in most patients both dysfunction forms coexist and the discrimination may appear unnecessary, the patients with preserved systolic and abnormal diastolic function may require a different therapeutic approach from patients with systolic HF.

The European Study Group on Diastolic Heart Failure requires for the diagnosis of diastolic HF the simultaneous presence of three conditions: (*i*) signs or symptoms of congestive HF, (*ii*) normal or only mildly abnormal LV systolic function, and (*iii*) evidence of abnormal LV diastolic function (69). The inclusion of the evidence of diastolic dysfunction raised criticism that is understandable given the diagnostic problems mentioned above. Alternative criteria for definitive diastolic HF still require (*i*) definitive evidence of HF (clinical symptoms and signs, supporting laboratory tests, and typical response to treatment with diuretics), (*ii*) LV EF ≥ 50% within 72 hours of the HF event, and (*iii*) objective evidence of LV diastolic dysfunction on cardiac catheterization. However, the criteria for probable and possible diastolic HF do not require evidence of diastolic dysfunction any more (81). There is indeed no convincing evidence that the detection of diastolic dysfunction is essential for the diagnosis of diastolic HF. When patients with history of HF and normal LV EF were studied by simultaneous cardiac catheterization and Doppler echocardiography, one or more of the indices of diastolic function were abnormal in every patient. Accordingly, the measurement of diastolic function serves to confirm rather than to establish the diagnosis of diastolic HF that can be made without these measurements (82).

Depending on the diagnostic method used, in cross-sectional population studies, the proportion of patients with preserved LV systolic function among HF patients varied between 39% and 71% (83). This proportion was consistently lower (24–55%, mean 41%) in hospitalized patient cohorts. In contrast to diastolic dysfunction, the prevalence of diastolic HF is much higher in women (84,85). In spite of the preserved LV systolic function, diastolic HF is not a benign condition. The reported annual mortality was reported in multiple studies to be about 5% to 9% (86). These figures seem to be lower than the 10% to 15% reported for patients with systolic HF but in a recent hospital cohort study no difference in mortality was found between systolic and diastolic HF (67,85). Symptoms and signs alone cannot differentiate systolic from diastolic HF. Factors that promote fluid retention and decompensation are also similar and include uncontrolled hypertension, atrial fibrillation, noncompliance with medication, myocardial ischemia, renal failure, use of nonsteroidal analgesics, and increased salt intake (67). In contrast to systolic HF, there is no established long-term therapy for chronic diastolic HF, and the results of several ongoing trials are awaited. In the meantime, treatment remains limited to alleviation or elimination of symptoms (5).

Acute Heart Failure

Acute HF is characterized by "rapid onset of symptoms and signs secondary to abnormal cardiac function" (6). Acute HF occurs either without or with a preexisting heart disease. The former condition represents acute "de novo" HF, the latter condition relates to acute decompensation of chronic HF. The common precipitating factors are listed in Table 1. The European Guidelines for Diagnosis and Treatment of Acute Heart Failure (6) distinguish six forms of acute HF (Table 2). Any of these forms of acute HF can occur in the perioperative period. Acute HF is usually a life-threatening condition that requires hospitalization and urgent therapy and has emerged as a major public health problem. In the U.S., hospitalizations for acute HF have increased over the last 20 years by 28% and represent the leading cause of hospital admission in patients over 60 years of age (7). The Acute Decompensated Heart Failure Registry (ADHERE) reported recently on 62,018 enrolled patients (87). The median age of the patients was 75.3 years and the majority of them had a history of HF. It is of note that 54% of the patients had preserved LV systolic function. The in-hospital mortality was 3.9%. Following a median hospital length of stay of 4.3 days, only 51% of patients were asymptomatic upon discharge (87). Even this limited success does not last long: Fifty percent of patients treated in hospital for acute HF are rehospitalized at least once and 15% at least twice within the next 12 months (88,89). Several studies have demonstrated the risks of perioperative volume overload and the superiority of restricted fluid regimen with regard to perioperative morbidity and mortality (90,91). Even patients with asymptomatic LV dysfunction undergoing surgery carry an increased risk of postoperative HF and pulmonary edema (92).

Not all cases of acute HF and pulmonary edema are caused by LV systolic dysfunction. Many patients have preserved LV systolic function, and the edema appears to be provoked by acute hypertension and exacerbation of LV diastolic dysfunction (93–95). Recently, acute ischemic mitral regurgitation has been identified as another cause of acute pulmonary edema (96). The critical period encompasses the time from discontinuation of positive pressure ventilation and onset of spontaneous breathing

TABLE 1 Common Causes of Acute HF or of Decompensation of Chronic Heart Failure

Cardiac
Arrhythmias
Atrial fibrillation/flutter
Ventricular tachycardia
Bradycardic rhythms
Acute coronary syndromes
Myocardial ischemia
Myocardial infarction
Complication of infarction
Valvular
New/increased regurgitation
Severe aortic stenosis
Prosthetic dysfunction
Trauma
Myocardial contusion
Myocarditis
Extra-cardiac
Hypertension
Volume overload
Increased salt intake
Noncompliance with prescribed drugs
Concomitant drugs (NSAIDs, glitazones)
Infection (sepsis)
Pulmonary embolism
Thyreotoxicosis
Anemia
Renal failure
Alcohol excess

Source: From Ref. 6.

to the time after extubation. Awakening from anesthesia, anxiety, pain perception, and increased venous return due to negative intrathoracic pressure can increase sympathetic tone, heart rate, systolic pressure, preload and afterload of the LV, and precipitate pulmonary edema (97). In patients with coronary artery disease, postoperative pulmonary edema can be precipitated by an episode of myocardial ischemia, which is common in patients with coronary artery disease during emergence (98).

Right Ventricular Failure

Most of the cases of RV failure are secondary to LV failure caused by ischemic, valvular, or primary cardiomyopathy. In these patients, RV dysfunction detected as low RV

TABLE 2 Forms of Acute HF According to Guidelines of European Society of Cardiology

Hypertensive acute HF
Pulmonary edema
Cardiogenic shock
High output failure (septic shock)
RV failure

Abbreviations: HF, heart failure; RV, right ventricular.
Source: From Ref. 6.

EF or RVFAC is an independent predictor of total and cardiovascular mortality and of HF (99,100). In a joint medical and surgical ICU, RV failure was found to be responsible for 18% of cases of hemodynamic instability and refractory hypotension (101). The mortality of RV failure occurring in ventilated critically ill patients can be as high as 44% (102). Most cases of primary RV failure are associated with acute or chronic pulmonary embolism, adult congenital heart disease, chronic obstructive lung disease (COLD), primary pulmonary hypertension, isolated RV myocardial infarction, RV arrhythmogenic dysplasia, heart transplantation, implantation of LV assist device, and adult respiratory distress syndrome (ARDS). The main causal factors involved in RV HF are *pressure overload* (e.g., in pulmonary hypertension), *volume overload* (e.g., ventricular septum defect), and *loss of contractile myocardium (RV infarction)*. As a low-pressure, high-volume pump, the RV is very sensitive to increases in afterload, which leads to increases in RV end-systolic volume and in fall in RV EF. The compensatory increase in RV end-diastolic volume and pressure can restore the RV stroke volume. However, the RV wall stress increases and promotes hypertrophy of the RV myocardium. Given enough time for adaptation to the elevated afterload, the RV is able to generate high, often systemic pressures. Elevated right atrial, RV end-diastolic and pulmonary artery pressures, high pulmonary vascular resistance, and high pressure gradient between right atrium and pulmonary artery characterize the hemodynamic profile. Elevated wall stress increases myocardial oxygen demand, whereas at the same time high intraventricular pressure interferes with myocardial perfusion. Because the dilatation of the RV free wall is limited by pericardium, the high diastolic pressure displaces the interventricular septum towards the left ventricle with the consequence of increased LV chamber stiffness and impaired LV filling. Echocardiography shows dilated and hypertrophied RV with reduced RV EF, leftward bulging of atrial and ventricular septum, paradoxical motion of ventricular septum, and tricuspid regurgitation (103). Clinically, there are signs of systemic venous hypertension such as hepatomegaly, edema, and ascites. Eventually, the RV fails. The impeding failure is signalized by right atrial pressure largely exceeding the left atrial pressure and a progressively decreasing difference between right atrial and RV systolic pressure. If a patent foramen ovale is present, a right to left shunt can develop and produce right-to-left shunt and severe hypoxemia. With acute massive central pulmonary embolism, the events described above can develop within hours or minutes because an RV, which is not adapted to pressure overload, is not able to sustain the sudden and excessive increase in afterload. In a retrospective study of documented massive acute pulmonary embolism, the diagnosis of RV dysfunction called *"acute cor pulmonale"* was based on echocardiographic evidence of RV dilatation (RV end-diastolic area/LV end-diastolic area > 0.6) and dyskinesia of ventricular septum (104). Acute cor pulmonale was found in 61% of the patients and carried an overall mortality of 23%. As long as the hemodynamics remained stable, with or without inotropic support, the mortality was low (3%) but rose to 59% in unstable patients who developed metabolic acidosis (104).

A different kind of RV failure develops secondary to a loss of RV myocardium due to isolated or predominant *RV myocardial infarction*, usually resulting from proximal occlusion of the right coronary artery (105). The ability of the infarcted RV to generate pressure can be markedly reduced and the difference between the high right atrial pressure and the peak systolic pressure is diminished. This right atrioventricular pressure gradient can be determined by measuring tricuspid regurgitant velocity with continuous-wave Doppler. Arrhythmias and conduction abnormalities are common in RV myocardial infarction (106). In cardiac surgery, the acute RV failure is relatively common and usually caused by inadequate intraoperative protection of the RV, RV

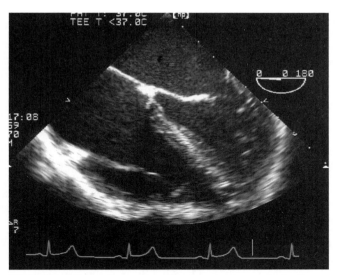

FIGURE 5 Midesophageal four-chamber view in a patient with coronary artery disease, history of inferior myocardial infarction, COLD, and acute postoperative RV failure. The echocardiogram shows a dilated right ventricle with an RV/LV area ratio of 1.2. The on-line measured RV EF was 28%, the RV free wall was hypokinetic, and the ventricular septum moved paradoxically towards the LV in diastole. *Abbreviations*: COLD, chronic obstructive lung disease; RV, right ventricular; LV, left ventricular; EF, ejection fraction.

ischemia, stunning, or coronary spasm (102). Another mechanism is an acute RV decompensation in patients with excessive pulmonary vascular resistance, e.g., after mitral valve surgery or following heart or lung transplantation. RV failure also frequently occurs after initiation of mechanical LV support (LV-assist device). Echocardiography shows dilated RV with extended zones of akinesia, usually including the infero-posterior LV wall, leftward shift, and paradoxic motion of the ventricular septum (Fig. 5). In all these situations, there is a striking difference between the pronounced systemic congestion and the clear lung fields. RV infarction has been shown to have more favorable long-term prognosis than LV infarction (105), but if it is responsible for cardiogenic shock (so-called *predominant RV shock*), the outcome (mortality of 53%) is comparable with that of LV shock. Patients with RV shock were shown to be younger, have lower prevalence of previous infarction and multivessel disease, and to exhibit a shorter time interval between infarction and onset of shock (107). In patients suffering from COLD, RV failure can develop secondary to pulmonary hypertension caused by rarefaction of the lung tissue and chronic hypoxemia and hypercapnia. Autopsy studies found RV hypertrophy in 7% to 10% of the patients with COLD as a sign of chronic cor pulmonale (108). The pulmonary hypertension of COLD is usually mild, evolves slowly, and the mean pulmonary artery pressure seldom exceeds 25 to 30 mmHg. Nevertheless, RV may fail when additional factors such as postoperative respiratory failure, pneumonia, or RV ischemia occur (108).

Approximately 25% of patients with acute ARDS mechanically ventilated in the ICU develop RV dysfunction that has also been designated as "acute cor pulmonale" (109). It is caused by a peripheral occlusive process in the pulmonary vasculature and the effects of mechanical ventilation, which increases RV afterload (110). The same echocardiographic criteria as described above are used. A ratio of RV to LV area of greater than 1.0 indicates the presence of a severe acute cor pulmonale. The development of acute cor pulmonale in ARDS is associated with pulmonary hypertension, tachycardia, decreased stroke volume, impaired LV diastolic function, and prolonged ventilatory support. The mortality rate of 32%, however, does not exceed the mortality of patients without acute cor pulmonale (109). RV function plays also an important role in cardiovascular adaptation to extended lung resection. If there is no or only an inadequate RV functional reserve, the postoperative increase in pulmonary vascular resistance will precipitate RV failure.

PREOPERATIVE RISK ASSESSMENT AND ANESTHESIA MANAGEMENT

Considering the stress that surgical trauma imposes on the heart, it is easy to understand that patients with ventricular dysfunction, reduced cardiac reserve, or HF are at serious risk of adverse postoperative cardiac outcomes. Large series have consistently noted that patients with severe LV dysfunction or evidence of HF have an increased perioperative risk (111–113). HF is not uncommon in surgical populations; for instance, 19% to 28% of the patients undergoing peripheral vascular surgery had history of previous HF and 7% to 9% of these patients developed acute HF after surgery (114).

The risk associated with HF is substantial. In patients undergoing vascular surgery, a history of HF less than one year before operation markedly increased risk of cardiac mortality, and if HF is present at surgery, the risk of cardiac death is 12 times higher than in patients without HF (115). In another study, 15% of patients presenting with overt HF at surgery developed postoperative pulmonary edema (116).

The available methods of preoperative risk evaluation are, however, not very helpful with regard to HF. This may be due to difficulty of discrimination between ischemic and nonischemic outcomes. As coronary artery disease is now responsible for up to 70% of all cases of HF, it is likely that many postoperative complications are diagnosed as ischemic even in the absence of positive proof of myocardial ischemia. In addition and not unexpectedly, the risk carried by both conditions is interrelated: HF increases the risk of perioperative myocardial infarction and vice versa (115). Nevertheless, in the classical Goldman Cardiac Risk Index, two signs of decompensated HF, third heart sound, or jugular venous distention were the top ranking risk factors, weighted even higher than recent myocardial infarction (117). The original index did not stand the test of time but was an important impulse for further research in preoperative risk stratification (118). In Detsky's Modified Multifactorial Index, the signs of HF were replaced by history of alveolar pulmonary edema and given much lower ratings than acute coronary syndromes (119). In the Revised Index, history of congestive HF is one of the six equivalent risk factors that are added in order to obtain the patient's risk (120). However, a comparison of these three indices did not reveal any convincing superiority of one index over the other and documented the persistent poor accuracy of preoperative cardiac risk prediction. Moreover, the prediction offered by ASA physical status classification of surgical mortality was shown to be not inferior to the other methods (120).

An important step forward was the introduction of ACC/AHA Guidelines for Perioperative Cardiovascular Evaluation for Noncardiac Surgery (47). These guidelines identify decompensated HF as a *major clinical predictor of risk*. According to the algorithm, the presence of such a major predictor should lead to postponement or canceling the elective noncardiac surgery, medical therapy, modification of risk factors, and further investigations, including coronary angiography if appropriate.

Compensated HF or a history thereof represents an *intermediate clinical predictor*. According to the guideline, this finding allows the practitioner to proceed with a low-risk surgical procedure but requires an estimation of the patient's functional capacity if moderate or high-risk surgery is planned. In contrast to the previous cardiac risk indices, these guidelines are also helpful in preoperative decision making. However, their utility in preoperative assessment of patients with HF still awaits confirmation in prospective studies. The guidelines leave it up to the anesthesiologist or consultant cardiologist to decide whether the patient has or had HF and to assess the severity. Here LV EF can be useful; although it does not correlate with the symptoms and is a poor predictor of ischemic outcomes, it predicts postoperative HF and cardiac death with reasonable accuracy. The risk of perioperative complications is particularly increased in patients with an LV EF of less than 35% (47).

As might be expected, there are no randomized studies of anesthetic techniques in patients with HF. Moreover, in most studies of cardiovascular effects of anesthesia, patients with HF and poor LV function were excluded. Nevertheless, it may be said that no anesthetic technique is superior to the others. Regional techniques offer many advantages but are not associated with better outcome (114,121). Patients with decompensated HF are likely to benefit from invasive hemodynamic monitoring to guide dosing with anesthetics and other drugs and to recognize and treat any deterioration of the hemodynamic function. However, evidence that invasive monitoring significantly improves outcome is still lacking (122). Parameters of peripheral perfusion such as arterial pH, base excess, gastric mucosal PCO_2, and mixed venous oxygen saturation may be useful to assess the degree of cardiovascular derangement. With regard to the differential diagnosis of different forms of acute HF, echocardiography is indispensable. It allows a distinction to be made between right and left or biventricular ventricular failure, the detection and quantification of valvular lesions, and the identification of other causes such as pericardial tamponade, LV outflow tract obstruction, aortic dissection, or cardiac trauma.

Patients with chronic or acute HF present with multiple comorbidities, including renal failure, diabetes, hypertension, peripheral vascular disease, COLD, and others. Unless optimally managed, these conditions can also contribute to perioperative morbidity and mortality. In addition, patients with chronic HF often exhibit sleep disorders. *Obstructive sleep apnea* or Cheyne–Stokes breathing with *central sleep apnea* has been detected in up to 50% of the patients with HF (123). Patients with HF tolerate obstructive sleep apnea poorly. Deeply negative intrathoracic pressure generated by inspiratory effort during the episodes of airway obstruction increases LV afterload. Hypoxia and hypercapnia increase pulmonary pressure and vascular resistance, activate the sympathoadrenergic system, and promote nocturnal hypertensive episodes. The disorder usually becomes worse in the postoperative period and requires close monitoring and efficient use of continuous positive airway pressure (124). Central sleep apnea is a sign of a bad prognosis and usually associated with end-stage HF (123).

THERAPY
Chronic Heart Failure

In the course of the last two decades, considerable success has been achieved in development of new and efficacious strategies for treatment of chronic HF (125–127). The goal of management of chronic HF is to prolong active life by improving symptoms, slowing or halting disease progression, and preventing major morbidity and sudden death (12,128). A broad therapeutic palette has now become available, allowing fine-tuning of pharmacologic treatment according to the individual needs of each patient, and avoiding untoward side effects. The established therapies in chronic HF include diuretics, nitrates, angiotensin-converting enzyme inhibitors, or angiotensin receptor (AT_1) antagonists, β-blockers, and aldosterone antagonists (127–129). There is a general agreement that therapy should not be abruptly discontinued because of surgery and that it should be carried on, with due dose adjustments, during the perioperative period. Furthermore, new therapy should be initiated in patients who did not receive it preoperatively if it is indisputably indicated. According to ADHERE Registry data, only 53% and 44% of patients hospitalized with acute HF were receiving β-blockers and ACE inhibitors, respectively. Upon discharge from the hospital, these figures were considerably improved (87). However, cardiac medications may also provoke complications when they interact with anesthetic agents (130).

The RAAS, together with the sympathoadrenergic and hypothalamus-hypophyseal (vasopressin) systems, is responsible for maintenance of adequate blood pressure and organ perfusion. In normovolemic states, the RAAS does not play a major role in the circulatory homeostasis (renin-independent state). In contrast, during major blood loss and severe hypovolemia, the circulation becomes renin (angiotensin)-dependent. In patients treated with ACE inhibitors or AT_1 antagonists, the anesthesiologist is confronted either with a risk of hypotension if the drug is continued, or with a possible deterioration of cardiovascular function if the drug is withdrawn. No important immediate rebound reactions have been described after preoperative withdrawal of these drugs. Hypotension, occasionally accompanied by bradycardia, has been repeatedly reported following induction of anesthesia. Most of these hypotensive episodes do respond to administration of fluids, however, some require administration of vasopressors. Occasionally, the hypotension may be refractory even to catecholamines, and vasopressin or terlipressin must be used (131,132). Therefore, it is advisable and safer to withdraw ACE inhibitors and AT_1 antagonists shortly (24–48 hours) before anesthesia and surgery and to reintroduce them after surgery as soon as possible.

The failing heart is exposed to increased adrenergic drive manifesting as increased plasma and coronary sinus noradrenaline and resulting in the downregulation of myocardial β-adrenoreceptors and reduced noradrenaline stores in myocardial tissue (133). Protection of the myocardium from the adverse effects of the adrenergic drive is the explanation for the favorable effects of β-blockers, including prolonged survival and reverse remodeling (134,135). Sympathoadrenergic activity can be inhibited by centrally acting sympatholytic agents such as clonidine or moxonidine. However, treatment with moxonidine resulted in decompensation and increased mortality in patients with chronic HF (133). Similarly, not all β-blockers exhibit beneficial effects in patients with chronic HF. The differences are related to their specific effects on the sympathoadrenergic system. For instance, xamoterol, a β-blocker with intrinsic $β_1$ sympatho-mimetic activity (ISA), was harmful in patients with chronic HF (133). In contrast, celiprolol, a drug with $β_2$ ISA is well-tolerated (136). Bucindolol reduces noradrenaline release by blocking the presynaptic $β_2$ and the $α_1$ adrenoceptors (137). In patients with severe chronic HF who were dependent on cardiac sympathetic drive, the powerful sympatholysis of bucindolol increased mortality (133,138). Carvedilol is a nonselective $β_1$–$β_2$ and $α_1$ blocker with an excellent record in chronic HF. Its efficacy may be explained by the combined $β_2$ and $α_1$ blockade in the presence of $β_1$ receptor down-regulation associated with chronic HF. In HF, the numbers of $β_2$ and $α_1$ adrenoceptors in the heart increase considerably and may also mediate the cytotoxic effects of noradrenaline (139).

All patients with chronic, stable HF and without contraindications should receive β-blockers. The β-blockers now recommended for use in chronic HF are metoprolol, bisoprolol, and carvedilol (140). In a direct comparison, carvedilol reduced mortality and prolonged survival significantly more than the β_1 selective metoprolol (139,141). Carvedilol appears to be more tightly bound to β_1 adrenoceptors than metoprolol and its effect persists for a longer time after discontinuation of the treatment. After long-term therapy, carvedilol but not metoprolol was able to completely suppress the hemodynamic response to dobutamine (142). The differences among the available β-blockers must be taken into account during perioperative management of patients with HF.

In the perioperative period, β-blockers improve outcomes in patients at high risk of cardiac complications and should not be withdrawn because of surgery (143,144). Effective β-blockade, however protective, means that the capacity of the cardiovascular system to increase its performance in response to increased oxygen demand (hypovolemia, anemia, postoperative stress, profound systemic vasodilation) is limited. β-Blockade can unveil myocardial depression caused by anesthetic agents or other drugs (145). High levels of endogenous or exogenous catecholamines in the presence of β-adrenoceptor blockade and unopposed α-adrenoceptor activity can lead to an excessive increase in systemic vascular resistance, LV failure, or coronary spasm (146). If patients on chronic β-blocker therapy need positive inotropic support, phosphodiesterase inhibitors or *levosimendan* should be used instead of dobutamine (142). Should an additional β-blockade become necessary (to treat inappropriate tachycardia or ischemia), the short acting *esmolol* is the β-blocker of first choice.

Amiodarone, the most effective antiarrhythmic agent, is used for treatment and prevention of both atrial and ventricular arrhythmias. It decreases systemic and coronary vascular resistance but has no clinically relevant negative inotropic effect. Therefore, amiodarone can be prescribed to patients with low EF and HF (5). However, in patients chronically treated with amiodarone, interaction with inhalation anesthetics, opioids, β-blockers, and calcium channel blockers (verapamil, diltiazem) can result in cardiovascular depression with hypotension, marked bradycardia, idioventricular rhythm, or even asystole (147). Given the long elimination halftime of amiodarone, the discontinuation shortly before surgery is not likely to reduce the risk of complications. Patients receiving chronic treatment with amiodarone may present with abnormal thyroid function (hypo- or hyperthyroidism) and, rarely, develop pulmonary complications.

The exogenous NO donors (isosorbide dinitrate, molsidomin) should be administered with the premedication and given as soon as possible after surgery. They can be replaced by intravenous nitroglycerine, particularly when a reduction in cardiac preload and filling pressures is desirable.

The potassium channel opener nicorandil can be managed in a similar manner to the oral nitrates. In comparison with the nitrates, it has a stronger effect on resistance vessels and can induce hypotension in the presence of unrecognized hypovolemia (148).

The use of digoxin is nowadays limited to control of ventricular rate in patients with chronic HF and atrial fibrillation. Under conditions of increased sympathetic tone, the rate control is often inadequate.

Despite any concerns about hypovolemia and ensuing hypotension, chronic diuretic treatment should be continued throughout the perioperative period in order to ensure adequate diuresis and to avoid fluid retention, pulmonary congestion, and postoperative HF. The replacement of the oral forms by intravenous loop diuretics (furosemide, torasemide) is necessary in most cases (5). In contrast to the saluretic agents, spironolactone should be stopped because of the risk of acute hyperpotassemia.

Statins are increasingly prescribed to patients with chronic HF because of their anti-inflammatory- and endothelium-protecting effects. In clinical trials, statins significantly reduced the incidence of cardiac death, myocardial infarction, recurrent ischemia, and HF (149). Any statin may induce myopathy or rhabdomyosis, particularly when its metabolism is markedly inhibited or when it is prescribed together with fibrates (gemfibrozil) or nicotinic acid (150). A withdrawal of statins in patients with acute myocardial ischemia was associated with increased incidence of death and nonfatal myocardial infarction as well as higher revascularization rate and higher troponin levels (151). This adverse effect, however, was not confirmed after abrupt discontinuation of statins in stable cardiac patients (152). Statin therapy before coronary artery surgery was associated with reduced hospital mortality and decreased incidence of adverse cardiovascular outcomes such as myocardial infarction, stroke, and atrial arrhythmias (153). Therefore, the protection offered by the statins should be maintained, and statins administration resumed as soon as possible during the perioperative period in both cardiac and noncardiac surgery (154).

About 8 to 30% of patients with chronic HF develop *anemia.* Its prevalence is higher in the elderly, in women, and patients with hypertension and/or renal failure. The degree of anemia increases with the severity of HF (155). Worsening of anemia over time was shown to be related to mortality and morbidity in patients with chronic HF (156). Whether correction of anemia in chronic HF, for instance, by darbepoetin and iron substitution, improves quality of life and outcome, is not known yet (157).

Patients with chronic HF exhibit impaired peripheral glucose utilization, which appears to be related to reduced insulin sensitivity (24). The antidiabetic drugs *thiazolidinediones* (glitazones) act as insulin sensitizers and are used to improve the functional capacity in chronic HF. However, thiazolidinediones can cause fluid retention, weight gain, and edema. The fluid retention usually responds to dose reduction and diuretics. However, in patients with ventricular dysfunction, it can precipitate acute HF. If this happens, the drug has to be discontinued and replaced by an alternate hypoglycemic drug (158).

Diabetes is a well-known risk factor of adverse perioperative cardiac outcomes and its presence in patients with HF further aggravates the risk (120). The recent reports on beneficial effects of insulin and of avoidance of hyperglycemia on morbidity and mortality in critically ill patients may also be applicable to surgical patients with HF. The positive inotropic effect of insulin may be a welcome side effect of the blood glucose control.

As several studies demonstrated increased mortality associated with administration of *positive inotropic agents*, they were banned from the treatment of chronic HF. Given the increasing numbers of patients with end-stage HF, it is not surprising that these drugs (dobutamine, milrinone) are again used for elective hospital or outpatient intermittent therapy. The goal is for the most part to improve the quality of life until the inevitable death. In some patients, it may serve as bridging to heart transplantation (159,160).

Patients with advanced HF, severe ischemic systolic LV dysfunction, and at high risk of sudden death benefit from implantation of *cardioverter defibrillators* (ICD). ICDs reduce mortality and were shown to prevent approximately half of all sudden deaths (161). A recent study demonstrated that ICDs are superior to amiodarone in prevention of sudden death (162). Nevertheless, the cost effectiveness of ICD devices used either alone or together with cardiac resynchronization therapy (see below) in chronic HF remains to be clarified.

Bundle branch and fascicular blocks are common findings in patients with chronic HF, presenting as interventricular or intraventricular conduction delay (<120 milliseconds). Left bundle branch block, the most common of the conduction abnormalities in this setting, can be detected in up to 40% of patients with advanced HF and is an important predictor of sudden death (163). Wide QRS complex with a left bundle branch block pattern is associated with delayed contraction of one portion of the LV relative to another, resulting in contractile dyssynchrony (164). Owing to altered propagation of action potentials, one portion of the LV myocardium is activated early, whereas the activation of the other portion is delayed. In the presence of poor LV function, such dyssynchrony will further compromise systolic function, reduce energetic efficiency, and elicit or worsen mitral regurgitation (164). It is possible to restore normal ventricular synchrony by properly timed biventricular pacing known as cardiac resynchronization therapy (165). Transvenous implantation of an LV lead is accomplished via the coronary sinus. Clinical investigations have demonstrated that resynchronization therapy in selected patients improves systolic function, cardiac output, mitral regurgitation, lowers pulmonary artery occlusion pressure, halts LV remodeling, and alleviates the symptoms of chronic HF (166,167). Optimal candidates for resynchronization therapy have dilated cardiomyopathy of an ischemic or nonischemic cause, an LV EF of 0.35 or less, QRS complexes greater than 120 milliseconds in duration, are in sinus rhythm, and are NYHA functional class III or IV despite maximal medical therapy for HF (168). Before surgery, the biventricular pacemaker must be programmed to asynchronous mode with appropriately increased pacing rate.

If a surgically correctable abnormality such as ischemia or hibernating myocardium is present, revascularization, possibly with concomitant mitral valve repair or aneurysmectomy, should be considered (169). Other surgical methods attempt to restore LV geometry by resecting the nonfunctional portion of LV wall in order to decrease wall stress, oxygen consumption, improve pump function, and prevent further dilatation (170). Surgical reduction or restoration of the LV may represent a solution for patients with no prospects for heart transplantation (171).

Acute Perioperative Heart Failure

The therapeutic approach to acute HF may vary according to the cause of HF but the principles are well established (Table 3). Morphine still remains the drug of first choice. By producing systemic venodilatation and central nervous system effects, morphine reduces pulmonary congestion, reduces anxiety, and relieves breathlessness. It also improves the tolerance of noninvasive ventilatory support (CPAP, BIPAP) administered by facemask (172,173). These techniques significantly reduce the need for tracheal intubation and mechanical ventilation. Patients suffering from acute coronary syndromes (perioperative infarction, unstable angina) and atrial fibrillation should receive heparin as soon as possible but the onset of heparinization may be delayed because of the risk of bleeding (6). Nitrates and diuretics are likely the most efficient drugs used to treat acute HF (128). Nesiritide, a recombinant human BNP, is a novel vasodilator drug. It is a venous, arterial, and coronary vasodilator, decreases preload and afterload, suppresses the RAAS and sympathetic system, and promotes sodium diuresis (174,175). It is administered in 2 µg/kg bolus doses, followed by continuous infusion (0.015–0.03 µg/kg) (176). According to a recent ADHERE report, patients with acute decompensated HF treated with intravenous nitroglycerine or nesiritide had lower in-hospital mortality than those treated with dobutamine or milrinone (177,178). These beneficial effects contrast with the recent report on worsening of renal function after nesiritide in patients with acute HF (179).

TABLE 3   Therapy of Acute Perioperative Heart Failure

Oxygen
Morphine
Diuretics
   Furosemide, torasemide
Nitrates
   Nitroglycerine
Natriuretic peptide
   Nesiritide
Ventilatory support
   Noninvasive
      Continuous positive airway
         pressure (CPAP), bilevel positive
         airway pressure (BiPAP) with
         face mask
   Tracheal intubation
      Mechanical ventilation + positive
         end-expiratory pressure (PEEP)
Inodilators
   Phosphodiesterase inhibitors
      Milrinone, enoximone
   Calcium sensitizers
      Levosimendan
Inotropes
   Dobutamine
Vasopressors (catecholamines)
   Adrenaline, noradrenaline
Pacing
   Atrial, dual, biventricular
Ultrafiltration
Surgical support
   Intra-aortic counterpulsation
   Ventricular assist device (VAD)
Emergency revascularization/
   valve surgery
Cardiopulmonary resuscitation

Intravenous loop diuretics (furosemide, torasemide) are indispensable in the management of acute HF. Their early relaxing effect on capacitance vessels contributes to the decrease in right and left filling pressures and reduction in pulmonary and systemic congestion. Occasionally, the patient can become resistant to loop diuretics. The resistance can be related to volume depletion, low cardiac output and renal blood flow, strong neurohormonal activation, renal failure, and concomitant use of nonsteroidal anti-inflammatory drugs. An addition of a thiazide diuretic, metolazone, spironolactone, or infusion of furosemide (5–40 mg/hr) is recommended as means to improve sensitivity to diuretics (5,6). The use of low-dose dopamine to increase renal blood flow and sodium excretion remains controversial.

β-Blockers can be useful in the treatment of acute HF as well, particularly in patients with pulmonary edema and signs of high sympathetic activity, tachycardia, hypertension, and preserved ventricular function (180). Usually given in combination with nitroglycerine, β-blockers improve LV filling and protect the myocardium from ischemia. Esmolol is also an effective antihypertensive drug, originally introduced for treatment of perioperative hypertension (181). The bolus dose of esmolol (0.5–1 mg/kg) can be repeated until the desired effect is achieved or administered as a continuous infusion (50–200 μg/kg/min).

Patients with systolic LV failure, inadequate peripheral perfusion, and hypotension will need inotropic support. The goal of the therapy with inotropes is to increase cardiac output, normalize its distribution, and improve oxygen supply without producing undesired side effects such as tachycardia or arrhythmias. Dobutamine is probably the mostly used inotrope in the perioperative setting (6). In cardiogenic and septic shock and similar life-threatening situations, the temporary use of vasopressors (adrenaline, noradrenaline, and vasopressin) becomes inevitable (6).

The introduction of inhibitors of the type III phosphodiesterase (PDEIs) proved to be a significant contribution to the short-term therapy of acute HF. The PDEIs (milrinone, enoximone) have positive inotropic, lusitropic, and peripheral vasodilatory effects: they are inodilators. They increase cardiac output, decrease filling pressures, and reduce both pulmonary and systemic vascular resistance (6). A simultaneous administration of a small dose of a vasopressor (e.g., noradrenaline) enhances the inotropic effect and prevents PDEI-induced hypotension. However, in patients with acutely decompensated HF, treatment with PDEIs resulted in higher mortality than the treatment with vasodilators and caused more side effects than placebo (178,182). On the other hand, the PDEIs may be preferable to dobutamine in patients on chronic β-blocker therapy (142).

Levosimendan is a new drug with inodilator profile used in acute HF (183,184). The positive inotropic effect of levosimendan is based on sensitization of contractile proteins to calcium while the vasodilatory effect stems from opening potassium channels in vascular smooth muscles. Treatment starts with a 10 to 15 µg/kg bolus given over 10 minutes, followed by continuous infusion (0.05–01 µg/kg/min) (185–187). Levosimendan is, similar to PDEIs, also effective in the presence of β-blockade (6). Before administration of levosimendan, hypovolemia must be ruled out or corrected and treatment delayed as long as hypotension is present.

Atrial flutter or acute atrial fibrillation with high ventricular rate and unstable hemodynamics should be cardioverted. Heart rate, atrioventricular conduction, and ventricular synchrony must be optimized by appropriate pacing modality. Amiodarone is the antiarrhythmic drug of first choice in the perioperative setting because in patients with HF it is safer and better tolerated than other agents (6,188,189).

A failing RV requires a judicious adjustment of preload (avoiding RV volume overload), inotropic support with inodilators, and reduction in pulmonary vascular resistance by nitric oxide or inhaled prostacycline (106). An adequate coronary perfusion pressure must be ensured (possibly with vasopressors) and the RV afterload associated with mechanical ventilation minimized by appropriate ventilator setting.

When an acute myocardial infarction is responsible for acute intra- or postoperative HF, mechanical support with intra-aortic counterpulsation and coronary angiography with prospect of successful percutaneous coronary angioplasty and stenting should be considered (190). The use of temporary mechanical circulatory assistance (VAD) is reasonable only if there is a realistic potential for recovery (6).

CONCLUSION

Increasing numbers of patients with HF now undergo surgery and are at considerable risk of adverse outcomes. The presence of HF and the associated limited cardiac reserve must be recognized preoperatively, and the perioperative management optimized. The necessary measures may include postponement of surgery, adjustment of medical therapy, and judicious planning of anesthetic and postoperative care. If acute HF occurs, its cause must be identified and the HF aggressively treated. The coordinated pre- and perioperative efforts of all professionals involved in the care of these patients should reduce the perioperative risk and possibly improve the long-term outcome as well.

REFERENCES

1. White PD Jr. Heart Disease. 4th ed. New York: McMillan, 1951:266–280.
2. Bundesamt für Statistik Todesursachenstatistik 14.3.1.1 Krankheiten. http.//www.bfs.admin.ch.
3. Cleland JG, McGowan J. Heart failure due to ischaemic heart disease: epidemiology, pathophysiology and progression. J Cardiovasc Pharmacol 1999; 33(suppl 3):S17–S29.
4. Guidelines for the diagnosis and treatment of chronic heart failure (Task Force Report). Eur Heart J 2001; 22:1327–1360.
5. European Society of Cardiology: guidelines for the diagnosis and treatment of chronic heart failure (update 2005). Eur Heart J 2005; 26:115–140.
6. The Task Force on Acute Heart Failure of the European Society of Cardiology: guidelines on the diagnosis and treatment of acute heart failure. Eur Heart J 2005; 26:384–416.
7. ACC/AHA 2005 Guideline update for the diagnosis and management of chronic heart failure in the adult—summary article. A Report of the American College of Cardiology/American Heart Association Task Force on Practice Guidelines (Writing Committee to Update the 2001 Guidelines for the Evaluation and Management of Heart Failure). www.american heart.org/www.acc.org.
8. Denolin H, Kuhn H, Krayenbuehl HP, et al. The definition of heart failure. Eur Heart J 1983; 4:445–448.
9. Cowie MR, Mostard A, Wood DA, et al. The epidemiology of heart failure. Eur Heart J 1997; 18:208–225.
10. Cowie MR, Wood DA, Coats AJ, et al. Incidence and aetiology of heart failure: a population-based study. Eur Heart J 1999; 20:421–428.
11. Massie BM, Shah NB. Evolving trends in the epidemiologic factors of heart failure: rationale for preventive strategies and comprehensive disease management. Am Heart J 1997; 133:703–712.
12. Cleland JGF. Heart Failure. London: Mosby Elsevier Ltd., 2004:29–75.
13. Lloyd-Jones DM, Larson MG, Leip EP, et al. Lifetime risk for developing congestive heart failure. Circulation 2002; 106:3068–3072.
14. Davis RC, Hobbs FDR, Lip GYH. ABC of heart failure: history and epidemiology. Br Med J 2000; 320:39–42.
15. McDonagh TA, Morrison CE, Lawrence A, et al. Symptomatic and asymptomatic left-ventricular systolic dysfunction in an urban population. Lancet 1997; 350:829–833.
16. Lip GYH, Gibbs CR, Beevers DG. ABC of heart failure: Aetiology. Br Med J 2000; 320:104–107.
17. Braunwald E, Ross J Jr, Sonnenblick EH. N Engl J Med, Medical Progress Series, Little, Brown and Company, Boston 1967, pages 165–176.
18. Lorell BH, Carabello BA. Left ventricular hypertrophy: pathogenesis, detection and prognosis. Circulation 2000; 102:470–479.
19. Remes J, Tikkanen I, Fyhrquist F. Neuroendocrine activity in untreated heart failure. Br Heart J 1991; 65:249–255.
20. Baig MK, Mahon N, McKenna WJ, et al. The pathophysiology of advanced heart failure. Am Heart J 1998; 135:S216–S230.
21. Jackson G, Gibbs CR, Davies MK. ABC of heart failure: pathophysiology. Br Med J 2000; 320:167–170.
22. Wei CM, Lerman A, Rodeheffer RJ, et al. Endothelin in human congestive heart failure. Circulation 1994; 89:1580–1586.
23. Wilson JR, Mancici DM, Dunkman WB. Exertional fatigue due to skeletal muscle dysfunction in patients with heart failure. Circulation 1993; 87:470–475.
24. Doehner W, Rauchhaus M, Davos CH, et al. Clinical significance of impaired insulin sensitivity in chronic heart failure. Circulation 2000; 102(suppl II):719.

25. Anker SD, von Haehling S. Inflammatory mediators in chronic heart failure: an overview. Heart 2004; 90:464–470.
26. Braunwald E, Bristow MR. Congestive heart failure: fifty years of progress. Circulation 2000; 102(suppl IV):14–23.
27. LeJemtel TH, Sonnenblick EH. Heart failure: adaptive and maladaptive processes. Circulation 1993; 87(suppl VII):1–4.
28. Cohn JN. Structural basis for heart failure: ventricular remodeling and its pharmacological inhibition. Circulation 1995; 91:2504–2507.
29. Yeh ETH. Life and death in the cardiovascular system. Circulation 1997; 95:782–786.
30. Weber KT. Extracellular matrix remodeling in heart failure. Circulation 1997; 96:4065–4082.
31. Iung B. Management of ischaemic mitral regurgitation. Heart 2003; 89:459–464.
32. Bursi F, Enriquez-Sarano M, Nkomo VT, et al. Heart failure and death after myocardial infarction in the community: emerging role of mitral regurgitation. Circulation 2005; 111:295–301.
33. Holte K, Sharrock NE, Kehlet H. Pathophysiology and clinical implications of perioperative fluid excess. Br J Anaesth 2002; 89:622–632.
34. Harlan WR, Oberman A, Grimm R, et al. Chronic congestive heart failure in coronary artery disease: clinical criteria. Ann Intern Med 1977; 86:133–138.
35. Davie AP, Love MP, McMurray JJ. Value of the electrocardiogram in identifying heart failure due to left ventricular dysfunction. Br Med J 1996; 313(7052):300–301.
36. Aurigemma GP, Gottdiener JS, Shemanski L, et al. Predictive value of systolic and diastolic function for incident congestive heart failure in the elderly. The Cardiovascular Health Study. J Am Coll Cardiol 2001; 37:1042–1048.
37. Grayburn PA, Appleton CP, DeMaria AN, et al. Echocardiographic predictors of morbidity and mortality in patients with advanced heart failure. J Am Coll Cardiol 2005; 45:1064–1071.
38. Skarvan K, Lambert A, Filipovic M, et al. Reference values for left ventricular function in subjects under general anaesthesia and controlled ventilation assessed by two-dimensional transoesophageal echocardiography. Eur J Anaesth 2001; 18:713–722.
39. Wang TJ, Larson MG, Levy D, et al. Plasma natriuretic peptide levels and the risk of cardiovascular events and death. N Engl J Med 2004; 350:655–663.
40. Haas M. Biomarker bei Herzinsuffizienz: Kardiologie Up2date 2005; 1:23–37.
41. Cowie MR, Struthers AD, Wood DA, et al. Value of natriuretic peptides in assessment of patients with possible new heart failure in primary care. Lancet 1997; 350:1349–1351.
42. Mueller T, Gegenhuber A, Poelz W, et al. Diagnostic accuracy of B type natriuretic peptide and amino terminal proBNP in the emergency diagnosis of heart failure. Heart 2005; 91:606–612.
43. Mueller C, Scholer A, Laule-Kilian K, et al. Use of B-type natriuretic peptide in the evaluation and management of acute dyspnea. N Engl J Med 2004; 350:647–654.
44. Latini R, Masson S, Anand IS, et al. The comparative prognostic value of plasma neurohormones at baseline in patients with heart failure enrolled in Val-HeFT. Eur Heart J 2004; 25:292–299.
45. Troughton RW, Frampton CM, Yandle TG, et al. Treatment of heart failure guided by plasma aminoterminal brain natriuretic peptide (N-BNP) concentrations. Lancet 2000; 355:1126–1133.
46. Older P, Hall A, Hader R. Cardiopulmonary exercise testing as a screening test for perioperative management of major surgery in elderly. Chest 1999; 116:355–362.
47. Eagle KA, Berger PB, Calkins H, et al. ACC/AHA Guideline Update for perioperative cardiovascular evaluation for noncardiac surgery. Circulation 2002; 105:1257–1267.
48. Biccard BM. Relationship between the inability to climb two flights of stairs and outcome after major non-cardiac surgery: implications for the pre-operative assessment of functional capacity. Anaesthesia 2005; 60:588–593.
49. Ingle L, Shelton RJ, Rigby AS, et al. The reproducibility and sensitivity of the 6-minutes walk test in elderly patients with heart failure. Eur Heart J 2005; 26:1742–1751.
50. Girish M, Trayner E, Dammann O, et al. Symptom-limited stair climbing as a predictor of postoperative cardiopulmonary complications after high-risk surgery. Chest 2001; 120:1147–1151.

51. Gitt A, Wassermann K, Kilkowski C, et al. Exercise anaerobic threshold and ventilatory efficiency identifies heart failure patients for high risk of early death. Circulation 2002; 106:3079–3084.
52. Kleber FX, Vietzke G, Wernecke KD, et al. Impairment of ventilatory efficiency in heart failure: prognostic impact. Circulation 2000; 101:2803–2809.
53. Gersh BJ. The epidemiology of atrial fibrillation and atrial flutter. In: DiMarco JP, Prystowsky EN, eds. Atrial Arrhythmias: State of the Art. American Heart Association Monograph Series. Armonk, NY: Futura Publishing Company, 1995:1–22.
54. Cleland JG, Chattopadhyay S, Khand A, et al. Prevalence and incidence of arrhythmias and sudden death in heart failure. Heart Fail Rev 2002; 7:229–242.
55. Maisel WH, Stevenson LW. Atrial fibrillation in heart failure: epidemiology, pathophysiology, and rationale for therapy. Am J Cardiol 2003; 91(suppl 6A):2D–8D.
56. Spencer KT, Mor-Avi V, Gorcsan J III, et al. Affects of aging on left atrial reservoir, conduit, and booster pump function. A Multi-institution Acoustic Quantification Study. Heart 2001; 85:272–277.
57. Hoit BD, Gabel M. Influence of left ventricular dysfunction on the role of atrial contraction. J Am Coll Cardiol 2000; 36:1713–1719.
58. Bauer F, Jones M, Qin JX, et al. Quantitative analysis of left atrial function during left ventricular ischemia with and without left atrial ischemia: a real-time 3-dimensional echocardiographic study. J Am Soc Echocardiogr 2005; 18:795–801.
59. Sparks PB, Jayaprakash S, Mond HG, et al. Left atrial mechanical function after brief duration atrial fibrillation. J Am Coll Cardiol 1999; 33:342–349.
60. Khan IA. Atrial stunning: determinants and cellular mechanisms. Am Heart J 2003; 145:787–794.
61. Oxorn D, Edelist G, Harrington E, et al. Echocardiographic assessment of left ventricular filling during isoflurane anaesthesia. Can J Anaesth 1996; 43:569–574.
62. Filipovic M, Wang J, Michaux I, et al. Effects of halothane, sevoflurane and propofol on left ventricular diastolic function in humans during spontaneous and mechanical ventilation. Br J Anaesth 2005; 94:186–192.
63. Douglas PS. The left atrium. J Am Coll Cardiol 2003; 42:1206–1207.
64. Tsang TSM, Barnes ME, Gersh BJ, et al. Prediction of risk for the first age-related cardiovascular events in an elderly population: the incremental value of echocardiography. J Am Coll Cardiol 2003; 42:1199–1205.
65. Kannel WB, Plehn JF, Cupples A. Cardiac failure and sudden death in the Framingham study. Am Heart J 1988; 115:869–875.
66. Pogwizd SM, McKenzie JP, Cain ME. Mechanisms underlying spontaneous and induced ventricular arrhythmias in patients with idiopathic dilated cardiomyopathy. Circulation 1998; 98:2404–2414.
67. Aurigemma GP, Gaasch WH. Diastolic heart failure. N Engl J Med 2004; 351:1097–1105.
68. Zile MR, Brutsaert DL. New concepts in diastolic dysfunction and diastolic heart failure, Part I. Circulation 2002; 105:1387–1393.
69. European Study Group on Diastolic Heart Failure. How to diagnose diastolic heart failure (Working Group Report). Eur Heart J 1998; 19:990–1003.
70. Brutsaert DL. Diagnosing primary diastolic heart failure. Eur Heart J 2000; 21:94–96.
71. Maurer MS, Spevack D, Burkhoff D, et al. Diastolic dysfunction: can it be diagnosed by Doppler echocardiography? J Am Coll Cardiol 2004; 44:1543–1549.
72. Lappas DG, Skubas NJ, Lappas GD, et al. Prevalence of left ventricular diastolic filling abnormalities in adult cardiac surgical patients: an intraoperative echocardiographic study. Semin Thorac Cardiovasc Surg 1999; 11:125–133.
73. Fischer M, Baessler A, Hense HW, et al. Prevalence of left ventricular diastolic dysfunction in the community. Eur Heart J 2003; 24:320–328.
74. Redfield MM, Jacobsen SJ, Burnett JC Jr, et al. Burden of systolic and diastolic ventricular dysfunction in the community. J Am Med Assoc 2003; 289:194–202.
75. Petrie MC, Hogg K, Caruana L, et al. Poor concordance of commonly used echocardiographic measures of left ventricular diastolic function in patients with suspected heart failure but preserved systolic function: is there a reliable echocardiographic measure of diastolic dysfunction? Heart 2004; 90:511–517.

76. Bella JN, Palmieri V, Roman MJ, et al. Mitral ratio of peak to late diastolic filling velocity as a predictor of mortality in middle-aged and elderly adults. Circulation 2002; 105:1928–1933.

77. Bernard F, Denault A, Babin D, et al. Diastolic dysfunction is predictive of difficult weaning from cardiopulmonary bypass. Anesth Anal 2001; 92:291–298.

78. Lattik R, Couture, Denault AY, et al. Mitral Doppler indices are superior to two-dimensional echocardiographic and hemodynamic variables in predicting responsiveness of cardiac output to a rapid intravenous infusion of colloid. Anesth Analg 2002; 94:1092–1099.

79. Steendijk P. Heart failure with preserved ejection fraction: diastolic dysfunction, subtle systolic dysfunction, systolic-ventricular and arterial stiffening, or misdiagnosis? Cardiovasc Res 2004; 64:9–11.

80. Baicu CF, Zile MR, Aurigemma GP, et al. Left ventricular systolic performance, function, and contractility in patients with diastolic heart failure. Circulation 2005; 111: 2306–2312.

81. Vasan RS, Levy D. Defining diastolic heart failure. Circulation 2000; 101:2118–2121.

82. Zile MR, Gaasch WH, Carroll JD, et al. Heart failure with a normal ejection fraction. Circulation 2001; 104:779–782.

83. Hogg K, Swedberg K, McMurray J. Heart failure with preserved left ventricular systolic function. J Am Coll Cardiol 2004; 43:317–327.

84. Masoudi FA, Havranek EP, Smith G, et al. Gender, age, and heart failure with preserved left ventricular systolic function. J Am Coll Cardiol 2003; 41:217–223.

85. Berry C, Hogg K, Norrie J, et al. Heart failure with preserved left ventricular systolic function: a hospital cohort study. Heart 2005; 91:907–913.

86. Vasan RS, Benjamin EJ, Levy D. Prevalence, clinical features and prognosis of diastolic heart failure: an epidemiologic perspective. J Am Coll Cardiol 1995; 26:1565–1574.

87. Fonarow GC. For the ADHERE scientific advisory committee overview of acutely decompensated congestive heart failure (ADHF): a report from the ADHERE registry. Heart Fail Rev 2004; 9:179–185.

88. Cleland JG, Swedberg K, Follath F, et al. The EuroHeart Failure survey programme: a survey on the quality of care among patients with heart failure in Europe. Part 1. Patient characteristics and diagnosis. Eur Heart J 2003; 24(5):442–463.

89. Krumholz HM, Parent EM, Tu N, et al. Readmission after hospitalization for congestive heart failure among Medicare beneficiaries. Arch Intern Med 1997; 157:99–104.

90. Lowell JA, Schifferdecker C, Driscoll DF, et al. Postoperative fluid overload: not a benign problem. Crit Care Med 1990; 18:728–733.

91. Brandstrup B, Tønnesen, Beier-Holgersen R, et al. Effects of intravenous fluid restriction on postoperative complications: comparison of two perioperative fluid regimens. Ann Surg 2003; 238:641–648.

92. Arieff AI. Fatal postoperative pulmonary edema. Chest 1999;115:1371–1377.

93. Desai DK, Moodley J, Naidoo DP, et al. Cardiac abnormalities in pulmonary oedema associated with hypertensive crises in pregnancy. Br J Obstet Gynaecol 1996; 103:523–528.

94. Gandhi SK, Powers JC, Nomeir A-M, et al. The pathogenesis of acute pulmonary edema associated with hypertension. N Engl J Med 2001; 344:17–22.

95. Bentacur AG, Rieck J, Koldanov R, et al. Acute pulmonary edema in the emergency department: clinical and echocardiographic survey in an aged population. Am J Med Sci 2002; 323:238–243.

96. Pierard LA, Lancellotti P. The role of ischemic mitral regurgitation in the pathogenesis of acute pulmonary edema. N Engl J Med 2004; 351:1627–1634.

97. Schmidt H, Rohr D, Bauer H. Changes in intrathoracic fluid volumes during weaning from mechanical ventilation in patients after coronary artery bypass grafting. J Crit Care 1997; 1:22–27.

98. Coriat P, Daloz M, Riche F, et al. Oedeme aigu pulmonaire postoperatoire chez le coronarien: incidence de l'ischemie myocardique. Presse Med 1983; 12:1591–1594.

99. de Groote P, Millaire A, Foucher-Hossein C, et al. Right ventricular ejection fraction is an independent predictor of survival in patients with moderate heart failure. J Am Coll Cardiol 1998; 32:948–954.

100. Zornoff LAM, Skali H, Pfeffer MA, et al., for the SAVE Investigators. Right ventricular dysfunction and risk of heart failure and mortality after myocardial infarction. J Am Coll Cardiol 2002; 39:1450–1455.
101. Heidenreich PA, Stainback RF, Redberg RF, et al. Transesophageal echocardiography predicts mortality in critically ill patients with unexplained hypotension. J Am Coll Cardiol 1995; 26:152–158.
102. Davila-Roman VG, Waggoner AD, Hopkins WE, et al. Right ventricular dysfunction in low output syndrome after cardiac operations: assessment by transesophageal echocardiography. Ann Thorac Surg 1995; 60:1081–1086.
103. Vieillard-Baron A, Prin S, Chergui K, et al. Echo-Doppler demonstration of acute cor pulmonale at the bedside in the medical intensive care unit. Am J Respir Crit Care Med 2002; 166:1310–1319.
104. Vieillard-Baron A, Page B, Augarde R, et al. Acute cor pulmonale in massive pulmonary embolism: incidence, echocardiographic pattern, clinical implications and recovery rate. Intensive Care Med 2001; 27:1481–1486.
105. Kinch JW. Right ventricular infarction. N Engl J Med 1994; 330:1211–1217.
106. Mebazaa A, Karpati P, Renaud E, et al. Acute right ventricular failure from pathophysiology to new treatments. Intensive Care Med 2004; 30:185–196.
107. Jacobs AK, Leopold JA, Bates E, et al. Cardiogenic shock caused by right ventricular infarction: a report from the SHOCK registry. J Am Coll Cardiol 2003; 41:1273–1279.
108. Macnee W. Pathophysiology of cor pulmonale in chronic obstructive pulmonary disease. Am J Respir Crit Care Med 1994; 150:833–852.
109. Vieillard-Baron A, Schmitt JM, Augarde R, et al. Acute cor pulmonale in acute respiratory distress syndrome submitted to protective ventilation: incidence, clinical implications, and prognosis. Crit Care Med 2001; 29:1551–1555.
110. Jardin F, Vieillard-Baron A. Right ventricular function and positive pressure ventilation in clinical practice: from hemodynamic subsets to respirator settings. Intensive Care Med 2003; 29:1426–1434.
111. Mangano DT. Assessment of the patient with cardiac disease. Anesthesiology 1999; 91:1521–1526.
112. Goldman L. Cardiac risk in noncardiac surgery: an update. Anesth Analg 1995; 80:810–820.
113. Mangano DT. Perioperative cardiac mortality. Anesthesiology 1990; 72:153–184.
114. Bode RH, Lewis KP, Zarich SW, et al. Cardiac outcome after peripheral vascular surgery: comparison of general and regional anesthesia. Anesthesiology 1996; 84:3–13.
115. Sprung J, Abdelmalak B, Gottlieb A, et al. Analysis of risk factors for myocardial infarction and cardiac mortality after major vascular surgery. Anesthesiology 2000; 93:129–140.
116. Larsen SF, Olesen KH, Jacobsen E, et al. Prediction of cardiac risk in noncardiac surgery. Eur Heart J 1987; 8:179–185.
117. Goldman L, Caldera DL, Nussbaum SR, et al. Multifactorial index of cardiac risk in noncardiac surgical procedures. N Engl J Med 1977; 297:845–850.
118. Jeffrey CC, Kunsman J, Cullen DJ, et al. A prospective evaluation of cardiac risk index. Anesthesiology 1983; 58:462–464.
119. Detsky AS, Abrams HB, Forbath N, et al. Cardiac assessment for patients undergoing noncardiac surgery: a multifactorial clinical risk index. Arch Intern Med 1986; 145:2131–2134.
120. Lee TH, Marcantonio ER, Mangione CM, et al. Derivation and prospective validation of a simple index for prediction of cardiac risk of major noncardiac surgery. Circulation 1999; 100:1043–1049.
121. Go AS, Browner WS. Cardiac outcomes after regional or general anesthesia: do we have the answer? Anesthesiology 1996; 84:1–2.
122. Sandham JD, Hull RD, Brant RF, et al., for the Canadian Critical Care Clinical Trials Group. A randomized, controlled trial of the use of pulmonary–artery catheters in high-risk surgical patients. N Engl J Med 2003; 348:5–14.
123. Gehlbach BK, Geppert E. The pulmonary manifestations of left heart failure. Chest 2004; 125:669–682.
124. Arzt M, Schulz M, Wensel R, et al. Nocturnal continuous positive airway pressure improves ventilatory efficiency during exercise in patients with chronic heart failure. Chest 2005; 127:794–802.

125. O'Connor CM, Gattis WA, Swedberg K. Current and novel pharmacologic approaches in advanced heart failure. Am Heart J 1998; 135:S249–S263.
126. Stevenson LW, Massie BM, Francis GS. Optimizing therapy for complex or refractory heart failure: a management algorithm. Am Heart J 1998; 135:S293–S309.
127. McMurray JJ, Pfeffer MA. Heart failure. Lancet 2005; 365:1877–1889.
128. Millane T, Jackson G, Gibbs CR, et al. ABC of heart failure: acute and chronic management strategies. Br Med J 2000; 320:559–562.
129. McMurray J, Cohen-Solal A, et al. Practical recommendations for the use of ACE inhibitors, beta-blockers, aldosterone antagonists and angiotensin receptor blockers in heart failure: putting guidelines into practice. Eur J Heart Fail 2005; 7: 710–721.
130. Makris R, Coriat P. Interactions between cardiovascular treatments and anaesthesia. Curr Opin Anaesthesiol 2001; 14:33–39.
131. Mets B, Michler RE, Delphin ED, et al. Refractory vasodilation after cardiopulmonary bypass for heart transplantation in recipients of combined amiodarone and angiotensin-converting enzyme inhibition therapy: a role for vasopressin administration. J Cardiothorac Vasc Anesth 1998; 12:326–329.
132. Meerschaert K, Brun L, Gourdin M, et al. Terlipressin-ephedrine versus ephedrine to treat hypotension at the induction of anesthesia in patients chronically treated with angiotensin converting-enzyme inhibitors: a prospective, randomized, double-blinded, crossover study. Anesth Analg 2002; 94:835–840.
133. Bristow M. Antiadrenergic therapy of chronic heart failure: surprises and new opportunities. Circulation 2003; 107:1100–1102.
134. Bristow MR, Gilbert EM, Abraham WT, et al. Carvedilol produces dose-related improvements in left ventricular function and survival in subjects with chronic heart failure. MOCHA Investigators. Circulation 1996; 94:2807–2816.
135. Bristow MR. Beta-adrenergic receptor blockade in chronic heart failure. Circulation 2000; 101:558–569.
136. Witchitz S, Cohen-Solal A, Dartois N, et al. Treatment of heart failure with celiprolol, a cardioselective β-blocker with β-2 agonist vasodilatory properties: the CELICARD Group. Am J Cardiol 2000; 85:1467–1471.
137. Silver MA, Carson P. BEST Investigators. Impact of nonfatal myocardial infarction on outcomes in patients with advanced heart failure and the effect of bucindolol therapy. Am J Cardiol 2005; 95:558–564.
138. Bristow MR, Krause-Steinrauf H, Nuzzo R, et al. Effect of baseline or changes in adrenergic activity on clinical outcomes in the beta-blocker evaluation of survival trial. Circulation 2004; 110:1437–1442.
139. Metra M, Dei Cas L, di Lenarda A, et al. Beta-blockers in heart failure: are pharmacological differences clinically important? Heart Fail Rev 2004; 9:123–130.
140. The Task Force on Beta-blockers of the European Society of Cardiology. Expert consensus document on β-adrenergic receptor blockers. Eur Heart J 2004; 25: 1341–1362.
141. Cleland JG. Comprehensive adrenergic receptor blockade with carvedilol is superior to beta-1-selective blockade with metoprolol in patients with heart failure: COMET. Curr Heart Fail Rep 2004; 1:82–88.
142. Metra M, Nodari S, D'Aloia A, et al. Beta-blocker therapy influences the hemodynamic response to inotropic agents in patients with heart failure: a randomized comparison of dobutamine and enoximone before and after chronic treatment with metoprolol or carvedilol. Am Coll Cardiol 2002; 40:1248–1258.
143. Akhtar S, Barash PG. Significance of beta-blockers in the perioperative period. Curr Opin Anesthesiol 2002; 15:27–35.
144. Auerbach AD, Goldman L. β-Blockers and reduction of cardiac events in noncardiac surgery. J Am Med Assoc 2002; 287:1435–1447.
145. Foex P, Francis CM, Cutfield GR. The interactions between β-blockers and anaesthetics: experimental observations. Acta Anaesth Scand Suppl 1982; 76(suppl):38–46.
146. Kern MJ, Ganz P, Horowitz JD, et al. Potentiation of coronary vasoconstriction by beta-adrenergic blockade in patients with coronary artery disease. Circulation 1983; 67: 1178–1185.

147. White CM. Dunn A, Tsikouris J, et al. An assessment of the safety of short-term amiodarone therapy in cardiac surgical patients with fentanyl-isoflurane anesthesia. Anesth Analg 1999; 89:585–589.
148. Markham A, Plosker GL, Goa KL. Nicorandil. Drugs 2000; 60:955–974.
149. Döhner W, von Haehling S, Anker SD. Chronische Herzinsuffizienz-eine metabolische Erkrankung: von der Pathophysiologie zu neuen Therapieansätzen. Kardiologie Up2date 2005; 1:45–58.
150. Corsini A. The safety of HMG-CoA reductase inhibitors in special populations at high cardiovascular risk. Cardiovasc Drugs Ther 2003; 17:265–285.
151. Heeschen C, Hamm CW, Laufs U, et al. Withdrawal of statins increases event rates in patients with acute coronary syndromes. Circulation 2002; 105:1446–1452.
152. McGowan MP. There is no evidence for an increase in acute coronary syndromes after short-term abrupt discontinuation of statins in stable cardiac patients. Circulation 2004; 110:2333–2335.
153. Pan W, Pintar T, Anton J, et al. Statins are associated with a reduced incidence of perioperative mortality after coronary artery bypass graft surgery. Circulation 2004; 110 (II, suppl 1):II45–II49.
154. Kreisler NS. Possible dangers of discontinuing statins preoperatively. Anesthesiology 2003; 98:1518.
155. Ezekowitz JA, McAlister FA, Armstrong PW. Anemia is common in heart failure and is associated with poor outcomes: insights from a cohort of 12,065 patients with new-onset heart failure. Circulation 2003; 107:223–225.
156. Anand IS, Kuskowski MA, Rector TS, et al. Anemia and change in hemoglobin over time related to mortality and morbidity in patients with chronic heart failure. Circulation 2005; 112:1121–1127.
157. Cleland JG, Sullivan JT, Ball S, et al. Once-monthly administration of darbepoetin alpha for the treatment of patients with chronic heart failure and anemia: a pharmacokinetic and pharmacodynamic investigation. J Cardiovasc Pharmacol 2005; 46:155–161.
158. Thiazolidinedione use, fluid retention, and congestive heart failure: a consensus statement from the American Heart Association and American Diabetes Association. Circulation 2003; 108:2941–2948.
159. Stevenson LW. Clinical use of inotropic therapy for heart failure: looking backward or forward? Part I. Inotropic infusions during hospitalization. Circulation 2003; 108:367–372.
160. Stevenson LW. Clinical use of inotropic therapy for heart failure: looking backward or forward? Part II. Chronic inotropic therapy. Circulation 2003, 108:492–497.
161. Connolly SJ, Hallstrom AP, Cappato R, et al. Meta-analysis of the implantable cardioverter defibrillator secondary prevention trials. AVID, CASH and CIDS Studies. Antiarrhythmics vs Implantable Defibrillator study. Cardiac Arrest Study Hamburg. Canadian Implantable Defibrillator Study. Eur Heart J 2000; 21:2071–2078.
162. Bardy GH, Lee KL, Mark DB, et al. The Sudden Cardiac Death in Heart Failure Trial (SCD-HeFT) Investigators. Amiodarone or an implantable cardioverter-defibrillator for congestive heart failure. N Engl J Med 2005; 352:225–237.
163. Baldasseroni S, Opasich C, Gorini M, et al. Left bundle branch-block is associated with increased 1-year sudden and total mortality rate in 5517 outpatients with congestive heart failure: a report from the Italian network on congestive heart failure. Am Heart J 2002; 143:398–405.
164. Kass DA. Pathophysiology of cardiac dyssynchrony and resynchronisation. In: Ellenbogen KA, Kay GN, Wilkoff BL, eds. Device Therapy for Congestive Heart Failure. Philadelphia: Saunders/Elsevier, 2004:27–46.
165. LeClercq C, Jass DA. Retiming the failing heart: principles and current clinical status of cardiac resynchronization. J Am Coll Cardiol 2002; 39:194–201.
166. Abraham WT, Fisher WG, Smith AL, et al. Cardiac resynchronisation in chronic heart failure. N Engl J Med 2002; 346:1845–1853.
167. Cleland JG, Daubert JC, Erdmann E, et al. Cardiac Resynchronisation-Heart Failure (CARE-HF) Study Investigators. The effect of cardiac resynchronisation on morbidity and mortality in heart failure. N Engl J Med 2005; 352:1539–1549.

168. Strickberger SA, Conti J, Daoud EG, et al. Patient selection for cardiac resynchronisation therapy. Circulation 2005; 111:2146–2150.
169. Cleland JG, Freemantle N, Ball SG, et al. The Heart Failure Revascularisation Trial (HEART): rationale, design and methodology. Eur J Heart Fail 2003; 5:295–303.
170. Acker MA. Surgical therapies for heart failure. J Card Fail 2004; 10(suppl 6):S220–S224.
171. Park SJ, Tector A, Piccioni W, et al. Left ventricular assist devices as destination therapy: a new look at survival. J Thorac Cardiovasc Surg 2005; 129:9–17.
172. Bersten AD, Holt AW, Vedig AE, et al. Treatment of severe cardiogenic pulmonary oedema with continuous positive airway pressure delivered by face mask. N Engl J Med 1991; 325:1825–1830.
173. Pang D, Keenan SP, Cook DJ, et al. The effect of positive pressure airway support on mortality and the need for intubation in cardiogenic pulmonary edema: a systematic review. Chest 1998; 114:85–92.
174. Skidmore KL, Russell IA. Brain natriuretic peptide: a diagnostic and treatment hormone for perioperative congestive heart failure. J Cardiothorac Vasc Anesth 2004; 18:780–787.
175. Wylie JV, Tsao L. Nesiritide for the treatment of decompensated heart failure. Expert Rev Cardiovasc Ther 2004; 2:803–813.
176. Colucci WS, Elkayam U, Horton DP, et al. Intravenous nesiritide, a natriuretic peptide, in the treatment of decompensated congestive heart failure. N Engl J Med 2000; 343:246–253.
177. Silver MA, Horton DP, Ghali JK, et al. Effects of nesiritide versus dobutamine on short-term outcomes in the treatment of patients with acutely decompensated heart failure. J Am Coll Cardiol 2002; 39:798–803.
178. Abraham WT, Adams KF, Fonarow GC, et al. In-hospital mortality in patients with acute decompensated heart failure requiring intravenous vasoactive medications. J Am Coll Cardiol 2005; 46:57–64.
179. Sackner-Bernstein J, Skopicky HA, Aaronson KD. Risk of worsening renal function with nesiritide in patients with acutely decompensated heart failure. Circulation 2005; 111:1487–1491.
180. Varon J, Marik PE. The diagnosis and management of hypertensive crises. Chest 2000; 118:214–227.
181. Gray RJ. Managing critically ill patients with esmolol: an ultra short-acting beta-adrenergic blocker. Chest 1988; 93:398–403.
182. Cuffe MS, Califf RM, Adams KF Jr, et al. Short-term intravenous milrinone for acute exacerbation of chronic heart failure. J Am Med Assoc 2002; 287:1541–1547.
183. Perrone SV, Kaplinsky EJ. Calcium sensitizer agents: a new class of inotropic agents in the treatment of decompensated heart failure. Int J Cardiol 2005; 103:248–255.
184. Haikala H, Pollesello P. Calcium sensitivity enhancers. Drugs 2000; 3:1199–1205.
185. Cleland JG, Takala A, Apajasalo M, et al. Intravenous levosimendan treatment is cost-effective compared with dobutamine in severe low-output heart failure: an analysis based on the international LIDO trial. Eur J Heart Fail 2003; 5:101–108.
186. Cleland JG, Nikitin N, McGowan. Levosimendan: first in a new class of inodilators for acute and chronic severe heart failure. Expert Rev Cardiovasc Ther 2004; 2:9–19.
187. Follath F, Cleland JG, Just H, et al. Steering committee and investigators of the levosimendan infusion versus dobutamine (LIDO) study. Efficacy and safety of intravenous levosimendan compared with dobutamine in severe low-output heart failure (the LIDO study): a randomized double-blind trial. Lancet 2002; 360:196–202.
188. Khand AU, Rankin AC, Kaye GC, et al. Systematic review of the management of atrial fibrillation in patients with heart failure. Eur Heart J 2000; 8:614–632.
189. Samuels LE, Holmes ES, Samuels FL. Selective use of amiodarone and early cardioversion for postoperative atrial fibrillation. Ann Thorac Surg 2005; 79:113–116.
190. Magner JJ, Royston D. Heart failure. Br J Anaesth 2004; 93:74–85.

13

Adult Congenital Heart Disease and the Surgical Patient

Matthew Barnard
The Heart Hospital, London, U.K.

INTRODUCTION

In the future, there will be more adults than children with congenital heart disease—this already applies to Tetralogy of Fallot which is the commonest of the cyanotic lesions. Fewer than 20% of patients with congenital heart disease would survive to adult life without treatment. As a result of modern medical and surgical techniques, nearly all deaths now occur in adults and not children. As a result, there is an increasing population of patients with adult congenital heart disease who require long-term follow-up and who may require medical and surgical interventions during the course of their lives.

The management of adults with congenital heart disease poses clinical, organizational, and logistical challenges including fundamental questions relating to the appropriate institutional environment, facilities, staff, training, and educational programs. There remains a lack of consensus as to whether this type of service should be organized at the local, regional, or supraregional level. Although many accept that complex cases benefit from concentration in specialized centers, there remains uncertainty over care boundaries for the larger number of patients with less complicated lesions (1). The complex medical and psychosocial problems of these patients requires support from a variety of specialists, and physicians who care for them must be trained in dealing with adults and acquired disorders, while maintaining invaluable input from pediatric cardiologists and surgeons (2).

Completely normal cardiovascular anatomy and physiology is rarely achieved by corrective surgery during childhood (3). One important principle is that patients have had their cardiac lesions *repaired—not cured* (4). Many patients will continue to manifest residua of their underlying pathology and or sequelae of therapeutic interventions.

CLASSIFICATION OF CONGENITAL HEART DISEASE

Congenital heart disease embraces a considerable number of complex conditions. A number of commonly used terms are brought together in Table 1. There are several ways of classifying adult congenital heart disease. The number of different lesions and heterogeneity within each lesion dictate that a reductionist approach is useful. One distinction is between cyanotic and noncyanotic patients. Cyanotic patients often have more comorbid medical problems and experience greater numbers of serious perioperative complications than noncyanotics (5). Lesions are often broadly categorized into simple, intermediate, and complex (Table 2). Although simplistic, this facilitates decisions about management, monitoring, and referral to specialist centers. Patients with simple lesions can be managed in most settings with minimal alterations to routine care other than antibiotic prophylaxis and anticoagulation. Complex patients should be referred to specialist units if sufficiently stable to

TABLE 1   Some Commonly Used Terms in Congenital Heart Disease

ASD	Atrial septal defect; commonly classified into ostium primum (partial AVSD), ostium secundum, sinus venosus Ostium primum are defects in the inferior septum and comprise the atrial component of AVSD; secundum defects are absences in the oval fossa region; sinus venosus defects occur around the superior atriocaval junction and are associated with pulmonary veins draining anomalously to the superior vena cava
AVSD	Atrioventricular septal defect, often called AV canal defect or endocardial cushion defect; defect including primum septal defect and separate atrioventricular orifices (partial) or primum septal defect and ventricular septal defect and common atrioventricular orifice (complete) or intermediate forms
Balanced circulation	Relatively equal systemic and pulmonary blood flow
Blalock Taussig shunt	Connection of subclavian artery to ipsilateral pulmonary artery; classical shunt involved transection of subclavian artery and end-to-side anastomosis to pulmonary artery; modified Blalock Taussig shunt uses synthetic interposition graft; used to increase pulmonary blood flow, albeit using inefficient recirculation of systemic blood
Concordance	Connection of two structures the same side morphologically—left atria to left ventricle or right ventricle to pulmonary artery
Discordance	Connection of morphologically left structure to morphologically right structure, e.g., left ventricle to pulmonary artery
Double inlet ventricle	Both atrioventricular valves (or greater than 50% of each) connect to one ventricle; usually left ventricle
Double outlet ventricle	Both great vessels (or greater than 50% of each) arise from one ventricle; usually right ventricle
Fenestration	Surgically created hole in atrial or ventricular septum or intracardiac baffle; diverts proportion of blood from right to left heart in situations where normal passage through the lungs is prevented by elevated pulmonary resistance; cardiac output thereby maintained or increased—at the expense of cyanosis
Fontan	Surgeon who described the Fontan procedure; now usually refers to circulatory arrangement whereby systemic veins are connected to the pulmonary arteries—without a right ventricle; the connection may be intracardiac or extracardiac
Glenn	Cavopulmonary shunt; connection of the superior vena cava to the pulmonary artery; bidirectional Glenn refers to connection to joined right and left pulmonary arteries
Hemitruncus	Right or left pulmonary artery from aorta
Konno	Enlargement of aortic annulus and left ventricular outflow tract
Left SVC	Persistence of connection between left subclavian vein and left internal jugular vein with coronary sinus; coronary sinus usually dilated, and if unroofed or fenestrated associated with intracardiac left to right shunt
Malposition	Malposition of the atrial or ventricular septum that results in valve overriding the septum

(Continued)

TABLE 1   Some Commonly Used Terms in Congenital Heart Disease *(Continued)*

Mustard	Intraatrial switch procedure for TGA; intraatrial baffles direct pulmonary venous blood to the right ventricle and systemic venous blood to the left ventricle; results in physiological appropriate but anatomically incorrect circulation
Overriding	Valve which is positioned over the ventricular septum
Rastelli	VSD closure incorporating baffling mitral inflow to (malpositioned) aorta; external conduit or homograft to connect right ventricle to pulmonary artery
Ross pulmonary autograft	Replacement of the aortic valve with native pulmonary valve; replacement of the pulmonary valve with cadaveric homograft
Senning	Similar to Mustard procedure; intra-atrial baffling to redirect venous blood to the opposite ventricle in TGA
Single outlet	Single vessel arising from the heart
Single ventricle	One functional ventricle, although there is usually a second vestigial ventricle
Straddling	Valve with attachments on both sides of the ventricular septum; limits anatomical repair
Transposition great arteries	Ventriculoarterial discordance; aorta from right ventricle, pulmonary artery from left ventricle
Truncus arteriosus	Single arterial vessel arises from the heart; systemic and pulmonary arteries branch from the single vessel
Univentricular connection	Both atria connected to one ventricle; connection is either via two valves in the absence of one of the atrioventricular valves and an ASD

Abbreviations: ASD, atrial septal defect; AVSD, atrioventricular septal defect; SVC, superior vena cava; TGA, transposition of the great arteries; VSD, ventricular septal defect.

be transferred. At least some patients with intermediate lesions will be managed in nonspecialist centers and so will pose the biggest challenge to general anesthetists and intensivists. Some specific and general conditions which suggest transfer to a specialist unit would be appropriate are listed in Table 3.

PATHOPHYSIOLOGY OF CONGENITAL HEART DISEASE

Congenital cardiac lesions run the gamut from simple septal defects to extremely complex anatomical rearrangements. All may be considered in terms of the primary effects of the cardiac lesion and the secondary effects seen as the condition evolves. Primary and secondary pathophysiological features of patients with congenital heart disease (CHD) are outlined in Table 4 and the effects of specific lesions are discussed in more detail later in this chapter. There are a number of important general considerations however.

Cyanosis and Hyperviscosity
Hypoxemia is caused by either right to left shunting or mixing of pulmonary and systemic venous blood in a common chamber. The main adaptive response to hypoxemia is secondary erythrocytosis. Blood viscosity increases almost exponentially with

TABLE 2 Classification of Congenital Heart Lesions

Complex (best managed in specialist unit)	Moderate (can often be managed in general hospitals; consider referral if noncardiac surgery is major, or recent cardiology review demonstrates complications)	Simple (can be managed in most settings using normal management principles)
Conduits	Aorta-LV fistulae	Isolated aortic valve disease
Cyanotic	Anomalous pulmonary veins	Isolated mitral valve disease
Double outlet ventricle	AV canal defects	Isolated ASD
Eisenmenger	Coarctation	Small VSD
Fontan	Ebsteins anomaly	Mild pulmonary stenosis
Mitral atresia	Infundibular RVOTO	Repaired PDA
Single ventricle	Primum ASD	Repaired ASD
Pulmonary atresia	Unclosed PDA	Repaired VSD
Pulmonary vascular disease	Pulmonary regurgitation (moderate/severe)	
Transposition great arteries	Pulmonary stenosis (moderate/severe)	
Tricuspid atresia	Sinus Valsalva fistula/aneurysm	
Truncus arteriosus	Sinus venosus ASD	
Other AV or VA connection abnormalities	Sub/supravalvar aortic stenosis	
	Tetralogy of Fallot	
	VSD with other lesion	

Abbreviations: LV, left ventricular; AV, atrioventricular; VA, ventricular arterial; ASD, atrial septal defect; PDA, patent ductus arteriosus; RVOTO, right ventricular outflow tract obstruction.

hematocrit. In the presence of iron deficiency, microcytosis results in erythrocyte rigidity. Increased viscosity should be borne in mind when considering optimal hematocrits for these patients. Venesection is used for the relief of symptoms but preoperative venesection is no longer practiced in the absence of symptomatic hyperviscosity (a constellation of hematological and neurological symptoms, including headaches, visual disturbances, and embolic complications) (1). Hemoglobin concentrations may be greater than 19 preoperatively, and a postoperative drop to approximately 14 would be acceptable. Coagulopathies and gallstones are other consequences of polycythemia.

TABLE 3 Abnormalities Best Treated in Specialist Congenital Heart Unit

Valvular atresia	Eisenmenger reaction
Double inlet/outlet ventricle	Pulmonary hypertension
Malposition of great arteries	Chronic hypoxemia
Fontan circulation	$Q_P:Q_S > 2:1$
Single/common ventricles	Ventricular outflow gradient >50 mmHg
Transposition of great arteries	↑PVR
Atrial switch procedure	Secondary polycythemia
Rastelli procedure	

Abbreviations: Q_p, pulmonary blood flow; Q_S, systemic blood flow; PVR, pulmonary vascular resistance.

TABLE 4 Features of Congenital Heart Disease

Primary	Secondary
Shunts	Arrhythmias
Stenotic lesions	Cyanosis
Regurgitant lesions	Infective endocarditis
	Myocardial ischemia
	Paradoxical emboli
	Polycythemia
	Pulmonary hypertension
	Ventricular dysfunction

Cyanosis in patients with congenital heart disease may be accompanied by congenital syndromes, airway and thoracic cage abnormalities, tracheobronchial compression, and kyphoscoliosis. Brain abscesses, impaired cognitive function, and chronic neurologic impairment are also recognized. Cyanosis may result in aortopulmonary collateral arteries, hematological abnormalities, renal impairment, and myocardial scarring (6). Collateral arteries may be acquired (e.g., bronchial) or congenital (e.g., complex pulmonary atresia). Cyanosis results in inadequate skin oxygenation, and acne or skin infections are common. This can be important in the context of surgical intervention. Cyanotic patients are frequently small or have an abnormal stature.

Decreased Pulmonary Blood Flow
In patients with diminished pulmonary blood flow, hypoxemia is minimized by adequate hydration, maintaining systemic arterial blood pressure, minimizing elevations in pulmonary vascular resistance (avoiding hypercarbia and acidosis), and minimizing total oxygen consumption.

In the presence of a systemic to pulmonary shunt (e.g., modified Blalock Taussig), pulmonary blood flow is dependent on the size of the shunt and the pressure gradient across the shunt (i.e., systolic arterial and pulmonary artery pressures).

Mixing Lesions and the Balanced Circulation
In the situation of mixing of systemic and pulmonary venous blood, the peripheral arterial oxygen saturation is dependent on the pulmonary: systemic flow ratio (Q_P:Q_S). This ratio can be estimated from saturation measurements using the equation

$$\frac{Q_P}{Q_S} = \frac{S_aO_2 - S_{SV}O_2}{S_{PV}O_2 - S_{PA}O_2}$$

where S_aO_2 is the arterial saturation, $S_{SV}O_2$ the systemic venous saturation, $S_{PV}O_2$ the pulmonary venous saturation, and $S_{PA}O_2$ the pulmonary artery saturation. (Note that $S_{PA}O_2$ is the S_aO_2 in patients with pulmonary blood flow (PBF) supplied through a Blalock Taussig shunt.)

In these patients when Q_P is greater than Q_S, S_aO_2 will be higher, but systemic cardiac output will be lower. When Q_S is greater than Q_P, systemic saturations will be lower but cardiac output higher. Thus, the systemic saturation can give a useful indication of Q_P:Q_S. However, these interpretations are subject to the limitation of knowing or estimating mixed venous oxygen saturations. A low S_aO_2 might be due to low pulmonary blood flow or there could be high pulmonary blood flow and a low systemic cardiac output with low mixed venous saturations. The relationship

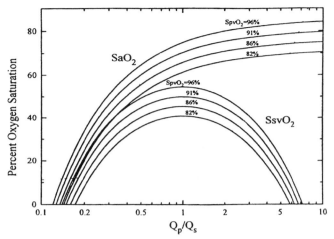

FIGURE 1 Arterial oxygen saturation (S_aO_2) and systemic venous oxygen saturation $(S_{SV}O_2)$ as a function of $Q_P{:}Q_S$ for different values of pulmonary venous oxygen saturation $(S_{PV}O_2)$. It is often assumed that $S_aO_2 \sim 75\%$ equates to the ideal $Q_P{:}Q_S$ of $\sim$1:1. This will be the case if there is good systemic perfusion (oxygen extraction resulting in $S_{SV}O_2 \sim 50\%$) and normal lung function $(S_{PV}O_2 \sim 100\%)$. However, an S_aO_2 of 75% may represent a $Q_P{:}Q_S$ 1:1 in certain situations.

between S_aO_2 and $Q_P{:}Q_S$ is hyperbolic, whereas that between systemic venous saturation $(S_{SV}O_2)$ and $Q_P{:}Q_S$ is parabolic (Fig. 1).

Elevated Q_P (and low Q_S) in a mixing type circulation will be suggested by the clinical picture of high S_aO_2, systemic hypotension, oliguria, acidosis, and increased serum lactate. A rapidly increasing metabolic acidosis is the first and sometimes dominant sign of pulmonary hyperperfusion. Elevated Q_P can decrease lung compliance, increase airway resistance, and work of breathing, and if left sufficiently long can, at an extreme, result in characteristic histological changes in the pulmonary vasculature (pulmonary vascular disease).

Ventricular Function

Systolic and diastolic ventricular dysfunctions are not infrequent. Right ventricle dysfunction is seen more commonly than in patients with acquired heart disease. Simple indices of ventricular function (e.g., ejection fraction) can be rendered inadequate by complex anatomy and loading conditions (7). Reduced ventricular compliance is a feature of some right-sided lesions such as Tetralogy of Fallot. An extreme of diastolic dysfunction is known as restrictive ventricular physiology. In this condition, due to the low compliance of the right ventricle, the pulmonary valve opens during diastole as a result of atrial contraction. Systemic ventricular impairment may be congenital (systemic right ventricle, hypertrophic cardiomyopathy) or acquired (previous surgery). The hemodynamic impact of dynamic left ventricular outflow obstruction may be reduced by a modest depression of ventricular function.

Arrythmias

Patients with diastolic dysfunction or restrictive physiology as well as those who have lesions which intrinsically limit ventricular filling (atrial switch procedures for transposition of great arteries—Mustard, Senning operations) tolerate loss of sinus rhythm or arrhythmias poorly (8). The latter can cause hemodynamic compromise in these patients more rapidly than in patients with acquired heart disease. The philosophy of treating arrhythmias is therefore relatively aggressive. An underlying hemodynamic cause (substrate) for the arrhythmia must be sought. Active measures to return sinus rhythm (including early DC cardioversion) are instituted.

PSYCHOSOCIAL CONSIDERATIONS

Adults with congenital heart disease are a well-informed population who have undergone previous major surgery and numerous hospital admissions. They may be faced with deteriorating cardiac function as young adults. Most patients function psychologically within the normal range, although low self-esteem, insecurity, and feelings of vulnerability occur. Three categories of morbidity are seen in adults with congenital heart disease—psychological, psychiatric, and neuropsychological (abnormalities due to cardiac dysfunction or interventions). Acute illness exacerbations can lead to profound psychological disturbances. The consequences of psychological problems include a lower proportion competing for higher education, increased unemployment, and many who underachieve due to a lack of self-confidence. Patients exhibit increased dependence on carers and greater immaturity. The effects of chronic illness on activity and social interactions can be pronounced. These effects are sometimes reinforced by inappropriate parental attitudes and "overprotection." Patients face problems with marriage, financial security, and worries over childbirth. Concern about genetic transmission of congenital defects is an issue when considering reproduction.

SPECIFIC LESIONS
Tetralogy of Fallot
Tetralogy of Fallot is the commonest cyanotic lesion in older patients. It comprises a ventricular septal defect (VSD), aortic overriding of the ventricular septum, and varying right ventricular outflow obstruction. The perimembranous outlet VSD allows right to left and bidirectional shunting and consequent cyanosis. The outflow obstruction results in right ventricular hypertrophy and may be subvalvar (infundibular), valvar, supravalvar (including branch pulmonary artery stenosis), or a combination. There may be a right aortic arch or atrial septal defect (ASD). The aortic annulus and aorta frequently dilate progressively with age. A small number of patients have anomalous coronary arteries (e.g., an anomalous left arterior descending (LAD) coronary artery arising from the right coronary artery).

Patients who present as adults will usually already have undergone surgery. Unoperated adults largely comprise those with anatomical features unsuitable for repair—usually abnormalities of the pulmonary arteries. Some adult patients will have undergone palliative procedures to improve pulmonary blood flow prior to definitive repair (Table 5).

Repair of tetralogy of fallot (TOF) has been performed for over 30 years, consequently older patients will be those individuals who underwent the earliest open heart surgery procedures. Repair involves closure of the VSD and relief of the outflow obstruction. The latter may involve resection of hypertrophic muscle as well as incision and enlargement of the outflow tract with a patch of pericardium or prosthetic material. If the patch needs to be extended beyond the outflow tract across the

TABLE 5   Key Features of the Tetralogy of Fallot

Anatomy	Anterior and cephalad deviation of the outlet septum
	Large subaortic VSD
	Right ventricular outflow obstruction
	Right ventricular hypertrophy
	±Branch pulmonary artery stenosis, ASD, right aortic arch
	Commonest cyanotic condition
Arrhythmias	Right bundle branch block
	Complete heart block
	Supraventricular and ventricular tachycardias
	More frequent in the presence of right ventricular failure
Palliation	Blalock Taussig/modified Blalock Taussig shunt (subclavian to pulmonary artery)
	Waterston shunt (ascending aorta to right pulmonary artery)
	Potts shunt (descending aorta to left pulmonary artery)
	Central or graft shunt (ascending aorta to main pulmonary artery)
	Brock procedure (infundibular resection and pulmonary valvotomy)
	Right ventricle to pulmonary artery conduit, leaving VSD alone or repairing with a fenestrated patch
Repair	Closure VSD
	Relief RVOTO
	Infundibular muscle resection
	Transannular patch
	Extracardiac conduit
	Pulmonary valve replacement
Outcome	30-yr actuarial survival 8.6% (90% expected)
	Sudden death 0–6%
Complications	Arrhythmias
	Right ventricular outflow tract obstruction
	Pulmonary and tricuspid regurgitation
	Diminished RV function
	Prosthetic complications
	Residual VSD

Abbreviations: VSD, ventricular septal defect; ASD, atrial septal defect; RV, right ventricular.

pulmonary valve (transannular), then pulmonary regurgitation is more likely, and homograft replacement of the pulmonary valve may be preferred. Other extracardiac conduits connecting the right ventricle to pulmonary artery are an alternative (e.g., Hancock prosthesis). Transatrial repair of VSDs has diminished myocardial complications from ventriculotomy. Twenty-year survival is 80% to 90%, whereas survival without surgical repair is poor.

Postrepair sequelae and residua include rhythm and conduction disorders, recurrent right ventricular outflow tract obstruction, right ventricular outflow tract aneurysm, recurrent VSD, pulmonary regurgitation, impaired right ventricular function, and tricuspid regurgitation. Functional capacity is usually good or normal, and left ventricular function is better with early operation. Reduced exercise ability is related mainly to right ventricular dysfunction consequent to pulmonary regurgitation. Arrhythmias are common. Ventricular ectopics occur in 40% to 50%, and become more frequent with age. A variety of arrhythmias and conduction abnormalities are described, including supraventricular tachycardia, ventricular tachycardia, right bundle branch block, and complete heart block; 15% of patients demonstrate inducible ventricular tachycardia during electrophysiological studies.

The preoperative management of these patients for noncardiac surgery depends on the nature of the repair or palliative operation that they have undergone, the extent of any residual disease, and the sequelae of the condition and of surgery. The clinician should obtain as much information about these as possible.

In assessing the patient with repaired tetralogy for noncardiac surgery, the key features to assess are the presence and severity of pulmonary regurgitation, right ventricular function, residual VSD, and arrhythmias. A patient with moderate or less pulmonary regurgitation and reasonable right ventricular function is likely to do well and can be managed with standard techniques and monitoring. A patient with significantly impaired right ventricular function needs careful attention to volume status and maintaining contractility. Central venous pressure monitoring is advisable and transesophageal echocardiography is useful for major surgery. Patients with very poor right ventricular function should be referred to a specialist unit.

The important aspects of the Tetralogy of Fallot are summarized in Table 5.

Atrial Septal Defect

ASD is the commonest previously undetected congenital heart lesion in adults. It comprises 7% of congenital heart disease overall, but 30% of adult congenital heart disease. Types include ostium secundum, sinus venosus, and coronary sinus defects. Ostium primum defects are discussed in a later section. They comprise the atrial component of the spectrum of atrioventricular septal defects (AVSDs) and are also referred to as partial AVSD.

Ostium secundum accounts for 70% of ASDs and manifests as an absence of the septum in the region of the oval fossa, usually 1 to 2 cm in diameter. It is distinct from patent foramen ovale in that the latter comprises a flap like slit, with no true septal deficiency. Superior sinus venosus defects account for 10% of the total, and occur around the superior atriocaval junction. They are associated with partial anomalous pulmonary venous drainage—usually with the right upper pulmonary veins draining directly into the superior vena cava. Defects occurring near the inferior vena cava junction do occur, but are rare.

The pathophysiology usually involves a predominant left-to-right shunt. Its magnitude is dependent on the size of the defect, relative ventricular compliances, and the ratio of systemic and pulmonary vascular resistances. The net effect is volume and pressure overload of the right heart, and increased pulmonary blood flow. If untreated, approximately 10% of patients would develop pulmonary vascular disease and eventually the Eisenmenger reaction (reversal of shunting consequent upon elevated pulmonary vascular resistance). Closure would then be contraindicated.

Many patients will be asymptomatic or have subtle clinical signs. However, 70% of patients will be symptomatic by 40 years, and many patients over the age of 60 years will be symptomatic. Symptoms when present consist of palpitations, fatigue, dyspnea, cough, and infection. Chest pain may reflect right ventricular ischemia. There is a preferential streaming of inferior vena caval blood to a secundum ASD, which places unoperated patients at risk of paradoxical emboli at any time, even if the shunt is almost entirely left to right. The decline in well being with age may reflect the onset of hypertension and coronary artery disease, which decrease left ventricular compliance and increase left-to-right shunting. Other causes of decreased left ventricular compliance such as mitral stenosis and mitral regurgitation will also increase shunt flow.

Physical examination demonstrates a prominent right ventricular impulse, loud S1, fixed and widely split S2. An ejection systolic murmur in the pulmonary area and a middiastolic tricuspid murmur are the result of increased (right heart) blood flow. Electrocardiography may show partial or complete right bundle branch block, right axis deviation, and an increased P–R interval. Echocardiography confirms the presence of a defect, and will often show dilated right atrium and ventricle, and paradoxical atrial septal motion.

The incidence of arrhythmias, ventricular dysfunction, and pulmonary vascular disease are related to the age at closure. If there are no arrhythmias prior to closure, there is a 5% to 10% late incidence of arrhythmias, whereas patients with a significant defect who exhibit arrhythmias preclosure virtually all have recurrent arrhythmias by 25 years. Thirty percent of patients with preoperative atrial fibrillation will retain sinus rhythm at late follow-up. Tachyarrhythmias become increasingly common after the fourth decade.

If surgical repair is delayed (e.g., beyond 40 years), elevation in pulmonary artery pressures may be observed. Owing to left ventricular volume and geometry changes, there is a small incidence of mitral regurgitation in adults with secundum ASD. If operation is carried out prior to 20 years of age in the presence of normal pulmonary vascular resistance, survival is the same as controls. These patients can effectively be treated as if they did not have congenital heart disease. Age at operation can affect (right) ventricular function. Similarly, ventricular end diastolic pressure increases in a minority of patients who undergo repair as adults, but those operated on when children do not exhibit left ventricular dysfunction.

Interestingly, the indications for repair continue to be debated. Traditionally intervention is advised if there is a significant left-to-right shunt (Q_p:Q_S more than 1.5:1) in order to avoid arrhythmias, infective endocarditis, pulmonary hypertension, and increased mortality. Modern echocardiographic techniques have improved detection of smaller defects in asymptomatic patients. Previous outcome data may not apply to this group, and at least one long-term follow-up of asymptomatic patients compared well with surgical treatment. In general, closure is advised for a "significant" defect which is defined as volume or pressure overload, exercise limitation, atrial arrhythmias, late right heart failure, or paradoxical embolism.

Transcatheter device closure is now routine. It is suitable for secundum defects less than approximately 30 mm, with a rim around the defect. Long-term comparisons of outcome with surgery are awaited. Endocarditis prophylaxis is not subsequently required.

Implications of nonoperated ASD include paradoxical embolism and elevated work of breathing due to decreased lung compliance. Late atrial arrhythmias may occur, and right heart failure or pulmonary vascular disease occurs in approximately 10%.

Patients who have undergone surgical closure should present few problems when undergoing noncardiac surgery, with arrhythmias being the commonest complication. Patients who have not undergone closure should be managed as normal, with specific attention paid to endocarditis prophylaxis and prevention of paradoxical embolism. Volume status should be maintained, to avoid increasing the magnitude of shunting. Theoretically, changes in pulmonary and systemic vascular resistance can alter the magnitude or even direction of shunting, but in the experience of this author this is of little clinical significance, because such alterations would have to be enormous to produce noticeable effects.

Transposition of the Great Arteries

Transposition of the great arteries (TGA) is defined as atrioventricular concordance and ventriculoarterial discordance—put simply, the atria are connected to the appropriate ventricle but the ventricles are connected to the "opposite" great artery. The aorta arises from the anatomical right ventricle and the pulmonary artery arises from the anatomical left ventricle. Blood flow, therefore, occurs in two parallel circulations rather than the normal series arrangement. Maintenance of life depends on a degree of mixing of oxygenated and deoxygenated blood between the two circulations. This can occur through an atrial or VSD, patent arterial duct, or atrial septostomy. Palliative intervention in the newborn to achieve mixing was originally achieved surgically (Blalock Hanlon septostomy) and subsequently by percutaneous balloon atrial septostomy (Rashkind). TGA is described as simple in the presence of an intact ventricular septum. Complex TGA involves the combination of TGA with VSD and possibly other abnormalities. The pulmonary artery overrides the ventricular septum, and if more than 50% is committed to the left ventricle the abnormality may be described as TGA with VSD, whereas if more than 50% of the pulmonary artery is committed to the right ventricle the correct terminology is double outlet right ventricle. Overall, 75% of TGA lesions are simple, 20% are combined with VSD, and 5% of patients have TGA with subpulmonary stenosis. Up to 28% demonstrate anomalies of the coronary arteries, which is important for surgical intervention in childhood.

TGA with VSD may be associated with unobstructed outflow; alternatively, deviation of the outlet septum causes outflow tract obstruction. Posterior deviation of the outlet septum restricts pulmonary blood flow, whereas anterior deviation results in subaortic stenosis. Complex TGA with subpulmonary stenosis presents early in life with severe cyanosis due to decreased pulmonary blood flow. Complex TGA with unobstructed aortic flow leads to gradual development of heart failure and may present later.

Adults with this circulation will usually have previously undergone surgery. Very occasionally a degree of subpulmonary stenosis can result in balanced flow which is compatible to survival to adult life without surgery. Surgical interventions are varied and have altered in response to the development of late complications. Simple TGA was originally and successfully treated with atrial redirection (atrial switch) operations, the Senning and Mustard procedures. These procedures redirect blood within the atria to the opposite ventricle, resulting in physiologically appropriate circulation pathways. The Rastelli operation was originally introduced for TGA, VSD, and left ventricular outflow obstruction (subpulmonary stenosis). It involves closing the VSD and thereby tunneling left ventricular blood to the aorta. Right ventricle to pulmonary artery continuity is achieved by placing a valved conduit between the two. The arterial switch operation involves transecting the aorta and pulmonary arteries and reconnecting them to the appropriate ventricle. The atrial or arterial switch procedures can be combined with VSD closure in the context of TGA, VSD, and unobstructed aortic flow. Finally, palliative atrial procedures involve redirection of blood at atrial level, while retaining or creating a VSD. This has been used in those patients who are unsuitable for physiological repair, usually because of pulmonary vascular abnormalities.

ATRIAL REPAIR

Although they are technically different, the Senning and Mustard procedures accomplish the same goal of redirecting blood flow at the atrial level. The Senning procedure utilizes native atrial tissue, whereas the Mustard incorporates autologous pericardium or synthetic material. The atrial septum if present is removed and the intraatrial baffle directs venous return to the appropriate ventricle. The atrial switch procedure was usually performed at 6 to 12 months of age. Survival to 25 years is approximately 65%, which can be subdivided into 80% survival for simple, and 45% for complex TGA. Sudden death accounts for 5% to 20% of late Mustard deaths. The atrial switch procedure is no longer routinely performed. However, the nonspecialist is likely to encounter adults with this morphology because (relatively) large numbers of operations were performed during the 1970s and 1980s. The author's institution alone has approximately 600 patients who are being followed-up.

There are some serious late complications associated with atrial redirection procedures. These include arrhythmias, atrial baffle obstruction, and leak and systemic (right) ventricular dysfunction. Systemic or pulmonary venous pathway obstruction occurs in 10% to 15%. Pulmonary venous obstruction is often well tolerated until severe and presents with dyspnea, orthopnea, and paroxysmal nocturnal dyspnea. Systemic venous obstruction manifests as peripheral and facial edema and ascites. Obstruction of a single limb of the baffle may be spontaneously relieved by azygous decompression, with resultant elevation in jugular venous pressure and hepatomegaly. Systemic venous obstruction is amenable to balloon dilation with stent insertion if required. Pulmonary venous obstruction is more difficult to treat with dilation. Either type of obstruction may require surgical intervention. Baffle leaks are detected with echocardiography. Closure is indicated if the shunt is severe, and can be achieved either by surgery or with transcatheter devices.

The systemic ventricle following atrial repair is a morphological right ventricle. There are important differences between the left and right ventricles, and the right ventricle sometimes fails to cope with the greater systemic workload. Impaired cardiopulmonary function, reduced exercise reserve, and declining ejection fraction can lead to right ventricular failure. An inability to increase ejection fraction during exercise occurs in over 50% of patients 5 to 15 years after Mustard procedures (6).

Arrhythmias are well recognized and are often poorly tolerated. The commonest are sinus node dysfunction with nodal or sinus bradycardia and recurrent atrial flutter and atrial fibrillation. Less than 50% will retain sinus rhythm at 20 years. Ventricular arrhythmias are less common. Treatment principles involve attempting to establish sinus rhythm, and if possible avoiding myocardial depressant antiarrhythmics. Pacemaker insertion is sometimes required for sick sinus syndrome; however, it may be technically difficult due to the baffles.

Other complications can occur at any time. Pulmonary outflow obstruction occurs, but the potentially stronger left ventricle copes until the obstruction is very severe. Systemic (tricuspid) atrioventricular valve insufficiency occurs rarely.

RASTELLI OPERATION

The Rastelli operation was introduced for TGA with VSD and left ventricular outflow obstruction. It involves closure of the VSD which incorporates left ventricle to aortic continuity and placement of a right ventricle to pulmonary artery conduit. It is used in patients who have an anatomically appropriate VSD and obstruction to pulmonary blood flow (left ventricular outflow obstruction) which makes them unsuitable for arterial switch operation. This operation pre-dates the arterial switch operation, and so older patients will be encountered. The conduit may subsequently degenerate with obstruction or regurgitation. There are a variety of conduit substitutes both synthetic and biological (homograft). Many conduits will subsequently require replacing at least once in the patients lifetime. Subaortic stenosis due to the tunnel formed by the VSD patch may occur and require revision.

ARTERIAL SWITCH OPERATION

The arterial switch has superseded the atrial switch operation. Normal physiology and anatomical connections are restored, and extensive intra-atrial surgery (and potential for arrhythmia generation) is avoided. The long-term effects are not yet completely defined. The pulmonary root becomes the aortic root. It requires reimplantation of the coronary ostia and leaves the native pulmonary valve as the systemic neoaortic valve. Neoaortic regurgitation is possible, and aortic root dilation has been reported. Similarly, there is the possibility of supravalvar stenosis of both great arteries, and physical obstruction or kinking of the reimplanted coronary arteries. Sudden death from myocardial infarction post-reimplantation has occurred, and there are particular risks if the arteries are intramural. Subpulmonary obstruction may require intervention such as balloon dilation. Long-term ventricular function may be better preserved than after atrial switch operation and arrhythmias may be less likely.

NONCARDIAC SURGERY IN PATIENTS WITH TRANSPOSITION OF THE GREAT ARTERIES

When undergoing noncardiac surgery, several factors need to be assessed. Patients who have undergone arterial switch operations are relatively rare at the moment (as most patients are still children), but will increase substantially over the next decade. The problems they will present are therefore still not completely determined, but the clinician should seek out coronary abnormalities (particularly ostial stenosis) and neoaortic regurgitation. If they appear well and have been given a clean bill of health from their cardiologist, normal management principles apply. Patients who have undergone atrial switch procedures should be assessed for venous pathway obstruction (elevated systemic venous pressures or history of pulmonary edema), arrhythmias, and impaired systemic ventricular function. Venous pathway obstruction mandates cardiology assessment prior to noncardiac surgery. Impaired ventricular function is managed in the same way as that produced by acquired heart disease, with invasive monitoring and minimizing myocardial depression. Inotropes such as phosphodiesterase inhibitors are useful if support is required, as there is a dominant diastolic impairment in many patients. Perioperative arrhythmias need to be treated aggressively because these patients are dependent on ventricular filling time. This usually means early DC cardioversion.

Patients who have undergone Rastelli operations should be assessed for left ventricular outflow gradients and residual VSD. In the absence of these, they can be managed along conventional lines. Significant gradients or residual VSD mandate referral to a specialist cardiologist prior to noncardiac surgery.

PALLIATIVE SURGERY

The palliative Mustard operation is undertaken in the situation where elevated pulmonary vascular resistance precludes physiological repair. It involves atrial baffle diversion while leaving or creating a VSD. The combination of Eisenmenger physiology with a systemic right ventricle and early hypoxia offered a reasonable chance of improved quality of life for 20 to 30 years, but survival is unlikely beyond the fifth decade.

Single Ventricle

Univentricular heart describes a number of variant conditions where one dominant and functionally useful ventricular chamber exists. There is usually a second small rudimentary ventricle. The characteristic feature of these hearts is that the majority of atrial mass is connected to one ventricle. The connection varies as either atrioventricular connection may be absent (e.g., tricuspid atresia), or more than 75% of the total atrioventricular junction is committed to the dominant ventricle (double inlet ventricle). Subpulmonary stenosis or atresia is common, and subaortic stenosis occurs occasionally. The physiological implication is mixing of systemic and pulmonary venous blood in the dominant ventricle. Pulmonary blood flow and hypoxemia are dependent on the presence and degree of pulmonary outlet obstruction.

Absent Atrioventricular Connection

Absent right atrioventricular connection is often referred to as tricuspid atresia, although there is no tricuspid valve tissue present. The left ventricle is large and dominant and receives all systemic and pulmonary venous blood. There is usually a VSD connecting a rudimentary right ventricle from which the pulmonary artery arises. This septal defect can be small and restrictive, in which case the pulmonary artery is small and pulmonary blood flow is limited. However, approximately 15% of cases demonstrate ventriculoarterial discordance (aorta from right ventricle, pulmonary artery from left ventricle), which may be associated with hypoplasia of the ascending aorta and arch. The left atrioventricular valve may be absent, although this is less common.

Double Inlet Ventricle

Double inlet ventricle implies that both (or more than 75% of the total) atrioventricular valves and junctions are committed to a dominant ventricle. The commonest form encountered is double inlet left ventricle with discordant ventriculoarterial connection (aorta from rudimentary right ventricle, pulmonary artery from left ventricle). Systemic blood flow is limited and aortic arch anomalies are common. Unless subpulmonary stenosis is present, pulmonary blood flow will be excessive resulting in pulmonary vascular occlusive disease. Occasionally pulmonary and systemic flows are balanced, and these patients may survive to adult life without surgery.

Twenty percent of double inlet ventricle hearts comprise double inlet right ventricle. These often involve a single common atrioventricular valve. This is usually associated with double outlet right ventricle. Chronic volume overload results in abnormal ventricular function which is also poorer if the dominant ventricle is of right morphology. Double inlet left ventricle is associated with a high incidence of congenital and surgical heart block and subaortic stenosis which may be progressive.

Treatment depends on the pulmonary blood flow. Ultimately this group of patients may be suitable for a cavopulmonary connection (see below) or possibly ventricular septation if there is adequate ventricular mass and two atrioventricular valves. Limited pulmonary blood flow can be increased with systemic pulmonary arterial shunts. Excessive pulmonary blood flow may be restricted with a pulmonary artery band. If systemic blood flow is naturally limited by a restrictive VSD or rudimentary right ventricle, left ventricular hypertrophy will develop, which will increase end-diastolic and left atrial pressures and thus compromise future cavopulmonary connections. Increasing systemic blood flow may prevent this, and can be achieved by enlarging the VSD or creating an aortopulmonary connection (aortopulmonary window or end-to-side pulmonary artery to aorta connection).

Noncardiac Surgery in Patients with Single Ventricles and Mixing Lesions

Patients with single ventricle physiology are a very complex group of patients, and their cardiac surgical management varies enormously as they are managed on an individual case-by-case basis. Essentially, however, they will fall into one of three broad groups. A few may be suitable for biventricular repair, in which case they are managed normally with attention paid to ventricular size and function. Some will be suitable for cavopulmonary connections, which are dealt with below. The remainder will have "mixing lesions," with systemic and pulmonary venous blood mixing in a common chamber. Pulmonary blood flow will depend on the individual anatomy. Some patients will have a natural blood supply either through pulmonary or collateral arteries. Others will have synthetic systemic to pulmonary shunts created surgically. These patients have to be assessed and managed on a case-by-case basis. These patients will be cyanotic and exhibit secondary erythrocytosis. Perioperative management for noncardiac surgery includes attention to coagulation and anticoagulation, endocarditis prophylaxis, and maintaining a balance between pulmonary and systemic blood flow. Ventricular impairment is common and should be managed with appropriate monitoring and by minimizing myocardial depression. Cyanotic single ventricle patients are at high risk for noncardiac surgery, and consideration of referral to a specialist unit should be made in all except minor surgical procedures.

Cavopulmonary Connections (e.g., Fontan and Glenn Circulations)

Essentially, any condition resulting in the absence or hypoplasia of a ventricular chamber, or the impossibility of biventricular repair, is a potential candidate for cavopulmonary connection. Originally described for tricuspid atresia, it has now been extended to a variety of lesions, including double inlet ventricle. It poses an alternative to (systemic) shunt-dependent pulmonary circulations which are less efficient due to recirculation of blood and also avoids cyanosis. Suitable candidates require a normal or low pulmonary vascular resistance, and normal left ventricular filling pressures.

The bidirectional Glenn shunt describes connection of the superior vena cava to the pulmonary artery. Inferior vena cava blood usually continues to reach the heart and maintains a right-to-left shunt with resultant hypoxemia. The palliative effect diminishes over time, and between 5 and 15 years over 40% require conversion to Fontan. Glenn patients can develop venous collaterals which communicate between the superior vena cava and the inferior vena cava (and provide natural decompression of the high superior vena cava pressures). Glenn procedures are generally unsuitable for adults due to the lower proportion of cardiac output returning via the superior vena cava. This results in inadequate pulmonary blood flow.

"Fontan circulation" is a term widely used to generically describe the final result of palliative procedures for patients who will ultimately be limited to a univentricular circulation. These involve diversion of all or part of the systemic venous return to the pulmonary circulation, usually without a subpulmonary ventricle. The aim is to separate the systemic and pulmonary circulations, with venous blood flowing directly to the lungs from the systemic veins. Flow across the lungs to the left atrium is dependent on the pressure gradient between the systemic veins and the left atrium.

The Fontan *operation* involves an atriopulmonary anastomosis which originally incorporated a valved connection. This was superseded by direct connection between the right atrial appendage and main pulmonary artery. Sophisticated physiological models demonstrated that the right atrium provided an insignificant contribution to forward flow through the lungs, and could actually be detrimental in terms of energy losses. As a result, the total cavopulmonary connection was developed. This involves connecting the end of the superior vena cava to the side of the right pulmonary artery, together with a conduit (either intracardiac or extracardiac) connecting the inferior vena cava to the inferior aspect of the right pulmonary artery. Exclusion of the right atrium results in less distension and diminished turbulence. This ought to improve forward flow, and the hope is that this will result in fewer arrhythmias and a lower incidence of right atrial thrombosis.

Partial or fenestrated intra-atrial conduits incorporate a fenestration that allows right-to-left shunting of blood at atrial level. This allows decompression of the systemic venous system and maintains or augments cardiac output at the expense of increased cyanosis (consequent upon the right-to-left shunt).

Continued survival depends on both low pulmonary vascular resistance and left atrial pressure. Pulmonary blood flow will diminish in the presence of elevated systemic ventricular end-diastolic pressure, elevations of pulmonary vascular resistance, atrioventricular valve regurgitation, and loss of sinus rhythm.

These patients have diminished reserve in terms of ability to increase cardiac output in response to exercise or stress. Cardiac index is decreased both at rest and during exercise. A patient with a completed Fontan circulation often has a peripheral arterial saturation of approximately 95% due to ventilation perfusion mismatching. Important factors that influence pulmonary vascular resistance (and hence cardiac output) include pCO_2, pO_2, arterial pH, mean airway pressure, positive end expiratory pressure, and extrinsic compression (pleural effusions). In practical terms, therefore, it is important to maintain central venous pressure, utilize positive pressure ventilation with caution, and to be aware that reduced contractility and loss of sinus rhythm are poorly tolerated. Cardiac performance may be evaluated with systemic venous oxygen saturation, lactate determination, clinical perfusion, urine output, and echocardiography. Diastolic function is frequently abnormal. Ventricular relaxation is incoordinate, with prolonged isovolumic relaxation, diminished early rapid filling, and dominant atrial systolic filling. Systolic performance can be within normal limits in the presence of markedly abnormal diastolic function.

Patients with a cardiopulmonary connection demonstrate high central, hepatic, mesenteric, and renal venous pressures. These may be important in the etiology of some late problems and complications which include arteriovenous fistulae, arrhythmias, thrombosis, peripheral edema, protein-losing enteropathy, and pathway obstruction. Up to 10% to 20% of patients who have had Glenn procedures develop pulmonary arteriovenous malformations. These may be multiple and diffuse, and result in right-to-left shunt and progressive cyanosis.

Arrhythmias are a major concern in the Fontan patient. All arrhythmias should provoke a search for underlying hemodynamic disturbances, such as pathway obstruction, decreased ventricular function, and valve regurgitation. Thrombosis and strokes are particular risks, especially when there are low flow areas within the heart. The right atrium is often large and dilated with marked "spontaneous contrast"—an echocardiographic appearance of "smoke" and swirling blood which is very low velocity or nearly static. An intrinsic thrombotic tendency exists in over 60% of patients which may be due to protein C deficiency. Ten to fifteen percent of patients will develop a protein losing enteropathy with hypoproteinemia by 10 years. Clinical features include hepatomegaly, ascites, cirrhosis, peripheral edema, and pleural and pericardial effusions. It carries a grim prognosis, with 50% of those affected dead at five years. Postoperative low cardiac output may be due to elevated pulmonary vascular resistance, myocardial dysfunction, hypovolemia, or inappropriate inotrope use.

Atrioventricular Septal Defect

AVSD describes lesions involving a maldevelopment of the atrioventricular septum. The embryologic region of the endocardial cushions comprises the inferior portion of the atrial septum, the atrioventricular valves, and the superior and posterior portion of the ventricular septum. A complete atrioventricular septal or atrioventricular canal defect comprises a common atrioventricular orifice together with a nonrestrictive VSD. Usually although not invariably a primum ASD is present. A partial AVSD almost always incorporates a primum ASD; there are separate atrioventricular orifices and no VSD. Intermediate forms comprise the spectrum between complete and partial defects.

AVSD may thus incorporate either atrial or VSDs or both. The VSD may be restrictive or nonrestrictive. The atrioventricular orifice may be common or separate. In all cases, the atrioventricular valve leaflets are of a typical morphological pattern. There are five leaflets: two right-sided leaflets (right anterosuperior and inferior), one left-sided leaflet (mural with 1/3 as opposed to 2/3 annular circumference attachment), and two bridging leaflets (superior and inferior) which join the right and left orifices. The left-sided commissure of the bridging leaflets frequently forms a separation—often referred to as a "cleft" (different from a true cleft of a single mitral valve leaflet). The absence of the true membranous and muscular atrioventricular septum results in "unwedging" of the aortic outflow tract from between the mitral and tricuspid valves. This in turn results in inlet/outlet disproportion of the left ventricle, and a narrowed or obstructed left ventricular outflow tract.

Clinical manifestations of AVSD are varied. There is a left-to-right shunt at atrial or ventricular level. The abnormal morphology of the atrioventricular valve frequently results in left-sided atrioventricular valve regurgitation through the "cleft" between the bridging leaflets. Arrhythmias or atrioventricular block may occur. Subaortic stenosis may be an integral anatomical feature as described above, or may be secondary to fibrous shelf formation consequent upon turbulent blood flow from broad left atrioventricular valve attachments. Nonrestrictive flow across the ventricular septum will lead to pulmonary hypertension and cyanosis if left untreated. This is particularly common in patients with trisomy 21. Forty percent of patients with trisomy 21 have congenital heart disease and of these approximately 40% have AVSD. Approximately 70% to 80% of children undergoing surgery for AVSD have trisomy 21.

Complete AVSD is usually repaired in childhood. The traditional approach was to band the pulmonary artery band as a neonate to reduce excessive pulmonary blood flow and undertake formal repair at two to three years of age. Currently, definitive repair is more often undertaken in the first year of life. If complete AVSD presents in adults, pulmonary vascular occlusive disease is very likely. Partial AVSD not uncommonly, however, presents in adult life, for example, during pregnancy.

Intervention in patients presenting in adult life is indicated for significant hemodynamic defects, left atrioventricular valve regurgitation causing symptoms, atrial arrhythmias, decreased ventricular function, or significant subaortic obstruction. After repair, residua and sequelae include residual septal defects, progressive atrioventricular valve regurgitation, heart block, arrhythmias, and left ventricular outflow obstruction.

Patients with AVSD presenting for noncardiac surgery have to be assessed on an individual basis, taking into account the anatomy of the defect, the magnitude and consequences of the left-to-right shunt and pulmonary blood flow, the nature of any repair or palliative operation, and the sequelae of the condition and any cardiac operations. Endocarditis prophylaxis must be employed. Patients with relatively small defects can be managed like an ASD. Patients with large untreated defects are uncommon, but could be encountered in the trisomy 21 population where surgery has not always been offered. Large defects predispose to heart failure and pulmonary hypertension. They should be referred to a specialist unit. Principles of management include minimizing heart failure, and balancing systemic and pulmonary blood flows with systemic vasoconstrictors and pulmonary vasodilators. Trisomy 21 patients with untreated AVSDs may demonstrate reactive pulmonary vasculature and pulmonary hypertensive "crises" similar to those commonly seen in infants. These are managed with heavy opioid sedation, ventilation to hypocapnia, and pulmonary vasodilators such as nitric oxide, inhaled prostacyclin, and phosphodiesterase inhibitors.

ASSESSMENT OF PATIENTS WITH CONGENITAL HEART DISEASE WHO REQUIRE NONCARDIAC SURGERY

A simple pathophysiologic approach to congenital heart disease involves four questions:

1. Is cyanosis present?
    This implies right-to-left shunting, although pulmonary blood flow is not necessarily reduced in all patients. Systemic oxygen saturation is determined by pulmonary venous saturation, systemic venous saturation, and the relative proportion of both types of venous blood represented in the arterial blood. In contrast to the situation in the normal circulation, factors that influence systemic venous saturation will affect arterial saturations.
2. If there is shunting of blood, what are its consequences?
    Shunting may be left to right, right to left, or mixing in a common chamber. This causes volume overload, chamber enlargement, hypertrophy, and decreased cardiac reserve. Pulmonary blood flow may be excessive or inadequate.
3. Is the pulmonary circulation dependent upon a shunt or connection?
    Such a connection may be a limiting factor when cardiac output or demand is increased. Systemic saturations will depend on pulmonary to systemic flow ratio and mixed venous oxygen saturation.

4. What are the structure and function of the systemic and pulmonary ventricles? There may be congenital and acquired abnormalities of ventricular structure and function. The systemic ventricle may be morphologically right or left.

Higher perioperative risk is probably conferred by chronic hypoxemia, a pulmonary to systemic blood flow ratio greater than 2:1, elevated pulmonary vascular resistance and secondary erythrocytosis, and ventricular outflow tract obstruction above 50 mmHg (9). Recent heart failure, syncope, or substantial deterioration in exercise tolerance are concerns. Pulmonary hypertension carries significant risks and surgery (including minor) is best avoided whenever possible. The functional status certainly plays a role in assessing risk, but using New York Heart Association class alone can be misleading, particularly in cyanotic patients. Endocarditis is a risk in nearly all corrected and uncorrected lesions, and appropriate antibiotic prophylaxis should be employed during noncardiac surgery (10).

Whenever possible, records of previous surgical procedures, anesthesia, and investigations should be obtained. Echocardiography is useful at confirming anatomy, detecting shunts and obstructions, and assessing ventricular performance. However,

TABLE 6 Sequelae of Surgery for Congenital Heart Disease

ASD	Residual shunt, septal aneurysm, device fracture
Coarctation of aorta	Systolic hypertension, residual gradient, inaccurate left arm BP (subclavian flap repair), aneurysm formation, dissection
PDA	Residual flow, recanalization, laryngeal nerve injury
TGA	Atrial switch Arrhythmias, systemic ventricular dysfunction, baffle leak, venous pathway obstruction Rastelli Residual VSD, ventricular dysfunction, LVOT obstruction, conduit failure Arterial switch Supravalvar AS/PS, aortic regurgitation, ventricular dysfunction, coronary artery stenosis
Tetralogy of Fallot	Residual VSD, RV outflow tract obstruction, RV dysfunction, pulmonary regurgitation, RBBB/AV block, ventricular arrhythmias; BT shunt—BP inaccurate
Single ventricle	Preload dependence, ventricular dysfunction, cyanosis (fenestration), protein-losing enteropathy, arrhythmias, diminished functional reserve

Abbreviations: ASD, atrial septal defect; PDA, patent ductus arteriosus; TGA, transposition of the great arteries; BP, blood pressure; VSD, ventricular septal defect; LVOT, left ventricular outflow tract obstruction; AS, aortic stenosis; PS, pulmonary stenosis; BT, Blalock Taussig; RBBB, right bundle branch block; AV, atrioventricular; RV, right ventricle.

it requires operators who have experience of congenital heart disease, which can be limited even among consultant cardiologists. Table 6 lists some long-term complications of surgery for different congenital lesions.

MANAGEMENT

In general, standard management principles for cardiac disease apply to most patients. For complex lesions, experience in the management of pulmonary vascular resistance, shunt lesions, and ventricular outflow tract obstruction is useful. If the clinician lacks relevant experience or appropriate cardiology support, then it is preferable to refer patients with complex lesions to specialist units (11).

If a prosthetic (Blalock Taussig) shunt is present, blood leaving the heart may travel in one of two parallel circulations: either to the systemic circulation via the aorta or to the pulmonary circulation via the shunt. The systemic and pulmonary vascular resistances and the resistance of the shunt determine the flow through each vascular bed. In general, the usual goal is to have a "balanced" circulation (i.e., $Q_P:Q_S = 1:1$). Depending on the mixed venous oxygen saturations, a balanced circulation is frequently associated with a systemic oxygen saturation of approximately 75% to 85%. Cyanotic patients should have serial hematocrit measurements.

If pulmonary blood flow is inadequate or appears to be falling, pulmonary vasodilators can be considered. These include control of arterial pCO_2, nitric oxide, prostacyclin, and phosphodiesterase inhibitors. Theoretically, they could be useful when lowering pulmonary vascular resistance is beneficial. This includes Fontan circulations, and any patient with chronic pulmonary hyperfusion and elevated pulmonary vascular resistance, for example, Eisenmengers. However, the response in adults is usually less impressive than in children, as pulmonary vascular resistance is more often "fixed." Cardiac medications are typically continued until the time of surgery. Nephrotoxic drugs (e.g., nonsteroidal anti-inflammatories, aminoglycosides) should be avoided in cyanotic patients.

The choice of anesthetic drugs is less important than appropriate hemodynamic goals, maintenance of ventricular performance, and avoidance of large alterations in $Q_P:Q_S$. Intravenous induction may be slow when the circulation time is prolonged. Right-to-left shunts theoretically prolong alveolar to arterial equilibration of volatile anesthetic gases, but this infrequently appears clinically important in adult (in whom shunts are not often torrential). Agents which cause vasodilation will increase right-to-left shunting and reduce S_aO_2, but again in clinical practice this is frequently offset by reductions in total oxygen consumption and consequent elevation of mixed venous oxygen saturation. Narcotic-based anesthesia is the choice of many in the presence of significant ventricular dysfunction.

Monitoring

The use of invasive monitoring is dependent on the magnitude of surgery, ventricular function, and underlying pathophysiology. Transesophageal echocardiography is useful for following ventricular performance, valvular function, and blood flow velocity. Some practical considerations are important. End-tidal CO_2 will underestimate $paCO_2$ in the presence of right-to-left shunting or common mixing. Vascular access may pose challenges. Interruption of the interior vena cava (IVC) or thrombosis following previous instrumentation may preclude femoral vein cannulation.

In the presence of a subclavian to right pulmonary artery (Blalock Taussig) shunt, the contralateral arm should be used for arterial pressure monitoring. Meticulous care must be taken to avoid venous air entrainment in patients with shunt lesions as systemic embolization can occur, even when shunting is considered to be predominantly left to right.

Pulmonary artery catheters do not have a significant role. Anatomical considerations dictate that placement can be technically difficult or even not possible (atrial baffle procedures—Mustard, Senning operations). Thermodilution cardiac output measurements will be inaccurate in patients with right-to-left shunting (12). In general, as outlined above, peripheral arterial oxygen saturation will give useful indications of trends in $Q_P:Q_S$. Finally, some suggest that catheters could actually be dangerous in the presence of pulmonary reactivity and there is a conservative approach to their use.

Some patients have direct connections between the systemic veins and pulmonary arteries. These cavopulmonary shunts (Glenn and Fontan) are at risk of venous thrombosis. Although pulmonary artery pressure monitoring with a superior vena cava line is often useful in this scenario, a single lumen line is preferable and is removed as early as possible.

Ventilation

Cardiopulmonary interaction is important, particularly in the context of cavopulmonary shunts (Fontan circulations) where pulmonary blood flow is passive, and depends on the pressure gradient between central veins and left atrium. In this situation, control of arterial blood gases (particularly $PaCO_2$) is an important influence on pulmonary blood flow and preventing elevation of pulmonary vascular resistance (12). While low airway pressures and early weaning from ventilation are beneficial to transpulmonary flow, the duration of the inspiratory phase during positive pressure ventilation is usually more important than the absolute level of peak inspiratory pressure. Indeed, shortening the inspiratory time (with consequent increase in peak inspiratory pressure) may be an appropriate strategy to maximize the expiratory phase and thus the time available for transpulmonary flow (11).

The ventilatory response to $PaCO_2$ is normal in hypoxic patients; hence, adequate analgesia and sedation are appropriate. This is particularly important in the presence of labile PA pressures.

Endocarditis

Twenty percent of adults with infective endocarditis have congenital heart disease. Infective endocarditis requires a susceptible substrate and a source of bacteremia. Lesions associated with major risk involve high blood flow velocities at sites of significant pressure gradients. Maximum deposition of organisms occurs at either the low-pressure "sink" beyond an orifice or at the site of jet impact. Congenital lesions associated with the highest risk include bicuspid aortic valve, restrictive VSD, tetralogy of Fallot, and high-pressure atrioventricular valve regurgitation. Postoperative lesions at particular risk are palliative shunt and prosthetic valves. Low-risk lesions include repaired septal defects and patent ducts. In general, antibiotic prophylaxis is recommended in the presence of prosthetic valves, previous endocarditis, systemic to pulmonary shunts, and most cardiac structural abnormalities.

FURTHER READING

Ammash NM, Connolly HM, Abel MD, Warnes CA. Noncardiac surgery in Eisenmenger syndrome. J Am Coll Cardiol 1999; 33:222–227.

Andropolous DB, Stayer SA, Skjonsby BS, et al. Anaesthetic and perioperative outcome of teenagers and adults with congenital heart disease. J Cardiothorac Vasc Anesth 2002; 16:731–736.

Baum VC, Stayer SA, Andropolous DB, Russell IA. Approach to the teenaged and adult patient. In: Andropoulos DB, Stayer SA, Russel IA, eds. Anesthesia for Congenital Heart Disease. Malden, MA: Blackwell Futura, 2005:210–222.

Brickner ME, Hillis LD, Lange RA. Congenital heart disease in adults: second of two parts. N Engl J Med 2000; 342:334–342.

Cassorla L. Preoperative evaluation and preparation: a physiologic approach. In: Andropoulos DB, Stayer SA, Russell IA, eds. Anesthesia for Congenital Heart Disease. Malden, MA: Blackwell Futura, 2005:175–196.

Deanfield J, Thaulow E, Warnes C, et al. Management of grown up congenital heart disease. Eur Heart J 2003; 24:1035–1084.

Fernandes SM, Landzberg MJ. Transitioning the young adult with congenital heart disease for life-long medical care. Pediatr Clin North Am 2004; 51:1739–1748.

Galli KK, Myers LB, Nicolson SC. Anesthesia for adult patients with congenital heart disease undergoing noncardiac surgery. Int Anesthesiol Clin 2001; 39:43–71.

Mott AR, Fraser CD, McKenzie ED, et al. Perioperative care of the adult with congenital heart disease in a free-standing tertiary pediatric facility. Pediatr Cardiol 2002; 23:624–630.

O'Kelly SW, Hayden-Smith J. Eisenmenger's syndrome: surgical perspectives and anaesthetic implications. Br J Hosp Med 1994; 51:150–153.

Perloff JK, Sangwan S. Noncardiac surgery. In: Perloff JK, Child JS, eds. Congenital Heart Disease in Adults. Philadelphia: WB Saunders, 1998:291–300.

Report of the British Cardiac Society Working Party. Grown-up congenital heart (GUCH) disease: current needs and provision of service for adolescents and adults with congenital heart disease in the UK. Heart 2002; 88(suppl 1):i1–i14.

Siu SC, Sermer M, Colman JM, et al. Prospective multicenter study of pregnancy outcomes in women with heart disease. Circulation 2001; 104:515–521.

Somerville J. Cardiac problems of adults with congenital heart disease. In: Moller JH, Hoffman JIE, eds. Pediatric Cardiovascular Medicine. New York: Churchill Livingstone, 2000; 200:688–705.

Srinathan SK, Bonser RS, Sethia B, et al. Changing practice of cardiac surgery in adult patients with congenital heart disease. Heart 2005; 91:207–212.

Stayer SA, Andropolous DB, Russell IA. Anesthetic management of the adult patient with congenital heart disease. Anesthesiol Clin North Am 2003; 21:653–673.

Warner MA, Lunn RJ, O'Leary PW, Schroeder DR. Outcomes of noncardiac surgical procedures in children and adults with congenital heart disease: Mayo Perioperative Outcomes Group. Mayo Clin Proc 1998; 73:728–734.

Warnes CA, Liberthson R, Danielson GK, et al. Task force 1: the changing profile of congenital heart disease in adult life. J Am Coll Cardiol 2001; 37:1170–1175.

Webb GW, Williams RG. 32nd Bethesda Conference: Care of the Adult with Congenital Heart Disease. JACC 2001; 37:1161–1119.

REFERENCES

1. Perloff JK, Warnes CA. Challenges posed by adults with repaired congenital heart disease. Circulation 2001; 103:2637–2643.
2. Therrien J, Webb G. Clinical update on adults with congenital heart disease. Lancet 2003; 362:1305–1313.
3. Drinkwater DC. The surgical management of congenital heart disease in the adult. Prog Paed Cardiol 2003; 17:81–89.
4. Rosenthal A. N Engl J Med 1993; 329(9):655–656.
5. Barnard MJ, Wright SJ, Deanfield JE, Cullen S, Tsang VT, Lees M. Characteristics and outcome of surgery for adult congenital heart disease. Anesth Analg 2003; 96:SCA80.

6. Findlow D, Doyle E. Congenital heart disease in adults. Br J Anaesth 1997; 78:416–413.
7. Brickner ME, Hillis LD, Lange RA. Congenital heart disease in adults. N Engl J Med 2001; 342:256–263.
8. Triedman JK. Arrhythmias in adults with congenital heart disease. Heart 2002; 87:383–389.
9. Mohindra R, Beebe DS, Belani KG. Anaesthetic management of patients with congenital heart disease presenting for non-cardiac surgery. Ann Cardiol Anesth 2002; 5:15–24.
10. Horstkotte D, Follath F, Gutschik, et al. Guidelines on prevention, diagnosis and treatment of infective endocarditis. Eur Heart J 2004; 5:267–276.
11. Barnard MJ. Adult congenital heart disease. In: Arrowsmith J, Simpson J, eds. Problems in Cardiothoracic Anaesthesia. London: Martin Dunitz Ltd., 2002.
12. Lovell AT. Anaesthetic implications of grown-up congenital heart disease. Br J Anaesth 1004; 93:129–139.

14 Management of Concomitant Carotid and Coronary Disease

Demosthenes Dellagrammaticas and Michael J. Gough
The Leeds Vascular Institute, The General Infirmary at Leeds, Leeds, U.K.

INTRODUCTION

The role for carotid endarterectomy in stroke prevention due to significant extracranial carotid atherosclerosis is well-defined, in both the neurologically symptomatic and asymptomatic populations. Similarly, patients with significant coronary artery atherosclerosis, particularly those with critical stenoses in three coronary vessels and/or left main-stem disease, are known to benefit from coronary artery bypass grafting. It is not unusual, given common underlying risk factors and pathophysiological mechanisms, to find patients where significant carotid and coronary disease coexist. They are often identified when patients are assessed for treatment of one or the other. The importance of this is obvious when it is considered that surgery for carotid disease carries a risk of cardiac complications, and coronary artery bypass surgery can be complicated by perioperative ischemic stroke. The challenge for specialists involved in the treatment of the patient with significant disease in both vascular territories is to minimize the risk of the cardiac and neurological complications of carotid and coronary surgery.

This review examines the evidence regarding the prevalence of concomitant significant carotid (asymptomatic or symptomatic) and coronary disease, and the strategies for the identification and management of such patients.

PREVALENCE AND IMPACT OF CORONARY DISEASE IN PATIENTS WITH CAROTID STENOSIS

Compared with the general population, patients who have suffered a stroke or TIA have a higher risk of myocardial infarction or nonstroke vascular death, each in the order of 2% per year (1). Further, anatomical studies have shown that carotid and coronary atherosclerosis may often coexist in an individual patient and the presence of asymptomatic carotid atherosclerosis is an independent risk factor for coronary disease. The prevalence of asymptomatic coronary disease is higher in patients with stroke attributable to large vessel atherosclerosis and increases with the severity of the carotid artery stenoses (1).

Some 25% to 60% of patients with carotid atherosclerotic disease have evidence of occult myocardial ischemia on the basis of noninvasive testing or coronary angiography (2). In the studies by Urbinati and colleagues (3) and Sconocchini and colleagues (4), 27 of 106 and 21 of 85 of patients, respectively, had silent coronary artery disease diagnosed on the basis of thallium scintigraphy and/or exercise ECG. Similarly, Chimowitz reported evidence of myocardial ischemia in approximately 60% (13 of 22) of patients studied using adenosine or exercise thallium imaging, (5) while Oki and colleagues[6] found carotid cross-sectional area to be independently associated with myocardial ischemia. Further, 24-hour ECG monitoring to identify ischaemic episodes in patients with carotid disease with and without known CHD demonstrated silent ischemia in 26% of patients in the latter group. Hertzer (7) reported the results of coronary angiography in 200 patients with evidence of extracranial carotid disease and no history of CHD. In this study, 40% of patients were identified as having severe CHD (defined as >70% stenosis of ≥1 coronary vessel) and only 14% had normal findings. Finally, the prevalence of nonflow limiting coronary stenosis in patients who are nevertheless at risk of acute MI or death from rupture of an atherosclerotic plaque is unknown, there being no reliable noninvasive technique to assess such lesions (2).

The association between carotid and coronary atherosclerotic disease may have particular importance in the setting of carotid endarterectomy, where the benefit of surgery is dependent on low perioperative morbidity and mortality. In the landmark trials of carotid endarterectomy for symptomatic carotid disease (ECST, NASCET), conducted mainly in the 1980s, the overall prevalence of a history of myocardial infarction or angina were 15.8% and 21.7%, respectively, while the 30-day postoperative myocardial infarction rates were 0.5% and 1%, respectively (3). Assessing patients undergoing CEA mainly in the 1990s, the Asymptomatic Carotid Surgery Trial (ACST) had an overall prevalence of ischaemic heart disease of 27% and a 30-day risk of myocardial infarction or sudden cardiac death of about 1% (9).

In all these studies, the majority of deaths during long-term follow-up, including patients not allocated to surgery, were due to ischaemic heart disease. Finally, retrospective analyses of large series of carotid endarterectomies have demonstrated a significant association between preoperative history of ischaemic heart disease and both early and late postoperative cardiac morbidity and mortality (2).

Assessment of Coronary Risk in the Patient with Carotid Disease

All patients with carotid disease requiring CEA should undergo preoperative assessment of their cardiac status. History and clinical examination, with particular reference to previous myocardial infarction, past or current angina or congestive heart failure, cardiac rhythm abnormalities, past cardiac interventions, as well as assessment of the current exercise tolerance, are mandatory. A routine baseline 12-lead ECG should also be performed since this may reveal evidence of past silent MI or demonstrate changes consistent with ischemia. The further cardiac investigation and risk stratification of patients presenting for noncardiac surgery is discussed elsewhere in this book. However, there are some additional points of note for patients presenting for carotid endarterectomy.

In a Veterans' Affairs study for asymptomatic carotid disease (10), patients had an increased long-term risk of myocardial events if they had evidence of diabetes, peripheral vascular disease, or intracranial occlusive disease. Over the four-year follow-up period, 36% of patients with one of these factors had a cardiac event, increasing to 42% of those with two factors and 69% when all three were present. During the same period, 43% of patients with known coronary artery disease had a cardiac event. Similarly, patients in NASCET with four or more of age more than 74 years, hypertension, diabetes, current smoking, creatinine >115 µmol/L, left ventricular hypertrophy on ECG or evidence of past MI on ECG had a 23.5% five-year risk of serious cardiac events, compared with 33.9% risk in patients with known CHD. In the absence of these risk factors and no history of CHD, the risk was 3.1% (11). It is therefore clear that despite a relatively low perioperative risk of cardiac events patients undergoing CEA should be assessed for cardiac disease and associated risk factors in order to reduce long-term cardiac morbidity. Appropriate intervention and/or referral for cardiological assessment should be considered for those at significant risk, and aggressive secondary prevention implemented for all.

The Impact of Carotid Disease on Stroke During and Following CABG

The risk of stroke during or following coronary artery surgery is on the order of 2%, a figure that has remained remarkably constant over the last 30 years. The risk increases with age (0.5% 50 years, up to 9%>80 years), and with increasing severity of carotid disease. Two-thirds of perioperative strokes occur after the first postoperative day and overall carry a mortality of approximately 23%. Patients with a history of past stroke or TIA are four times more likely to suffer a further stroke following CABG (12).

Identification of patients with an increased risk of CABG-related stroke may be difficult. However, patients with a carotid bruit have an estimated risk of 5.6%, a four-fold excess risk compared with patients without bruit (12). While suggestive, it is not certain that a carotid bruit reflects the presence of internal carotid artery disease (bruits may arise from the external carotid artery or be transmitted from other vessels), although it is certainly a marker for advanced vascular disease. Thus, carotid bruit has been identified as the only significant predictor for aortic arch atheroma (13), itself a significant risk factor for post-CABG stroke (14,15).

The association of age with increasing stroke risk may reflect increasing prevalence of severe atherosclerosis. Other factors associated with stroke post-CABG include emergency surgery, peripheral vascular disease, hypertension, intraoperative hypotension, prolonged aortic cross-clamp time, poor left ventricular function, and the need for α-adrenergic drugs or a balloon pump in the postoperative period (16,17).

The true prevalence of carotid disease in patients presenting for CABG is difficult to establish because different studies have used different modalities (duplex ultrasound, catheter angiography, magnetic resonance angiography) to establish this. Furthermore, many studies combine reports of significant stenosis and carotid occlusion, the latter not being amenable to surgical intervention. Finally, the available data may be skewed, as patients with coronary symptoms requiring urgent CABG (presenting with triple-vessel or left main stem disease and potentially at a higher risk of carotid atherosclerosis) may have been excluded from reports.

From the available evidence, it is estimated that some 90% of patients requiring CABG have a less than 50% stenosis of one or both internal carotid arteries and about 6% of patients have an 80% to 99% stenosis or occlusion. Although it is clear that the prevalence of carotid disease increases with age, the risk of stroke is also dependent on the severity of the stenosis (12). This is estimated at 1.9% in patients with no significant carotid disease, 6.7% to 8.4% in patients with 50% to 99% carotid stenosis, and 7% to 11% in patients with carotid occlusion (12). Most of these data are derived from asymptomatic patients, although one study identified a stroke risk of 18% and 26% in neurologically symptomatic patients with unilateral and bilateral carotid disease, respectively (18). Although these data indicate an association between carotid disease and post-CABG stroke, there is considerable heterogeneity among the studies that have been reported and thus it is not easy to accurately assess the risk.

Despite the association between the severity of carotid disease and the increasing stroke risk following CABG, a review of several small studies suggests that carotid disease alone is unlikely to be the sole cause of about 50% to 60% of strokes. Thus, about 50% of stroke sufferers do not have evidence of significant carotid disease, and CT/autopsy data of the pattern of cerebral infarction and carotid disease identified that up to 59% of strokes were not due to carotid thromboembolism alone (12). It is therefore important to realize that prophylactic carotid endarterectomy may only prevent 40% to 50% of CABG-related strokes.

Screening for Carotid Disease Prior to CABG

Although some investigators have suggested that nonselective screening for carotid disease in patients undergoing coronary surgery may be of benefit, and indeed this is routine practice in some institutions, it is unlikely to be cost-effective given that the majority of patients will not have a surgically significant carotid stenosis. It would therefore seem more sensible to selectively screen a subset of patients at higher risk for carotid stenosis. Unfortunately, there is no consensus as to the criteria for such screening. Age greater than 65 and a history of symptomatic peripheral or cerebrovascular disease are fairly consistently reported as predictors of significant carotid stenosis. Other potential factors include the presence of a carotid bruit, diabetes, smoking, hypercholesterolemia, and hypertension (18–25). Clearly, inclusion of all these putative criteria will result in screening most, if not all CABG patients.

The gold standard for carotid artery imaging remains digital subtraction angiography (DSA). This technique was used for assessment of stenosis in the landmark trials (ECST, NASCET) for symptomatic carotid disease. However, the invasive nature and serious complication rate (including stroke) of 1% to 4% renders conventional angiography unsuitable as a screening tool. Indeed, even in patients suspected of having symptomatic carotid disease, primary assessment is almost always performed noninvasively using duplex ultrasound (DUS) and may be the only modality used to determine the severity of stenosis and plan surgery as highlighted by ACST.

The measurement of stenosis depends on assessment of blood flow velocity in conjunction with the color-flow and gray-scale images, and it permits assessment of the character of the atherosclerotic plaque (Fig. 1). DUS is widely available and relatively inexpensive. Further, its sensitivity and specificity, compared with DSA, is acceptable (26), and thus despite some limitations (different measurement criteria, operator dependence), it is a highly suitable tool for screening CABG patients preoperatively. While magnetic resonance angiography is gaining in popularity, with a reported sensitivity and specificity comparable to DSA for the detection of 70% to 99% stenosis and carotid occlusion (26,27), its availability and cost do not make it suitable as a screening modality.

Selection of Patients Requiring Carotid Endarterectomy

There are no clear guidelines that indicate which patients with a carotid stenosis should be considered for surgery when CABG is also required. Clearly, for patients with a symptomatic stenosis of greater than 70%, the decision to undertake carotid endarterectomy can be made on the basis of current evidence. However the majority of CABG patients will have an asymptomatic stenosis. Although ACST has shown a benefit to surgery in patients with a greater than 50% stenosis, this is relatively small, and may not justify the increased risk associated with combined CABG and carotid endarterectomy (see subsequently). A review of the literature (28) indicates that the risk of ipsilateral stroke or ipsilateral stroke and death is 3.9% and 4.9%, respectively, for CABG patients with a unilateral stenosis of 50% to 99%, which suggests that CEA is unlikely to be of benefit for these patients. In contrast, the risks for

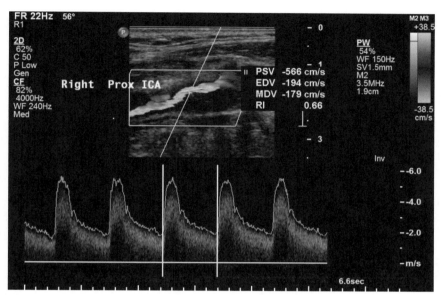

FIGURE 1   Duplex ultrasound scan of an 80% to 99% internal carotid artery stenosis.

patients with bilateral stenoses of 50% to 99% are 3.9% and 12.3%. It is therefore logical to consider CEA in these patients with surgery being performed upon the ICA with the maximum stenosis, or, if these are similar, then to the ICA supplying the dominant hemisphere. As a rule of thumb, it would seem appropriate to advise CEA in patients with an aggregate ICA stenosis of ≥160%. This protocol is summarized in Figure 2.

Management of the Patient Requiring Surgery for an Asymptomatic Carotid Stenosis and Coronary Artery Bypass Grafting

The optimum approach to the management of a patient requiring both carotid endarterectomy and coronary surgery is a matter of controversy. Three approaches have been suggested: simultaneous CEA and CABG, staged CEA then CABG, or reverse-staged CABG then CEA.

The combined approach was first reported in 1972 (29) and has gained popularity in many centers, with the majority of surgeons performing CEA immediately prior to institution of cardiopulmonary bypass. Harvesting of the great saphenous vein is often performed simultaneously. Alternatively, some surgeons perform CEA during hypothermic (25–30°C) cardiopulmonary bypass, citing the potential neuroprotective effect of this technique (30,31). The main disadvantage of this strategy is the significant increase in on-pump time. During a combined procedure, the neck wound is usually closed following CABG and reversal of the much higher doses of heparin that are required during cardiopulmonary bypass.

The alternative to combined CEA and CABG is to stage the two procedures. Logically, CEA is performed first, followed by CABG as a separate operation after a suitable interval. In previous reports, this has varied from a few days to six months, although two to four weeks seems most appropriate. Alternatively, staging may be

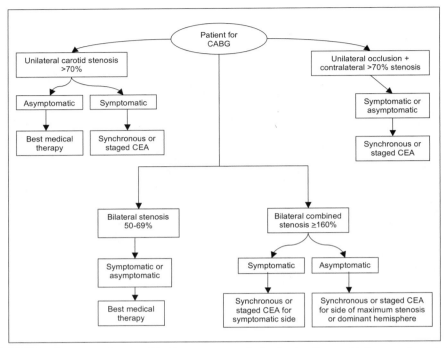

FIGURE 2 A suggested protocol for the management of patients with carotid disease who require coronary artery bypass grafting.

reversed with CABG performed before CEA. Although this may reduce the cardiac risk of CEA, it clearly will not impact upon the risk of stroke during CABG.

When staged CEA is undertaken prior to CABG, it is especially important to avoid hemodynamic instability, and increased use of invasive hemodynamic monitoring has been recommended (16). Many surgeons advocate CEA using local anesthesia in order to minimize cardiac risk, as several nonrandomized studies have suggested a 50% relative reduction in serious cardiac complications when this technique is used (32). Other advantages of the LA technique are preservation of cerebral autoregulation and the facility for awake neurological testing to guide the selective use of a carotid shunt to preserve ipsilateral cerebral blood flow (33). Although robust data from randomized studies have yet to confirm an advantage for LA, the ongoing GALA Trial (general vs. local anaesthesia for carotid endarterectomy) should provide definitive information about this.

If performing CABG prior to CEA, relatively higher perfusion pressures during cardiopulmonary bypass (60–80 mmHg) are employed. Pulsatile flow, which may avoid systemic vasoconstriction, and careful attention to acid–base balance using the alpha-stat method of pH management, which is effective in matching cerebral blood flow to metabolic demand, have both been recommended (16). Again, hypothermic cardiopulmonary bypass is often advocated by virtue of its potential neuroprotective effect.

In recent years, data for off-pump CABG (OPCAB) suggest that it may be associated with fewer neurological sequelae, probably by avoidance of aortic cross-clamping and thus reducing the risk of embolization from aortic arch atherosclerosis. However, a recent meta-analysis of the randomized trials of on- versus off-pump CABG, while demonstrating a number of advantages (lower rates of atrial fibrillation and respiratory infection, reduced ventilation time and intensive care stay, decreased transfusion requirement, and inotrope use), failed to show any differences in the main outcomes of mortality, stroke, myocardial infarction, and renal failure (34). Although a more recent review of nonrandomized studies in the elderly (age>70 years) has suggested a reduction in mortality (OR 0.48) and stroke (OR 0.19) for OPCAB (35), it must be recognized that nonrandomized studies are associated with publication and a number of other biases.

Unfortunately, despite numerous published studies, there is no consensus as to the ideal approach for patients with combined carotid and coronary artery disease. This is reflected in the excellent systematic review by Naylor and colleagues (28), which assesses the reported outcomes in 97 studies (8972 procedures) spanning the last three decades. Approximately 60% of patients were neurologically asymptomatic, and 37% had bilateral carotid stenosis of more than 50% or a contralateral occlusion. The highest operative mortality was seen following synchronous procedures (4.6%), while for staged and reverse-staged procedures, the combined mortality of the two procedures was 3.9% and 2%, respectively. For operative stroke (ipsilateral or contralateral), the risk in synchronous procedures was 4.6%, in staged procedures 2.7%, and in reverse-staged procedures 6.3%. The risk of myocardial infarction was highest in the staged procedures (6.5%), while MI occurred in 3.6% and 0.9% of synchronous and reverse-staged procedures, respectively. The overall cardiovascular risk (death or stroke or MI) was 11.5% for synchronous carotid endarterectomy and coronary artery bypass grafting, 10.2% in staged surgery, and 5.0% for reverse-staged surgery. The risk of stroke or death was 8.7%, 6.1% and 7.3%, respectively. While these figures suggest that mortality is highest with synchronous procedures, the risk of stroke was highest with reverse-staged procedures and of MI highest with staged surgery. Importantly, the 95% confidence intervals for all these outcomes overlapped, suggesting no significant difference in outcome between these strategies.

Although the overall cardiovascular risk was lowest for reverse-staged procedures, only a small number of studies have been published (11 studies of 302 patients). Significant heterogeneity was evident for the majority of the end-points analyzed, suggesting no consistency in event reporting between the studies. Further, it is worth noting that outcome events were either recorded in-hospital or within 30 days of either procedure, so the true incidence of outcomes may be underreported. Finally, while the overall risk of death/stroke/MI in staged or synchronous procedures was 10% to 12%, there is no systematic review documenting this risk in patients with carotid stenosis undergoing CABG alone, although Naylor and colleagues suggest that this may be in the order of 12% to 15% (28).

The fundamental problem in interpreting data from different studies is that it is difficult to ensure that patient populations are comparable, as most surgeons will instinctively prioritize the management of concomitant carotid and coronary disease according to the severity of presenting symptoms. For staged procedures, it is possible that a significant adverse event in the first procedure may have caused the second procedure to be abandoned, leading to underreporting of outcomes using this approach. Until more robust data becomes available, there remains no evidence to suggest that a synchronous or a staged approach to carotid and coronary revascularization is preferable. While a synchronous procedure may be more cost-effective (36), it is likely that patients requiring both procedures will be managed according to individual circumstances, taking particular account of the severity of carotid or coronary artery disease.

Management of Patients Requiring Surgery for a Symptomatic Stenosis and Coronary Artery Bypass Grafting

For patients who present with a symptomatic carotid stenosis, due consideration should be given to the timing of carotid surgery in relation to the presenting neurological symptoms. Analysis of the combined data from ECST and NASCET (8), together with evidence from the Oxford Vascular Study (37), suggest that the highest risk of stroke is within two weeks of the initial neurological event, and that the maximum benefit of CEA in terms of stroke prevention is also within this time. Thus, both carotid and coronary assessment should be expedited for these patients. The surgical options are either staged CEA followed by CABG or a synchronous procedure, depending on the severity of the coronary disease. Clearly, in the presence of symptomatic carotid disease, a reverse-staged procedure has no role.

The Role of Minimally Invasive Procedures

It would be impossible to cover this topic adequately without a brief discussion of the developments in endovascular techniques for coronary and carotid disease. Both carotid and coronary angioplasty and stenting are becoming more widespread in their use.

Coronary artery stenting is increasingly used in the management of disease patterns that have been traditionally treated by surgery (triple-vessel disease or left main-stem lesions) (38). In comparison to CABG, however, re-intervention rates may be higher while the incidence of serious complications has not convincingly been shown to be lower. Further, an effect on long-term survival has yet to be demonstrated (39). The effect of certain processes of care such as the use of newer antiplatelet agents, glycoprotein IIb/IIIa inhibitors, and drug-eluting stents are still to be fully evaluated. Nonetheless, coronary artery stenting would appear to be a useful option for patients requiring surgery for a critical symptomatic carotid stenosis who also present with active cardiac symptoms.

Angioplasty and stenting of the carotid arteries (CAS) is advocated by a number of authors. However, there is no evidence base for this, particularly in patients with a symptomatic carotid stenosis, and it has yet to be shown to be either as good as or superior to carotid endarterectomy, both in terms of reducing morbidity and mortality or in long-term durability (40). Furthermore, the ICAROS study (41) showed that patients with echolucent plaques with a low grey-scale median on ultrasound (a feature of plaque instability) had a higher risk of stroke. Thus, in the patient with symptomatic carotid disease, CAS should only be considered when there is concurrent symptomatic severe coronary disease precluding anaesthesia. In contrast, if CAS does have a role in the management of carotid atherosclerosis, it might be considered in the neurologically asymptomatic patients requiring CABG, as these patients are more likely to have a stable carotid plaque.

CONCLUSIONS

The management of coexistent carotid and coronary disease remains a matter of controversy. Regardless of the dominant presentation, the emphasis must be placed on reducing the overall risk of death, stroke, and MI both in the perioperative period and in the long term. Patients with carotid and coronary disease should undergo careful evaluation to assess the severity of disease in both vascular territories, and the treatment strategy should be tailored appropriately. This may include the consideration of synchronous or staged CEA and CABG. The superiority of either approach has yet to be determined. In the absence of a randomized controlled trial, our knowledge on this difficult issue would be improved by greater consistency in reporting the results of the various treatment options.

REFERENCES

1. Touzé E, Varenne O, Chatellier G, Peyrard S, Rothwell PM, Mas J-L. Risk of myocardial infarction and vascular death after transient ischemic attack and ischemic stroke. Stroke 2005; 36:2748–2755.
2. Adams RJ, Chimowitz MI, Alpert JS, Awad IA, Cerqueria MD, Fayad P, et al. Coronary risk evaluation in patients with transient ischemic attack and ischemic stroke. A scientific statement for healthcare professionals from the Stroke Council and the Council on Clinical Cardiology of the American Heart Association/American Stroke Association. Stroke 2003; 34:2310–2322.
3. Urbinati S, Di Pasquale G, Andreoli A, Lusa AM, Ruffini M, Lanzino G, et al. Frequency and prognostic significance of silent coronary artery disease in patients with cerebral ischemia undergoing carotid endarterectomy. Am J Cardiol 1992; 69(14):1166–1170.
4. Sconocchini C, Racco F, Pratillo G, Alesi C, Zappelli L. Patients with carotid stenosis and clinical history negative for coronary disease. Usefulness of the ergometric test for the identification of ischemic myocardial disease. Minerva Medica 1997; 88(5):173–181.
5. Chimowitz MI, Poole RM, Starling MR, Schwaiger M, Gross MD. Frequency and severity of asymptomatic coronary disease in patients with different causes of stroke. Stroke 1997; 28(5):941–945.
6. Okin PM, Roman MJ, Schwartz JE, Pickering TG, Devereux RB. Relation of exercise-induced myocardial ischemia to cardiac and carotid structure. Hypertension 1997; 30(6):1382–1388.
7. Hertzer NR, Young JR, Beven EG, Graor RA, O'Hara PJ, Ruschhaupt WF III, et al. Coronary angiography in 506 patients with extracranial cerebrovascular disease. Arch Int Med 1985; 145(5):849–852.
8. Rothwell PM, Eliasziw M, Gutnikov SA, Warlow CP, Barnett HJ, Carotid Endarterectomy Trialists Collaboration. Endarterectomy for symptomatic carotid stenosis in relation to clinical subgroups and timing of surgery. Lancet 2004; 363(9413):915–924.
9. Halliday A, Mansfield A, Marro J, Peto C, Peto R, Potter J, et al. Prevention of disabling and fatal strokes by successful carotid endarterectomy in patients without recent neurological symptoms: randomised controlled trial. Lancet 2004; 363(9420):1491–1502.
10. Chimowitz MI, Weiss DG, Cohen SL, Starling MR, Hobson RW II. Cardiac prognosis of patients with carotid stenosis and no history of coronary artery disease. Veterans Affairs Cooperative Study Group 167. Stroke 1994; 25(4):759–765.
11. Gates PC, Eliasziw M, Algra A, Barnett HJM, Gunton RW, North American Symptomatic Carotid Endarterectomy Trial G. Identifying patients with symptomatic carotid artery disease at high and low risk of severe myocardial infarction and cardiac death. Stroke 2002; 33(10):2413–2416.
12. Naylor AR, Mehta Z, Rothwell PM, Bell PRF. Carotid artery disease and stroke during coronary artery bypass: a critical review of the literature. Eur J Vasc Endovasc Surg 2002; 23(4):283–294.
13. Katz ES, Tunick PA, Rusinek H, Ribakove G, Spencer FC, Kronzon I. Protruding aortic atheromas predict stroke in elderly patients undergoing cardiopulmonary bypass: experience with intraoperative transesophageal echocardiography. J Am Coll Cardiol 1992; 20(1):70–77.
14. Mickleborough LL, Walker PM, Takagi Y, Ohashi M, Ivanov J, Tamariz M. Risk factors for stroke in patients undergoing coronary artery bypass grafting. J Thorac Cardiovasc Surg 1996; 112(5):1250–1258.

15. Roach GW, Kanchuger M, Mangano CM, Newman M, Nussmeier N, Wolman R, et al. Adverse cerebral outcomes after coronary bypass surgery. Multicenter Study of Perioperative Ischemia Research Group and the Ischemia Research and Education Foundation Investigators. N Engl J Med 1996; 335(25):1857–1863.

16. Renton S, Hornick P, Taylor KM, Grace PA. Rational approach to combined carotid and ischaemic heart disease. Br J Surg 1997; 84(11):1503–1510.

17. Das SK, Brow TD, Pepper J. Continuing controversy in the management of concomitant coronary and carotid disease: an overview. Int J Cardiol 2000; 74(1):47–65.

18. D'Agostino RS, Svensson LG, Neumann DJ, Balkhy HH, Williamson WA, Shahian DM. Screening carotid ultrasonography and risk factors for stroke in coronary artery surgery patients. Ann Thorac Surg 1996; 62(6):1714–1723.

19. Berens ES, Kouchoukos NT, Murphy SF, Wareing TH. Preoperative carotid artery screening in elderly patients undergoing cardiac surgery. J Vasc Surg 1992; 15(2):313–321.

20. Salasidis GC, Latter DA, Steinmetz OK, Blair JF, Graham AM. Carotid artery duplex scanning in preoperative assessment for coronary artery revascularization: the association between peripheral vascular disease, carotid artery stenosis, and stroke. J Vasc Surg 1995; 21(1):154–160.

21. Walker WA, Harvey WR, Gaschen JR, Appling NA, Pate JW, Weiman DS. Is routine carotid screening for coronary surgery needed? Am Surg 1996; 62(4):308–310.

22. Hill AB, Obrand D, Steinmetz OK. The utility of selective screening for carotid stenosis in cardiac surgery patients. J Cardiovasc Surg 1999; 40(6):829–836.

23. Qureshi AI, Janardhan V, Bennett SE, Luft AR, Hopkins LN, Guterman LR. Who should be screened for asymptomatic carotid artery stenosis? Experience from the Western New York Stroke Screening Program. J Neuroimaging 2001; 11(2):105–111.

24. Ascher E, Hingorani A, Yorkovich W, Ramsey PJ, Salles-Cunha S. Routine preoperative carotid duplex scanning in patients undergoing open heart surgery: is it worthwhile? Ann Vasc Surg 2001; 15(6):669–678.

25. Durand DJ, Perler BA, Roseborough GS, Grega MA, Borowicz LM Jr, Baumgartner WA, et al. Mandatory versus selective preoperative carotid screening: a retrospective analysis. Ann Thorac Surg 2004; 78(1):159–166.

26. Long A, Lepoutre A, Corbillon E, Branchereau A. Critical review of non- or minimally invasive methods (duplex ultrasonography, MR- and CT-angiography) for evaluating stenosis of the proximal internal carotid artery. Eur J Vasc Endovasc Surg 2002; 24(1): 43–52.

27. Nederkoorn PJ, van der Graaf Y, Hunink MGM. Duplex ultrasound and magnetic resonance angiography compared with digital subtraction angiography in carotid artery stenosis: a systematic review. Stroke 2003; 34(5):1324–1332.

28. Naylor AR, Cuffe RL, Rothwell PM, Bell PRF. A systematic review of outcomes following staged and synchronous carotid endarterectomy and coronary artery bypass. Eur J Vasc Endovasc Surg 2003; 25(5):380–389.

29. Bernhard VM, Johnson WD, Peterson JJ. Carotid artery stenosis. Association with surgery for coronary artery disease. Arch Surg 1972; 105(6):837–840.

30. Khaitan L, Sutter FP, Goldman SM, Chamogeorgakis T, Wertan MA, Priest BP, et al. Simultaneous carotid endarterectomy and coronary revascularization. Ann Thorac Surg 2000; 69(2):421–424.

31. Minami K, Fukahara K, Boethig D, Bairaktaris A, Fritzsche D, Koerfer R. Long-term results of simultaneous carotid endarterectomy and myocardial revascularization with cardiopulmonary bypass used for both procedures. J Thorac Cardiovasc Surg 2000; 119(4 Pt 1):764–773.

32. Rerkasem K, Bond R, Rothwell PM. Local versus general anaesthesia for carotid endarterectomy. Cochrane Datab Syst Rev 2004(2):CD000126.

33. McCleary AJ, Maritati G, Gough MJ. Carotid endarterectomy; local or general anaesthesia? Eur J Vasc Endovasc Surg 2001; 22(1):1–12.

34. Cheng DC, Bainbridge D, Martin JE, Novick RJ, The Evidence-Based Perioperative Clinical Outcomes Research Group. Does off-pump coronary artery bypass reduce mortality, morbidity, and resource utilization when compared with conventional coronary artery bypass? A meta-analysis of randomized trials. Anesthesiology 2005; 102:188–203.

35. Panesar SS, Athanasiou T, Nair S, Rao C, Jones C, Nicolaou M, et al. Early outcomes in the elderly: a meta-analysis of 4921 patients undergoing coronary artery bypass grafting—a comparison between off-pump and on-pump techniques. Heart 2006:hrt.2006.088450.

36. Daily PO, Freeman RK, Dembitsky WP, Adamson RM, Moreno-Cabral RJ, Marcus S, et al. Cost reduction by combined carotid endarterectomy and coronary artery bypass grafting. J Thorac Cardiovasc Surg 1996; 111(6):1185–1192.

37. Coull AJ, Lovett JK, Rothwell PM. Population based study of early risk of stroke after transient ischaemic attack or minor stroke: implications for public education and organisation of services. BMJ 2004; 328(7435):326.

38. Arjomand H, Turi ZG, McCormick D, Goldberg S. Percutaneous coronary intervention: historical perspectives, current status, and future directions. Am Heart J 2003; 146(5): 787–796.

39. Bakhai A, Hill RA, Dundar Y, Dickson R, Walley T. Percutaneous transluminal coronary angioplasty with stents versus coronary artery bypass grafting for people with stable angina or acute coronary syndromes. Cochrane Datab Syst Rev 2005(1):CD004588.

40. Coward LJ, Featherstone RL, Brown MM. Percutaneous transluminal angioplasty and stenting for carotid artery stenosis. Cochrane Datab Syst Rev 2004(2):CD000515.

41. Biasi GM, Froio A, Diethrich EB, Deleo G, Galimberti S, Mingazzini P, et al. Carotid plaque echolucency increases the risk of stroke in carotid stenting: the Imaging in Carotid Angioplasty and Risk of Stroke (ICAROS) study. Circulation 2004; 110(6):756–762.

15 Urgent or Semiurgent Surgery in Patients with Severe Coronary Artery Disease

Pierre-Guy Chassot and Carlo Marcucci
Department of Anesthesiology, University Hospital of Lausanne (CHUV), Lausanne, Switzerland

Donat R. Spahn
University Hospital Zurich, Zurich, Switzerland

INTRODUCTION AND DEFINITIONS

More and more frequently, the trend towards invasive management of severe coronary events by cardiologists and towards liberal indications to noncardiac operations by surgeons places the anesthesiologist in front of a difficult situation: how to manage a patient with severe coronary artery disease (CAD) or an acute coronary syndrome (ACS) who requires urgent surgery? In the algorithm for assessing patients with or at risk of CAD presented elsewhere in this book (chap. 7, Fig. 2), this patient will be allotted to the intermediate-risk or to the high-risk group. Most of the time, patients in these groups should be investigated and prepared for surgery, and frequently revascularized. The surgical situations we are dealing with in this chapter are defined by their urgent or vital character, and the delays imposed by such investigations and treatments cannot be tolerated. Therefore, some solution must be found to protect these patients from ischemic complications during the perioperative period. The literature concerning noncardiac surgery for these patients is scarce and consists mostly of nonrandomized series, observational data, or expert opinions. The rationale of the perioperative care for CAD patients with urgent or semiurgent operations is thus largely based on studies from the cardiology domain and extrapolated from the recommendations for their medical treatment. The decisions are the result of the application of the precaution principle rather than being the result of firm scientific evidence.

Before embarking on the discussion of the different possible strategies, it is necessary to rely on clear definitions of the clinical situations from a cardiological point of view.

STABLE CHRONIC CORONARY ARTERY DISEASE

According to the algorithms published in the recent literature (1–3), patients with chronic and stable coronary disease belong to the intermediate-risk category. Patients in this category suffer from documented but medically controlled CAD; they may be asymptomatic under optimal treatment, or have episodes of angina Canadian class I or II (Table 1). Intermediate-risk category comprises also silent ischemia (by Holter monitoring), patients asymptomatic after infarction or revascularization but only while receiving maximal therapy, and patients more than six weeks and less than three months after myocardial infarction (MI) or revascularization without sequelae or threatened myocardium. These patients have a global perioperative cardiac complication rate of 2% to 6% (2). Chronic stable CAD is said to be severe when the patient

TABLE 1 Canadian Cardiovascular Society Functional Classification of Angina Pectoris

Class	Definition
I	Angina occurs with strenuous, rapid, or prolonged exertion at work or recreation; ordinary physical activity (e.g., walking and climbing stairs) does not cause angina
II	Slight limitation of ordinary activity; angina occurs on walking or climbing stairs rapidly; walking uphill; walking or stair climbing after meals, in cold, in wind, or under emotional stress; walking more than two blocks on the level at a normal pace and in normal conditions, or climbing more than one flight of ordinary stairs at a normal pace and in normal conditions
III	Marked limitation of ordinary physical activity; angina may occur after walking one to two blocks on the level or climbing one flight of stairs at a normal pace and in normal conditions
IV	Angina may be present at rest

Source: From Ref. 4.

is suffering from the following: (*i*) three-vessel disease, (*ii*) multiple stenoses on two or three vessels, (*iii*) positive stress test, (*iv*) ventricular dysfunction [ejection fraction (EF) <0.35], or (*v*) insulin-dependent diabetes mellitus.

ACUTE CORONARY SYNDROMES (UNSTABLE ANGINA AND EVOLVING MYOCARDIAL INFARCTION)

Disruption of coronary plaques is now considered to be the common pathophysiologic substrate of ACS. Such a plaque disruption exposes tissue factor bearing cells to the blood components, and is associated with a high risk of a local thrombus formation. When completely occlusive, this will lead to necrosis involving the full or nearly full thickness of the ventricular wall, and typically produce increased troponin levels and ST elevation on the electrocardiogram (ECG) (STEMI: ST-elevation myocardial infarction). One-quarter of the patients presenting with ACS are in this situation; most of them will develop a Q-wave on subsequent ECG; they require urgent reperfusion (Fig. 1) (5). Three-quarters of the patients with ACS have unstable angina (UA) or non-ST elevation myocardial infarction (N-STEMI), which is mainly caused by a subtotal arterial occlusion; among them, 40% have evidence of myocardial necrosis, usually subendocardial, with elevated troponin; they develop a non-Q-wave MI. Reperfusion is the mainstay of therapy in case of elevated troponin and impending infarction, whereas medical treatment is recommended for UA without elevated troponin.

UA (Canadian class IV) is characterized by angina at rest, recently appeared symptoms, a change in previous symptoms, or attacks lasting more than 20 minutes, occurring more than twice a day, and resistant to nitroglycerin. There are several independent risk factors for adverse outcome associated with UA and N-STEMI that have been identified as independent predictors (6,7): age older than 65 years, ST deviation greater than 0.5 mm, elevated cardiac markers (troponin, CK-MB), more than two episodes of angina in the last 24 hours, aspirin prophylaxis within the prior week, low systolic blood pressure, signs of heart failure, and severe two- or three-vessel disease on coronary angiogram. These predictors can be integrated in a comprehensive score for clinical use (5,8). When less than three predictors are present (score <3), the patients are in a low-risk category, where medical and invasive (revascularization) treatment give equivalent results (9,10). The presence of more predictors defines intermediate-risk (score 3–4) and high-risk (score 5 or more) categories, where revascularization gives significantly better results than medical therapy in a

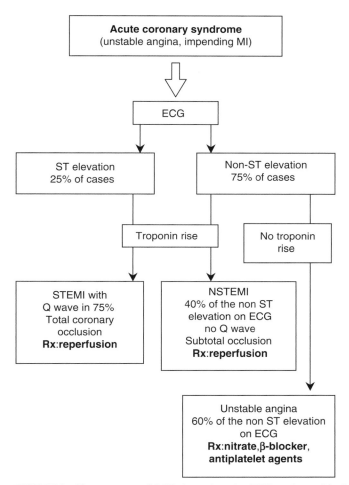

FIGURE 1 Management of ACSs based on the ECG performed in the emergency room. ST elevation is the marker of a transmural necrosis due to total occlusion of the culprit coronary artery. Non-ST-elevation, or ST depression, is the marker of a subendocardial lesion or of UA. The level of troponin indicates the presence of necrosis. *Abbreviations*: ACS, acute coronary syndrome; MI, myocardial infarction; STEMI, ST-elevation myocardial infarction; N-STEMI, non-ST-elevation myocardial infarction; UA, unstable angina. *Source*: From Ref. 5.

nonsurgical setting (death and nonfatal MI: 9% vs. 15%, respectively) (11). Therefore, patients with clinically low-risk UA should be investigated with dobutamine echocardiography or with thallium-dipyridamole perfusion scan (12); if the test does not induce significant new wall motion abnormalities (WMA), medical treatment can be started with β-blockers, antiplatelet agents [acetylsalicylic acid (ASA) and clopidogrel], nitrate, angiotensin-converting enzyme inhibitors (ACEI), and statins. If new WMA appear during the test, the patient should be revascularized, as should those who are in the intermediate- or high-risk groups (score 3 or more) (8). This management is summarized in an algorithm illustrated in Fig. 2.

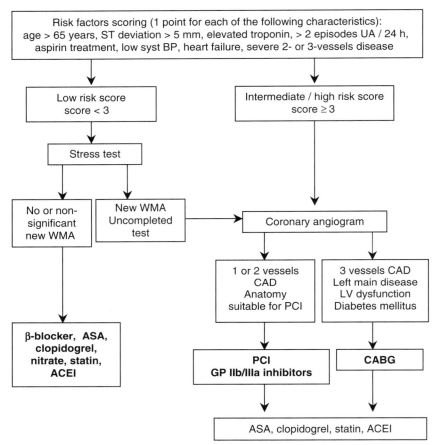

FIGURE 2 Management of UA with a scoring system based on clinical characteristics. Low-risk patients are managed with medical treatment, whereas intermediate and high-risk patients are revascularized. In each situation, they are protected by antiplatelet drugs: lifelong ASA and clopidogrel for 6 weeks to 6 months depending of the revascularization technique. *Abbreviations*: UA, unstable angina; CAD, coronary artery disease; WMA, wall motion abnormality; ASA, acetylsalicylic acid; ACEI, angiotensin-converting enzyme inhibitor; PCI, percutaneous coronary intervention; CABG, coronary artery bypass graft. *Source*: From Ref. 8.

RISK FACTORS OF THE OPERATION

Surgical procedures are usually stratified into three categories (Table 2 in chap. 7) (2,3). Minor procedures include ambulatory and superficial operations such as herniorrhaphy, eye surgery, plastic surgery, or endoscopic procedures. Intermediate operations comprise abdominal and thoracic procedures, orthopedics, neurosurgery, otorhino-laryngeological and urologic operations (as long as they are not complicated by unusual duration), hemorrhage, large volume shifts, or emergency. Minor peripheral vascular surgery and carotid endarterectomy belong to this category. Major procedures include aortic and major vascular surgery, prolonged surgical procedures with large fluid shifts or hemorrhage, intermediate operations in emergency, and unstable hemodynamic situations. The average cardiac complication rate in general population is less than 1% with minor procedures, 1% to 5% with intermediate operations, and more than 5% in case of major surgery (2).

In the context of severe or unstable CAD, as well as shortly after revascularization, it is more useful to classify surgical procedures according to their degree of emergency or maximum possible delays. A nonexhaustive list of examples is given for each category.

1. Life-saving procedures (within four hours): ruptured abdominal aortic aneurysm, aortic dissection type A, surgical acute hemorrhage, acute tamponade, polytrauma
2. Emergencies within 48 hours: same as above but in a stable condition, intracranial compression (space-occupying lesion, hemorrhage), open fracture, limb dislocation, appendectomy, bowel occlusion, or perforation
3. Delay less than two weeks: rapidly spreading tumors, impending aneurysm rupture, infections requiring surgical drainage or resection (abscess, infected wound, sigmoiditis, cholecystitis), disabling bone fractures
4. Delay of more than two weeks clinically acceptable: moderately invasive and slowly evolving tumors, fistula for dialysis, lesions causing intractable pain, chronic limb ischemia, hernial disc

The surgical pathologies in the first three categories share the common feature of being an obvious priority in the patient's management. In these cases, the cardiological management must be adapted to the timing of the surgical procedure. It is exactly the opposite from the usual care of purely elective situations, where the timing of the operation is decided by the type of cardiological intervention. Therefore, a new algorithm must be established for the management of these peculiar situations. Before proposing different strategies, we shall briefly review the different possibilities to protect the myocardium from ischemia during the perioperative period.

PERIOPERATIVE CARDIOPROTECTION

The perioperative myocardial protection is based on the pathophysiological principles of prevention of thrombosis in unstable coronary lesions, stabilization of atheromatous plaques, and optimization of the oxygen demand/oxygen consumption balance. Most patients presenting for urgent or semiurgent surgery with known CAD are, or should be, treated with antiplatelet drugs, β-adrenergic antagonists, nitrates, ACEI, cholesterol-lowering agents, and possibly revascularization (Table 2). The use of nitrates, ACEI, and cholesterol-lowering agents is beyond the scope of this chapter but, in the perioperative context, it is important to note that their withdrawal does not induce a rebound effect. Therefore, we will concentrate on antiplatelet drugs and β-adrenergic antagonists, because they have an outstanding position in the therapy of acute and severe CAD, and because they present dangerous rebound effects when stopped abruptly.

ANTITHROMBOTIC DRUGS

Antiplatelet drugs protect high-risk patients against MI, stroke, and vascular death (13). Three classes of antiplatelet agents are currently used in the treatment of patients with CAD: aspirin or ASA, adenosine-5'-diphosphate (ADP) receptor antagonists (tienopyridines), and glycoprotein (GP) IIb/IIIa receptor antagonists.

TABLE 2 Anti-ischemic Treatments Before Urgent or Semiurgent Noncardiac Surgery

Criteria for use of β-blockers	Criteria for use of antiplatelet agents	Criteria for revascularization
Stable angina (class I–II)	ASA/aspirin	Untractable angina
Use of antianginal medical treatment	Previous MI, PCI, or CABG (lifelong treatment)	Coronary lesion threatening a large area of myocardium
Silent ischemia on ECG	Documented ischemia	Mandatory delays for surgery
Q-wave on ECG	Clopidogrel	PCI (+ bare metal stent)
Documented previous ischemia or MI	UA (class IV)	Delay for surgery >6 wk
Positive stress tests	Impending infarction	PTCA (no stent)
PCI or CABG <3 mo but >6 wk	PCI or MI <6 wk to 12 mo	Delay for surgery >2 wk
PCI or CABG >3 mo if complications		IIb/IIIa inhibitors
Diabetes requiring insulin therapy		PCI < 48 hr
Renal insufficiency (creatine > 200 mmol/L)		
History of stroke		
Vascular surgery		

Note: If indicated, β-blocker and antiplatelet treatments should be started as soon as possible. They must not be withdrawn before surgery. β-Blockade should be tailored to achieve a heart rate of 60 to 65 bpm. ASA dosage: 100 to 300 mg/day. Clopidogrel dosage: loading dose of 300 mg, followed by 75 mg/day.
Abbreviations: UA, unstable angina; PCI, percutaneous coronary intervention; PTCA, percutaneous transluminal coronary angioplasty; CABG, coronary artery bypass graft; ASA, acetylsalicilic acid; MI, myocardial infarction; ECG, electrocardiogram.

A good understanding of their pharmacodynamic and pharmacokinetic profiles will help in establishing a strategy for the use of these drugs in the perioperative setting.

Aspirin or Acetylsalicylic Acid

ASA irreversibly acetylates platelet cyclooxygenase-1 (COX-1), inhibiting the synthesis of the potent platelet aggregator and vasoconstrictor thromboxane-A2 (TxA2). Fifteen to twenty minutes after oral intake, ASA is metabolized to its inactive metabolite salicylate. The terminal half-lives of ASA and salicylate are 0.4 and 2.1 hours, respectively (14). As platelets are unable to regenerate COX-1, restoration of platelet COX-1 activity depends on the generation of fresh platelets. Serum TX B2 levels normalize after 12 to 14 days. Yet within two to four days after ASA cessation, the ability for platelets to aggregate in the presence of a strong stimulus, such as arachidonic acid or collagen, is restored (14). As the inhibition of COX-1 is irreversible, there is no antidote to ASA. Rapid reversal of the antiplatelet effect can only be obtained by platelet transfusion. However, because ASA is characterized by a rather weak inhibition of platelet function, platelet replacement is rarely indicated (15). ASA inhibition of platelet function can be detected by arachidonic acid or collagen-induced aggregation. ASA rarely prolongs bleeding time.

Tienopyridines (Clopidogrel and Ticlopidine)

The tienopyridines are inhibitors of the platelets ADP receptor. Both clopidogrel and ticlopidine are inactive precursors that require hepatic metabolization by the cytochrome P450 1A2 complex. The active metabolite irreversibly modifies the platelet ADP receptor and thus inhibits granule release and aggregation by other agonists such as thromboxane, platelet-activating factor, collagen, and low concentrations of thrombin (16,17). The effect of clopidogrel is dose- and time-dependent, reaching the maximum inhibition of 40% to 60% after three to seven days of therapy. After clopidogrel cessation, platelet function recovers gradually and reaches normal levels seven days after the last dose (16,17). Ticlopidine has largely been abandoned because of serious side effects, and clopidogrel remains the only drug of its type in use. Clopidogrel prolongs bleeding time 1.5 to 3-fold of baseline after three to seven days of treatment. Clopidogrel as monotherapy has a weak-to-moderate, but irreversible, antiplatelet action. Platelet transfusion, although seldom indicated, is the only way to rapidly restore platelet function.

GPIIb/IIIa Inhibitors (Abciximab, Tirofiban, Eptifibatide)

The GPIIb/IIIa receptor antagonists are potent antiplatelet agents that are administered intravenously after percutaneous coronary interventions (PCIs). Abciximab is a human–murine monoclonal antibody fragment that binds to GPIIb/IIIa with high affinity. A 50% block of the GPIIb/IIIa receptors produces significant inhibition of platelet aggregation and an 80% block is considered necessary to prevent stent thrombosis after PCI. Minutes after an intravenous bolus, most of the molecules are bound, and free drug is eliminated. Plasma half-life of unbound abciximab is 26 minutes (18). At steady state, during abciximab infusion, 4% of the total dose circulates unbound. This fraction decreases rapidly after interruption of the infusion (19). GPIIb/IIIa-bound abciximab, on the other hand, is eliminated much more slowly due to its high affinity. Twelve and twenty-three hours after discontinuation, receptor occupation decreases to 70% and 50%, respectively. After seven days, a 25% residual GPIIb/IIIa block can still be measured. Moreover, seven days after discontinuation, the degree of receptor occupation is the same for all circulating platelets. This indicates that the abciximab molecules are redistributed among circulating, newly formed, and probably transfused platelets (18).

Eptifibatide and tirofiban are agents with considerably lower affinity for the GPIIb/IIIa receptor than abciximab. Their antiaggregant effect is time- and dose-dependent and they are characterized by rapid plasma clearance of 2.5 and 2 hours, respectively. Eighty percent inhibition of aggregation is obtained after a bolus dose followed by an infusion, and, respectively, six and four hours after cessation of the infusion platelet aggregation recovers to 50%. The fast recovery of platelet function makes antidote strategy unnecessary for eptifibatide and tirofiban. Because of the redistribution of abciximab molecules, platelet transfusion can theoretically be used to antagonize its antiaggregant effect, but no data are available on either the necessity nor the efficacy of such a strategy.

Unfractionated Heparin (UFH) and Low Molecular Weight Heparin (LMWH)

Heparin is a glycosaminoglycane that binds to circulating antithrombin III (ATIII) and accelerates the latter's capacity of inhibiting the coagulation factors IIa, IXa, and Xa 2000-fold. Its capacity for inhibiting factors Xa and IIa is in the ratio of 1:1. After intravenous administration, UFH has an immediate effect. UFH is absorbed and metabolized in the reticuloendothelial system, and its half-life is dose-dependent: one hour for a 100 U/kg bolus and 2.5 hours for a 400 U/kg dose. LMWHs are fractions of the longer heparin chain, and have a much weaker anti-IIa effect. The capacity of inhibition of factors Xa and IIa is in the ratio 2–4:1. After intravenous administration, it takes 20 to 60 minutes for the LMWHs to be effective, but they have much more predictable pharmacodynamic and pharmacokinetic profiles than unfractionated heparin (UFH). Because of its unpredictability, the effect of UFH has to be monitored by apt or activated clotting time (ACT) essays. Therapy with LWMH does not require monitoring of coagulation parameters. The effect of UFH can be completely reversed by protamine.

Use of Antithrombotic Drugs in Patients with CAD

Lifelong ASA therapy is a grade 1A recommendation for chronic stable CAD, acute non-ST-elevation (NSTE) coronary syndrome, and other ACS or post-MI (20). A meta-analysis of randomized trials of antiplatelet therapy (13) demonstrated that the use of ASA leads to a proportional risk reduction for serious vascular events of 33% and 46% for patients with stable and UA, respectively. For patients with a history of MI, a mean duration of 27 months of ASA therapy results in a highly significant reduction in nonfatal reinfarction (18 fewer per 1000) and vascular death (14 fewer per 1000). In all the patient groups, the net benefits were substantially larger than the excess risk for major extracranial bleeds caused by the antiplatelet drugs. The optimal dose range for ASA is 75 to 150 mg/day. Higher doses do not increase myocardial protection but may increase the risk for major extracranial hemorrhage (21).

In the CAPRIE trial, ASA (325 mg/day) was compared to clopidogrel (75 mg/day) for its efficacy in preventing ischemic events and for its side effects. It showed clopidogrel to be more efficacious in the prevention of ischemic stroke, MI, and vascular death. The relative risk reduction for patients receiving clopidogrel compared to ASA was 7.9% for the overall study population. This benefit increases in high-risk subgroups: 9.7% in patients with hypercholesterolemia, 10.0% in patients with a history of ischemic events, 12.5% in patients with diabetes, and 28.9% for patients with previous CABG. The risk of bleeding, and other side effects, was similar in both groups (22). Initiation of clopidogrel therapy requires an oral loading dose of 300 mg followed by a daily dose of 75 mg.

The combination of ASA and clopidogrel is a grade 1A recommendation in N-STEMI and UA in whom diagnostic catheterization will be delayed or when coronary bypass surgery will not occur until more than five days following coronary angiography, and in patients with chronic stable CAD with a high-risk profile of developing acute MI (20). Dual antiplatelet therapy in patients with UA results in a further reduction of death from cardiovascular causes, nonfatal MI, and stroke compared to ASA alone (23,24). But the CURE trial showed that dual antiplatelet therapy results in a significantly higher incidence of major hemorrhage (3.7%) compared to ASA monotherapy (2.7%) (23). The benefit that can be gained of combining two different types of antiplatelet agents thus must be weighed against the risk on hemorrhage for different patient groups.

One group in which the advantages clearly outweigh the side effects is the group of patients that undergo PCI for ACSs. Because of the interruption of endothelial continuity provoked by the dilation of the coronary vessel during the procedure, a highly thrombogenic lesion is created. The risk of intracoronary thrombosis remains extremely high until re-endothelialization is completed. The time needed for re-endothelialization depends on the procedure performed. In simple percutaneous transluminal coronary angioplasty (PTCA) without placement of an intracoronary stent, two weeks are considered sufficient. When a stent is deployed in the artery, the highly thrombogenic metal has to be completely covered with newly formed endothelium for the risk of thrombosis to decrease. For a bare metal stent, the process of re-endothelialization takes six to eight weeks (2,25). The inflammation induced by an intracoronary stent causes hypertrophy of the newly formed intima, neointimal hyperplasia. This process is responsible for late stent stenosis. To avoid this, drug-eluting stents have been developed. These stents slowly release antimitogen drugs, inhibiting cell proliferation in the adjacent coronary artery wall. Thereby restenosis is prevented but, at the same time, the process of re-endothelialization is delayed, thus prolonging the period during which the patients is at high risk of in-stent thrombosis. Because of the success of these devices in preventing hyperplastic stent stenosis, 85% of all intracoronary stents used in PCI today are drug-eluting stents (26).

In the PCI-CURE study, patients undergoing PCI were treated with either ASA alone or with a combination of ASA and clopidogrel. The incidence of cardiovascular death, MI, or urgent target vessel revascularization was significantly reduced in the ASA-clopidogrel group immediately after the intervention and at long-term follow-up (27). Dual antiplatelet therapy is recommended for four to six weeks after insertion of a bare metal stent, and for three or six months after stenting with a sirolimus or paclitaxel-eluting stent, respectively. The ACCP Conference on Antithrombotic and Thrombolytic Therapy even recommends 9 to 12 months of clopidogrel 75 mg/day in addition to ASA (28). The interruption of dual antiplatelet therapy earlier than the recommended delay, for any reason, will put the patient at an unacceptably high risk of myocardial ischemia.

UFH and LMWH can be used in combination with ASA for the treatment of ACS (20). Only one study compared UFH to ASA as monotherapy and found that both drugs reduced the occurrence of refractory angina and MI with a trend in favor of UFH (29). Several trials investigated the combination of ASA and UFH in the treatment of ACS. Although not statistically significant, a consistent trend favors combined therapy for its ability to reduce death or MI in ACS (30–32). The combination of ASA and LMWH improves the outcome of patients with non-ST-elevation ACS as compared to UFH (20). The only recommendation for heparin is its use in combination with ASA in the treatment of NSTE ACS (grade 1A) with a preference for the use of LMWH over UFH (grade 1B). If UFH is used, an initial bolus of 60 to 70 U/kg followed by an initial infusion of 12 to 15 U/kg/hr titrated to a target aPTT of 50 to 75 seconds is recommended (12). Lower aPTT values (50–60 seconds) result in less hemorrhagic complications and, interestingly, longer aPTT values are associated with an increase in a 30-day death or reinfarction (33). In the treatment of ACS, the relationship between high levels of heparin anticoagulation and death has indeed been consistently reported (34–36), and is not related to hemorrhage but probably to an increase in thrombogenicity due to activation of protein C and heparin-induced platelet activation (37,38). When heparin treatment is ended, gradual decrease rather than abrupt interruption may reduce rebound thrombin generation and ischemic/thrombotic events.

Urgent Surgery and Antiplatelet Drugs

Treatment with antiplatelet agents before surgery generates a difficult dilemma: maintaining the treatment increases the risk of bleeding, but stopping it increases the risk of acute ischemic syndromes. In many surgical disciplines, it is standard practice to interrupt all antiplatelet therapy before the intervention, aiming to minimize perioperative blood loss. A review of the literature reveals a surprising paucity of level I studies exploring the influence of antiplatelet agents on perioperative bleeding and outcome (39). Three studies in vascular surgery showed no increase of perioperative blood loss when ASA was used (40–42). In two of these (carotic surgery and femoro-popliteal bypass), a significant reduction in cerebrovascular accidents was noted (40,41). In abdominal and gynecologic surgery, the use of ASA was associated with an increase in perioperative bleeding, but this was found to be of no clinical relevance (43,44). In one study on 52 patients undergoing emergency abdominal surgery, ASA did not cause any bleeding complications (45). In orthopedic surgery, the use of ASA was not associated with a higher perioperative blood loss or with a clinically significant increase in perioperative bleeding (46–48). Patients treated with different types and different combinations of anticoagulant drugs did not present major bleeding complications when they underwent different types of hemorrhagic surgery within 60 days of PCI (49). Although in this study 33% of patients received red blood cell or platelet transfusion, there was no association between transfusion requirements and time of discontinuation of antiplatelet and anticoagulant therapy. For surgical disciplines such as ophthalmology, otorhino-laryngeology, dermatology, and urology, or for invasive that may be associated with bleeding procedures, there is a lack of high-level evidence, but the available literature indicates that the perioperative use of antiplatelet agents does not increase the risk of clinically important bleeding complications (39). The average increase in surgical bleeding is 2.5% to 10% with ASA (40) and 25% with clopidogrel (23). Antiplatelet agents did not lead to an increase in bleeding after colonoscopic polypectomy in one study (50), and clopidogrel alone or in combination with ASA did not increase bleeding complications when given to animals undergoing transbronchial lung biopsy (51).

Increased perioperative blood loss due to antiaggregants can result in severe anemia, which may not be tolerated by the coronary artery patient. Patients with acute MI have increased mortality rates if admission hemoglobin (Hb) levels are lower than $10\,g/dL$ (52,53). In contrast, transfusing patients with ACS who have a hematocrit of 30 or more results in excess mortality (54). In addition, patients with stable CAD have been shown to tolerate normovolemic hemodilution to Hb levels of 9.9 to $0.2\,g/dL$, without sings of ischemia or heart failure (55), and Hebert et al. (56) found in a subgroup of the TRICC trial that patients with CAD did not benefit from a liberal (Hb transfusion trigger of $9.0\,g/dL$) as compared to a restrictive (Hb transfusion trigger of $7.0\,g/dL$) transfusion strategy. Most patients with severe CAD will thus tolerate perioperative hemoglobin values of $8.0\,g/dL$ well (57). In addition, anemia-related myocardial ischemia can reliably be treated with minimal blood transfusion (58,59).

On the other hand, interruption of antiplatelet agents used for primary or secondary prevention of cardiovascular disease puts the patients at high risk of coronary thrombosis with possible catastrophic outcomes. Defective compliance or withdrawal of aspirin in patients with stable coronary disease has been shown to be associated with a fourfold increase in the rate of death compared with patients appropriately treated (60). Cessation of antiplatelet therapy is also associated with a 20% incidence of thrombosis of an uncoated stent implanted on average 15 months previously (61). It is clear that withdrawing oral antiplatelet drugs during the period of stent endothelialization may have dramatic consequences, with perioperative mortality rates from 20% up to 86% (62–64). In addition, premature antiplatelet therapy discontinuation has been identified as the major independent predictor of drug-eluting stent thrombosis (hazard ration 89.8), with a fatality rate of 45% (65). After withdrawal of antiplatelet agents, thrombotic stent occlusion resulting in MI has been reported as late as 375 days post-PCI for a sirolimus-eluting stent and 442 days post-PCI for a paclitaxel-eluting stent (66).

A retrospective analysis of 475 consecutive patients, admitted for acute MI, identified 11 patients who interrupted chronic ASA therapy within 15 days prior to admission (67). All of them had been stable and free from acute coronary events for an average of 3.8 years before ASA cessation. All coronary angiographies showed complete thrombotic occlusion of the culprit coronary artery. In a subsequent prospective cohort study on 1358 patients admitted for ACSs, Collet et al. (68) found 73 patients (5.4%) who stopped ASA within two weeks before the event (recent withdrawers) and compared their outcomes with the patients who did not interrupt antiplatelet therapy (prior users) and with nonusers of antiplatelet dugs. Two-thirds of the recent withdrawers interrupted their antiplatelet therapy prior to scheduled surgery. Even if a replacement therapy with LMWH was initiated, the recent withdrawers had a twofold increased mortality (19.2% vs. 9.9%) and MI rate (21.9% vs. 12.4%) compared to prior users or nonusers.

Several factors influence the interaction between ASA cessation and coronary thrombosis. When ASA treatment is interrupted, rebound hyperactivity of platelets is described (69). In addition, CAD patients exhibit enhanced generation of thrombin and increased thrombin- and ADP-induced platelet aggregation (70–72). Thaulow et al. (71) studied a cohort of 487 healthy adult males, with no signs of CAD. Long-term follow-up at 13.5 years showed that annual total and cardiac mortality increased with platelet concentration at baseline. Cardiac mortality was 2.5 times higher in the 25% of subjects with the highest platelet count. Subjects with an ADP-induced platelet aggregation rate above the median had a significantly higher cardiac mortality than those with an aggregation rate below the median level. Another study on patients with known CAD showed that selective thrombin-induced platelet hyperaggregability is associated with a 2.5-fold increase in the likelihood of progression of coronary artery sclerosis, as assessed by coronary angiogram (72). The enhanced platelet sensitivity leads to a significant reduction of survival over a follow-up period of only four years, even in the absence of angiographic progression of the stenosis.

Withdrawing antiplatelet agents before surgery, combined with the postoperative state of hypercoagulability, thus, puts the surgical patient with severe or unstable CAD in a very precarious position. This practice should be revised (70). Assuming that the perioperative use of antiplatelet agents should not lead to clinically significant hemorrhage, we consider the cessation of antiaggregant agents to minimize bleeding unjustified for almost all surgical procedures in patients with severe or unstable CAD. The only possible exception is surgery for intracranial pathology, where even minor hemorrhagic complications can lead to dramatic outcomes. For this group of patients, interruption of antiaggregants is probably indicated provided all other measures of myocardial protection have been instituted (β-blockers, statins, etc.).

β-ADRENERGIC ANTAGONISTS

β-Adrenergic antagonists (β-blockers) are first-line agents in the treatment of hypertension and cardiovascular diseases. The mechanisms by which they provide myocardial protection are complex (73). β-Blockers have a positive impact on cardiac bioenergetics by decreasing oxygen requirement and increasing oxygen supply. By reducing tachycardia, they diminish myocardial oxygen consumption and shear stress on the atheromatous plaque; they prolong duration of diastole and increase the net blood flow to myocardial cells. They alter gene expression and signal transmission in the cardiomyocyte. They influence platelet aggregability and cardiac cell apoptosis and necrosis. They decrease the release of proinflammatory cytokines and endothelin E1 (74,75).

Several trials have shown tremendous reductions in cardiac morbidity and in short- and long-term mortality with the use of β-receptor antagonists. Mangano et al. (76) found a reduction of 65% in cardiac mortality in patients at risk for CAD, who were scheduled to undergo elective surgery if they were treated with atenolol in the perioperative period. Poldermans used bisoprolol and reported a 90% reduction of 30-day death in a selected subgroup of high-risk vascular patients.

Thus, do all the patients benefit from β-blockers? Several studies aim at answering this question. Using a modified cardiac risk index (77) in combination with the results of dobutamine stress echocardiography (DSE), Boersma et al. (78) attempted to predict the efficacy of perioperative β-blockade in patients undergoing major vascular surgery. In a retrospective study of 1351 patients scheduled for vascular operations, the combination of three categories of clinical scores (no risk factors, fewer than three risk factors, three or more risk factors) and the results of DSE (no WMA, WMA in one to four segments, WMA in five or more segments) stratifies the patients into five risk groups (Fig. 3). The first group comprises the patients with no risk factors; cardiac event rates were comparably low in patients receiving and patients not receiving β-blockers. The three intermediate groups are patients with increasingly severe CAD. The protection offered by β-blockers increased in parallel with the degree of coronary disease, with a 3- to 10-fold decrease in the incidence of cardiac complications in β-blocked patients. Finally, the group of highest risk (>3 risk factors and WMA in ≥5 segments) showed no difference between patients under β-blockers or not. These data suggest that perioperative β-blockers represent outstanding perioperative cardioprotection for CAD patients, particularly in the intermediate-risk groups; the worse the coronary disease, the more efficient they are. They may not be beneficial in the very-low-risk (28% of the total cohort) and in very-high-risk patients (2% of the total cohort). In this last category, patients require revascularization and not medical treatment, and the cardiac complication rate during noncardiac surgery is 36% (78).

In a retrospective cohort of 663,635 patients from 329 hospitals, 122,338 of whom were β-blocked, the relationship between β-blockade and mortality varied directly with the cardiac risk index (79). In low-risk patients (cardiac risk index score of 0 or 1), β-blockade was associated with an increased mortality. In intermediate- and high-risk patients (cardiac risk index score of 2, 3, and 4 or more), the adjusted odds ratio for in-hospital death in β-blocked patients were 0.88, 0.71, and 0.57, respectively. The cardioprotective effect of β-blockers seemed therefore to be limited to patients with an intermediate- or high-risk score of cardiac adverse events; they might be harmful on very low-risk cases, and do not replace revascularization in highly unstable coronary syndromes.

A third study included 31 vascular surgery patients, with positive stress tests or positive coronary angiogram, who underwent noncardiac surgery without prior surgical or percutaneous revascularization (80). Of 31 patients, 12 had multiple areas at risk for myocardial ischemia and seven had ventricular EF >40%. This cohort represents a group of very-high-risk patients that may have been excluded in other studies. All patients were β-blocked in the perioperative period with metoprolol or labetalol according to a very rigorous protocol aiming at a heart rate of 70 bpm or less.

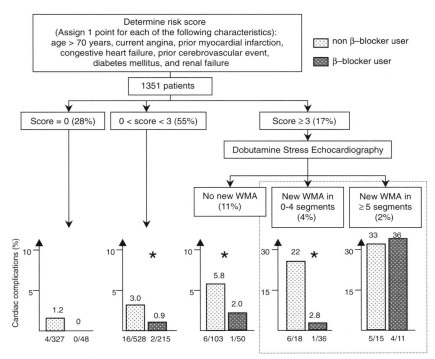

FIGURE 3 Reduction of cardiac complication rate by β-blockers in subgroups of patients with increasing ischemic risk. Numbers in brackets are the percentage of patients in each category of the 1351 patients. Numbers below the bars are the number of patients in each subgroup. Numbers above the bars are the percentage of cardiac complications in each subgroup. The two subgroups at right (clear area) represent patients with severe and/or unstable CAD; they are at a different scale. *The differences are statistically significant. *Abbreviation*: WMA: wall motion abnormality. *Source*: From Ref. 78.

In patients who were not chronically β-blocked, oral metoprolol was started a mean of two days before the operation. Supplemental intravenous metoprolol was titrated before endotracheal intubation and throughout surgery, and oral β-blockade was continued postoperatively in an effort to maintain heart rate ≤70 bpm. None of the patients suffered from MI, congestive heart failure, or cardiac death. This study illustrates that, even in very-high-risk patients, the cardiac complication rate can be very low if β-blockers are titrated in the individual patient in a rigorous and sustained way.

In contrast to first-generation β-blockers, which were not tolerated by 20% of patients, the new β-blockers are characterized by a drug tolerability of 90% to 100% and a very low complication rate. Most randomized trials did not find an increase in complications related to β-blockers compared to controls, although a review of the literature identified bradycardia as the only adverse reaction that was significantly increased (81). Patients with relative contraindications for β-blockers (obstructive pulmonary disease, peripheral vascular disease, congestive heart failure, diabetes) tolerate β_1-selective β-blockers (atenolol, bisoprolol, metoprolol) very well. Considering the efficacy of β-blockers in patients with severe or unstable CAD in improving perioperative cardiac outcome, only severe active asthma or chronic obstructive lung disease with a strong reactive component, vasospastic CAD, and high-grade heart block in the absence of a pacemaker can be considered as contraindications (74). Although the efficacy of perioperative β-blockade for the protection of the intermediate and high-risk patient has now clearly been established, and although it is recommended by the ACC/AHA Perioperative Guidelines (2), several authors report that β-AAs are still largely underutilized or that they are used in an inaccurate way (82–85).

Patients chronically taking β-blockers are not always protected against intraoperative ischemia. In a retrospective analysis of 6948 vascular surgery patients, there was no difference in intraoperative extremes of heart rate between patients on β-blocker therapy and those not receiving therapy, implying inadequate β-blockade in a high number of patients (86). Because the upregulation of β-adrenergic receptors during the chronic β-blockade leaves the myocardium hypersensitive to endogenous catecholamines (87), there is a trend towards an overreaction to noxious sympathetic stimulation with excessive tachycardia, hypertension, and myocardial oxygen demand. In addition, the risk of a postoperative ischemic event is increased fourfold in patients in whom chronic β-blocker therapy was discontinued preoperatively (88). After major vascular operations, this difference is even larger. In one study, the mortality of patients in whom β-blockers were withdrawn preoperatively was 50% as compared with a mortality of 1.5% in patients with uninterrupted β-blockade (89). It is therefore of the utmost importance to continue the treatment throughout the perioperative period. Frequently, β-blockade needs to be reinforced during the critical intraoperative and postoperative periods by the administration of shorter acting drugs in order to maintain the heart rate at 60 to 65 bpm (90). Slow heart rate is a good marker of an adequate β-blockade, and intraoperative tachycardia and hypertension are independently associated with adverse outcome in noncardiac surgery (91).

CORONARY REVASCULARIZATION

Coronary revascularization is the first choice therapy for severe CAD and unstable coronary syndromes. A successful revascularization places patients in a low-risk category, as if the CAD was cured, as long as they are asymptomatic without treatment besides ASA. Among patients who underwent coronary artery bypass graft (CABG), the infarction rate (0.8%) and the mortality (1.7%) after major noncardiac surgery are identical to those of patients without CAD; beyond six years after CABG, the infarction rate raises again (2.2%) (92). After PCI, the same benefit is present only in patients with normal ventricular function, and for a shorter period of four years (93). The goal of revascularization is to salvage threatened myocardium and to increase long-term survival. It does not offer prophylactic protection before noncardiac surgery for two reasons: (*i*) Revascularization has its own mortality rate (1–6% for CABG and 0.1–1% for PCI) and a certain infarction rate (2–5% for CABG and 1–3% for PCI) (94–96), the highest values being in vascular patients; these values must be added to the mortality and complication rate of the noncardiac surgery, which are around 5% in major vascular surgery (97). (*ii*) Every instrumentation of the coronary arteries results in a lesion of the endothelium which is unstable until it is covered by a newly formed endothelium.

Anastomoses and bare-metal stents are covered by a proliferation of endothelium within six to eight weeks (25). During this time period, the situation in the grafted or stented coronary artery is equivalent to an unstable lesion; if noncardiac surgery is performed during this period of time, the mortality rate (20%) and the risk of infarction (30%) are exceedingly high (49,62–64,98). Within 40 days of PCI, patients are nearly three times more likely to have adverse cardiac events than normal controls. Their cardiac outcome is improved compared to nonrevascularized patients only beyond 90 days after PCI and stenting with bare-metal stents (64). With the new drug-eluting stents becoming standard PCI therapy, it goes without saying that revascularization, despite its ability to treat the coronary disease, is a solution poorly adapted to the patients who need urgent or vital surgery within tight delays.

ALGORITHM

In the algorithm we propose (Fig. 4), the patients are divided into two categories based on the degree of urgency of the planned operation. For urgent operations, and when

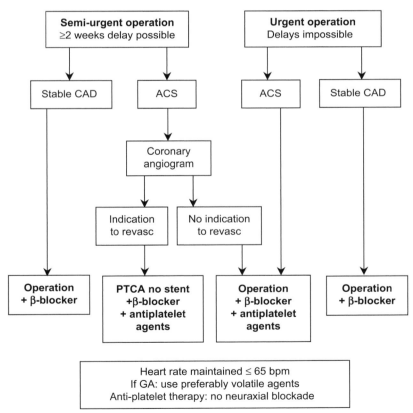

FIGURE 4 General algorithm for evaluating patients suffering from severe CAD and requiring urgent or semiurgent surgery. In case of positive stress tests, a coronary angiogram may be indicated in severe stable CAD if a revascularization is possible. *Abbreviations*: ACS, acute coronary syndrome; PTCA, percutaneous transluminal coronary angioplasty; GA, general anesthesia.

surgery is mandatory within two weeks, coronary revascularization is not an option. PTCA, PCI, and CABG are not conceivable because the perioperative mortality and the infarction rates after noncardiac surgery are dramatically increased during the first weeks following the coronary procedure (49,62–64). Cardiac outcome is at least five times worse than without revascularization, whereas the use of perioperative β-blockade decreases the cardiac mortality from 3.9% to 0.8% and the nonfatal infarction rate from 5% to 0.9% in this category (99). Cardiological tests such as dobutamine echocardiography or thallium-dipyridamole scan are used to select the patients who need a revascularization. They are useless if the noncardiac operation cannot wait for at least six to eight weeks, because it will never be possible to enforce the therapeutic propositions drawn from the tests. Coronary angiography is not indicated if PCI or CABG is not feasible. Patients will be treated according to the degree of their CAD and their tolerance of β-blockade. Patients with stable CAD should be β-blocked in the perioperative period; if they cannot tolerate β-blockade initially, it should be initiated as soon as their hemodynamic status allows to. The treatment should be continued throughout hospital stay.

Patients presenting with an ACS, on the other hand, are at very high risk. Their postoperative cardiac complication rate is above 20% (up to 36%) (78). According to conventional medical management (Fig. 2), these patients should be revascularized. This is obviously not possible in case of life-saving or urgent operations or in case of delays less than two weeks. The only alternative is treatment with an antiplatelet agent (clopidogrel) on top of the β-blockers. If the surgical pathology does not allow antiplatelet therapy to be started before surgery, it should be started as soon as possible, preferentially within six hours postoperatively.

When surgery can be postponed for two to six weeks, the evaluation of functional capacity and the risk associated with the surgical procedure will be crucial in further stratifying the patients. Patients with stable CAD who have good functional capacity and low-risk scores can undergo surgery without further investigation. Patients with poor functional capacity scheduled for any type of surgery, and patients with good functional capacity undergoing major surgery, may be investigated by stress tests (2,3). All patients should be β-blocked preoperatively. If they are already on β-blockade, additional preoperative β-blockade should be considered, the aim being a heart rate of less than 65 bpm. Coronary angiography should be performed for patients with stable CAD if a stress test indicates this is appropriate, and for patients presenting with an ACS. If, on coronary angiography, there is no indication for coronary revascularization, perioperative antiplatelet therapy may be added to the β-blocker therapy. If, on the other hand, coronary revascularization is needed, the cardiologist should consider the delay to surgery imposed by the type of coronary intervention performed. PTCA without stenting may allow noncardiac surgery as soon as two weeks after the revascularization. The use of an intracoronary stent is feasible only if cardiac surgery can be delayed for more than six weeks. These different options will be detailed in the next section. In daily practice, it will most of the time be very difficult to organize invasive testing and coronary angiograms without further delaying the operation. It generally takes two to five days before the revascularization is performed, and the minimal delay after PTCA is two full weeks. As stated before, for these patients, the strategy of perioperative cardioprotection is dictated by the degree of urgency of the noncardiac surgery. If stress testing and angiograms cannot be organized without delay, one should proceed with surgery under β-blockade and possibly antiplatelet agents.

STRATEGIES FOR URGENT OR SEMIURGENT OPERATIONS

In real-life, the anesthesiologist may be facing many different scenarios which can be summarized in a few typical strategies combining the degree of urgency of the procedure, the indication to revascularization, and the risk of operating under medical treatment only. The possible strategies will be laid out according to the grade of emergency of the surgical disease.

LIFE-SAVING PROCEDURES

Some emergencies require an immediate (within four hours) intervention, such as ruptured abdominal aortic aneurysm, aortic dissection type A, acute surgical hemorrhage, acute tamponade, or polytrauma. Nothing can be done specifically to treat the CAD. Maintaining an adequate perfusion pressure and normal oxygen transport, while avoiding very high heart rates, are the principal goals in this situation. β-Blockade may not be well tolerated intraoperatively, but should be reconsidered in the postoperative period as soon as possible. The priority is to relieve the cause of the shock state. Intra-aortic balloon pumping might help to increase the diastolic coronary perfusion and to decrease the left ventricular afterload; however, it is feasible only if the aorta is normal; it is inefficient when the patient is hypovolemic or when the arterial resistance is low.

EMERGENCIES REQUIRING SURGERY WITHIN 48 HOURS

The situations described above may present a less dramatic form when the patient is hemodynamically stable in the emergency room. The procedure is still imperative, but there is more time to optimize the patient's condition. Intracranial compression, by a space-occupying lesion or by a hemorrhage, open fracture, and bowel occlusion or perforation are examples of surgical emergencies falling into this category. There is no time for comprehensive assessment or coronary revascularization. The only justifiable test, if necessary, is transthoracic echocardiography to rule out a significant valvulopathy and determine the ventricular function.

Patients with Severe Chronic CAD

In most cases, these patients are already on full medication. However, it has usually not been taken during the last hours. This interruption is not dangerous for substances without rebound effect, such as statins, angiotensin-converting enzyme (ACE) inhibitors, or calcium entry blockers. However, treatment interruption might precipitate ischemic events in the case of antiplatelet agents and β-blockers. Stent thrombosis and ACSs appear most frequently 5 to 20 days after withdrawal of aspirin (61,68); with drug-eluting stents, this may happen more than a year after stent placement (66). It may seem innocuous to stop the medication two days before the operation, because platelet adhesiveness is still reduced for a week; however, the increased risk of thrombosis will manifest in the postoperative period, during the phase of increased platelet adhesiveness and decreased fibrinolysis. Therefore, antiplatelet treatment should be restarted as soon as possible after completion of the surgical procedure.

Interruption of the β-blockers is immediately harmful, because of an important rebound effect due to the upregulation of β-adrenergic receptors. In order to keep the heart rate at 60 to 65 bpm, it is frequently necessary to adjust the β-blockade to the surgical stimuli by adding intravenous short-acting drugs. Esmolol in repeated bolus (10 mg) or by perfusion (0.1–0.3 mg/kg/min) is an easy way to regulate the hemodynamic response during surgery, although tachyphylaxis is frequent. The main advantage of esmolol is the very high rate of drug elimination, with the effect wearing off a few minutes after interruption of the infusion. If the patient is too unstable for β-blockade before induction, the treatment should be initiated once the patient has stabilized, because ischemia is more common during emergence than during induction of anesthesia. Metoprolol (5–15 mg iv 2–4 times/24 hours) is practical for the postoperative period until the patient is able to take oral medication. In patients not chronically β-blocked and presenting for emergency surgery, intravenous atenolol or metoprolol can be titrated before induction of anesthesia, and continued throughout the perioperative period. For patients with heart failure, very low EFs, acute hypovolemia, or sepsis, β-blockers are not absolutely contraindicated but should be administered with caution.

Patients Shortly After Revascularization

Patients may present with surgical disease requiring emergency operation shortly after coronary revascularization. Aspirin and clopidogrel are mandatory during the re-endothelialization period of the stents. Their interruption during the first three weeks after PCI with stenting leads to an average mortality of 20% (63,64). Drug-eluting stents require antiplatelet treatment for at least three months (paclitaxel stents) or six months (sirolimus stents), but preferentially 9 to 12 months (28). Therefore, antiplatelet agents should be administered as usual, even with the premedication. This practice might increase surgical bleeding by 2.5% to 10% for ASA (100) and 25% for clopidogrel (23). This is acceptable for abdominal or orthopedic surgery, but might be excessive for intracranial surgery. It is up to the anesthesiologist and the surgeon to decide what is best for the patient in each situation, by pondering the risk of bleeding versus the risk of coronary thrombosis. The evidence collected in the recent literature supports a continuation of antiplatelet drugs even at the cost of a slightly elevated risk of bleeding and transfusion. One or two units of transfused blood may be less deleterious than acute myocardial ischemia with infarction.

Patients with Untreated ACS

When patients with untreated ACS present for urgent surgery, revascularization is obviously not an option. The recommended treatment of ACS consists then of nitrate, β-blocker, antiplatelet agents (aspirin and clopidogrel), ACE inhibitors, and statins. The physician should consider introducing antiplatelet therapy for the whole perioperative period. Aspirin should be started at doses between 100 and 300 mg and clopidogrel at 75 mg daily after one loading dose of 300 mg. The effect of clopidogrel cannot easily be interrupted nor antagonized if a hemorrhagic operation requires reversing its action. Therefore, some surgeons would prefer to operate on patients treated by heparin instead of antiplatelet agents. Unfortunately, heparin is a poor choice as a monotherapy, because of its unpredictability in the individual patient. Heparin alone is not recommended by the ACCP guidelines as a therapy for ACS (28). On the other hand, the combination of aspirin and heparin adjusted to an aPTT kept between 1.5 and 2 times the control value (50–70 seconds) has given results similar to aspirin and clopidogrel (27,101). Only a combination of heparin and aspirin can replace dual antiplatelet therapy.

OPERATIONS WITHIN 48 HOURS OF A PERCUTANEOUS CORONARY INTERVENTION OR THROMBOLYSIS

Operations carried out shortly after a PCI or a thrombolysis mainly fall under two headings: (*i*) femoral arteriotomy bleeding or pseudoaneurysmal lesions and (*ii*) intracranial or visceral hemorrhage. Intracranial hemorrhage is the most serious complication of fibrinolytic therapy; its overall incidence is less than 1%, but it varies between 0.3% and 4% depending on the number of risk factors of the patient (102). The principal risk factors are older age, hypertension, history of stroke, and low body weight (103). Operating less than two days after a PCI is certainly a dangerous situation, because the mortality and the incidence of ischemic complications are at least 20% and 30%, respectively, during the first two weeks. However, these numbers come from studies where the antiplatelet drugs were stopped a few days before surgery. This is not the case in the present situation. There are no studies on which we can base recommendations.

The patients may bleed profusely because of the persisting effect of the thrombolytic agent or because they are treated with GPIIb/IIIa inhibitor after PCI. The half-life of tirofiban and eptifibatide is only two hours, whereas it is 23 hours for abciximab. Therefore, platelet transfusions are necessary in case of operation within 24 hours of abciximab to prevent massive blood losses (104); in contrast, six hours after administration of tirofiban or eptifibatide, the hemorrhagic risk is no longer increased (105,106).

When administering platelets, the anesthesiologist must take care not to overshoot and increase the risk of coronary thrombosis. Today physicians cannot rely on standardized platelet function assays to estimate the need for interruption or reversal of antiplatelet therapy. Bleeding time was considered the most useful test of platelet function until the 1990s. But it is poorly reproducible, insensitive, and time-consuming; moreover, it does not correlate with bleeding tendency, platelet inhibition by ASA, and does not predict MI or ischemic stroke (107). Several new assays have been developed and commercialized, some of which have been shown to correlate well to platelet inhibition by non-steroidal anti-inflammatory drugs (NSAIDs) and clopidogrel, and might, in the future, be used for preoperative evaluation of platelet function in order to determine the therapeutical strategy (107,108).

OPERATIONS WITH A DELAY OF TWO WEEKS OR LESS

This situation is frequently encountered in oncology, general surgery, and orthopedics. The prevailing rule is not to revascularize the patient, because the delay is too short to be safe and corresponds to the maximal risk. The only alternative is an optimal medical treatment: in chronic CAD, continuation of the established therapy, including β-blocker and aspirin; in ACS, preparation with a β-blocker and an antiplatelet agent for 5 to 10 days. Atenolol, metoprolol, and bisoprolol have all been investigated for this purpose (2). The dosage is adapted to reach an average heart rate of 60 to 65 bpm. A seven-day preoperative treatment is ideal (99). Aspirin (100–325 mg/day) and clopidogrel (75 mg/day) are the main antiplatelet drugs in use (5,8). All these medications must be maintained without interruption during the perioperative period.

It is useless to perform stress tests or coronary angiography in this situation. They might help to quantify the risk, but their result will not modify the therapeutic choice. If it has not been done recently, a simple transthoracic echocardiography will determine the ventricular function and rule out associated valvulopathy. Its results might influence the choice of the anesthesia technique.

OPERATIONS WITH A DELAY BETWEEN TWO AND SIX WEEKS

If a delay of two weeks or more is possible, a coronary arteriography might be justified in some cases of ACS because revascularization is conceivable under certain circumstances. When the coronary flow is extremely unstable, when the stenosis is extremely tight and proximal, and when the amount of threatened myocardium is large, it is possible to consider a PTCA without stenting. In two studies from the Mayo Clinic performed before the era of coronary stents, major vascular surgery was performed on average 9 to 10 days after simple coronary angioplasty (109,110); overall mortality of surgery was halved and infarction rate five times less in the groups having previous PTCA compared with nonrevascularized patients. After a median interval of 11 days between PTCA without stenting and vascular surgery, Gottlieb et al. (111) reported an infarction and mortality rate of only 0.5%. In a review of 345 patients who underwent different types of noncardiac surgery within 60 days of balloon angioplasty without stenting (PTCA), global mortality and nonfatal MI rates were 0.3% and 0.6%, respectively (112). Among 188 patients who underwent surgery within two weeks of PTCA, only three major adverse cardiac events (one death and two MIs) were noted. Only nine patients needed target vessel revascularization within the seven-week postoperative period. Therefore, PTCA without stenting may be a safe means of revascularization for patients who need a surgical operation within two to six weeks (112).

The absence of stent reduces the thrombotic risk and avoids the mandatory delay of six weeks. It allows the patient to undergo a noncardiac operation much earlier after revascularization, and is not necessarily a second best choice treatment for the patient. A recent meta-analysis reveals that, when optimal coronary dilatation is obtained with simple balloon angioplasty, the rates of major adverse cardiac events, repeat revascularization, and death up to 12 months are similar between PTCA without stenting and PCI with immediate routine bare-metal stents (113). Nevertheless, the patients should be placed under aspirin and clopidogrel therapy during the whole perioperative period. Coronary revascularization makes sense only if there is an impending infarction threatening a large area of myocardium, whose mortality, in case of noncardiac surgery, would be more than 20%; this would be higher than the mortality of an operation performed within six weeks of a PCI or CABG, which is 10% to 20%. It is worth noting, although, that these conditions usually correspond to tight proximal stenoses, which are an indication for CABG rather than to PCI (Fig. 2). The situation is therefore more complex, because the surgical pathology might contraindicate revascularization on bypass with full heparinization, for example, an intracranial tumor. Off-pump coronary artery surgery could be a more appropriate solution in these cases (114). This is fortunately a rare situation, because it arises in less than 2% of the patients scheduled for vascular surgery, who have the highest incidence of CAD of all the surgical population (78).

ANESTHESIA CARE

The objective of protecting the heart from ischemia continues during the intraoperative period. The technique of anesthesia is dominated by the priority of reducing myocardial oxygen consumption (VO_2) and increasing oxygen delivery (DO_2). There are many techniques for maintaining the DO_2/VO_2 ratio and for reducing noxious stimuli and sympathetic stimulation. However, two important facts deserve a special mention because they concern directly the management of patients with severe ischemic heart disease undergoing urgent or vital noncardiac surgery: the use of neuraxial blockade and the importance of volatile halogenated agents.

NEURAXIAL BLOCKADE

In the preoperative period, sympatholysis with a β-blocker and platelet aggregation prevention with aspirin and clopidogrel are additive cardioprotective treatments of severe CAD and unstable coronary syndromes. During the intraoperative period, however, sympatholysis can be completed by neuraxial blockade with epidural or intrathecal anesthesia, but these techniques are contraindicated with concomitant antiplatelet therapy. The anesthetist is forced to choose between two different options: (*i*) maintaining the protective effect of clopidogrel on unstable plaques and uncovered stents and proceeding with conventional general anesthesia or (*ii*) stopping clopidogrel for at least 10 days before the operation in order to perform epidural or combined anesthesia and benefit from its sympatholytic and analgesic effects. Both solutions have their advocates.

Neuraxial sympatholysis is beneficial on the ischemic myocardium as long as the cardiac nerves are blocked; therefore, the reduction in the incidence of intraoperative ischemia and postoperative MI is significant only with high thoracic epidural anesthesia, where it has been recorded as high as 40% (115–117). It does not reach significance with low thoracic or lumbar epidural anesthesia, nor with an intrathecal technique (115,118,119). Epidural anesthesia, alone or in combination with general anesthesia, did not modify mortality nor infarction rate in a meta-analysis of 11 randomized trials (1173 patients) (115). Almost all comparative clinical studies have related a significant improvement in postoperative analgesia with epidural anesthesia, regardless of analgesic agent or location of the catheter, and despite a failure rate of up to 30% for thoracic epidural analgesia (120,121). Neuraxial blockade has an antithrombotic effect: it slightly reduces the incidence of postoperative pulmonary embolism (122) and the rate of thrombosis after peripheral arterial surgery (123). Unfortunately, these advantages are possible only at the cost of withdrawing the antiplatelet agents two weeks before the operation.

In ACS and during the re-endothelialization phase of coronary stents, this withdrawal is associated with a two to five times increase in mortality and infarction rate (60,62,65,68). This is much higher than the 40% decrease in MI observed with high thoracic (and only high thoracic) epidurals. As the intra- and postoperative "acute-phase syndrome" is accompanied by increased platelet adhesiveness and decreased fibrinolysis (124), it is not surprising that the risk of native coronary or stent thrombosis is particularly high when the protection of antiplatelet agents is removed. Of note, there is no study showing that the antithrombotic effect of epidural anesthesia might be superior to the effect of clopidogrel and aspirin.

In ACS due to unstable coronary plaques and during the early phase after coronary stenting, it seems therefore safer to continue aspirin and clopidogrel throughout the operative period and to forgo using neuraxial blockade. The intraoperative sympatholysis of epidural anesthesia can be realized as well with intravenous substances such as β-blockers, α-agonists, and higher dosages of opioids (125). The only real disadvantage is a lack of equivalence in the quality of postoperative analgesia and comfort for the patient.

VOLATILE AGENTS

It has been argued for more than 15 years that the choice of the primary agent of anesthesia did not modify the outcome after coronary artery surgery (126,127). This dogma was extrapolated to noncardiac surgery. The recent discovery of the preconditioning effect of halogenated agents may replace this concept of equivalence of anesthesia techniques by the idea that the anesthetist himself can substantially influence the ischemic process by choosing the right substance. Preconditioning, defined as improvement of tolerance to ischemia by brief ischemic bouts followed by reperfusion, is an attractive experimental technique for protecting the myocardium (chap. 7) (128). It can also be induced pharmacologically. Experimental studies have shown that volatile anesthetics such as isoflurane, sevoflurane, or desflurane protect the myocardium against ischemic and reperfusion lesions by activation of a preconditioning-like mechanism when administered at 1.5 minimum alveolar concentrations at least 30 minutes prior to the ischemic insult (129,130). In CABG surgery, the use of isoflurane or sevoflurane as the main anesthetic agent is associated with a better preservation of left ventricular function, with a lower postoperative release of troponin I, and with a shorter length of stay in postoperative intensive care compared to a total intravenous anesthetic regimen (131–134). The cardioprotective effect is most apparent when the agent is administered throughout the entire surgical procedure (135). Experimental data have revealed that halogenated agents may produce a second window of cardioprotection at 24 hours, lasting up to 72 hours (136,137). Collectively, these observations tend to indicate that administration of halogenated anesthetic gases may limit the adverse effects of intra- and postoperative ischemic myocardial damage.

There are no prospective studies on the impact of halogenated agents in noncardiac surgery, but some retrospective data on abdominal aortic operations seem to show a trend towards a lower postoperative troponin I release when a volatile anesthetic is used (138). To the best of our knowledge, it seems therefore reasonable to prefer the use of isoflurane, sevoflurane, or desflurane as the main anesthetic agent for the patient suffering from CAD.

In contrast to halogenated agents, other volatiles have a detrimental effect on cardiac outcome. Two trials have disclosed that nitrous oxide increases the incidence of intraoperative and postoperative myocardial ischemia (139,140); it also increases homocysteine levels postoperatively, which may negatively influence platelet reactivity and endothelial function (140). As nitrous oxide is a poor anesthetic agent, it should be completely avoided in anesthesia for patients suffering from myocardial ischemia.

POSTOPERATIVE CARE

The greatest risk of ischemia and infarction occurs during the first days after surgery. Postoperative MI is known to be associated with early postoperative long-lasting episodes of ischemia, which are silent most of the time, and therefore difficult to diagnose (141,142). Half of the postoperative infarctions after aortic abdominal surgery occurs with an average delay of 74 hours in individuals who have had a discrete but constant increase in troponin levels since the first postoperative hours (143). In surgical intensive care units, it has been shown that any increase in the troponin level, even below the threshold for myocardial necrosis, is a powerful predictor correlated with long-term mortality (144). Therefore, routine monitoring of cardiac enzymes in patients at risk may be useful to unmask silent ischemia during the postoperative period. A slightly elevated troponin level should therefore alert the physician of an ongoing ischemia. Maximal cardioprotection should be offered to the patient by regulating heart rate and myocardial oxygen consumption with β-blockers, α-agonists, antihypertensive agents, and adequate analgesia.

Continuous ST segment monitoring is potentially valuable during the first postoperative days in patients at risk. Outside intensive care units, it is best realized by telemetry. In the event of ST elevation, it may be appropriate to take the patient to the cardiac catheter lab for a coronary angiogram and a PCI. Unfortunately, it is not possible to use IIb/IIIa inhibitors in the first 24 to 48 hours after surgery, because of the risk of catastrophic bleeding. Treatment of chronic CAD or ACSs must be restarted as soon as possible after the operation, not only with β-blockers and antihypertensive drugs but also with antiplatelet agents, such as ASA and clopidogrel. This is particularly important because of the postoperative state of hyperaggregability and decreased fibrinolysis.

CONCLUSIONS

The management of patients with severe CAD or unstable coronary syndrome requiring urgent or semiurgent surgery is governed by a few principles which differ from the standard perioperative care. They can be summarized in the following headlines.

- β-Blockade is imperative; if the patient is already under chronic β-blocker therapy, the treatment needs to be adjusted to meticulously achieve a heart rate of 60 to 65 bpm; stopping β-blocker induces a dangerous rebound effect.
- ASA is a lifelong therapy for CAD patients; the risk of coronary thrombosis due to its interruption is higher than the risk of bleeding.
- Clopidogrel is indicated in ACS and during endothelialization of stents; early withdrawal is associated with an unacceptable increase in the risk of coronary thrombosis; this risk is further increased by the state of hypercoagulability characteristic of the postoperative period. Despite the risk of augmented bleeding, it should be continued during the perioperative period, with the probable exception of intracranial surgery. Heparin alone is not an efficacious alternative.
- When surgery must be performed within two weeks, revascularization is not possible, and coronary angiogram or stress tests are useless. Patients with chronic severe CAD must be β-blocked and their usual medication maintained. Patients with ACS should also be β-blocked, but in addition clopidogrel should be initiated and continued throughout the perioperative period.
- Revascularization is possible only if it is acceptable to delay surgery, and only if the coronary stenosis is highly unstable and/or threatens a large area of myocardium. If surgery can be delayed for more than six weeks, a PCI with bare-metal stent is possible; if the delay is two weeks, a PTCA without stenting is conceivable; in both cases, the protection of clopidogrel must continue throughout the perioperative period.
- Central neuraxial blockade (epidural and intrathecal) is feasible under low-dose ASA (≤300 mg), but contraindicated in patients receiving clopidogrel;

nevertheless, the risk/benefit ratio leans in favor of continuing antiplatelet therapy and thus not performing central neuraxial blocks.

■ General anesthesia, if indicated, should be performed with halogenated agents.

■ Careful anesthesia with tight control of heart rate and maximized perioperative anti-ischemic therapy should maintain the cardiac complication rate at an acceptable level in these high-risk situations.

REFERENCES

1. Guidelines for assessing and managing the perioperative risk from coronary artery disease associated with major noncardiac surgery. American College of Physicians. Ann Intern Med 1997; 127(4):309–312.
2. Eagle KA, Berger PB, Calkins H, et al. ACC/AHA guideline update for perioperative cardiovascular evaluation for noncardiac surgery—executive summary. A Report of the American College of Cardiology/American Heart Association Task Force on Practice Guidelines (Committee to Update the 1996 Guidelines on Perioperative Cardiovascular Evaluation for Noncardiac Surgery). Circulation 2002; 105(10):1257–1267.
3. Chassot PG, Delabays A, Spahn DR. Preoperative evaluation of patients with, or at risk of, coronary artery disease undergoing non-cardiac surgery. Br J Anaesth 2002; 89(5):747–759.
4. Campeau L. Grading in angina pactoris. Circulation 1976; 54:522–524.
5. Cannon CP, Braunwald E. Unstable angina and non-ST elevation myocardial infarction. In: Zipes DP, Libby P, Bonow RO, Braunwald E, eds. Braunwald's Heart Disease: A Textbook of Cardiovascular Medicine. Philadelphia: Elsevier/Saunders, 2005:1243–1279.
6. Antman EM, Cohen M, Bernink PJ, et al. The TIMI risk score for unstable angina/non-ST elevation MI: a method for prognostication and therapeutic decision making. J Am Med Assoc 2000; 284(7):835–842.
7. Boersma E, Pieper KS, Steyerberg EW, et al. Predictors of outcome in patients with acute coronary syndromes without persistent ST-segment elevation. Results from an international trial of 9461 patients: the pursuit investigators. Circulation 2000; 101(22): 2557–2567.
8. Braunwald E. Application of current guidelines to the management of unstable angina and non-ST-elevation myocardial infarction. Circulation 2003; 108(16, suppl 1):III28–III37.
9. Cannon CP, Weintraub WS, Demopoulos LA, et al. Comparison of early invasive and conservative strategies in patients with unstable coronary syndromes treated with the glycoprotein IIb/IIIa inhibitor tirofiban. N Engl J Med 2001; 344(25):1879–1887.
10. Mehta SR, Cannon CP, Fox KA, et al. Routine vs selective invasive strategies in patients with acute coronary syndromes: a collaborative meta-analysis of randomized trials. J Am Med Assoc 2005; 293(23):2908–2917.
11. Fox KA, Poole-Wilson PA, Henderson RA, et al. Interventional versus conservative treatment for patients with unstable angina or non-ST-elevation myocardial infarction. The British Heart Foundation RITA 3 randomised trial: randomized intervention trial of unstable angina. Lancet 2002; 360(9335):743–751.
12. Braunwald E, Antman EM, Beasley JW, et al. ACC/AHA guideline update for the management of patients with unstable angina and non-ST-segment elevation myocardial infarction 2002: summary article. A Report of the American College of Cardiology/American Heart Association Task Force on Practice Guidelines (Committee on the Management of Patients with Unstable Angina). Circulation 2002; 106(14):1893–1900.
13. Collaboration AT. Collaborative meta-analysis of randomised trials of antiplatelet therapy for prevention of death, myocardial infarction, and stroke in high risk patients. Br Med J 2002; 324(7329):71–86.
14. Patrono C. Aspirin as an antiplatelet drug. N Engl J Med 1994; 330(18):1287–1294.
15. Harder S, Klinkhardt U, Alvarez JM. Avoidance of bleeding during surgery in patients receiving anticoagulant and/or antiplatelet therapy: pharmacokinetic and pharmacodynamic considerations. Clin Pharmacokinet 2004; 43(14):963–981.

16. Heptinstall S, May JA, Glenn JR, et al. Effects of ticlopidine administered to healthy volunteers on platelet function in whole blood. Thromb Haemost 1995; 74(5):1310–1315.
17. Weber AA, Braun M, Hohlfeld T, et al. Recovery of platelet function after discontinuation of clopidogrel treatment in healthy volunteers. Br J Clin Pharmacol 2001; 52(3):333–336.
18. Kleiman NS. Pharmacokinetics and pharmacodynamics of glycoprotein IIb–IIIa inhibitors. Am Heart J 1999; 138(4, pt 2):263–275.
19. Faulds D, Sorkin EM. Abciximab (c7E3 Fab): a review of its pharmacology and therapeutic potential in ischaemic heart disease. Drugs 1994; 48(4):583–598.
20. Harrington RA, Becker RC, Ezekowitz M, et al. Antithrombotic therapy for coronary artery disease: the Seventh ACCP Conference on Antithrombotic and Thrombolytic Therapy. Chest 2004; 126(suppl 3):513S–548S.
21. Peters RJ, Mehta SR, Fox KA, et al. Effects of aspirin dose when used alone or in combination with clopidogrel in patients with acute coronary syndromes: observations from the clopidogrel in unstable angina to prevent recurrent events (CURE) study. Circulation 2003; 108(14):1682–1687.
22. A randomised, blinded, trial of clopidogrel versus aspirin in patients at risk of ischaemic events (CAPRIE). CAPRIE Steering Committee. Lancet 1996; 348(9038):1329–1339.
23. Yusuf S, Zhao F, Mehta SR, et al. Effects of clopidogrel in addition to aspirin in patients with acute coronary syndromes without ST-segment elevation. N Engl J Med 2001; 345(7):494–502.
24. Hirsh J, Bhatt DL. Comparative benefits of clopidogrel and aspirin in high-risk patient populations: lessons from the CAPRIE and CURE studies. Arch Intern Med 2004; 164(19):2106–2110.
25. Ueda Y, Nanto S, Komamura K, et al. Neointimal coverage of stents in human coronary arteries observed by angioscopy. J Am Coll Cardiol 1994; 23(2):341–346.
26. Kastrati A, Dibra A, Eberle S, et al. Sirolimus-eluting stents vs paclitaxel-eluting stents in patients with coronary artery disease: meta-analysis of randomized trials. J Am Med Assoc 2005; 294(7):819–825.
27. Mehta SR, Yusuf S, Peters RJ, et al. Effects of pretreatment with clopidogrel and aspirin followed by long-term therapy in patients undergoing percutaneous coronary intervention: the PCI-CURE study. Lancet 2001; 358(9281):527–533.
28. Popma JJ, Berger P, Ohman EM, et al. Antithrombotic therapy during percutaneous coronary intervention: the Seventh ACCP Conference on Antithrombotic and Thrombolytic Therapy. Chest 2004; 126(suppl 3):576S–599S.
29. Theroux P, Ouimet H, McCans J, et al. Aspirin, heparin or both to treat acute unstable angina. N Engl J Med 1988; 319(17):1105–1111.
30. Cohen M, Adams PC, Hawkins L, et al. Usefulness of antithrombotic therapy in resting angina pectoris or non-Q-wave myocardial infarction in preventing death and myocardial infarction (A Pilot Study from the Antithrombotic Therapy in Acute Coronary Syndromes Study Group). Am J Cardiol 1990; 66(19):1287–1292.
31. Cohen M, Adams PC, Parry G, et al. Combination antithrombotic therapy in unstable rest angina and non-Q-wave infarction in nonprior aspirin users: primary end points analysis from the ATACS trial. Antithrombotic Therapy in Acute Coronary Syndromes Research Group. Circulation 1994; 89(1):81–88.
32. Risk of myocardial infarction and death during treatment with low dose aspirin and intravenous heparin in men with unstable coronary artery disease. The RISC Group. Lancet 1990; 336(8719):827–830.
33. Lee MS, Wali AU, Menon V, et al. The determinants of activated partial thromboplastin time, relation of activated partial thromboplastin time to clinical outcomes, and optimal dosing regimens for heparin treated patients with acute coronary syndromes: a review of GUSTO-IIb. J Thromb Thrombolysis 2002; 14(2):91–101.
34. Granger CB, Hirsh J, Califf RM, et al. Activated partial thromboplastin time and outcome after thrombolytic therapy for acute myocardial infarction: results from the GUSTO-I trial. Circulation 1996; 93(5):870–878.
35. Arnout J, Simoons M, de Bono D, et al. Correlation between level of heparinization and patency of the infarct-related coronary artery after treatment of acute myocardial infarction with alteplase (rt-PA). J Am Coll Cardiol 1992; 20(3):513–519.

36. Bozovich GE, Gurfinkel EP, Antman EM, et al. Superiority of enoxaparin versus unfractionated heparin for unstable angina/non-Q-wave myocardial infarction regardless of activated partial thromboplastin time. Am Heart J 2000; 140(4):637–642.

37. De Cristofaro R, De Candia E, Landolfi R. Effect of high- and low-molecular-weight heparins on thrombin–thrombomodulin interaction and protein C activation. Circulation 1998; 98(13):1297–1301.

38. Warkentin TE. Heparin-induced thrombocytopenia: IgG-mediated platelet activation, platelet microparticle generation, and altered procoagulant/anticoagulant balance in the pathogenesis of thrombosis and venous limb gangrene complicating heparin-induced thrombocytopenia. Transfus Med Rev 1996; 10(4):249–258.

39. Fijnheer R, Urbanus RT, Nieuwenhuis HK. Withdrawing the use of acetylsalicyclic acid prior to an operation usually not necessary. Ned Tijdschr Geneeskd 2003; 147(1):21–25.

40. Lindblad B, Persson NH, Takolander R, et al. Does low-dose acetylsalicylic acid prevent stroke after carotid surgery? A double-blind, placebo-controlled randomized trial. Stroke 1993; 24(8):1125–1128.

41. McCollum C, Alexander C, Kenchington G, et al. Antiplatelet drugs in femoropopliteal vein bypasses: a multicenter trial. J Vasc Surg 1991; 13(1):150–161; discussion 161–152.

42. Findlay JM, Lougheed WM, Gentili F, et al. Effect of perioperative platelet inhibition on postcarotid endarterectomy mural thrombus formation: results of a prospective randomized controlled trial using aspirin and dipyridamole in humans. J Neurosurg 1985; 63(5):693–698.

43. Kitchen L, Erichson RB, Sideropoulos H. Effect of drug-induced platelet dysfunction on surgical bleeding. Am J Surg 1982; 143(2):215–217.

44. CLASP: a randomised trial of low-dose aspirin for the prevention and treatment of preeclampsia among 9364 pregnant women. CLASP (Collaborative Low-dose Aspirin Study in Pregnancy) Collaborative Group. Lancet 1994; 343(8898):619–629.

45. Ferraris VA, Swanson E. Aspirin usage and perioperative blood loss in patients undergoing unexpected operations. Surg Gynecol Obstet 1983; 156(4):439–442.

46. Horlocker TT, Wedel DJ, Schroeder DR, et al. Preoperative antiplatelet therapy does not increase the risk of spinal hematoma associated with regional anesthesia. Anesth Analg 1995; 80(2):303–309.

47. Harris WH, Salzman EW, Athanasoulis CA, et al. Aspirin prophylaxis of venous thromboembolism after total hip replacement. N Engl J Med 1977; 297(23):1246–1249.

48. Amrein PC, Ellman L, Harris WH. Aspirin-induced prolongation of bleeding time and perioperative blood loss. J Am Med Assoc 1981; 245(18):1825–1828.

49. Wilson SH, Fasseas P, Orford JL, et al. Clinical outcome of patients undergoing noncardiac surgery in the two months following coronary stenting. J Am Coll Cardiol 2003; 42(2):234–240.

50. Hui AJ, Wong RM, Ching JY, et al. Risk of colonoscopic polypectomy bleeding with anticoagulants and antiplatelet agents: analysis of 1657 cases. Gastrointest Endosc 2004; 59(1):44–48.

51. Wahidi MM, Garland R, Feller-Kopman D, et al. Effect of clopidogrel with and without aspirin on bleeding following transbronchial lung biopsy. Chest 2005; 127(3):961–964.

52. Lipsic E, van der Horst IC, Voors AA, et al. Hemoglobin levels and 30-day mortality in patients after myocardial infarction. Int J Cardiol 2005; 100(2):289–292.

53. Wu WC, Rathore SS, Wang Y, et al. Blood transfusion in elderly patients with acute myocardial infarction. N Engl J Med 2001; 345(17):1230–1236.

54. Rao SV, Jollis JG, Harrington RA, et al. Relationship of blood transfusion and clinical outcomes in patients with acute coronary syndromes. J Am Med Assoc 2004; 292(13):1555–1562.

55. Spahn DR, Schmid ER, Seifert B, et al. Hemodilution tolerance in patients with coronary artery disease who are receiving chronic beta-adrenergic blocker therapy. Anesth Analg 1996; 82(4):687–694.

56. Hebert PC, Wells G, Blajchman MA, et al. A multicenter, randomized, controlled clinical trial of transfusion requirements in critical care. Transfusion Requirements in Critical Care Investigators, Canadian Critical Care Trials Group. N Engl J Med 1999; 340(6):409–417.

57. Spahn DR, Dettori N, Kocian R, et al. Transfusion in the cardiac patient. Crit Care Clin 2004; 20(2):269–279.

58. Spahn DR, Smith LR, Veronee CD, et al. Acute isovolemic hemodilution and blood transfusion: effects on regional function and metabolism in myocardium with compromised coronary blood flow. J Thorac Cardiovasc Surg 1993; 105(4):694–704.

59. Zollinger A, Hager P, Singer T, et al. Extreme hemodilution due to massive blood loss in tumor surgery. Anesthesiology 1997; 87(4):985–987.

60. Allen LaPointe NM, Kramer JM, DeLong ER, et al. Patient-reported frequency of taking aspirin in a population with coronary artery disease. Am J Cardiol 2002; 89(9):1042–1046.

61. Ferrari E, Benhamou M, Cerboni P, et al. Coronary syndromes following aspirin withdrawal: a special risk for late stent thrombosis. J Am Coll Cardiol 2005; 45(3):456–459.

62. Sharma AK, Ajani AE, Hamwi SM, et al. Major noncardiac surgery following coronary stenting: when is it safe to operate? Catheter Cardiovasc Interv 2004; 63(2):141–145.

63. Kaluza GL, Joseph J, Lee JR, et al. Catastrophic outcomes of noncardiac surgery soon after coronary stenting. J Am Coll Cardiol 2000; 35(5):1288–1294.

64. Posner KL, Van Norman GA, Chan V. Adverse cardiac outcomes after noncardiac surgery in patients with prior percutaneous transluminal coronary angioplasty. Anesth Analg 1999; 89(3):553–560.

65. Iakovou I, Schmidt T, Bonizzoni E, et al. Incidence, predictors, and outcome of thrombosis after successful implantation of drug-eluting stents. J Am Med Assoc 2005; 293(17): 2126–2130.

66. McFadden EP, Stabile E, Regar E, et al. Late thrombosis in drug-eluting coronary stents after discontinuation of antiplatelet therapy. Lancet 2004; 364(9444):1519–1521.

67. Collet JP, Himbet F, Steg PG. Myocardial infarction after aspirin cessation in stable coronary artery disease patients. Int J Cardiol 2000; 76(2–3):257–258.

68. Collet JP, Montalescot G, Blanchet B, et al. Impact of prior use or recent withdrawal of oral antiplatelet agents on acute coronary syndromes. Circulation 2004; 110(16):2361–2367.

69. Vial JH, McLeod LJ, Roberts MS. Rebound elevation in urinary thromboxane B2 and 6-keto-PGF1 alpha excretion after aspirin withdrawal. Adv Prostaglandin Thromboxane Leukot Res 1991; 21A:157–160.

70. Samama CM, Thiry D, Elalamy I, et al. Perioperative activation of hemostasis in vascular surgery patients. Anesthesiology 2001; 94(1):74–78.

71. Thaulow E, Erikssen J, Sandvik L, et al. Blood platelet count and function are related to total and cardiovascular death in apparently healthy men. Circulation 1991; 84(2):613–617.

72. Lam JY, Latour JG, Lesperance J, et al. Platelet aggregation, coronary artery disease progression and future coronary events. Am J Cardiol 1994; 73(5):333–338.

73. Zaugg M, Schaub MC, Pasch T, et al. Modulation of beta-adrenergic receptor subtype activities in perioperative medicine: mechanisms and sites of action. Br J Anaesth 2002; 88(1):101–123.

74. London MJ, Zaugg M, Schaub MC, et al. Perioperative beta-adrenergic receptor blockade: physiologic foundations and clinical controversies. Anesthesiology 2004; 100(1):170–175.

75. Yeager MP, Fillinger MP, Hettleman BD, et al. Perioperative beta-blockade and late cardiac outcomes: a complementary hypothesis. J Cardiothorac Vasc Anesth 2005; 19(2):237–241.

76. Mangano DT, Layug EL, Wallace A, et al. Effect of atenolol on mortality and cardiovascular morbidity after noncardiac surgery. Multicenter Study of Perioperative Ischemia Research Group. N Engl J Med 1996; 335(23):1713–1720.

77. Lee TH, Marcantonio ER, Mangione CM, et al. Derivation and prospective validation of a simple index for prediction of cardiac risk of major noncardiac surgery. Circulation 1999; 100(10):1043–1049.

78. Boersma E, Poldermans D, Bax JJ, et al. Predictors of cardiac events after major vascular surgery: role of clinical characteristics, dobutamine echocardiography, and beta-blocker therapy. J Am Med Assoc 2001; 285(14):1865–1873.

79. Lindenauer PK, Pekow P, Wang K, et al. Perioperative beta-blocker therapy and mortality after major noncardiac surgery. N Engl J Med 2005; 353(4):349–361.

80. Park KW, Subramaniam K, Mahmood F, et al. Patients with positive preoperative stress tests undergoing vascular surgery. J Cardiothorac Vasc Anesth 2005; 19(4):494–498.

81. Yang HR, Butler K, Parlow R, Roberts J, Tech R. Metoprolol after Vascular Surgery. Can J Anaesth 2004; 51:A7 (abstract).

82. Kertai MD, Bax JJ, Klein J, et al. Is there any reason to withhold beta blockers from high-risk patients with coronary artery disease during surgery? Anesthesiology 2004; 100(1):4–7.

83. Akhtar S, Amin M, Tantawy H, et al. Preoperative beta-blocker use: is titration to a heart rate of 60 beats per minute a consistently attainable goal? J Clin Anesth 2005; 17(3):191–197.

84. Warltier DC. Beta-adrenergic-blocking drugs: incredibly useful, incredibly underutilized. Anesthesiology 1998; 88(1):2–5.

85. Siddiqui AK, Ahmed S, Delbeau H, et al. Lack of physician concordance with guidelines on the perioperative use of beta-blockers. Arch Intern Med 2004; 164(6):664–667.

86. Sprung J, Abdelmalak B, Gottlieb A, et al. Analysis of risk factors for myocardial infarction and cardiac mortality after major vascular surgery. Anesthesiology 2000; 93(1):129–140.

87. Brodde OE, Daul A, Michel MC. Subtype-selective modulation of human beta 1- and beta 2-adrenoceptor function by beta-adrenoceptor agonists and antagonists. Clin Physiol Biochem 1990; 8(suppl 2):11–17.

88. Psaty BM, Koepsell TD, Wagner EH, et al. The relative risk of incident coronary heart disease associated with recently stopping the use of beta-blockers. J Am Med Assoc 1990; 263(12):1653–1657.

89. Shammash JB, Trost JC, Gold JM, et al. Perioperative beta-blocker withdrawal and mortality in vascular surgical patients. Am Heart J 2001; 141(1):148–153.

90. Giles JW, Sear JW, Foex P. Effect of chronic beta-blockade on peri-operative outcome in patients undergoing non-cardiac surgery: an analysis of observational and case control studies. Anaesthesia 2004; 59(6):574–583.

91. Reich DL, Bennett-Guerrero E, Bodian CA, et al. Intraoperative tachycardia and hypertension are independently associated with adverse outcome in noncardiac surgery of long duration. Anesth Analg 2002; 95(2):273–277, table of contents.

92. Eagle KA, Rihal CS, Mickel MC, et al. Cardiac risk of noncardiac surgery: influence of coronary disease and type of surgery in 3368 operations. CASS Investigators and University of Michigan Heart Care Program: Coronary Artery Surgery Study. Circulation 1997; 96(6):1882–1887.

93. Hassan SA, Hlatky MA, Boothroyd DB, et al. Outcomes of noncardiac surgery after coronary bypass surgery or coronary angioplasty in the Bypass Angioplasty Revascularization Investigation (BARI). Am J Med 2001; 110(4):260–266.

94. Cutlip DE, Baim DS, Ho KK, et al. Stent thrombosis in the modern era: a pooled analysis of multicenter coronary stent clinical trials. Circulation 2001; 103(15):1967–1971.

95. Nalysnyk L, Fahrbach K, Reynolds MW, et al. Adverse events in coronary artery bypass graft (CABG) trials: a systematic review and analysis. Heart 2003; 89(7):767–772.

96. Rihal CS, Sutton-Tyrrell K, Guo P, et al. Increased incidence of periprocedural complications among patients with peripheral vascular disease undergoing myocardial revascularization in the bypass angioplasty revascularization investigation. Circulation 1999; 100(2):171–177.

97. Khuri SF, Daley J, Henderson W, et al. The National Veterans Administration Surgical Risk Study: risk adjustment for the comparative assessment of the quality of surgical care. J Am Coll Surg 1995; 180(5):519–531.

98. Breen P, Lee JW, Pomposelli F, et al. Timing of high-risk vascular surgery following coronary artery bypass surgery: a 10-year experience from an academic medical centre. Anaesthesia 2004; 59(5):422–427.

99. Stevens RD, Burri H, Tramer MR. Pharmacologic myocardial protection in patients undergoing noncardiac surgery: a quantitative systematic review. Anesth Analg 2003; 97(3):623–633.

100. Ridker PM, Cushman M, Stampfer MJ, et al. Inflammation, aspirin, and the risk of cardiovascular disease in apparently healthy men. N Engl J Med 1997; 336(14):973–979.

101. Oler A, Whooley MA, Oler J, et al. Adding heparin to aspirin reduces the incidence of myocardial infarction and death in patients with unstable angina: a meta-analysis. J Am Med Assoc 1996; 276(10):811–815.

102. Brass LM, Lichtman JH, Wang Y, et al. Intracranial hemorrhage associated with throm-

bolytic therapy for elderly patients with acute myocardial infarction: results from the Cooperative Cardiovascular Project. Stroke 2000; 31(8):1802–1811.

103. Sloan MA, Giugliano RP, Thompson SL, et al. Prediction of intracranial hemorrhage in the InTIME-II trial. J Am Coll Cardiol 2001; 37(suppl A):372A.

104. Juergens CP, Yeung AC, Oesterle SN. Routine platelet transfusion in patients undergoing emergency coronary bypass surgery after receiving abciximab. Am J Cardiol 1997; 80(1):74–75.

105. Dyke CM, Bhatia D, Lorenz TJ, et al. Immediate coronary artery bypass surgery after platelet inhibition with eptifibatide: results from PURSUIT. Platelet Glycoprotein IIb/IIIa in Unstable Angina: Receptor Suppression Using Integrelin Therapy. Ann Thorac Surg 2000; 70(3):866–871; discussion 871–862.

106. Genoni M, Zeller D, Bertel O, et al. Tirofiban therapy does not increase the risk of hemorrhage after emergency coronary surgery. J Thorac Cardiovasc Surg 2001; 122(3):630–632.

107. Harrison P. Platelet function analysis. Blood Rev 2005; 19(2):111–123.

108. Craft RM, Chavez JJ, Snider CC, et al. Comparison of modified thrombelastograph and platelet works whole blood assays to optical platelet aggregation for monitoring reversal of clopidogrel inhibition in elective surgery patients. J Lab Clin Med 2005; 145(6):309–315.

109. Huber KC, Evans MA, Bresnahan JF, et al. Outcome of noncardiac operations in patients with severe coronary artery disease successfully treated preoperatively with coronary angioplasty. Mayo Clin Proc 1992; 67(1):15–21.

110. Elmore JR, Hallett JW Jr, Gibbons RJ, et al. Myocardial revascularization before abdominal aortic aneurysmorrhaphy: effect of coronary angioplasty. Mayo Clin Proc 1993; 68(7):637–641.

111. Gottlieb A, Banoub M, Sprung J, et al. Perioperative cardiovascular morbidity in patients with coronary artery disease undergoing vascular surgery after percutaneous transluminal coronary angioplasty. J Cardiothorac Vasc Anesth 1998; 12(5):501–506.

112. Brilakis ES, Orford JL, Fasseas P, et al. Outcome of patients undergoing balloon angioplasty in the two months prior to noncardiac surgery. Am J Cardiol 2005; 96(4):512–514.

113. Agostini P, Biodi-Zoccai GGL, Gasparini GL, et al. Is bare-metal stenting superior to balloon angioplasty for small vessel coronary artery disease? Evidence from a meta-analysis of randomised trials. Eur Heart J 2005; 26:881–889.

114. Woo YJ, Grand T, Valettas N. Off-pump coronary artery bypass grafting attenuates postoperative bleeding associated with preoperative clopidogrel administration. Heart Surg Forum 2003; 6(5):282–285.

115. Beattie WS, Badner NH, Choi P. Epidural analgesia reduces postoperative myocardial infarction: a meta-analysis. Anesth Analg 2001; 93(4):853–858.

116. Rodgers A, Walker N, Schug S, et al. Reduction of postoperative mortality and morbidity with epidural or spinal anaesthesia: results from overview of randomised trials. Br Med J 2000; 321(7275):1493.

117. Park WY, Thompson JS, Lee KK. Effect of epidural anesthesia and analgesia on perioperative outcome: a randomized, controlled Veterans Affairs Cooperative Study. Ann Surg 2001; 234(4):560–569; discussion 569–571.

118. O'Hara DA, Duff A, Berlin JA, et al. The effect of anesthetic technique on postoperative outcomes in hip fracture repair. Anesthesiology 2000; 92(4):947–957.

119. Norris EJ, Beattie C, Perler BA, et al. Double-masked randomized trial comparing alternate combinations of intraoperative anesthesia and postoperative analgesia in abdominal aortic surgery. Anesthesiology 2001; 95(5):1054–1067.

120. Block BM, Liu SS, Rowlingson AJ, et al. Efficacy of postoperative epidural analgesia: a meta-analysis. J Am Med Assoc 2003; 290(18):2455–2463.

121. McLeod G, Davies H, Munnoch N, et al. Postoperative pain relief using thoracic epidural analgesia: outstanding success and disappointing failures. Anaesthesia 2001; 56(1):75–81.

122. Urwin SC, Parker MJ, Griffiths R. General versus regional anaesthesia for hip fracture surgery: a meta-analysis of randomized trials. Br J Anaesth 2000; 84(4):450–455.

123. Christopherson R, Beattie C, Frank SM, et al. Perioperative morbidity in patients randomized to epidural or general anesthesia for lower extremity vascular surgery: Perioperative Ischemia Randomized Anesthesia Trial Study Group. Anesthesiology 1993; 79(3):422–434.

124. Brown MJ, Nicholson ML, Bell PR, et al. The systemic inflammatory response syndrome, organ failure, and mortality after abdominal aortic aneurysm repair. J Vasc Surg 2003; 37(3):600–606.
125. Liu SS, Block BM, Wu CL. Effects of perioperative central neuraxial analgesia on outcome after coronary artery bypass surgery: a meta-analysis. Anesthesiology 2004; 101(1):153–161.
126. Slogoff S, Keats AS. Randomized trial of primary anesthetic agents on outcome of coronary artery bypass operations. Anesthesiology 1989; 70(2):179–188.
127. Tuman KJ, McCarthy RJ, Spiess BD, et al. Does choice of anesthetic agent significantly affect outcome after coronary artery surgery? Anesthesiology 1989; 70(2):189–198.
128. Kloner RA, Jennings RB. Consequences of brief ischemia: stunning, preconditioning, and their clinical implications: part 1. Circulation 2001; 104(24):2981–2989.
129. Zaugg M, Lucchinetti E, Spahn DR, et al. Differential effects of anesthetics on mitochondrial K(ATP) channel activity and cardiomyocyte protection. Anesthesiology 2002; 97(1):15–23.
130. Zaugg M, Schaub MC, Foex P. Myocardial injury and its prevention in the perioperative setting. Br J Anaesth 2004; 93(1):21–33.
131. Julier K, da Silva R, Garcia C, et al. Preconditioning by sevoflurane decreases biochemical markers for myocardial and renal dysfunction in coronary artery bypass graft surgery: a double-blinded, placebo-controlled, multicenter study. Anesthesiology 2003; 98(6):1315–1327.
132. De Hert SG, Cromheecke S, ten Broecke PW, et al. Effects of propofol, desflurane, and sevoflurane on recovery of myocardial function after coronary surgery in elderly high-risk patients. Anesthesiology 2003; 99(2):314–323.
133. Conzen PF, Fischer S, Detter C, et al. Sevoflurane provides greater protection of the myocardium than propofol in patients undergoing off-pump coronary artery bypass surgery. Anesthesiology 2003; 99(4):826–833.
134. De Hert SG, Van der Linden PJ, Cromheecke S, et al. Choice of primary anesthetic regimen can influence intensive care unit length of stay after coronary surgery with cardiopulmonary bypass. Anesthesiology 2004; 101(1):9–20.
135. De Hert SG, Van der Linden PJ, Cromheecke S, et al. Cardioprotective properties of sevoflurane in patients undergoing coronary surgery with cardiopulmonary bypass are related to the modalities of its administration. Anesthesiology 2004; 101(2):299–310.
136. Takahashi MW, Otani H, Nakao S, et al. The optimal dose, the time window, and the mechanism of delayed cardioprotection by isoflurane. Anesthesiology 2004; 101 [Abstract].
137. De Hert SG, Turani F, Mathur S, et al. Cardioprotection with volatile anesthetics: mechanisms and clinical implications. Anesth Analg 2005; 100(6):1584–1593.
138. De Hert SG, Longrois D, Yang H, et al. Do volatile anesthetics attenuate troponin I release after vascular surgery? Anesthesiology 2004; 101:A287.
139. Hohner P, Backman C, Diamond G, et al. Anaesthesia for abdominal aortic surgery in patients with coronary artery disease. Part II. Effects of nitrous oxide on systemic and coronary haemodynamics, regional ventricular function and incidence of myocardial ischaemia. Acta Anaesthesiol Scand 1994; 38(8):793–804.
140. Badner NH, Beattie WS, Freeman D, et al. Nitrous oxide-induced increased homocysteine concentrations are associated with increased postoperative myocardial ischemia in patients undergoing carotid endarterectomy. Anesth Analg 2000; 91(5):1073–1079.
141. Mangano DT, Browner WS, Hollenberg M, et al. Association of perioperative myocardial ischemia with cardiac morbidity and mortality in men undergoing noncardiac surgery. The Study of Perioperative Ischemia Research Group. N Engl J Med 1990; 323(26):1781–1788.
142. Landesberg G, Mosseri M, Zahger D, et al. Myocardial infarction after vascular surgery: the role of prolonged stress-induced, ST depression-type ischemia. J Am Coll Cardiol 2001; 37(7):1839–1845.
143. Le Manach Y, Perel A, Coriat P, et al. Early and delayed myocardial infarction after abdominal aortic surgery. Anesthesiology 2005; 102(5):885–891.
144. Landesberg G, Vesselov Y, Einav S, et al. Myocardial ischemia, cardiac troponin, and long-term survival of high-cardiac risk critically ill intensive care unit patients. Crit Care Med 2005; 33(6):1281–1287.

Anesthetic Management of Patients with Valvular Heart Disease in Noncardiac Surgery

Kim A. Boost and Bernhard Zwissler

Department of Anesthesiology, Intensive Care, and Pain Therapy, Johann Wolfgang Goethe-University, Frankfurt, Germany

INTRODUCTION

Valvular heart diseases are accompanied by burdening of the right or left ventricle or atrium with volume or pressure overload, often followed by hemodynamic alterations. The impact of the hemodynamic changes can eventually lead to cardiac muscle dysfunction, congestive heart failure, arrhythmias, and sudden death. The cardiovascular consequences of valvular heart diseases may be aggravated in patients who have to undergo general or regional anesthesia. The perioperative management of patients with valvular heart diseases in noncardiac surgery, therefore, requires a profound understanding of the changes in the cardiovascular system. Accurate preoperative evaluation of the hemodynamic situation may minimize the patient's perioperative morbidity. The following chapter summarizes the specific anesthetic considerations in patients with valvular heart disease undergoing noncardiac surgery.

In general, heart murmurs that are detected during a physical examination require detailed evaluation whether or not the patient is scheduled for surgery. Although systolic heart murmurs are frequently not associated with valvular cardiac disease and often are related to physiological increases in blood flow velocity, a heart murmur (especially if it occurs in the diastole) can be an important clue to the diagnosis of severe undetected heart diseases.

Basic investigations for all those patients are a preoperative electrocardiogram (ECG) and the chest X ray. Patients with unknown diastolic, continuous, or holo- and late-systolic heart murmurs of grade 3/6 or greater should always be additionally evaluated with Doppler echocardiography; patients with midsystolic murmurs of grade 3/6 require further evaluation only when additional cardiac symptoms are present.

The absence of ventricular hypertrophy, abnormal P-waves, arrhythmias, or an abnormal heart silhouette on the chest X ray does not completely exclude serious valvular diseases, but makes them unlikely (1). Patients with symptomatic valvular stenosis are at increased risk of ventricular fibrillation and shock. Percutaneous valvulotomy or surgical valvular replacement prior to elective noncardiac interventions can reduce perioperative cardiac risk in these patients (2).

The choice of the anesthetic regimen in patients with valvular heart disease should always take into account the hemodynamic interaction of the anesthetic method (e.g., variations in heart rate, heart rhythm, blood pressure, and peripheral vascular resistance) with the pathophysiology of the functionally compromised valve. Most valve lesions cannot be treated sufficiently by drugs. Therefore, the major anesthetic goal in most patients should be the maintenance of a stable hemodynamic situation.

AORTIC STENOSIS
Pathophysiology
Major causes of aortic stenosis include the idiopathic degeneration and calcification of the aortic leaflets, long-term consequences of arterial hypertension, rheumatic fever, or morphological abnormalities (e.g., bicuspid aortic valve). The obstruction of the aortic orifice increases left ventricular pressure in order to maintain stroke volume. Over time, hypertrophy of the left ventricular myocardium develops. The oxygen demand of the left heart is elevated due to both the increase of muscular mass and intraventricular hypertension. Simultaneously, the increased pressure in the left ventricle compresses the subendocardial vessels, thereby impairing coronary blood flow and, hence, oxygen delivery to the muscle cells. This explains why angina pectoris may occur in 50% to 70% of all patients with aortic stenosis, although often no critical coronary stenosis can be verified during angiography. Fifteen to thirty percent of patients with aortic stenosis suffer from syncope.

Patients with symptoms of hemodynamic alterations (dyspnea, syncope, or angina pectoris) generally have an aortic valve orifice area less than $1\,cm^2$ and a transvalvular pressure gradient of greater than $50\,mmHg$. After onset of symptoms, average survival is limited to less than two to three years (3). Therefore, the development of symptoms marks a critical point in the course of aortic stenosis.

Decompensation of aortic stenosis is characterized by clinical symptoms of left ventricular insufficiency which may include acute ventricular dilatation and pulmonary edema followed by consecutive right heart failure. Severe aortic stenosis represents the single most important factor predicting perioperative cardiac complications in noncardiac surgery. Aortic sclerosis occurs in 30% of older patients and increases cardiovascular mortality in the perioperative period from 6.1% to 10.1%.

The severity of aortic stenosis can be divided into three groups:

1. Severe: orifice area of the aortic valve $\leq 1\,cm^2$
2. Moderate: orifice area of the aortic valve 1 to $1.5\,cm^2$
3. Mild: orifice area of the aortic valve $>1.5\,cm^2$

Perioperative Management
Preoperative Assessment and Medication
Preoperative assessment of the severity of aortic stenosis should always include auscultation, ECG, chest X ray, and echocardiography with Doppler examination of the aortic valve. Auscultation in patients with aortic stenosis will typically reveal a holosystolic heart murmur and mostly an early-systolic ejection click. Additionally, the ECG can show signs of left ventricular hypertrophy including a Sokolow-Lyon Index $>3.5\,mV$. Echocardiography in the evaluation of aortic stenosis can provide information about

1. the mobility of the valve,
2. thickness and calcifications of the aortic leaflets,
3. the orifice area of the aortic valve,
4. the transvalvular pressure gradient,
5. the presence of ventricular hypertrophy, and
6. left ventricular ejection fraction (estimation).

If echocardiography cannot adequately determine the severity of aortic stenosis, left heart catheterization may be necessary.

TABLE 1 Perioperative Antibiotic Prophylaxis in Cardiac Risk Patients

	Gastrointestinal or urologic surgery	Oral, dental airway or esophageal surgery
High risk		
Valve replacement (mechanical, biologic, homograft)	Ampicillin + gentamicin	Amoxicillin
Following bacterial endocarditis; complex and cyanotic heart defect	alternative: teicoplonin+ gentamicin	alternative: clindamycin or cephalosporin
Medium risk		
Other congenital heart defects	Amoxicillin or ampicillin	Azithromycin or clarithromycin
Acquired valvular diseases	alternative: vancomycin	
Hypertrophic cardiomyopathy		
Mitral valve prolapse (accompanied with regurgitation and/or thickened leaflets)		
Low risk		
After occlusion of ASD, VSD, or ductus botalli		
After coronary bypass surgery		
Mitral valve prolapse (without regurgitation)		
Functional heart murmur		
Implanted pace maker/defibrillator		

Abbreviations: ASD, atrial septal defect; VSD, ventricular septal defect.

Prophylactic antibiotic therapy must be given preoperatively to diminish the risk of infective endocarditis in patients with aortic stenosis (Table 1). The patient should receive adequate preoperative sedation for the avoidance of stress-related tachycardia.

Anesthetic Management

The main aim of anesthesia for noncardiac surgery in patients with aortic stenosis must be to avoid any events which may further decrease cardiac output (Table 2). Epidural or spinal anesthesia may result in the undesirable combination of profound hypotension due to sympathetic nervous system blockade and reflex tachycardia. Although case reports describe the safe use of neuroaxial blockade even in patients with severe aortic stenosis, general anesthesia is the anesthetic method preferred by most practitioners. There is, however, no scientific evidence of the superiority of this method. If neuroaxial blockade is chosen, epidural anesthesia should be preferred due to the fact that onset of sympathetic blockade and hypotension is better controlled than in spinal anesthesia.

TABLE 2 Hemodynamic Goals in Patients with Aortic Stenosis

Prevention of tachycardia (aim: heart rate 50–70 bpm)
Prevention of peripheral vasodilatation and hypotension
Optimization of intravascular fluid volume in order to maintain left ventricular filling
Maintenance of myocardial contractility

For the optimal management of general anesthesia, the specific pathophysiology of aortic stenosis must be considered:

1. The increased left ventricular pressure is due to the stenotic orifice of the aortic valve. Hence, any decrease in arterial blood pressure will have little beneficial effects on left ventricular afterload, but will seriously impair coronary blood flow and increase the risk of subendocardial ischemia or myocardial infarction. Thus, anesthetic management must aim at preventing systemic hypotension through a careful fluid administration and administration of vasopressors such as norepinephrine.

2. Left ventricular compliance is decreased in patients with aortic stenosis. Therefore, adequate fluid replacement is essential in order to maintain adequate venous return and ventricular filling (i.e., preload).

3. The choice of anesthetic drugs for induction and maintenance of general anesthesia must take into account drug-specific hemodynamic side effects, i.e., myocardial depression, hypotension, tachycardia, or arrhythmias. As basically all potent anesthetic drugs have negative inotropic properties, an opioid-based technique of general anesthesia has been recommended in patients with marked impairment of left ventricular function related to aortic stenosis. Depression of the sinoatrial node by volatile anesthetics may lead to junctional rhythm and loss of properly synchronized atrial contractions. Accordingly, patients should only receive the minimal required concentration on volatile anesthetics for inhibition of consciousness, supplemented with adequate doses of opioids. Nondepolarizing neuromuscular-blocking drugs may be used safely because of their minimal effects on systemic blood pressure.

4. Sudden bradycardia during anesthesia requires prompt treatment with atropine due to the inability of the left ventricle to accommodate to the acute fluid overload by increasing stroke volume. In patients with persistent bradycardia or junctional rhythm, treatment with a temporary pacemaker should be considered. Persistent tachycardia is also detrimental in patients with aortic stenosis because it reduces the diastolic filling time, thereby compromising coronary perfusion. Carefully titrated administration of β-adrenoceptor blockers may be an option for treatment but must take into account that patients with aortic stenosis may be dependent on their endogenous β-adrenergic stimulation. Ventricular tachycardia and acute atrial fibrillation should be terminated pharmacologically or by cardioversion. The termination of new atrial fibrillation is especially important as atrial contraction contributes by 40% to left ventricular filling.

Specific Monitoring
Besides standard monitoring (ECG, S_aO_2), monitoring of blood pressure through an intra-arterial catheter is of value to detect sudden hemodynamic alterations and should be instituted prior to induction of anesthesia in patients with severe aortic stenosis undergoing major surgery. The indications for monitoring by a pulmonary artery catheter are limited because severe catheter-induced arrhythmias may occur in the hypertrophic heart, and no benefits of the Swan Ganz catheter have been demonstrated in patients with valvular heart disease.

AORTIC REGURGITATION
Pathophysiology

Aortic regurgitation is characterized by diastolic reflux of blood from the aorta into the left ventricle, due to the incomplete closing of the aortic valve. Severe aortic insufficiency is characterized by a regurgitation fraction of more than 50% of stroke volume. Causes of aortic regurgitation include: rheumatic fever, infective endocarditis, and diseases of the aortic root (idiopathic root dilatation, thoracic aortic dissection, Marfan's syndrome, and collagen vascular diseases). These lead to distortion or disruption of the aortic leaflets followed by the impaired and incomplete closing of the valve.

The diastolic reflux of blood through the aortic valve determines the degree of hemodynamic compromise in patients with aortic regurgitation. The extent of the regurgitant volume depends on:

1. the orifice area of the incompletely closing valve,
2. the diastolic pressure gradient between aorta and the left ventricle (which depends on the systemic vascular resistance), and
3. the duration of the diastole (which depends on the heart rate).

Chronic aortic regurgitation results in combined volume and pressure overload of the left ventricle, left ventricular hypertrophy, and increased myocardial oxygen consumption. As with aortic stenosis, angina pectoris can occur in these patients due to the disproportion between increased myocardial oxygen demand and decreased coronary blood flow caused by ventricular hypertrophy and reduced aortic diastolic pressure. Tachycardia and a wide pulse pressure are pathognomonic for aortic regurgitation.

In contrast to the chronic state, acute aortic regurgitation is only poorly compensated by the left ventricle due to a sudden large volume load which is imposed on a normal-sized, nonaccommodated left ventricle. A rapid drop in cardiac output and systemic hypotension necessitate immediate surgical valvular replacement. Such patients frequently present with pulmonary edema or in cardiogenic shock.

Interestingly, chronic treatment with vasodilators does not prevent the progression of the severe aortic regurgitation (4).

Perioperative Management
Preoperative Assessment and Medication

Preoperative assessment of the severity of aortic regurgitation should always include auscultation, ECG, chest X ray, and echocardiography with Doppler examination of the aortic valve. Auscultation usually reveals a diastolic heart murmur which starts immediately after the second heart sound. The ECG is characterized by signs of left ventricular hypertrophy (Sokolow-Lyon Index >3.5 mV) and the chest X ray reveals an enlarged heart shadow.

The patient's perioperative risk is determined by severity and duration of the left ventricular dysfunction and increases with the decrease of exercise tolerance. Several echocardiographic parameters are associated with increased mortality in patients with aortic regurgitation after surgical intervention. These include a shortening fraction of less than 25%, an end-diastolic left ventricular diameter greater than 55 mm and an ejection fraction less than 40% to 50% (5).

Prophylactic antibiotics must be given to diminish the risk of developing infective endocarditis in patients with aortic regurgitation (Table 1).

TABLE 3   Hemodynamic Goals in Patients with Aortic Regurgitation

Moderate tachycardia (80–100 bpm)
Reduction of systemic resistance
Optimized left-ventricular filling
Stable myocardial contractility

Anesthetic Management
The anesthesiologic and hemodynamic management should emphasize the maintenance of the forward left ventricular stroke volume and should be based on the
following pathophysiologic considerations (Table 3):

1. Primary goal of the hemodynamic management should be the reduction of
   the regurgitation volume by shortening diastole through moderate tachycardia and by reduction of systemic vascular resistance. Although regional
   anesthesia may offer benefits from the sympathetic blockade, general
   anesthesia is often preferred in severe aortic insufficiency. If a neuroaxial
   blockade is chosen, epidural anesthesia can achieve adequate anesthesia by
   allowing titration of the dose of local anesthetic and hence may offer better
   hemodynamic stability than to spinal anesthesia.
2. Intravenous drugs such as etomidate, benzodiazepines, or opioids are
   useful for induction of anesthesia in patients with aortic regurgitation.
   The administration of ketamine provides the advantage of moderately
   accelerating heart rate, but concurrently increases the systemic resistance and
   so may increase the left ventricular regurgitation volume. All nondepolarizing
   drugs have been safely used in this setting, but succinylcholine is undesirable
   due to its potential to induce profound bradycardia.
3. Maintenance of anesthesia may be provided with volatile anesthetics which
   lower systemic resistance and so may improve stroke volume. In patients with
   severe heart failure, only small concentrations of volatile anesthetics should be
   administered due to their negative inotropic effect, and these should be
   supplemented with higher doses of opioids. When left ventricular function
   is severely compromised, afterload should be additionally decreased by
   administration of peripheral vasodilators such as nitroglycerin or sodium
   nitroprusside. In addition, positive inotropic support (e.g., by dobutamine or
   dopamine) may be required (6).
4. Bradycardia and junctional rhythms require prompt treatment with atropine.
5. Hyperventilation should be avoided, because hypocapnia increases peripheral
   vasoconstriction thereby potentially aggravating regurgitation.

Specific Monitoring
Patients with asymptomatic aortic regurgitation undergoing minor surgical interventions do not require invasive monitoring. In contrast, patients with severely
impaired left ventricular function must be monitored with an intra-arterial catheter,
which should be inserted before the induction of anesthesia. A central venous catheter
is indicated in cases where significant blood loss is expected. Intraoperative monitoring with transesophageal echocardiography (TEE) can be helpful to assess left
ventricular function.

MITRAL STENOSIS
Pathophysiology
As with most cardiac valve lesions, rheumatic fever is the major cause of mitral stenosis (6,7). Less common causes include congenital mitral stenosis, systemic lupus erythematosus, rheumatoid arthritis, atrial myxoma, and bacterial endocarditis. Clinical symptoms of mitral stenosis usually include orthopnea, dyspnea on exertion, or paroxysmal nocturnal dyspnea as a sign of left ventricular dysfunction. The underlying pathophysiology is a chronic impairment of left ventricular diastolic filling secondary to progressive decrease in the orifice area of the mitral valve. As a consequence, there is a rise in left atrial and pulmonary venous pressures. Left ventricular stroke volume is further compromised by tachycardia or if an effective atrial contraction is missing, e.g., in atrial fibrillation.

The orifice area of the valve determines the severity of mitral stenosis. Three degrees of severity have been defined:

1. Mild: 1.5 to 2.5 cm^2
2. Moderate: 1 to 1.5 cm^2
3. Severe: <1 cm^2

The normal area of the mitral valve orifice is 4 to 6 cm^2. When this area is reduced to 2 cm^2, an increase in left atrial pressure is necessary for normal transvalvular flow to occur. Most patients remain asymptomatic at this stage of disease. When the orifice area of the valve decreases to 1.5 cm^2 or smaller, clinical symptoms such as dyspnea and fatigue occur. Critical mitral stenosis occurs when the opening of the valve is reduced to 1 cm^2 or less. At this stage, a left atrial pressure of 25 mmHg is required to maintain a normal cardiac output at rest. This increase in left atrial pressure elevates pulmonary venous and capillary pressures, resulting in transudation of fluid into the pulmonary interstitium followed by decreased pulmonary compliance and increased work of breathing. Acute cardiac decompensation occurs in patients when stress such as sepsis, atrial fibrillation, pulmonary embolism, or pregnancy appears. Owing to the elevated pulmonary pressure and the delayed left ventricular filling, any rapid decrease in systemic resistance and/or increase in left atrial pressure are only poorly tolerated. During the progress of mitral stenosis, chronic elevation of left atrial pressure leads to pulmonary hypertension, tricuspid and pulmonary valve incompetence, and finally right heart failure.

Perioperative Management
Preoperative Assessment and Medication
Echocardiography with Doppler examination is the primary noninvasive diagnostic tool to assess the severity of mitral stenosis and to permit the measurement of the transvalvular gradient, the ejection fraction, and the calculation of the valve area. Preoperative assessment should include auscultation, ECG, and chest X ray. Auscultation of patients with mitral stenosis typically reveals a diastolic (decrescendo) heart murmur, starting with a mitral opening sound. The ECG may display signs of right ventricular hypertrophy (Sokolow-Lyon Index for right heart hypertrophy: ≥1.05 mV).

Prophylactic antibiotic therapy is essential to reduce the risk of infective endocarditis (Table 1). Preoperative medication with benzodiazepines decreases anxiety. However, only moderate dosages should be administered, because patients are susceptible to the ventilatory depressant effects of benzodiazepines and the subsequent

TABLE 4 Hemodynamic Goals in Patients with Mitral Stenosis

Avoidance of sinus tachycardia (60–70 bpm) (prevention of shortened diastole).
Control of heart rate during atrial fibrillation with rapid ventricular response.
Optimized left ventricular filling/avoidance of rapid increases in central venous blood volume, as associated with overtransfusion or head-down position.
Stable systemic vascular resistance (careful administration of catecholamines, if necessary).
Stable pulmonary venous resistance (avoidance of hypoxemia or hypercapnia that may exacerbate the pulmonary venous resistance and provoke right ventricular failure).

hypercapnia can increase pulmonary venous resistance. If anticholinergic drugs are needed, scopolamine or glycopyrrolate have less chronotropic effects than atropine and hence should be preferred. Atrial fibrillation is present in 30% of patients and a rapid ventricular response should be controlled during acute onset of atrial fibrillation by electrical cardioversion. During chronic atrial fibrillation, intro-atrial thrombus formation must be excluded by electrocardiography to prevent embolism and strokes prior to electrical or pharmacological cardioversion. For pharmacological cardioversion, medication with β-blockers, calcium antagonists, amiodarone or digoxin can be administered to control rapid ventricular response CA2I. Preexisting antiarrhythmic medication should be continued during the perioperative period. Anticoagulant therapy with warfarin should be continued until three to five days before surgery and then converted to heparin, which will be discontinued two to three hours preoperatively (3) (Tables 7 and 8). The timing of the resumption of anticoagulant therapy depends on the form of surgical intervention and the risk of postoperative bleeding (3).

Anesthetic Management
The anesthetic and hemodynamic management of patients with mitral stenosis should aim to maintain stroke volume and cardiac output (Table 4):

1. For induction of anesthesia, anesthetic drugs such as etomidate with less hypotensive potential should be preferred. Ketamine should be avoided because of possible alterations in heart rate.
2. Muscle relaxants are useful that cause little histamine release and so have minimal effects on heart rate and systemic blood pressure. The frequency of histamine-related reactions decreases as follows: succinylcholine > rocuronium > pancuronium > vecuronium > mivacurium > atracurium > cisatracurium (8).
3. An opioid-based technique for the maintenance of anesthesia is recommended. Both volatile anesthetics and propofol may be used to provide narcosis. Dosages or concentrations should be kept as small as possible, in order to avoid major decreases in systemic vascular resistance.
4. Profound arterial hypotension due to systemic vasodilation requires immediate vasopressor therapy (e.g., norepinephrine).
5. In patients with existing pulmonary hypertension, hypoxemia or hypercapnia can generate right heart failure.
6. In case of right heart failure, the administration of positive inotropic drugs such as catecholamines or phosphodiesterase III inhibitors, e.g., milrinone, enoximone may be required.
7. Intraoperative volume management requires care as patients with mitral stenosis are susceptible to left atrial overexpansion, e.g., related to intraoperative fluid

overload, head-down position, autotransfusion during postpartal uterus contraction, or bradycardia.

Specific Monitoring
In asymptomatic patients, standard monitoring may be sufficient. Use of invasive monitoring depends on the degree of cardiovascular impairment and the complexity of the surgical intervention. In patients with symptomatic mitral stenosis, continuous measurement of intra-arterial pressures is indicated. Additionally, direct monitoring of ventricular function by TEE may be useful in these patients during surgery.

MITRAL REGURGITATION
Pathophysiology
While acute mitral regurgitation is normally caused by dysfunction or rupture of a papillary muscle (e.g., due to myocardial infarction) or bacterial endocarditis, the chronic form is caused by rheumatic fever. Mitral regurgitation is characterized by systolic blood flow from the left ventricle to the left atrium generated by incomplete valvular closing. Therefore, left atrial volume overload is the major pathophysiologic change.

Left atrial volume overload directly depends on the size of the closing defect, the transvalvular pressure gradient, and the duration of the systole as determined by the heart rate. Mitral regurgitation reduces forward left ventricular stroke volume and may result in pulmonary hypertension and pulmonary edema. Once the regurgitation volume exceeds 50% of the stroke volume, mitral regurgitation is considered to be severe and immediate surgical repair of the mitral valve is indicated.

In cases of acute mitral insufficiency, the left atrium is not able to accommodate to the sudden volume overload. In these patients, acute pulmonary edema with pulmonary hypertension and consecutive right heart failure can occur. Patients with left atrial dilatation frequently present with atrial fibrillation and require anticoagulation with warfarin, which has to be converted preoperatively to heparin (Tables 7 and 8). Patients with isolated mitral insufficiency are less dependent on properly timed atrial contractions for ventricular filling as compared to patients with mitral or aortic stenosis. Therefore, conversion from atrial fibrillation to normal sinus rhythm produces only minor changes in cardiac output. In patients with combined mitral regurgitation and mitral stenosis, symptoms of cardiac dysfunction develop earlier than in those with isolated mitral regurgitation.

Perioperative Management
Preoperative Assessment and Medication
Preoperative assessment of the severity of mitral regurgitation should always include auscultation ECG, chest X ray, and echocardiography with Doppler examination of the mitral valve. The auscultation of patients with mitral regurgitation characteristically reveals a holosystolic heart murmur (decrescendo), starting with the first heart sound. The ECG shows signs of left ventricular hypertrophy (P mitral). The chest X ray may show an increase in size of the left atrium and ventricle. Prophylactic antibiotic therapy is essential because of the risk of infective endocarditis (Table 1). Adequate preoperative sedation should be administered to avoid stress-related tachycardia.

TABLE 5   Hemodynamic Goals in Patients with Mitral Regurgitation

Normal to slightly increased heart rate (aim: 85–100 bpm)
Avoidance of sudden decreases in heart rate
Avoidance of sudden increases in systemic or pulmonary vascular resistance
Stable myocardial contractility
Stable left-ventricular preload
Minimized drug induced myocardial depression

Anesthetic Management
The anesthesiologic and hemodynamic management of patients with mitral regurgitation includes the prevention of events that may further decrease cardiac output (Table 5). A moderate decrease in systemic vascular resistance may be beneficial by lowering left ventricular afterload thereby promoting forward flow, whereas a sudden and long-lasting decrease in systemic resistance can provoke sustained hemodynamic alterations and hence should be avoided. As spinal anesthesia and, to a lesser extent epidural anesthesia, may be associated with a profound reduction in systemic vascular resistance, general anesthesia is the technique preferred by many practitioners.

1. For induction of anesthesia, any of the commonly used intravenous anesthetics can be used safely if their hemodynamic side effects are borne in mind, and measures are taken to avoid sudden and excessive changes in systemic vascular resistance.
2. Succinylcholine should be avoided due to its potential to induce bradycardia.
3. In patients without severe left ventricular dysfunction, anesthesia can be maintained using volatile anesthetics and opioids in normal doses. Although volatile anesthetics may be of benefit in mitral regurgitation due to their vasodilatory properties, patients with severe left ventricular dysfunction should not receive more than 1 MAC of volatile anesthetics due to their cardiodepressant effects. A further deterioration of myocardial contractility can provoke severe left ventricular dysfunction and failure.
4. If required, positive inotropic drugs can be administered to improve left ventricular stroke volume and to decrease regurgitation volume through contraction of the mitral valve area. Dobutamine may be specifically beneficial, since it increases both heart rate and decreases left ventricular afterload.

Specific Monitoring
Asymptomatic patients with mitral regurgitation do not require invasive monitoring during minor operations. For patients with severe mitral regurgitation and left ventricular dysfunction, monitoring of intra-arterial pressures and central venous pressures is essential and facilitates the detection of myocardial depression and pulmonary hypertension. A Swan Ganz catheter may be helpful in monitoring the degree of mitral regurgitation by assessing the magnitude and alterations of V-waves in the pulmonary artery occlusion pressure curve (9). However, TEE is a less invasive and more powerful tool for intraoperative visualization of mitral valve function, myocardial contractility, and intravascular fluid volume.

MITRAL VALVE PROLAPSE
Pathophysiology
Prolapse of the mitral valve is characterized by systolic bulging of mitral valve leaflets into the left atrium. It is frequently observed in young women. Its prevalence

ranges between 2% and 6% (3). The echocardiographic findings include bulging of the posterior or both mitral leaflets during systole into the left atrium of more than 2 mm with or without regurgitation (10,11). Thickened leaflets (>5 mm) can also be found and the ECG often shows abnormal T-waves. Many patients are completely asymptomatic. Supraventricular and ventricular arrhythmias may occur, but in general do not require therapeutic intervention. Angina pectoris and sudden cardiac death due to malignant arrhythmias are extremely rare.

Perioperative Management
Preoperative Assessment and Medication
The preoperative assessment in patients with mitral prolapse follows that of patients with mitral regurgitation (see "Preoperative Assessment and Medication"). Patients who have a systolic murmur and have confirmed mitral valve prolapse with regurgitation or thickened leaflets should receive preoperative prophylactic antibiotic therapy to reduce the risk of infective endocarditis (Table 1).

Anesthetic Management
Perioperative risk in patients with asymptomatic mitral valve prolapse is not increased and there are no specific anesthetic considerations. Symptomatic patients have regurgitation through the mitral valve, leading to progressive dilatation of left ventricle and atrium. Left atrial dilatation may result in atrial fibrillation and moderate-to-severe mitral regurgitation may finally result in left ventricular dysfunction and development of congestive heart failure. Therefore, management of symptomatic patients depends on the severity of any mitral regurgitation and patients should be managed as outlined above in the section on mitral regurgitation (see "Anesthetic Management").

TRICUSPID STENOSIS
Pathophysiology and Perioperative Management
Isolated tricuspid stenosis is rare. If the orifice area of the tricuspid valve is reduced to less than $1.5\,cm^2$ (normal: 7–$9\,cm^2$), symptoms of central venous congestion such as hepatomegaly, ascites, or jugular venous congestion occur. For the management of patients with tricuspid stenosis, the principles outlined in the section on mitral stenosis can be applied (see "Perioperative Management").

TRICUSPID REGURGITATION
Pathophysiology
Infective endocarditis—frequently found in drug addicts—is the most common cause for isolated tricuspid regurgitation. In addition, tricuspid regurgitation is frequently found as a consequence of other valvular lesions such as aortic or mitral valve disease and results from dilatation of the right ventricle due to pulmonary hypertension. The hemodynamic changes during isolated progressive tricuspid regurgitation include right atrial volume overload, which is in general well tolerated due to the high compliance of the right atrium and the vena cava. Left ventricular dysfunction during tricuspid regurgitation occurs, when the regurgitated volume is high enough to significantly decrease pulmonary blood flow and, hence, left ventricular stroke volume. A similar situation occurs, when venous filling of the right atrium decreases due to insufficient fluid replacement or increased blood loss.

TABLE 6   Hemodynamic Goals in Patients with Tricuspid Regurgitation

Moderate tachycardia (80–100 bpm)
High normal right ventricular preload
Stable myocardial contractility
Stable systemic vascular resistance
Reduction of pulmonary vascular resistance

Perioperative Management

Preoperative Assessment and Medication

The preoperative assessment in patients with tricuspid regurgitation includes auscultation, ECG, and chest X ray and follows the recommendations applicable in patients with mitral regurgitation (see "Preoperative Assessment and Management"). Patients should receive preoperative prophylactic antibiotic therapy to reduce the risk of infective endocarditis (Table 1).

Anesthetic Management

The primary concern of the anesthetic management is the avoidance of inadequate venous return into the right atrium and increased right ventricular afterload (Table 6). High intrathoracic pressures generated by high-positive pressure ventilation, hypovolemia, or drug-induced venodilation should therefore be prevented. Similarly, any elevation of pulmonary vascular resistance (e.g., by hypoxia, acidosis, hypercapnia, or nitrous oxide) should be avoided.

To improve myocardial contractility, inodilators such as dobutamine and phosphodiesterase III inhibitors can be administered, as they both increase contractility and reduce right ventricular afterload by pulmonary vasodilation. Inhaled vasodila-

TABLE 7   Perioperative Management of Patients Chemically Treated with Anticoagulants

Patient on long-term warfarin	Discontinue warfarin 72 hrs preoperatively
	Restart warfarin at the evening of surgical intervention, except in case of active bleeding
Patient on long-term acetylsalicylic acid (ASS)	Discontinue ASS 1 week preoperatively
	Restart on the first postoperative day

Abbreviation: ASS, acetylsalicylic acid.

TABLE 8   Perioperative Coagulation Management in Anticoagulated Patients

High risk of embolism (history of thromboembolism, atrial fibrillation, left ventricular dysfunction, mechanical valve, hypercoagulobility)	Discontinue warfarin 72 hrs preoperatively
	Start heparin, if INR < 2.0
	Heparin-dosage: PTT 55–70 sec
	Discontinue heparin 6 hrs preoperatively
	Restart heparin within 24 hrs postoperatively
	Restart warfarin, except in case of bleeding
	Discontinue heparin, when INR > 2.0
Minimal risk of perioperative bleeding	Continue anticoagulation, monitor risk of bleeding

Abbreviations: INR, international normalized ratio; LV, left ventricular; PTT, partial thromboplastin time.

tors may also be efficient in lowering pulmonary vascular tone, but have not been approved for this indication.

MANAGEMENT OF PATIENTS WITH PROSTHETIC VALVES

There are some special considerations for the anesthetic management of patients with prosthetic valves or after reconstruction of valves. First, the mechanical repair of a destroyed valve itself does not necessarily reverse the pathophysiological changes that have developed in the heart over years (e.g., hypertrophy, dilatation, impaired contractility). Secondly, perioperative antibiotic prophylaxis is mandatory in most of these patients. Thirdly, prophylactic anticoagulation with warfarin (target value: INR 2.0–3.5) is obligatory in all patients with mechanical valves and takes places for at least three months in patients with biological valves. Additional low-dose aspirin may further reduce the risk of thromboembolism. It is important to know in this context that each day without sufficient anticoagulation, for example, because elective noncardiac surgery is planned, is associated with a 0.02% to 0.05% risk of developing new thromboembolism. This risk has to be carefully weighed against the risk of perioperative bleeding. An algorithm for the perioperative management of patients who are chronically treated with anticoagulants is given in Tables 7 and 8.

REFERENCES

1. Eagle KA, Berger PB, Calkins H, et al. ACC/AHA guideline aspects for perioperative cardiovascular evaluation for non-cardiac surgery-executive summary. Anesth Amalg 2002.
2. Auerbach AD, Goldmann L. β-Blockers and reduction of cardiac events in noncardiac surgery: scientific review. J Am Med Assoc 2002; 287:1435–1444.
3. Bonow RO, Carabello B, Karu C, et al. ACC/AHA Guidelines for the Management of Patients with Valvular Heart Disease. A Report of the American College of Cardiology/American Heart Association Task Force on Practice Guidelines (Committee on Management of Patients with Valvular Heart Disease). Circulation 2006; 114:284–291.
4. Evangelista A, Tornos P, Sambola A, Permanyer-Miralda G, Soler-Soler J. Long-term vasodilator therapy in patients with severe aortic regurgitation. N Engl J Med 2005; 353:1342–1349.
5. Stone JG, Hoar PF, Calabro JR, et al. Afterload reduction and preload augmentation improve the anesthetic management of patients with cardiac failure and valvular regurgitation. Anesth Analg 1980; 59:737–742.
6. Carabello BA, Crawford FA. Valvular heart disease. N Engl J Med 1997; 337:32–41.
7. Kinare SG, Kulkarni HL. Quantitative study of mitral valve in chronic rheumatic heart disease. Int J Cardiol 1987; 16:271–284.
8. Laxenaire MC, Mertes PM. Anaphylaxis during anesthesia: results of a two-year survey in France. Br J Anaesth 2001; 87:549–558.
9. Greenberg BH, Rahimtoola SH. Vasodilator therapy for valvular heart disease. J Am Med Assoc 1981; 246:269–272.
10. Nishimura RA, McGoon MD. Perspectives on mitral-valve prolapse. N Engl J Med 1999; 341:48–50.
11. Freed LA, Levy D, Levine RA, et al. Prevalence and clinical outcome of mitral-valve prolapse. N Engl J Med 1999; 341:1–7.
12. Fuster V, Ryden LE, Asinger RW, et al. ACC/AHA/ESC guidelines for the Management of patients with atrial fibrillation. Circulation 2001; 104:2118–2150.

17 Primary and Secondary Prevention of Coronary Heart Disease

Deoraj Zamvar and Alistair S. Hall

C-NET Research Group, The General Infirmary at Leeds, Leeds, U.K.

INTRODUCTION

Cardiovascular disease (CVD) is the leading cause of death in developed countries, although mortality rates have fallen in the last 30 years (Fig. 1) (1–3). However, the increasing prevalence of obesity appears to be slowing the decline in the incidence of coronary disease possibly via the development of type 2 diabetes mellitus with its associated features. Reductions in major risk factors and improvements in medical therapies have contributed substantially to the fall in mortality, further emphasizing the importance of preventive strategies (1,5). Primary prevention strategies are aimed at delaying or preventing new-onset coronary heart disease. Secondary prevention denotes therapy to reduce recurrent coronary heart disease events and decrease coronary mortality in patients with established coronary heart disease. Some patients without known CVD have a risk of subsequent cardiovascular events that is comparable to that seen in patients with established disease. There is, therefore, only a slim distinction between secondary prevention and high-risk primary prevention. Both groups of people require aggressive management with a combination of effective lifestyle modification and medication.

CARDIOVASCULAR RISK ESTIMATION

Numerous mathematical models have been developed for estimating the risk of cardiovascular events based upon assessment of various risk factors. Most of the frequently used models [e.g., Joint British Societies (6) and Framingham Risk Score (7)] are based on data gathered in the Framingham Heart Study. These models incorporate age, sex, low-density lipoprotein (LDL)-cholesterol, high-density lipoprotein (HDL)-cholesterol, blood pressure, diabetes, and smoking to derive an estimated risk of developing coronary heart disease within 10 years (Fig. 2). The Second Joint British Societies Guidelines have opted to further extend their model to include prediction of all cardiovascular endpoints (stroke and myocardial infarction) as this is of clear clinical relevance. Furthermore, the concept of treating global or total risk has now emerged, as compared to earlier focus on isolated disease states. Any person with a total risk of ≥20% over 10 years is defined as "high risk" and requires professional intervention and, where appropriate, drug therapies to achieve the lifestyle and risk factor targets. These models can sometimes falsely reassure persons deemed to be at low risk who may have a strong family history of CVD or a number of marginal abnormalities (8,9). In addition, these models identify people who are likely to develop CVD within a 10-year period—but do not consider lifetime risk—which might often be substantially higher and highly amenable to risk factor reduction (8,10–12).

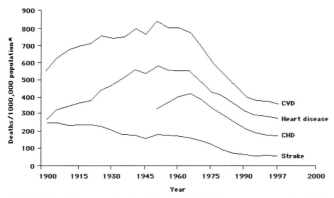

FIGURE 1   Changes in death from CVD. Rates are age-adjusted to 2000 standard. *Abbreviation*: CVD, cardiovascular disease. *Source*: From Ref. 4.

PREVENTION OF CARDIOVASCULAR DISEASE

Prevention of CVD requires intensive lifestyle intervention and appropriate use of drug therapy in order to reduce the overall cardiovascular risk. This imperative relates particularly to patients with:

1. clinical evidence of atherosclerotic CVD,
2. known diabetes mellitus (type 1 or 2),
3. a global CVD risk of 20% or more over 10 years,
4. elevated blood pressure ≥160 mmHg systolic or ≥100 mmHg diastolic, or lesser degrees of blood pressure elevation with target organ damage,
5. elevated total cholesterol to HDL-cholesterol ratio ≥6.0 mmol/L, and
6. diagnosis of a familial dyslipidemia, for example, familial hypercholesterolemia or familial combined hyperlipidemia.

LIFESTYLE MODIFICATION

Lifestyle modification plays a key role in the prevention of CVD. It includes changing habits with regards to smoking, body weight, diet, and physical activities (Table 1). Lifestyle intervention is the only approach that can be offered for CVD prevention for many people whose total CVD risk is not sufficiently high to justify pharmacotherapy, a situation that applies to most of the adult population in developed and now also in developing countries.

Smoking

Smoking is an major independent risk factor for CVD and the incidence of a myocardial infarction is increased substantially in people who smoke compared to subjects who have never smoked (13,14). In addition, it increases all-cause and cardiovascular mortality (15,16). Patients with established coronary heart disease who continue to smoke have an increased risk of further cardiac ischemic events including sudden cardiac death (17,18). Smoking adversely effects the lipid profile (19) and increases insulin resistance (20,21). It activates the sympathetic nervous system, producing

Framingham Risk Score

Joint British Societies Tables

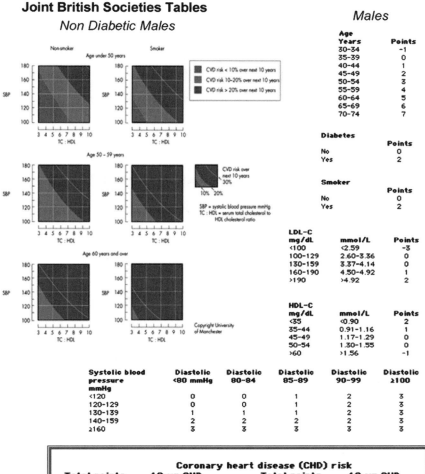

FIGURE 2 Framingham and Joint British Societies Risk Charts. To calculate risk from Framingham tables, use set appropriate to gender and add points based on the presence or absence of risk factors to determine 10-year risk of coronary heart disease. To calculate risk from JBS-2 charts, use set appropriate to gender, smoking status, and age—locate level of systolic blood pressure and LDLc/HDLc ratio to determine 10-year risk of CVD. *Abbreviations*: JBS, Joint British Society; LDL, low-density lipoprotein; HDL, high-density lipoprotein. *Source*: From Refs. 6, 7.

TABLE 1   Recommended Targets for Lifestyle Factors

Do not smoke
Maintain ideal body weight for adults (body mass index 20) and avoid central obesity (waist cir-
    cumference in white Caucasians <102 cm in men and <88 cm in women, and in Asians <90 cm
    in men and <80 cm in women)
Keep total dietary intake of fat to 30% of total energy intake
Keep the intake of saturated fats to 10% of total fat intake
Keep the intake of dietary cholesterol to <300 mg/day
Replace saturated fats by an increased intake of monounsaturated fats
Increase the intake of fresh fruit and vegetables to at least five portions per day
Regular intake of fish and other sources of ω-3 fatty acids (at least two servings of fish per week)
Limit alcohol intake to <21 units/week for men or <14 units/week for women
Limit the intake of salt to <100 mmol/L day (<6 g of sodium chloride or <2.4 g of sodium per day)
Regular aerobic physical activity of at least 30 min/day, most days of the week, should be taken
    (e.g., fast walking/swimming)

Source: From Ref. 6.

an increase in heart rate and blood pressure, and cutaneous and possibly coronary
vasoconstriction (22–24). In addition, it damages the vascular wall and enhances the
prothrombotic state.

   Smoking cessation can be followed by a rapid decline in the risk of coronary
heart disease in people with and without known coronary heart disease (25,26). It
also improves outcomes in patients who have had a myocardial infarction (18,27,28).
The cardiac risks associated with cigarette smoking diminish soon after smoking cessation and continue to fall with passage of time. Smokers should be encouraged by
physicians and indeed all health professionals to stop smoking completely. There are
a number of ways that physicians can actively intervene against smoking. Behav-
ioral therapy, nicotine replacement, and the use of antidepressant medications may
all improve the quit rate.

Weight Reduction

Obesity is a risk factor for coronary heart disease (29,30) and heart failure (31). It is
associated with other risk factors including adverse lipid profile, elevated blood
pressure, insulin resistance, and type 2 diabetes (32). This clustering of risk factors
is commonly referred to as the metabolic syndrome. Weight reduction has a beneficial effect on blood pressure (33), lipid profile (34), and an improvement in other
elements of the metabolic syndrome such as hyperinsulinemia and hyperglycemia
(35). Body mass index (BMI) is calculated from a person's weight and height. BMI
correlates to direct measures of body fat. The most practical marker of abdominal
obesity is the measurement of waist circumference. All patients with CVD should
have measurement of waist circumference and calculation of BMI. The target BMI is
18.5 to 24.9 kg/m² (36,37).

   Overweight individuals have BMI of greater than 25, whereas BMI above 30
constitutes obesity. Patients with an increased waist circumference (greater than
102 cm in men and greater than 88 cm in women in Caucasians) should undergo evaluation for the metabolic syndrome and implementation of weight reduction strategies that include behavior modification, dietary therapy, exercise, drug therapy, and
surgery. Caloric intake can be reduced by reducing the consumption of high-energy
foods and some alcoholic drinks. Fat intake should be less than a third of the total
energy intake. Increased consumption of vegetables, fruit, and cereal products

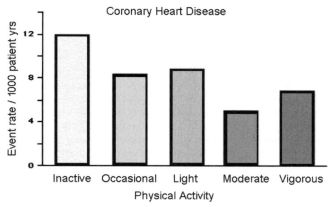

FIGURE 3   Physical exercise and CVD. Study of 5159 men aged 40 to 49 years followed for an average of 19 years showing age-adjusted rate per 1000 person years for coronary heart disease. *Abbreviation*: CVD, cardiovascular disease. *Source:* From Ref. 39.

should be encouraged in place of food with high fat content. Regular exercise can play an important role in losing weight. Antiobesity medications act by inhibiting intestinal fat absorption, suppressing appetite, or increasing thermogenesis. These include orlistat, an inhibitor of fat absorption, and sibutramine, a centrally acting medication. Several surgical approaches have been used to treat severe obesity (BMI > 40 kg/m²) that has not responded to the above approaches.

Physical Activity
Inadequate physical activity has been recognized as an independent risk factor for premature development of coronary heart disease (Fig. 3) (38). There is a strong inverse relationship between physical activity and the risk of coronary disease and death (40,41). In addition to reducing weight, exercise improves lipid profile and reduces in blood pressure. It also reduces inflammation as there is increasing evidence that inflammation, as manifested in part by elevations in serum C-reactive protein, plays an important role in atherosclerosis (42). Exercise training programs decrease insulin resistance and lower the rate of progression to overt type 2 diabetes. Exercise is beneficial in people with established coronary heart disease (39,43,44). Exercise rehabilitation programs have shown to significantly reduce all-cause mortality and in recurrent myocardial infarction among patients with coronary disease (43). An exercise program should be associated with control of other risk factors.

Diet
There is substantial evidence that healthy diets that include unsaturated fats, whole grains, fruits, vegetables, and ω-3 fatty acids offer protection against coronary heart disease (45). The type of fat consumed is more important than the amount of total fat. *Trans*-Fatty acids, derived from industrial hydrogenation of monounsaturated and polyunsaturated trans-fatty acids, increase risk of CHD (46,47), whereas polyunsaturated fat and monounsaturated fat decrease risk (48). Plant stenols or sterols incorporated into food reduce the absorption of cholesterol from the gut and lower blood cholesterol values. In observational studies, people who eat more fish generally have

a lower risk of CHD and CHD mortality. Beneficial effects of fish consumption may be related to intake of n-3 fatty acids, which have been shown in randomized trials of supplements to decrease subsequent CVD (49). Randomized controlled trials in people with established coronary disease of increased fish consumption and supplementation with eicosapentenoic acid and docosahexenoic acid have shown reductions in coronary and total mortality (49–51). A reduction of sodium intake, especially in the form of sodium chloride, also reduces blood pressure (52).

Individuals who consume small-to-moderate amounts of alcohol between 1 and 3 units per day have lower risks of CVD, including reduced cardiovascular mortality (53,54). Drinking should be strongly discouraged for individuals under the age of 40 who are at low risk of CHD, because the risks are likely to outweigh the benefits in this group (55). Higher consumption of alcohol is associated with increase in the systolic and diastolic blood pressures, the risk of cardiac arrhythmias, cardiomyopathy, and sudden death (56–58). It is recommended that all high-risk people including those with established CHD and people with diabetes should be given professional support to make lifestyle changes to prevent atherosclerotic events.

HYPERTENSION

Hypertension is a well-established risk factor for adverse cardiovascular outcomes (59,60). Risk is determined by both the level of blood pressure and the presence of other risk factors for atherosclerotic disease (61,62). Antihypertensive therapy is effective at reducing this risk and the benefit is greatest in those at highest risk (63–66). Hypertension is defined as a systolic blood pressure of 140 mmHg or greater or a diastolic blood pressure of 90 mmHg or greater. Grades of hypertension are defined in Table 2 (6,61). Blood pressure should be measured in all individuals over the age of 40 years. For people already on antihypertensive drug therapy, the blood pressure level before drug treatment was started should be used to estimate risk of CVD.

Blood Pressure Thresholds for Intervention with Drug Therapy

All people with elevated blood pressure or with high–normal blood pressures or a family history of hypertension should receive lifestyle advice to help reduce their blood

TABLE 2   Grades of Hypertension

Blood pressure (BP) category	Systolic BP (mmHg)	Diastolic BP (mmHg)	Lifestyle intervention	Drug therapy
Normal	<120	<80	—	—
High–normal	135–139	85–89	Yes	Consider[a]
Mild hypertension (grade 1)	140–159	90–99	Yes	Consider[b]
Moderate hypertension (grade 2)	160–179	100–109	Yes	Yes
Severe hypertension (grade 3)	≥180	≥110	Yes	Yes

[a]Drug therapy may be indicated for people with established CVD, chronic renal disease, or diabetes with complications at BP levels > 130/80 mmHg.
[b]Drug therapy is recommended for people with established CVD or diabetes or evidence of target organ damage or a 10-year cardiovascular risk ≥20%.
Abbreviation: CVD, cardiovascular disease.
Source: From Ref. 6.

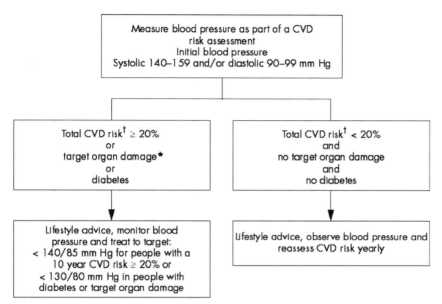

FIGURE 4 Joint British Society Guidance for management of systemic hypertension when assessed as part of a cardiovascular risk assessment. *Abbreviation*: CVD, cardiovascular disease. *Source:* From Ref. 6.

pressure and CVD risk (61). This can reduce blood pressure and obviate the need for drug therapy in people with mild hypertension, or reduce the number of drugs required to control blood pressure in people with treated hypertension (61,67). Blood pressure thresholds for intervention with drug therapy are outlined in Figure 4. People with persistent blood pressure elevation with a systolic pressure of 160 mmHg or more or a diastolic pressure of 100 mmHg or more are at sufficiently high risk of CVD risk on the basis of blood pressure levels alone to require drug therapy to reduce their blood pressure. People with sustained systolic blood pressures between 140 and 159 mmHg systolic and/or diastolic blood pressures between 90 and 99 mmHg (grade 1 hypertension) and clinical evidence of CVD, diabetes, or target organ damage or a total CVD risk of 20% or more should be considered for blood-pressure-lowering drug therapy (61,67). However, those without CVD, diabetes, target organ damage, and with a total CVD risk of less than 20% should continue with lifestyle strategies and have their blood pressure and total CVD risk reassessed annually (61,67). The threshold for treating blood pressure is lower—a systolic pressure of greater than 130 mmHg or diastolic of greater than 80 mmHg in some people at very high cardiovascular risk, for example, following a myocardial infarction, stroke, or transient ischemic attack (TIA), or people with established chronic renal disease or those with diabetes with complications (61,64).

Selection of Drug Therapy
In general, once-daily preparations that provide full 24-hour blood pressure control are preferred. The main benefit from antihypertensive therapy is blood pressure lowering, and various drug classes are considered to be equally effective at reducing cardiovascular morbidity and mortality per unit fall in blood pressure (63–68). There is

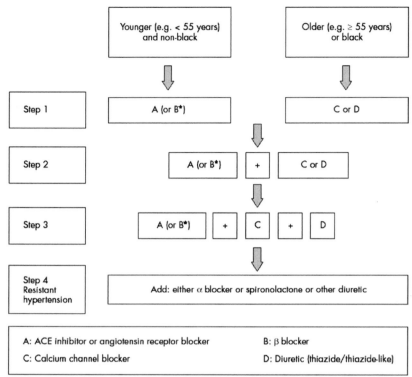

FIGURE 5 Joint British Society Guidance for drug therapy of patients with established systemic hypertension. *Source:* From Ref. 6.

an increasing recognition that monotherapy is usually insufficient for hypertension and that for most people with high blood pressure will require multiple drug therapy. The British Hypertension Society in its recent guideline suggested the AB/CD treatment algorithm (Fig. 5) on sequencing and combinations of drug therapy for the treatment of hypertension (61,69).

The theory behind the AB/CD algorithm is that hypertension can be broadly classified as *"high renin"* or *"low renin"* and is therefore best treated initially with one of two categories of antihypertensive drug: those that inhibit the renin–angiotensin system [ACE inhibitors or angiotensin receptor blockers (A) or β-blockers (B)], and those that do not [calcium channel blockers (C) or thiazide and thiazide-like diuretics (D)]. People who are younger, that is, aged under 55 years, and white tend to have higher renin concentrations than older people or those of African descent. A or B drugs are therefore generally more effective as initial blood-pressure-lowering treatment in younger white patients than C or D drugs. However, C or D drugs are more effective first-line agents for older white people or black people of any age. The AB/CD algorithm has four steps. Step 1 is a single drug: A or B or C or D, depending on age and ethnic group, titrated up to the highest recommended dose if tolerated. When

TABLE 3 Reasons to Select Drugs for Treatment of Hypertension

Class of drug	Compelling indications	Possible indications	Caution	Compelling contraindications
α-Blockers	Benign prostatic hypertrophy		Postural hypertension[a]	Urinary incontinence
ACE inhibitors	Heart failure, LV dysfunction, post-MI, or established CHD, type I diabetic nephropathy, 2° stroke prevention	Chronic renal disease[b], type II diabetic nephropathy, proteinuric renal disease	Renal impairment[b], PVD[c]	Pregnancy, renovascular disease[d]
ARBs	ACE inhibitor intolerance, type II diabetic nephropathy, hypertension with LVH, heart failure in ACE-intolerant people, post-MI	LV dysfunction post-MI, intolerance of other antihypertensive disease, chronic renal disease, heart failure[a]	Renal impairment[b], PVD[c]	Pregnancy, renovascular disease[d]
β-Blockers	MI, angina	Heart failure[e]	Heart failure[e], PVD, diabetes (except with CHD)	Asthma/COPD, heart block
CCBs (dihydropyridine), CCBs (rate limiting)	Elderly, ISH, angina, CHD	Elderly, angina, MI	—	
Thiazide/thiazide-like diuretics	Elderly, ISH, heart failure, 2° stroke prevention			Gout[f]

[a]HF when used as monotherapy.

[b]ACE inhibitors or ARBs may be beneficial in chronic renal failure but should only be used with caution, close supervision, and specialist advice.

[c]Caution with ACE inhibitors and ARBs in peripheral vascular disease because of the association with renovascular disease.

[d]ACE inhibitors and ARBs are sometimes used in people with renovascular disease under specialist supervision; in combination with a thiazide/thiazide-like diuretic.

[e]β-Blockers are increasingly used to treat stable heart failure; however, β-blockers may worsen heart failure.

[f]Thiazide and thiazide-like diuretics may sometimes be necessary to control BP in people with a history of gout, ideally used in combination with allopurinol.

Abbreviations: ACE, angiotensin-converting enzyme; ARBs, angiotensin II receptor blockers; CHD, coronary heart disease; COPD, chronic obstructive pulmonary disease; ISH, isolated hypertension; LVH, left ventricular hypertrophy; MI, myocardial infarction; PVD, peripheral vascular disease.

Source: From Ref. 6.

the first drug is well-tolerated but the response is small and insufficient, substitution of an alternative drug is appropriate if hypertension is mild (grade 1) and uncomplicated. In more severe or complicated hypertension, it is safer to add drugs stepwise until blood pressure is controlled.

In this algorithm, B (β-blockade) is bracketed. This is because several trials, including the largest randomized comparison of β-blocker/thiazide against CCB/ACE in primary prevention of CVD have all revealed an increased risk of developing diabetes in people treated with β-blockers, especially when combined with thiazide and thiazide-like diuretics (70,71). As diabetes further increases the risk of CVD, it is advisable to limit the dose of β-blockers and not to combine this class with a diuretic, particularly in people at high risk of developing diabetes.

For each major class of antihypertensive drug, there are compelling indications and contraindications for use (Table 3). When none of the special considerations apply, initial drug selection should follow step 1 of the AB/CD algorithm. When there are compelling indications for a specific drug class, the AB/CD algorithm can still be used to identify optimal drug combinations with the caveat that the drugs with compelling indications should be part of the treatment regimen, and ones with compelling contraindications should not.

HYPERLIPIDEMIA

CVD risk increases with increasing concentrations of cholesterol (72–74). Modifying lipids is an essential component of cardiovascular risk management. An adverse lipid profile continues to be a risk factor in patients with established CVD and the lowering of cholesterol by any means, decreases this risk (75–81).

Several large-scale randomized primary prevention trials have demonstrated a benefit of lowering cholesterol in patients without clinical evidence of coronary heart disease. The West of Scotland Coronary Prevention Study (WOSCOPS) showed that pravastatin reduced the number of coronary events and coronary mortality in middle-aged men with a serum LDL-cholesterol concentration above 4.0 mmol/L (155 mg/dL) (82). The Air Force/Texas Coronary Atherosclerosis Prevention Study (AFCAPS/TexCAPS) similarly showed a reduction in the incidence of a first major coronary event with lovastatin in low-risk individual without clinical evidence of CVD and LDL-cholesterol levels near the average for the general population [3.9 mmol/L (150 mg/dL)], but low HDL (83).

Several large randomized trials have demonstrated the benefit of lipid lowering for secondary prevention in patients with prior cardiovascular events. These are in patients with hypercholesterolemia as in the 4S trial (84) as well as in patients with "average" serum cholesterol as in the CARE and LIPID trials and the Heart Protection Study (85,86). The PROVE IT-TIMI 22 trial demonstrated a benefit of lowering cholesterol to a target below 2.6 mmol/L (100 mg/dL) (87). Similarly, the Treatment to New Targets (TNT) trial showed benefit of lowering cholesterol to 1.9 mmol/L (75 mg/dL) (88). A meta-analysis of 58 randomized trials of cholesterol lowering by any means showed a significant reduction in coronary death and nonfatal myocardial infarction in a graded fashion. The greater the reduction in LDL-cholesterol and the longer the duration of treatment, the greater was the reduction in CHD events (89). The recent Cholesterol Trialists' Collaboration, a meta-analysis of data from more than 90,000 participants in 14 randomized trials of statins, has shown that statin therapy can reduce the five-year incidence of major coronary events, coronary revascularization, and stroke by about one-fifth per mmol/L reduction in LDL-cholesterol

(90). This reduction in cardiovascular events per mmol/L reduction in LDL-cholesterol was largely independent of the presenting LDL level and that the benefit of absolute LDL reduction is present across a wide range of baseline LDL-cholesterol values. Fibrates and nicotinic acid studies have also reported a substantial reduction in the risk of major coronary events (91,92).

Lipid Assessment

All asymptomatic individuals aged over 40 years should have their total cholesterol and HDL-cholesterol measured to estimate total cardiovascular risk. For people already on lipid-lowering therapy, the total cholesterol value before diet and drug treatment was started should be used to estimate risk. Total cholesterol and HDL-cholesterol can be measured in a nonfasting state. However, all people who are found to be at high risk should have a full fasting lipid profile including total cholesterol, HDL- and LDL-cholesterol, and triglycerides. Secondary causes of hyperlipidemia including alcohol abuse, diabetes, renal disease, liver disease, and inadequately treated hypothyroidism should be investigated before drug treatment is given. At the time of myocardial infarction as well as following major surgery, total cholesterol, LDL-cholesterol, and HDL-cholesterol can decrease; this reduction may last for six to eight weeks. However, a lipid measurement as soon as possible following myocardial infarction will give a reasonable indication of the total cholesterol and HDL-cholesterol values before the acute event. Creatine phosphokinase (CK) and alanine or aspartate transaminase (ALT or AST) is generally measured before starting treatment with a statin as some people may have high values that are physiological. A rise in ALT or AST to three times, and CK to 5 to 10 times, the upper limit of normal can be acceptable in patients on statin therapy.

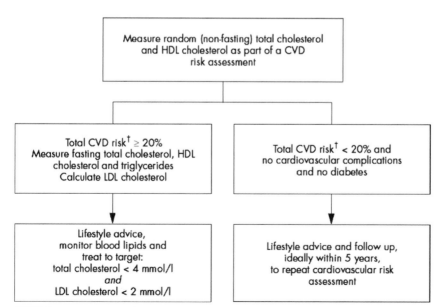

FIGURE 6 Joint British Society Guidance for assessment of hyperlipidemia when assessed as part of a cardiovascular risk assessment. *Abbreviation*: CVD, cardiovascular disease. *Source:* From Ref. 6.

Triglycerides, HDL-Cholesterol, and Non-HDL-Cholesterol

The primary target for lipid management in high-risk people, as well as those with mixed dyslipidemia, elevated triglycerides, and low HDL-cholesterol, is LDL-cholesterol. HDL-cholesterol is inversely related to risk of CVD and for this reason the ratio of total cholesterol to HDL-cholesterol is used for CVD risk assessment. Individuals with hypertriglyceridemia (>1.7 mmol/L) have a higher CVD risk. HDL-cholesterol can be increased by a variety of drugs including statins, fibrates, nicotinic acid, and ω-3 fatty acid, whereas fibrates and ω-3 fatty acid reduce triglycerides. Low HDL-cholesterol and high triglycerides each appear to contribute independently to cardiovascular risk. Non-HDL-cholesterol is defined as the difference between the total cholesterol and HDL-cholesterol and it represents the total of cholesterol circulating on apoprotein B particles (both LDL- and triglyceride-rich lipoproteins). A desirable value for non-HDL-cholesterol is less than 3 mmol/L.

Management of Blood Lipids

The following groups of people should be treated with lipid-lowering drug therapy in addition to lifestyle advice to modify their lipoproteins favorably and reduce their cardiovascular risk (Fig. 6).

1. Patients with established atherosclerotic disease
2. Those who are aged 40 years or more with either type 1 or 2 diabetes or younger diabetic who have poor glycemic control, complications of the disease, or other risk factors for CVD
3. Those at high total risk (CVD risk greater than 20% over 10 years)

In addition to LDL-cholesterol, other lipid parameters including HDL-cholesterol and triglycerides should be targeted, especially in people with a mixed dyslipidemia which is generally seen in diabetics and those with metabolic syndrome.

HYPERLIPIDEMIA DRUG THERAPY

There are various classes of drugs that have a favorable effect on the lipid profile. These include inhibitors of 3-hydroxy-3-methylglutaryl coenzyme A (HMG-CoA) reductase (statins), fibrates, anion exchange resins, nicotinic acid and its derivatives, fish oils, and an inhibitor of cholesterol absorption.

Statins

Statins act by inhibiting HMG-CoA reductase and are the most potent of the lipid-lowering drugs, lowering both total and LDL-cholesterol. They also raise HDL-cholesterol and lower triglycerides to some extent. Statin therapy also reduces C-reactive protein (CRP) and has been associated with clinical benefit independent of its lipid-lowering effect. These groups of drugs are generally safe and the annual risk of myopathy is about 0.001%. CK needs to be checked if the patient experiences unexplained muscle pains. Other lipid-lowering drugs will be needed in some people, usually in combination with a statin, if statins are unable to achieve the desired therapeutic effect, or in place of a statin when the primary lipid abnormality is severe hypertriglyceridemia (>10 mmol/L), or when the patient is intolerant of statins.

Fibrates

Fibrates primarily raise HDL-cholesterol and lower triglycerides and are indicated for the management of mixed lipemia and hypertriglyceridemia (93). Fibrates (apart from gemfibrozil) may be added to statin therapy on specialist advice where hypertriglyceridemia and low HDL persist after LDL-cholesterol has been treated to target (94).

Anion Exchange Resins

Cholestyramine and colestipol bind bile acids in the intestine and increase LDL receptor activity in the liver which results in the clearance of LDL-cholesterol from plasma. They can substantially reduce cholesterol and are indicated in patients with familial hypercholesterolemia.

Cholesterol Absorption Inhibitors

Ezetimibe inhibits cholesterol absorption in the gut and can lower LDL-cholesterol by around 15% to 20% when added to diet, or by 20% to 25% when added to diet with a statin (95). It can be used as monotherapy in patients intolerant to statins.

Nicotinic Acid

Nicotinic acid raises HDL-cholesterol and reduces triglycerides by inhibiting adipose tissue lipolysis, and hepatic triglyceride synthesis.

ω-3 (n-3) Fatty Acids

ω-3 (n-3) Fatty acids lower triglycerides and are licensed for the prevention of CHD. They can be used with statins or with other lipid-lowering therapies.

The current recommended target for total cholesterol and LDL-cholesterol is less than 4.0 and less than 2.0 mmol/L, respectively, or a 25% reduction in total cholesterol and a 30% reduction in LDL-cholesterol, whichever is lower. The recent AHA/ACC update on secondary prevention for patient with coronary and other

TABLE 4   Diagnosis of Diabetes

	Fasting plasma glucose (FPG) test (preferred)[a]	Random plasma glucose test	Oral glucose tolerance test (OGTT)
Diabetes	FPG ≥ 7.0 mmol/L plus symptoms[b]	Random plasma glucose ≥ 11.1 mmol/L plus symptoms[c]	Two-hr plasma glucose ≥ 11.1 mmol/L[d]
Impaired glucose regulation	IFG ≥ 6.1 and < 7.0 mmol/L		IGT = 2 hr PG ≥ 7.8 and < 11.1 mmol/L
Normal	FPG ≥ 6.0 mmol/L		Two-hr PG ≥ 7.8 mmol/L

[a]The FPG is the preferred test for diagnosis, but any one of the three listed is acceptable. In the absence of unequivocal hyperglycemia with acute metabolic decompensation, one of these three tests should be repeated on a different day to confirm diagnosis. Venous plasma samples are used (symptoms are the classic ones of polyuria, polydipsia, and unexplained weight loss).
[b]Fasting is defined as no caloric intake for at least eight hours. Water is allowed.
[c]Random = any time of day without regard for time since last meal.
[d]OGTT should be performed using a glucose load containing the equivalent of 75 g anhydrous glucose dissolved in water.
Source: JBS 2: Joint British Societies' guidelines on prevention of CVD in clinical practice British Cardiac Society, British Hypertension Society, Diabetes U.K., HEART U.K., Primary Care Cardiovascular Society, The Stroke Association (6).

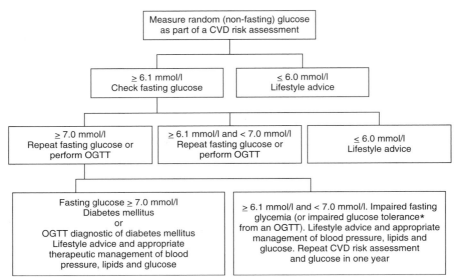

FIGURE 7   Joint British Society Guidance—Hyperglycemia. Risk thresholds and targets for plasma blood glucose in asymptomatic people without CVD. *Impaired glucose tolerance: two-hour glucose in an OGTT ≥7.8 and ≤11.0 mmol/L. *Abbreviation*: OGTT, oral glucose tolerance test. *Source:* From Ref. 6.

vascular disease recommends LDL-C of less than 2.6 mmol/L and certain groups of patients less than 1.8 mmol/L.

DIABETES AND BLOOD GLUCOSE

Hyperglycemia increases the risk of developing CVD. The absolute risk of CVD associated with any level of glycemia is also determined by the presence of other risk factors (96). In individuals with impaired glucose tolerance, the relative risk of developing CVD is 1.5 compared to individuals with normal glucose tolerance (97), whereas in those with diabetes it is two- to fourfold (98,99). Impaired glucose regulation and diabetes mellitus are both underdiagnosed in clinical practice.

Assessment of Plasma Glucose

All adults aged over 40 years should have a random blood glucose measured. Diabetes can be diagnosed on the basis of fasting or random glucose or oral glucose tolerance test as shown in Table 4. Individuals with impaired glucose regulation and a CVD risk of 20% or more over 10 years should receive appropriate lifestyle and risk factor intervention, including the use of cardiovascular-protective drug therapies. If CVD risk is less than 20%, then appropriate lifestyle advice should be given and their CVD risk and fasting glucose measured on an annual basis. In people who present with an acute CVD event, fasting glucose should be measured during the acute phase of the illness and, if there is evidence of impaired fasting glycemia or an indication of diabetes, a fasting glucose measurement should be repeated on two occasions between 8 and 12 weeks following discharge from hospital. Those with impaired glucose regulation should have fasting glucose, and all other cardiovascular risk factors, measured on an annual basis (Table 4).

Prevention of Diabetes

In people with impaired glucose tolerance (IGT), clinical trials have shown that progression to diabetes can be prevented or postponed by lifestyle intervention (100). Other treatments that reduce progression to diabetes include acarbose for IGT and orlistat for obese individuals with normal or IGT (101,102). A significant increase in new cases of diabetes was associated with use of β-blockers and diuretics in a recent trial of antihypertensive treatment (71,103).

BLOOD PRESSURE, LIPIDS, AND GLUCOSE IN DIABETES
Blood Pressure

Hypertension is twice as common in diabetics and greatly increases CVD risk in people with diabetes. Intensive treatment of hypertension in patients with diabetes reduces the risk of stroke and myocardial infarction (104). The blood pressure target for people with diabetes is lower than for those without diabetes at a pressure of less than 130/80 mmHg, as studies have shown that the greater the blood pressure lowering, the greater the benefit in terms of cardiovascular events. Sometimes, especially in the elderly it may be difficult to achieve this target and in this situation one must aim for a blood pressure of 140/80 mmHg. Generally, patients with diabetes and hypertension will require a combination of antihypertensive medications to achieve the recommended blood pressure targets. These include ACE inhibitors or angiotensin receptor blockers, thiazide and thiazide-like diuretics, longer acting calcium channels blockers, α-blockers, or low-dose spironolactone (105).

Lipids

Several trials of statins have shown significant reductions in coronary and cardiovascular events in people with diabetes comparable to that seen in those without diabetes (92,106–109). This treatment effect is independent of baseline cholesterol. Statin treatment is effective for primary prevention of CVD in patients with diabetes mellitus (110). Statins are recommended in patients 40 years or more with either type 1 or 2 diabetes; and in younger diabetics who have other risk factors for CVD, poorly controlled diabetes or target organ damage due to diabetes. Statins are the drug of choice in diabetes even though the most common form of dyslipidemia is low HDL-cholesterol and elevated triglycerides.

Glycemic Control in Diabetes

Good glycemic control has been shown to prevent microvascular complications in both type 1 and 2 diabetes (111–113), thus reducing the risk of stroke and myocardial infarction (114). Ideally, one should aim for normoglycemia (a fasting glucose of 6.0 mmol/L or less) and normal HbA1c% (<6.0%), with the avoidance of hypoglycemia and decompensated hyperglycemia. However, the practical HbA1c% target is 6.5% or less. In type 1 diabetes, glucose control requires insulin therapy along with dietary and lifestyle modifications. In type 2 diabetes, nonpharmacological means of controlling blood glucose including adherence to appropriate diet, weight reduction, and increased physical activity should be the first approach. If these measures fail, then oral hypoglycemic drugs (biguanide, sulfonylurea, thiazolidinediones, or a combination) or insulin need to be added to the treatment regimen. In overweight and obese people with a BMI of 25 kg/m^2 or more, metformin is the drug of first choice. Insulin treatment should be considered if treatment with oral agents fails

TABLE 5   Clinical Diagnosis of Metabolic Syndrome

Clinical identification of the syndrome can be made if three of the following are met:
Central obesity: waist circumference >88 cm (women) and >102 cm (men) in Caucasians
Blood pressure ≥130/≥85 mmHg
Fasting glucose ≥6.1 mmol/L
Serum triglycerides ≥1.7 mmol/L
HDL-cholesterol <1.3 mmol/L (women) and <1.0 mmol/L (men)

to achieve HbA1c of 7.5% or less. Effective care in diabetes involves a multidisciplinary approach and close involvement of the patient.

ASPIRIN THERAPY

Aspirin or other platelet-modifying drugs should be given to all people with established CVD. It significantly reduces all-cause mortality, vascular mortality, nonfatal myocardial reinfarction, and nonfatal stroke in people with unstable angina, acute myocardial infarction, stroke, or TIAs (115,116). It has fewer side effects at lower doses and is generally prescribed at 75 mg/day. In patients with acute coronary disease, unstable angina or non-ST segment elevation myocardial infarction, a combination of clopidogrel and aspirin has been shown to be beneficial in terms of reducing further cardiovascular events. Aspirin is recommended for all people with type 2 diabetes who are 50 years of age or more, and in younger patients who have had the disease for more than 10 years or who are already receiving treatment for hypertension or have evidence of target organ damage. It is also recommended in asymptomatic high-risk patients (risk 20% or more over 10 years) as long as the blood pressure has been controlled.

PRIMARY PREVENTION OF CHD BASED ON FAMILY HISTORY

Asians in the United Kingdom are at increased risk of coronary heart disease and CVD as compared to the indigenous local population (117–119). It is primarily due to the high prevalence of metabolic syndrome in this population (Table 5). In the African-Caribbean population, coronary heart disease mortality is nearly half that of white Caucasians. However, these people have high rates of hypertension and stroke. CVD risk also increases in person with a family history of premature coronary heart disease defined as having a male or female first-degree relative (parent or sibling) affected by overt vascular disease prior to the age of 65 years.

Although there are a number of sophisticated methods for quantifying familial risk, few of these are able to improve upon the more simple estimation of a ratio of affected to unaffected first-degree relatives. So, for example, if one member of a family of four were affected, this would be a ratio of 1/4 or 0.25. If two parents in a family of four were affected that would be a ratio of 0.5 representing a stronger familial risk. Additional weight might also be attached to the occurrence of early fatalities from CVD and also when female family members have been affected as this implies a higher underlying genetic burden. Although guidelines for primary prevention in such families have not yet been developed, current clinical practice would be to strongly advise lifestyle changes and to consider use of one or more of three drugs capable of risk reduction. These are aspirin, statins, and ACE inhibitors. Indications for use should be borderline hypertension (ACE inhibitors), hyperlipidemia (statins), and age over 50 years (aspirin).

ANESTHETISTS IN PRIMARY AND SECONDARY PREVENTION

The often transient nature of contact between anesthetists and patients with overt or subclinical cardiovascular risk limits the opportunity for beneficial intervention. However, the occurrence of a major life event such as elective or acute surgery or admission to an intensive care facility serves to focus the minds of both patients and their friends and families with regard to the issue of clinical risk. Consequently, it can act as a potent catalyst for smoking cessation, weight reduction, exercise—whether in the preoperative or postoperative phase. Furthermore, the prevention of perioperative cardiovascular events is a major priority that is helped by maximizing cardiovascular risk reduction strategies as outlined in this chapter.

REFERENCES

1. Capewell S, Morrison CE, McMurray JJ. Contribution of modern cardiovascular treatment and risk factor changes to the decline in coronary heart disease mortality in Scotland between 1975 and 1994. Heart 1999; 81(4):380–386.
2. Kuulasmaa K, Tunstall-Pedoe H, Dobson A, et al. Estimation of contribution of changes in classic risk factors to trends in coronary-event rates across the WHO MONICA Project populations. Lancet 2000; 355(9205):675–687.
3. McGovern PG, Pankow JS, Shahar E, et al. Recent trends in acute coronary heart disease—mortality, morbidity, medical care, and risk factors. The Minnesota Heart Survey Investigators. N Engl J Med 1996; 334(14):884–890.
4. Cooper, R, et al. Circulation 2000; 102; 31375.
5. Capewell S, Beaglehole R, Seddon M, et al. Explanation for the decline in coronary heart disease mortality rates in Auckland, New Zealand, between 1982 and 1993. Circulation 2000; 102(13):1511–1516.
6. JBS 2: Joint British Societies' guidelines on prevention of cardiovascular disease in clinical practice. Heart 2005; 91(suppl 5):v1–v52.
7. Wilson PW, D'Agostino RB, Levy D, et al. Prediction of coronary heart disease using risk factor categories. Circulation 1998; 97(18):1837–1847.
8. Lloyd-Jones DM, Leip EP, Larson MG, et al. Prediction of lifetime risk for cardiovascular disease by risk factor burden at 50 years of age. Circulation 2006; 113(6):791–798.
9. Vasan RS, Sullivan LM, Wilson PW, et al. Relative importance of borderline and elevated levels of coronary heart disease risk factors. Ann Intern Med 2005; 142(6):393–402.
10. Vasan RS, D'Agostino RB Sr. Age and time need not and should not be eliminated from the coronary risk prediction models. Circulation 2005; 111(5):542–545.
11. Ridker PM, Cook N. Should age and time be eliminated from cardiovascular risk prediction models? Rationale for the creation of a new national risk detection program. Circulation 2005; 111(5):657–658.
12. Executive Summary of the Third Report of the National Cholesterol Education Program (NCEP) Expert Panel on Detection, Evaluation, and Treatment of High Blood Cholesterol in Adults (Adult Treatment Panel III). J Am Med Assoc 2001; 285(19):2486–2497.
13. Njolstad I, Arnesen E, Lund-Larsen PG. Smoking, serum lipids, blood pressure, and sex differences in myocardial infarction: a 12-year follow-up of the Finnmark Study. Circulation 1996; 93(3):450–456.
14. Prescott E, Hippe M, Schnohr P, et al. Smoking and risk of myocardial infarction in women and men: longitudinal population study. Br Med J 1998; 316(7137):1043–1047.
15. Qiao Q, Tervahauta M, Nissinen A, et al. Mortality from all causes and from coronary heart disease related to smoking and changes in smoking during a 35-year follow-up of middle-aged Finnish men. Eur Heart J 2000; 21(19):1621–1626.
16. Foody JM, Cole CR, Blackstone EH, et al. A propensity analysis of cigarette smoking and mortality with consideration of the effects of alcohol. Am J Cardiol 2001; 87(6): 706–711.
17. Tofler GH, Muller JE, Stone PH, et al. Comparison of long-term outcome after acute myocardial infarction in patients never graduated from high school with that in more educated

patients. Multicenter Investigation of the Limitation of Infarct Size (MILIS). Am J Cardiol 1993; 71(12):1031–1035.

18. Goldenberg I, Jonas M, Tenenbaum A, et al. Current smoking, smoking cessation, and the risk of sudden cardiac death in patients with coronary artery disease. Arch Intern Med 2003; 163(19):2301–2305.

19. Craig WY, Palomaki GE, Haddow JE. Cigarette smoking and serum lipid and lipoprotein concentrations: an analysis of published data. Br Med J 1989; 298(6676):784–788.

20. Facchini FS, Hollenbeck CB, Jeppesen J, et al. Insulin resistance and cigarette smoking. Lancet 1992; 339(8802):1128–1130.

21. Reaven G, Tsao PS. Insulin resistance and compensatory hyperinsulinemia: the key player between cigarette smoking and cardiovascular disease? J Am Coll Cardiol 2003; 41(6):1044–1047.

22. Cryer PE, Haymond MW, Santiago JV, et al. Norepinephrine and epinephrine release and adrenergic mediation of smoking-associated hemodynamic and metabolic events. N Engl J Med 1976; 295(11):573–577.

23. Winniford MD, Wheelan KR, Kremers MS, et al. Smoking-induced coronary vasoconstriction in patients with atherosclerotic coronary artery disease: evidence for adrenergically mediated alterations in coronary artery tone. Circulation 1986; 73(4):662–667.

24. Narkiewicz K, van de Borne PJ, Hausberg M, et al. Cigarette smoking increases sympathetic outflow in humans. Circulation 1998; 98(6):528–534.

25. Rose G, Hamilton PJ, Colwell L, et al. A randomised controlled trial of anti-smoking advice: 10-year results. J Epidemiol Community Health 1982; 36(2):102–108.

26. Multiple Risk Factor Intervention Trial. Risk factor changes and mortality results. Multiple Risk Factor Intervention Trial Research Group. J Am Med Assoc 1982; 248(12): 1465–1477.

27. Wilson K, Gibson N, Willan A, et al. Effect of smoking cessation on mortality after myocardial infarction: meta-analysis of cohort studies. Arch Intern Med 2000; 160(7):939–944.

28. Rea TD, Heckbert SR, Kaplan RC, et al. Smoking status and risk for recurrent coronary events after myocardial infarction. Ann Intern Med 2002; 137(6):494–500.

29. Krauss RM, Winston M, Fletcher BJ, et al. Obesity: impact on cardiovascular disease. Circulation 1998; 98(14):1472–1476.

30. Willett WC, Manson JE, Stampfer MJ, et al. Weight, weight change, and coronary heart disease in women: risk within the 'normal' weight range. J Am Med Assoc 1995; 273(6):461–465.

31. Kenchaiah S, Evans JC, Levy D, et al. Obesity and the risk of heart failure. N Engl J Med 2002; 347(5):305–313.

32. Grundy SM. Metabolic complications of obesity. Endocrine 2000; 13(2):155–165.

33. Neter JE, Stam BE, Kok FJ, et al. Influence of weight reduction on blood pressure: a meta-analysis of randomized controlled trials. Hypertension 2003; 42(5):878–884.

34. Dattilo AM, Kris-Etherton PM. Effects of weight reduction on blood lipids and lipoproteins: a meta-analysis. Am J Clin Nutr 1992; 56(2):320–328.

35. Anderson JW, Konz EC. Obesity and disease management: effects of weight loss on comorbid conditions. Obes Res 2001; 9(suppl 4):326S–334S.

36. Antman EM, Anbe DT, Armstrong PW, et al. ACC/AHA guidelines for the management of patients with ST-elevation myocardial infarction—executive summary. A Report of the American College of Cardiology/American Heart Association Task Force on Practice Guidelines (Writing Committee to Revise the 1999 Guidelines for the Management of Patients With Acute Myocardial Infarction). Circulation 2004; 110(5):588–636.

37. Smith SC Jr, Blair SN, Bonow RO, et al. AHA/ACC Scientific Statement: AHA/ACC guidelines for preventing heart attack and death in patients with atherosclerotic cardiovascular disease—2001 update: a statement for healthcare professionals from the American Heart Association and the American College of Cardiology. Circulation 2001; 104(13):1577–1579.

38. Powell KE, Thompson PD, Caspersen CJ, et al. Physical activity and the incidence of coronary heart disease. Annu Rev Public Health 1987; 8:253–287.

39. Wannamethee SG, Shaper AG, Walker M. Physical activity and mortality in older men with diagnosed coronary heart disease. Circulation 2000; 102(12):1358–1363.

40. Sesso HD, Paffenbarger RS Jr, Lee IM. Physical activity and coronary heart disease in men: The Harvard Alumni Health Study. Circulation 2000; 102(9):975–980.

41. Ekelund LG, Haskell WL, Johnson JL, et al. Physical fitness as a predictor of cardiovascular mortality in asymptomatic North American men: The Lipid Research Clinics Mortality Follow-up Study. N Engl J Med 1988; 319(21):1379–1384.

42. Smith JK, Dykes R, Douglas JE, et al. Long-term exercise and atherogenic activity of blood mononuclear cells in persons at risk of developing ischemic heart disease. J Am Med Assoc 1999; 281(18):1722–1727.

43. Clark AM, Hartling L, Vandermeer B, et al. Meta-analysis: secondary prevention programs for patients with coronary artery disease. Ann Intern Med 2005; 143(9):659–672.

44. Taylor RS, Brown A, Ebrahim S, et al. Exercise-based rehabilitation for patients with coronary heart disease: systematic review and meta-analysis of randomized controlled trials. Am J Med 2004; 116(10):682–692.

45. Hu FB, Willett WC. Optimal diets for prevention of coronary heart disease. J Am Med Assoc 2002; 288(20):2569–2578.

46. Trans fatty acids and coronary heart disease risk: Report of the expert panel on *trans* fatty acids and coronary heart disease. Am J Clin Nutr 1995; 62(3):655S–708S; discussion 518–526.

47. Ascherio A, Hennekens CH, Buring JE, et al. *trans*-Fatty acids intake and risk of myocardial infarction. Circulation 1994; 89(1):94–101.

48. Ascherio A, Rimm EB, Giovannucci EL, et al. Dietary fat and risk of coronary heart disease in men: cohort follow up study in the United States. Br Med J 1996; 313(7049):84–90.

49. Dietary supplementation with n-3 polyunsaturated fatty acids and vitamin E after myocardial infarction: results of the GISSI-Prevenzione trial. Gruppo Italiano per lo Studio della Sopravvivenza nell'Infarto miocardico. Lancet 1999; 354(9177):447–455.

50. Burr ML, Fehily AM, Gilbert JF, et al. Effects of changes in fat, fish, and fibre intakes on death and myocardial reinfarction: diet and reinfarction trial (DART). Lancet 1989; 2(8666):757–761.

51. Marchioli R, Barzi F, Bomba E, et al. Early protection against sudden death by n-3 polyunsaturated fatty acids after myocardial infarction: time-course analysis of the results of the Gruppo Italiano per lo Studio della Sopravvivenza nell'Infarto Miocardico (GISSI)-Prevenzione. Circulation 2002; 105(16):1897–1903.

52. Hooper L, Bartlett C, Davey Smith G, et al. Systematic review of long term effects of advice to reduce dietary salt in adults. Br Med J 2002; 325(7365):628.

53. Rimm EB. Alcohol consumption and coronary heart disease: good habits may be more important than just good wine. Am J Epidemiol 1996; 143(11):1094–1098; discussion 1099.

54. Thun MJ, Peto R, Lopez AD, et al. Alcohol consumption and mortality among middle-aged and elderly U.S. adults. N Engl J Med 1997; 337(24):1705–1714.

55. Jackson R, Beaglehole R. Alcohol consumption guidelines: relative safety vs absolute risks and benefits. Lancet 1995; 346(8977):716.

56. Power C, Rodgers B, Hope S. U-shaped relation for alcohol consumption and health in early adulthood and implications for mortality. Lancet 1998; 352(9131):877.

57. Britton A, McKee M. The relation between alcohol and cardiovascular disease in Eastern Europe: explaining the paradox. J Epidemiol Community Health 2000; 54(5):328–332.

58. Klatsky AL. Alcohol, coronary disease, and hypertension. Annu Rev Med 1996; 47:149–160.

59. Chobanian AV, Bakris GL, Black HR, et al. The Seventh Report of the Joint National Committee on Prevention, Detection, Evaluation, and Treatment of High Blood Pressure: the JNC 7 report. J Am Med Assoc 2003; 289(19):2560–2572.

60. Brown DW, Giles WH, Croft JB. Left ventricular hypertrophy as a predictor of coronary heart disease mortality and the effect of hypertension. Am Heart J 2000; 140(6):848–856.

61. Williams B, Poulter NR, Brown MJ, et al. Guidelines for management of hypertension: report of the fourth working party of the British Hypertension Society, 2004-BHS IV. J Hum Hypertens 2004; 18(3):139–185.

62. Williams B, Poulter NR, Brown MJ, et al. British Hypertension Society guidelines for hypertension management 2004 (BHS-IV): summary. Br Med J 2004; 328(7440):634–640.

63. Turnbull F. Effects of different blood-pressure-lowering regimens on major cardiovascular events: results of prospectively-designed overviews of randomised trials. Lancet 2003; 362(9395):1527–1535.
64. 2003 European Society of Hypertension—European Society of Cardiology guidelines for the management of arterial hypertension. J Hypertens 2003; 21(6):1011–1053.
65. Staessen JA, Wang JG, Thijs L. Cardiovascular prevention and blood pressure reduction: a quantitative overview updated until 1 March 2003. J Hypertens 2003; 21(6):1055–1076.
66. Williams B. Recent hypertension trials: implications and controversies. J Am Coll Cardiol 2005; 45(6):813–827.
67. National Institute of Clinical Excellence (NICE) Clinical Guideline 18—Management of hypertension in adults in primary care. London: NICE, 2004.
68. Psaty BM, Lumley T, Furberg CD, et al. Health outcomes associated with various antihypertensive therapies used as first-line agents: a network meta-analysis. J Am Med Assoc 2003; 289(19):2534–2544.
69. Brown MJ, Cruickshank JK, Dominiczak AF, et al. Better blood pressure control: how to combine drugs. J Hum Hypertens 2003; 17(2):81–86.
70. Dahlof B, Devereux RB, Kjeldsen SE, et al. Cardiovascular morbidity and mortality in the Losartan Intervention for Endpoint reduction in hypertension study (LIFE): a randomised trial against atenolol. Lancet 2002; 359(9311):995–1003.
71. Dahlof B, Sever PS, Poulter NR, et al. Prevention of cardiovascular events with an antihypertensive regimen of amlodipine adding perindopril as required versus atenolol adding bendroflumethiazide as required, in the Anglo-Scandinavian Cardiac Outcomes Trial-Blood Pressure Lowering Arm (ASCOT-BPLA): a multicentre randomised controlled trial. Lancet 2005; 366(9489):895–906.
72. Neaton JD, Wentworth D. Serum cholesterol, blood pressure, cigarette smoking, and death from coronary heart disease: overall findings and differences by age for 316,099 white men. Multiple Risk Factor Intervention Trial Research Group. Arch Intern Med 1992; 152(1):56–64.
73. Smith GD, Shipley MJ, Marmot MG, et al. Plasma cholesterol concentration and mortality: The Whitehall Study. J Am Med Assoc 1992; 267(1):70–76.
74. Neaton JD, Blackburn H, Jacobs D, et al. Serum cholesterol level and mortality findings for men screened in the Multiple Risk Factor Intervention Trial: Multiple Risk Factor Intervention Trial Research Group. Arch Intern Med 1992; 152(7):1490–1500.
75. Muldoon MF, Manuck SB, Matthews KA. Lowering cholesterol concentrations and mortality: a quantitative review of primary prevention trials. Br Med J 1990; 301(6747): 309–314.
76. Holme I. An analysis of randomized trials evaluating the effect of cholesterol reduction on total mortality and coronary heart disease incidence. Circulation 1990; 82(6):1916–1924.
77. Antman EM, Lau J, Kupelnick B, et al. A comparison of results of meta-analyses of randomized control trials and recommendations of clinical experts: treatments for myocardial infarction. J Am Med Assoc 1992; 268(2):240–248.
78. Superko HR, Krauss RM. Coronary artery disease regression: convincing evidence for the benefit of aggressive lipoprotein management. Circulation 1994; 90(2):1056–1069.
79. Gould AL, Rossouw JE, Santanello NC, et al. Cholesterol reduction yields clinical benefit: a new look at old data. Circulation 1995; 91(8):2274–2282.
80. Bucher HC, Griffith LE, Guyatt GH. Systematic review on the risk and benefit of different cholesterol-lowering interventions. Arterioscler Thromb Vasc Biol 1999; 19(2):187–195.
81. Cholesterol, diastolic blood pressure, and stroke: 13,000 strokes in 450,000 people in 45 prospective cohorts. Prospective studies collaboration. Lancet 1995; 346(8991–8992): 1647–1653.
82. Shepherd J, Cobbe SM, Ford I, et al. Prevention of coronary heart disease with pravastatin in men with hypercholesterolemia. West of Scotland Coronary Prevention Study Group. N Engl J Med 1995; 333(20):1301–1307.
83. Downs JR, Clearfield M, Weis S, et al. Primary prevention of acute coronary events with lovastatin in men and women with average cholesterol levels: results of AFCAPS/TexCAPS. Air Force/Texas Coronary Atherosclerosis Prevention Study. J Am Med Assoc 1998; 279(20):1615–1622.

84. Randomised trial of cholesterol lowering in 4444 patients with coronary heart disease: the Scandinavian Simvastatin Survival Study (4S). Lancet 1994; 344(8934):1383–1389.
85. Sacks FM, Pfeffer MA, Moye LA, et al. The effect of pravastatin on coronary events after myocardial infarction in patients with average cholesterol levels: Cholesterol and Recurrent Events Trial Investigators. N Engl J Med 1996; 335(14):1001–1009.
86. Tonkin AM, Colquhoun D, Emberson J, et al. Effects of pravastatin in 3260 patients with unstable angina: results from the LIPID study. Lancet 2000; 356(9245):1871–1875.
87. Cannon CP, Braunwald E, McCabe CH, et al. Intensive versus moderate lipid lowering with statins after acute coronary syndromes. N Engl J Med 2004; 350(15):1495–1504.
88. LaRosa JC, Grundy SM, Waters DD, et al. Intensive lipid lowering with atorvastatin in patients with stable coronary disease. N Engl J Med 2005; 352(14):1425–1435.
89. Law MR, Wald NJ, Rudnicka AR. Quantifying effect of statins on low density lipoprotein cholesterol, ischaemic heart disease, and stroke: systematic review and meta-analysis. Br Med J 2003; 326(7404):1423.
90. Baigent C, Keech A, Kearney PM, et al. Efficacy and safety of cholesterol-lowering treatment: prospective meta-analysis of data from 90,056 participants in 14 randomised trials of statins. Lancet 2005; 366(9493):1267–1278.
91. Robins SJ, Rubins HB, Faas FH, et al. Insulin resistance and cardiovascular events with low HDL cholesterol: the Veterans Affairs HDL Intervention Trial (VA-HIT). Diabetes Care 2003; 26(5):1513–1517.
92. Frick MH, Elo O, Haapa K, et al. Helsinki Heart Study: primary-prevention trial with gemfibrozil in middle-aged men with dyslipidemia: safety of treatment, changes in risk factors, and incidence of coronary heart disease. N Engl J Med 1987; 317(20):1237–1245.
93. Sacks FM. The role of high-density lipoprotein (HDL) cholesterol in the prevention and treatment of coronary heart disease: expert group recommendations. Am J Cardiol 2002; 90(2):139–143.
94. Wierzbicki AS, Mikhailidis DP, Wray R, et al. Statin–fibrate combination: therapy for hyperlipidemia: a review. Curr Med Res Opin 2003; 19(3):155–168.
95. Pearson TA, Denke MA, McBride PE, et al. A community-based, randomized trial of ezetimibe added to statin therapy to attain NCEP ATP III goals for LDL cholesterol in hypercholesterolemic patients: the ezetimibe add-on to statin for effectiveness (EASE) trial. Mayo Clin Proc 2005; 80(5):587–595.
96. Stamler J, Vaccaro O, Neaton JD, et al. Diabetes, other risk factors, and 12-yr cardiovascular mortality for men screened in the Multiple Risk Factor Intervention Trial. Diabetes Care 1993; 16(2):434–444.
97. Glucose tolerance and cardiovascular mortality: comparison of fasting and 2-hour diagnostic criteria. Arch Intern Med 2001; 161(3):397–405.
98. Haffner SM, Lehto S, Ronnemaa T, et al. Mortality from coronary heart disease in subjects with type 2 diabetes and in nondiabetic subjects with and without prior myocardial infarction. N Engl J Med 1998; 339(4):229–234.
99. Adlerberth AM, Rosengren A, Wilhelmsen L. Diabetes and long-term risk of mortality from coronary and other causes in middle-aged Swedish men: a general population study. Diabetes Care 1998; 21(4):539–545.
100. Tuomilehto J, Lindstrom J, Eriksson JG, et al. Prevention of type 2 diabetes mellitus by changes in lifestyle among subjects with impaired glucose tolerance. N Engl J Med 2001; 344(18):1343–1350.
101. Chiasson JL, Josse RG, Gomis R, et al. Acarbose for prevention of type 2 diabetes mellitus: the STOP-NIDDM randomised trial. Lancet 2002; 359(9323):2072–2077.
102. Torgerson JS, Hauptman J, Boldrin MN, et al. XENical in the prevention of diabetes in obese subjects (XENDOS) study: a randomized study of orlistat as an adjunct to lifestyle changes for the prevention of type 2 diabetes in obese patients. Diabetes Care 2004; 27(1):155–161.
103. Lindholm LH, Ibsen H, Dahlof B, et al. Cardiovascular morbidity and mortality in patients with diabetes in the Losartan Intervention For Endpoint reduction in hypertension study (LIFE): a randomised trial against atenolol. Lancet 2002; 359(9311):1004–1010.
104. Tight blood pressure control and risk of macrovascular and microvascular complications in type 2 diabetes: UKPDS 38. UK Prospective Diabetes Study Group. Br Med J 1998; 317(7160):703–713.

105. Curb JD, Pressel SL, Cutler JA, et al. Effect of diuretic-based antihypertensive treatment on cardiovascular disease risk in older diabetic patients with isolated systolic hypertension. Systolic Hypertension in the Elderly Program Cooperative Research Group. J Am Med Assoc 1996; 276(23):1886–1892.

106. Pyorala K, Pedersen TR, Kjekshus J, et al. Cholesterol lowering with simvastatin improves prognosis of diabetic patients with coronary heart disease. A subgroup analysis of the Scandinavian Simvastatin Survival Study (4S). Diabetes Care 1997; 20(4):614–620.

107. Lewis SJ, Moye LA, Sacks FM, et al. Effect of pravastatin on cardiovascular events in older patients with myocardial infarction and cholesterol levels in the average range: Results of the Cholesterol and Recurrent Events (CARE) trial. Ann Intern Med 1998; 129(9):681–689.

108. Prevention of cardiovascular events and death with pravastatin in patients with coronary heart disease and a broad range of initial cholesterol levels: The Long-Term Intervention with Pravastatin in Ischaemic Disease (LIPID) Study Group. N Engl J Med 1998; 339(19):1349–1357.

109. Rubins HB, Robins SJ, Collins D, et al. Gemfibrozil for the secondary prevention of coronary heart disease in men with low levels of high-density lipoprotein cholesterol: Veterans Affairs High-Density Lipoprotein Cholesterol Intervention Trial Study Group. N Engl J Med 1999; 341(6):410–418.

110. Colhoun HM, Betteridge DJ, Durrington PN, et al. Primary prevention of cardiovascular disease with atorvastatin in type 2 diabetes in the Collaborative Atorvastatin Diabetes Study (CARDS): multicentre randomised placebo-controlled trial. Lancet 2004; 364(9435):685–696.

111. Stratton IM, Adler AI, Neil HA, et al. Association of glycaemia with macrovascular and microvascular complications of type 2 diabetes (UKPDS 35): prospective observational study. Br Med J 2000; 321(7258):405–412.

112. The effect of intensive treatment of diabetes on the development and progression of long-term complications in insulin-dependent diabetes mellitus: The Diabetes Control and Complications Trial Research Group. N Engl J Med 1993; 329(14):977–986.

113. Intensive blood-glucose control with sulphonylureas or insulin compared with conventional treatment and risk of complications in patients with type 2 diabetes (UKPDS 33): UK Prospective Diabetes Study (UKPDS) Group. Lancet 1998; 352(9131):837–853.

114. Turner RC, Cull CA, Frighi V, et al. Glycemic control with diet, sulfonylurea, metformin, or insulin in patients with type 2 diabetes mellitus: progressive requirement for multiple therapies (UKPDS 49): UK Prospective Diabetes Study (UKPDS) Group. J Am Med Assoc 1999; 281(21):2005–2012.

115. Collaborative overview of randomised trials of antiplatelet therapy-I: prevention of death, myocardial infarction, and stroke by prolonged antiplatelet therapy in various categories of patients. Antiplatelet Trialists' Collaboration. Br Med J 1994; 308(6921):81–106.

116. Collaborative meta-analysis of randomised trials of antiplatelet therapy for prevention of death, myocardial infarction, and stroke in high risk patients. Br Med J 2002; 324(7329): 71–86.

117. McKeigue PM, Miller GJ, Marmot MG. Coronary heart disease in south Asians overseas: a review. J Clin Epidemiol 1989; 42(7):597–609.

118. Shaukat N, de Bono DP. Are Indo-origin people especially susceptible to coronary artery disease? Postgrad Med J 1994; 70(823):315–318.

119. Enas EA, Yusuf S, Mehta JL. Prevalence of coronary artery disease in Asian Indians. Am J Cardiol 1992; 70(9):945–949.

18 | Conclusions and the Future

Simon Howell
University of Leeds, Leeds, U.K.

Chris Pepper
The General Infirmary at Leeds, Leeds, U.K.

Donat R. Spahn
University Hospital Zurich, Zurich, Switzerland

Two decades ago, perioperative myocardial infarction was thought to be primarily a result of myocardial oxygen supply–demand imbalance. All anesthetists could do to protect the heart of the patient was to avoid cardiovascular instability and hope for the best. That view has changed almost beyond recognition. As described in chapter 2, from the 1980s onwards there has been an explosion of knowledge about the pathophysiology of coronary artery disease. It has become clear that in the non-surgical setting, myocardial infarction results from atherosclerotic plaque rupture, thrombosis, and embolization and that this is a dynamic and complex process. We have come to understand that the environment produced by surgery can facilitate this pernicious process; both the release of inflammatory mediators and the activation of the coagulation system can help to fuel the fire of inflammation and thrombus formation on an active coronary plaque. This is discussed in depth in chapter 4. Our changing understanding of the pathophysiology of myocardial infarction has been matched by a changing view of the natural history of myocardial infarction and angina. Previously, myocardial infarction was seen as a dichotomous event; patients had either suffered an infarction or not. A patient who presented with chest pain but no ECG changes would have his cardiac enzymes checked and if these were normal he would be sent on his way with a reassurance that he had not had a heart attack. The development of the cardiac troponin assays over the past 10 years has changed this. It is now understood that there is a spectrum of myocardial injury characterized by increasing levels of cardiac troponin release. The acute coronary syndromes embrace a range of conditions from unstable angina, through non-ST segment myocardial infarction to full blown "Q-wave" infarction. It has become clear that even a small amount of cardiac troponin release portends future problems and means that the patient is likely to suffer further cardiac events in the future. This is discussed in more depth in chapter 3 by Smith and Pepper.

All of this has led to a reconsideration of the nature of perioperative myocardial infarction. There is an ongoing debate about the nature of perioperative infarction; is it the result of myocardial supply–demand imbalance or coronary plaque rupture? Does an increasing ischemic load eventually result in myocardial infarction or is infarction an "out of the blue" event? There is evidence to support both these models and it may be that one process predominates in some patients and the other in the remainder. Priebe, in his chapter on the mechanisms of perioperative myocardial infarction, suggests a model that may unify the two views. The increased sympathetic tone produced by surgery could cause paradoxical vasoconstriction in abnormal coronary arteries with diseased endothelium. The combination of low flow in the coronary artery and the thrombogenic environment produced by surgery could lead to thrombus formation at the site of coronary plaque, that is to say, coronary thrombosis could be produced by low flow conditions rather than vice versa. The persistence of the coronary thrombus and the severity of the resulting injury would depend on the balance between thrombus formation and lysis and the flow conditions. The validity of this model has yet to be tested and examining the dynamics of thrombus formation and myocardial injury in real-time may seem challenging indeed. However, new biomarkers that reveal both myocardial ischemia and injury may offer considerable insights into the relationship between myocardial ischemia and infarction.

The range of clinical manifestations of acute coronary syndromes has been alluded to above. As with the nonsurgical setting, patients undergoing noncardiac surgery may suffer not only full-blown myocardial infarction with substantially elevated serum troponin levels and marked ECG changes such as ST segment elevation and the appearance of new Q-waves, but also lesser degrees of perioperative troponin release that may or may not be accompanied by ECG changes and clinical signs of myocardial injury. In the nonsurgical setting, a patient who presents with chest pain and small cardiac troponin rise is considered to be at increased risk of further cardiac events and will undergo further cardiac evaluation that may include an exercise test, noninvasive cardiac imaging, and, if indicated, coronary angiography. It is now well established that perioperative cardiac troponin release is associated with a worsened long-term prognosis and an increased risk of subsequent death. This association is discussed in chapter 1. The optimal management of patients who have suffered some perioperative cardiac troponin release but have no other evidence of myocardial injury is far from clear. Should these patients undergo formal risk stratification? This would be a considerable extra work load for health services, but would be justified if it led to improved outcome in a substantial number of patients. This is an area where further studies are badly needed.

It has become clear that not only may the conduct of anesthesia affect the outcome from perioperative myocardial ischemia and infarction, but also that the very drugs that we use may have an effect. The observations of Reimer and by Murry that short periods of ischemia may protect the myocardium from subsequent ischemic injury was surprising enough. These observations have now been confirmed many times over and, as described by Foëx and Biccard in chapter 5, the mechanisms of this protection are gradually being elucidated. More surprising still was the discovery of pharmacological preconditioning, the observation that exposure to volatile anesthetic agents, even for a short period, will protect the heart from the effects of a subsequent ischemic insult. The clinical benefit of volatile agents in reducing cardiac troponin release in the setting of cardiac surgery has now been confirmed in a number of small studies. The place of anesthetic preconditioning in the setting of noncardiac surgery has yet to be defined. Studies will be difficult to conduct in this setting, but not impossible, the obvious comparators are total intravenous anesthesia and regional anesthesia.

Both ischemic and anesthetic preconditioning have to be applied before the ischemic insult. This is possible in settings where ischemia might be expected, such as coronary artery bypass grafting (CABG) or percutaneous coronary intervention (PCI), but generally the aim of the perioperative physician is to avoid myocardial ischemia in the first place. The phenomenon of postconditioning offers the prospect of myocardial protection after the ischemic insult has occurred. Zhao and colleagues first demonstrated that the short period of ischemia during myocardial reperfusion could reduce the severity of myocardial injury. This observation has been confirmed in subsequent studies and there is some evidence that anesthetic agents may confer a degree of myocardial protection after an ischemic insult. There are now also substantial data to support the existence of remote preconditioning, the phenomenon whereby ischemia of a distant organ or limb may protect the heart from the effects of myocardial ischemia. The clinical roles of postconditioning and remote conditioning have yet to be clearly defined, but both offer the possibility of significant myocardial protection in clinically challenging settings.

Although the volatile anesthetic agents seem to hold out considerable promise for protecting the heart, the role of β-blockers for perioperative myocardial protection is now less clear than it was even five years ago. The effectiveness of β-blockers in preventing perioperative myocardial ischemia has been known for many years. Two studies, that of Mangano et al. (1) published in 1996 and that of Poldermans et al. (2) published in 1999, seemed to confirm that not only were β-blockers effective at preventing myocardial ischemia, but that they also offer a significant benefit in preventing perioperative cardiac complications. Since then, broad applicability of these studies has been questioned. The study by Mangano et al. has a number of weaknesses, chief among them being the exclusion of in-hospital deaths from the analysis and a preponderance of cardiac comorbidity in the placebo group. The study by Poldermans et al., which randomized only the highest risk patients out of a large vascular surgery population, was unblinded and did not use a placebo and yielded a benefit from β-blockers which some suggested was implausibly high. Subsequent studies including the study by Yang and colleagues, the POBBLE study, and the DIPOM study have not shown an outcome benefit from preoperative β-blockade (3–5). Nevertheless, this remains a plausible intervention which undoubtedly reduces perioperative myocardial ischemia. Patients who have a primary cardiological indication for the prescription of β-blockers, such as angina or secondary prevention after myocardial infarction, may be prescribed a β-blocker on the basis of this indication if not contraindicated, and care should be taken to ensure that treatment is maintained after surgery. It is well established that withdrawing β-blockers prior to surgery is associated with an increased incidence of cardiac complications and every care should be taken to ensure that this does not happen (6). The use of perioperative β-blockade in selected patients is supported by an updated guideline from the American College of Cardiology and the American Heart Association (7). It remains unclear if all patients with cardiac disease or evidence of cardiac disease should receive β-blockers in the perioperative period. A number of small studies have failed to support this and at the time of going to press the results of a large study that is currently in progress are awaited (8).

The doubts expressed above about perioperative β-blockade should not allow us to dismiss all pharmacological interventions out of hand. A number of studies have suggested that statins may reduce perioperative cardiac morbidity and mortality (9–12). This would be consistent with their benefits in the nonsurgical setting. As with perioperative β-blockade it is important not to "jump the gun" and recommend perioperative statins to all patients without a robust evidence base to support this. Further studies are required. However, the preliminary data are promising and many, if not all, patients who are at risk of perioperative cardiac complications will have an indication for the prescription of statins. There is evidence from the nonsurgical setting that the withdrawal of statins is associated with an increased risk of cardiac events and it seems appropriate to ensure that patients who are receiving statins remain on these drugs through the perioperative period (13). Very similar considerations apply to aspirin. Collet et al. (14) produced data from the nonsurgical setting suggesting that aspirin withdrawal from patients with known cardiac disease is associated with worse outcome in patients who suffer a subsequent myocardial infarction. Worryingly, many of the patients in Collet's study had had aspirin withdrawn in preparation for surgery.

It is now generally accepted that patients should not undergo prophylactic coronary revascularization. That is to say that coronary angioplasty or CABG should not be performed only to reduce the risk of noncardiac surgery. Although there is evidence that patients who have undergone revascularization are at reduced risk of perioperative complications, there are a number of studies that suggest that the cumulative risk associated with coronary angiography, revascularization, and then noncardiac surgery outweighs the risk of proceeding directly to noncardiac surgery. A randomized controlled trial conducted by McFalls et al. (15) and published in 2004 supports this conclusion. Patients in whom one or more major coronary arteries had a stenosis of at least 70% were randomized either to undergo coronary revascularization by PCI or CABG, or to proceed directly to surgery. Five hundred and ten patients were randomized. There was no difference in 30-day or long-term outcome between the patients who had undergone revascularization and those who had not. Although this study supports the current strategy, it has been criticized on the grounds that its design did not conform to the preoperative assessment strategy described in the ACC/AHA guidelines and that some of the patients studied would be classified as being at low risk after noninvasive cardiac testing. These are matters of debate. The study was designed before the ACC/AHA guidelines were published and so could not be based on this algorithm. The authors of the study contend that many of the patients studied were indeed at high risk. Moscucci and Eagle suggested that the high mortality rate of 23% seen after less than three years follow-up is such that further studies are required to assess the value of revascularization and other therapies in high-risk patients (16–18).

The McFalls study, while well conducted, does not address the question of how best to manage surgical patients who have been found to have significant coronary artery disease upon noninvasive testing. The risk of cardiac complications following noncardiac surgery is elevated for many weeks or months after PCI or CABG. The view of this author is that high-risk patients should undergo rigorous preassessment, but that the use of invasive cardiac testing and coronary angiography should take into account the urgency of the proposed noncardiac surgery. CABG and PCI with the use of stenting produce a thrombogenic surface in the coronary artery. It may be weeks or months after CABG or coronary angioplasty before the risk of cardiac complications associated with noncardiac surgery to falls to an acceptable level. This may take three months or longer after PCI (19–21). It may be appropriate to use noninvasive cardiac testing and coronary angiography in assessing a patient presenting for noncardiac surgery if these are indicated because of evidence of coronary artery disease that may require intervention. It may be appropriate to perform a noninvasive test to gain further information about the risk of surgery and counsel the patient and the surgeon about this. Before the patient is subjected to coronary angiography, it must be decided if the non-cardiac surgery can be delayed for several months to allow healing of the coronary artery endothelium if a primary indication for coronary revascularization is found. Further studies are indeed required, but they will need to be large multicenter studies in which patients are stratified both according to their cardiac risk and the urgency of surgery.

A closely related debate is the management of anticoagulation and antiplatelet therapy in patients who have undergone PCI with coronary stenting and are now to undergo noncardiac surgery. The presence of a coronary stent delays re-endothe-lization after angioplasty especially if it is a drug-eluting stent. (Indeed, slowing proliferation is the function of these devices for they are intended to prevent coronary restenosis of after angioplasty.) The result is a thrombogenic surface in the coronary artery at the site of the angioplasty. Patients receive heparin and antiplatelet agents immediately after angioplasty and are generally maintained on aspirin and clopidogrel after the procedure. As already stated, it is well reported that patients who undergo noncardiac surgery soon after coronary stenting are at increased risk of perioperative cardiac complications. In recent study by Vicenzi et al. (20), patients who had undergone coronary stenting within 35 days of non-cardiac surgery had a more than twofold increased risk of cardiac complications after surgery (OR 2.11, 95% CI 1.11–4.33). The dilemma for the anesthetist and the surgeon is how best to manage antiplatetet therapy in these patients, especially if they are on both aspirin and clopidogrel. Continuing with both drugs through the perioperative period is likely to lead to increased surgical bleeding; stopping one or both of the drugs may predispose the patient to the risk of in-stent thrombosis and perioperative myocardial infarction. In an editorial that accompanied the Vin-cenzi paper, Spahn et al. (22) advocated maintaining the established antiplatelet regimen in almost all cases (neurosurgery being a possible exception). However, they acknowledged the need for further studies in this area.

In chapter 17, Zamvar and Hall discuss the role of the perioperative physician in the primary and secondary prevention of cardiac disease. For many surgical patients who have cardiac risk factors or even active cardiac disease, their preoper-ative assessment may be the first time that they undergo a formal cardiac assessment. If the opportunity for the prevention of cardiac disease is seized, be it primary or sec-ondary prevention, this may have as big an impact on the patient's life expectancy as the surgery itself. As discussed in chapter 1, patients who do suffer a perioperative cardiac event are more likely to die in the months and years after surgery. Although perioperative myocardial injury is to be avoided if at all possible, patients who do suffer such an event are candidates both for formal cardiac assessment and for secondary cardiac prevention. Ideally this should be arranged before the patient is discharged from the care of the surgeon and the anesthetist.

In chapter 7, Wacker, Schaub, and Zaugg discuss the genetic variability of adrenergic receptors. They highlight a number of polymorphisms as being potentially clinically relevant. To list but a few described in more detail in their chapter, the 301 to 303 deletion of the postsynaptic α_{2B}-adrenergic receptor may produce increased coronary vasoconstriction and so cause myocardial ischemia. The 322 to 325 deletion in the presynaptic α_{2C}-adrenergic receptor is associated with an increased risk of the early development and progression of heart failure. The combination of this deletion and the deletion of arginine at position 389 in the β_1-adrenergic receptor greatly increases the heart failure risk. They also identify other polymorphisms that may have functional relevance. They make the point that genetic variation may impact on the effectiveness of drug treatments. In the Beta-Blocker Evaluation Survival Trial (BEST) study of β-blockade in heart failure, bucindolol significantly increased mor-tality among Afro-Americans, while there was a tendency towards mortality reduc-tion among the non-Afro-Americans at termination of the study. Their work points to a future in which genotyping is an essential aspect of the design of clinical trials and of patient management.

As indicated in chapter 1, the surgical population is growing older and more high-risk patients are undergoing surgery. The realization that not only myocardial infarction but any perioperative troponin release has prognostic implications has expanded the population of patients who may be considered to have suffered a perioperative cardiac event. Although there are exciting new therapies and the future holds much promise, there is still much to be done before the scourge of perioperative cardiac complications is defeated.

REFERENCES

1. Mangano DT, Layug EL, Wallace A, Tateo I. Effect of atenolol on mortality and cardiovascular morbidity after noncardiac surgery. Multicenter Study of Perioperative Ischemia Research Group. N Engl J Med 1996; 335:1713–1720.
2. Poldermans D, Boersma E, Bax JJ, et al. The effect of bisoprolol on perioperative mortality and myocardial infarction in high-risk patients undergoing vascular surgery. Dutch Echocardiographic Cardiac Risk Evaluation Applying Stress Echocardiography Study Group. N Engl J Med 1999; 341:1789–1794.
3. Brady AR, Gibbs JS, Greenhalgh RM, Powell JT, Sydes MR. Perioperative beta-blockade (POBBLE) for patients undergoing infrarenal vascular surgery: results of a randomized double-blind controlled trial. J Vasc Surg 2005; 41:602–609.
4. Yang H, Raymer K, Butler R, Parlow J, Roberts R. Metoprolol after vascular surgery. Can J Anaesth 2004; 51:A7.
5. Juul AB, Wetterslev J, Gluud C, et al. Effect of perioperative beta blockade in patients with diabetes undergoing major non-cardiac surgery: randomised placebo controlled, blinded multicentre trial. Br Med J 2006; 332:1482.
6. Shammash JB, Trost JC, Gold JM, Berlin JA, Golden MA, Kimmel SE. Perioperative beta-blocker withdrawal and mortality in vascular surgical patients. Am Heart J 2001; 141: 148–153.
7. Fleisher LA, Beckman JA, Brown KA, et al. ACC/AHA 2006 guideline update on perioperative cardiovascular evaluation for noncardiac surgery: focused update on perioperative beta-blocker therapy. A Report of the American College of Cardiology/American Heart Association Task Force on Practice Guidelines (Writing Committee to Update the 2002 Guidelines on Perioperative Cardiovascular Evaluation for Noncardiac Surgery): developed in collaboration with the American Society of Echocardiography, American Society of Nuclear Cardiology, Heart Rhythm Society, Society of Cardiovascular Anesthesiologists, Society for Cardiovascular Angiography and Interventions, and Society for Vascular Medicine and Biology. Circulation 2006; 113:2662–2674.
8. Devereaux PJ, Yang H, Guyatt GH, et al. Rationale, design, and organization of the PeriOperative ISchemic Evaluation (POISE) trial: a randomized controlled trial of metoprolol versus placebo in patients undergoing noncardiac surgery. Am Heart J 2006; 152:223–230.
9. Durazzo AE, Machado FS, Ikeoka DT, et al. Reduction in cardiovascular events after vascular surgery with atorvastatin: a randomized trial. J Vasc Surg 2004; 39:967–975; discussion 975–976.
10. Kertai MD, Boersma E, Westerhout CM, et al. A combination of statins and beta-blockers is independently associated with a reduction in the incidence of perioperative mortality and nonfatal myocardial infarction in patients undergoing abdominal aortic aneurysm surgery. Eur J Vasc Endovasc Surg 2004; 28:343–352.
11. Kertai MD, Boersma E, Westerhout CM, et al. Association between long-term statin use and mortality after successful abdominal aortic aneurysm surgery. Am J Med 2004; 116:96–103.
12. Lindenauer PK, Pekow P, Wang K, Gutierrez B, Benjamin EM. Lipid-lowering therapy and in-hospital mortality following major noncardiac surgery. J Am Med Assoc 2004; 291:2092–2099.
13. Heeschen C, Hamm CW, Laufs U, Snapinn S, Bohm M, White HD. Withdrawal of statins increases event rates in patients with acute coronary syndromes. Circulation 2002; 105:1446–1452.
14. Collet JP, Montalescot G, Blanchet B, et al. Impact of prior use or recent withdrawal of oral antiplatelet agents on acute coronary syndromes. Circulation 2004; 110:2361–2367.

15. McFalls EO, Ward HB, Moritz TE, et al. Coronary–artery revascularization before elective major vascular surgery. N Engl J Med 2004; 351:2795–2804.

16. Moscucci M, Eagle KA. Coronary revascularization before noncardiac surgery. N Engl J Med 2004; 351:2861–2863.

17. Brett AS. Coronary revascularization before vascular surgery. N Engl J Med 2005; 352:1492–1495.

18. Landesberg G, Mosseri M, Fleisher LA. Coronary revascularization before vascular surgery. N Engl J Med 2005; 352:1492–1495.

19. Kaluza GL, Joseph J, Lee JR, Raizner ME, Raizner AE. Catastrophic outcomes of noncardiac surgery soon after coronary stenting. J Am Coll Cardiol 2000; 35:1288–1294.

20. Vicenzi MN, Meislitzer T, Heitzinger B, Halaj M, Fleisher LA, Metzler H. Coronary artery stenting and non-cardiac surgery—a prospective outcome study. Br J Anaesth 2006; 96:686–693.

21. Wilson SH, Fasseas P, Orford JL, et al. Clinical outcome of patients undergoing noncardiac surgery in the two months following coronary stenting. J Am Coll Cardiol 2003; 42:234–240.

22. Spahn DR, Howell SJ, Delabays A, Chassot PG. Coronary stents and perioperative antiplatelet regimen: dilemma of bleeding and stent thrombosis. Br J Anaesth 2006; 96: 675–677.

Index